WAIMH

HANDBOOK OF

Infant
Mental Health

VOLUME TWO

Early Intervention, Evaluation,
and Assessment

WAIMH

HANDBOOK OF

Infant
Mental Health

Joy D. Osofsky and Hiram E. Fitzgerald / Editors

VOLUME TWO

Early Intervention, Evaluation, and Assessment

WORLD ASSOCIATION FOR INFANT MENTAL HEALTH

John Wiley & Sons, Inc.

New York • Chichester • Weinheim • Brisbane • Singapore • Toronto

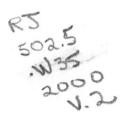

This book is printed on acid-free paper. ∞

This publication is designed to provide accurate and authoritative information in regard to the subject matter covered. It is sold with the understanding that the publisher is not engaged in rendering professional services. If legal, accounting, medical, psychological or any other expert assistance is required, the services of a competent professional person should be sought.

Library of Congress Cataloging-in-Publication Data:
WAIMH Handbook of infant mental health / World Association for Infant Mental Health ; edited by
   Joy D. Osofsky and Hiram E. Fitzgerald.
    p.   cm.
   Includes bibliographical references and indexes.
   Contents: v. 1. Perspectives on infant mental health — v. 2. Early intervention, evaluation, and assessment — v. 3. Parenting and child care — v. 4. Infant mental health groups at high risk.
   Other title: WAIMH handbook of infant mental health.
   ISBN 0-471-18988-X (set : alk. paper). — ISBN 0-471-18941-3 (v. 1 : cloth : alk. paper) — ISBN 0-471-18944-8 (v. 2 : cloth : alk. paper). — ISBN 0-471-18946-4 (v. 3 : cloth : alk. paper). — ISBN 0-471-18947-2 (v. 4 : cloth : alk. paper)
   1. Infants—Mental health Handbooks, manuals, etc.   2. Infant psychiatry Handbooks, manuals, etc.   3. Child psychopathology—Prevention Handbooks, manuals, etc.   I. Osofsky, Joy D.   II. Fitzgerald, Hiram E.   III. World Association for Infant Mental Health.   IV. Title: WAIMH handbook of infant mental health.
   [DNLM: 1. Child Development. 2. Infant. 3. Child Psychology. 4. Parenting. 5. Early Intervention (Education) 6. Developmental Disabilities—prevention & control. WS 105 H2363 2000]
RJ502.5.H362 2000
618.92′89—dc21
                                             99-11893
                                              CIP

Printed in the United States of America.

10 9 8 7 6 5 4 3 2 1

Contributors

ANNE BENHAM, M.D.
Stanford University School of Medicine, Stanford, California

T. BERRY BRAZELTON, M.D.
Child Development Unit, Children's Hospital Medical Center, Boston, Massachusetts

MARIA CORDEIRO, M.D.
Hospital de D. Estefania, Departmento de Pedopsi Quiatria, Unidade da Primeira Infantia, Lisboa, Portugal

BERTRAND CRAMER, M.D.
Hopitaux Univeritaires de Geneve (HUG), Clinique de Psychiatrie Infantile, Geneva, Switzerland

SALLY DOULIS, MSW
Hincks/Dellcrest Children's Mental Health Centre, Toronto, Ontario, Canada

ROBERT EMDE, M.D.
Department of Psychiatry, University of Colorado School of Medicine, Denver, Colorado

KAREN FRANKEL, PH.D.
Division of Child Psychiatry, University of Colorado, Health Sciences Department, Denver, Colorado

LINDA GILKERSON, PH.D.
Erikson Institute, Chicago, Illinois

STANLEY I. GREENSPAN, M.D.
George Washington University Medical Center, Bethesda, Maryland

KAREN A. GUSKIN, PH.D.
St. Louis University School of Medicine, St. Louis, Missouri

ROBERT J. HARMON, M.D.
Division of Child Psychiatry, University of Colorado, Health Sciences Department, Denver, Colorado

JOHN KORFMACHER, PH.D.
Erickson Institute, Chicago, Illinois

LORRAINE F. KUBICEK, PH.D.
Department of Psychiatry, University of Colorado Health Sciences Center, Denver, Colorado

SARAH LANDY, PH.D.
Hincks/Dellcrest Treatment Centre, Toronto, Ontario, Canada

SUSAN MCDONOUGH, MSW, PH.D.
School of Social Work, University of Michigan, Ann Arbor, Michigan

KLAUS MINDE, M.D.
Division of Child Psychiatry, McGill University, Montreal, Quebec, Canada

J. KEVIN NUGENT, PH.D.
Child Development Unit, Children's Hospital Medical Center, Boston, Massachusetts

JEREE H. PAWL, PH.D.
Infant Parent Program, San Francisco General Hospital, San Francisco, California

CONTRIBUTORS

JUDITH H. PEKARSKY, PH.D.
Infant Parent Program, San Francisco General Hospital, San Francisco, California

CHRISTIANE ROBERT-TISSOT, PH.D.
Hopitaux Univeritaires de Geneve (HUG), Clinique de Psychiatrie Infantile, Geneva, Switzerland

REBECCA SHAHMOON-SHANOK, MSW, PH.D.
Early Childhood Group Therapy Program and Institute for Clinical Studies of Infants, Toddlers and Parents, Child Development Center, Jewish Board of Family & Children's Services, New York, New York

MARIA ST. JOHN, MFCC
Infant Parent Program, San Francisco General Hospital, San Francisco, California

FRANCES STOTT, PH.D.
Erikson Institute, Chicago, Illinois

JEAN M. THOMAS, M.D.
St. Louis University School of Medicine, St. Louis, Missouri

ELIZABETH TUTERS, MSW, CSW
Hincks/Dellcrest Children's Mental Health Centre, Toronto, Ontario, Canada

DEBORAH J. WEATHERSTON, MA
Infant Mental Health Program, Merrill-Palmer Institute, Wayne State University, Detroit, Michigan

SERENA WIEDER, PH.D.
Private Practice, Silver Spring, Maryland

JOHN WOROBEY, PH.D.
Department of Nutritional Sciences, Rutgers University, New Brunswick, New Jersey

Contents

CONTENTS

Contents

CONTENTS

Contents

CONTENTS

Contents

Foreword

Yvon Gauthier

I had the privilege to participate in the first international congress of the World Association for Infant Mental Health, then the World Association of Infant Psychiatry, held in Portugal in 1980. There was a very special feeling throughout this congress, a feeling that researchers and clinicians from several countries were for the first time putting together their observations about infants, and discovering their importance. Most probably, these people knew one another's writings and had met before in other situations, but there was, in their presentations and discussions an emotional tone that I personally felt intensely. And I often heard others talk about it in similar terms over the years. Can we say that this was the beginning of an infant mental health movement? We evidently need more historical facts before answering this question. But as I look back on it, this 1980 congress stands in my mind as a historical mark in terms of an international beginning of knowledge transfer in the infant mental health domain. The publication of this WAIMH handbook 20 years later is an international attempt, sponsored by WAIMH, to mark the progress made during those two decades, and to propose important directions in many areas of this most dynamic field.

In many parts of the world, ideas and practices concerned with infants and young families are gaining in importance. We may note that Spitz's and Bowlby's early works gradually had an influence on practices of institutional life and adoption all over the world, and that foster homes have become standard practice in many countries, in spite of their frequent inadequacies. Attachment-exploration phenomena are being studied in several countries, with findings that show cultural variations in infant care (see Bretherton and Waters, 1985; Waters, Vaughn, Posada, & Kondo-Ikemura, 1995). Can we predict that this movement will continue to have a considerable influence all over the world, particularly in less developed countries? It is very interesting and important that several chapters of this handbook develop cross-cultural perspectives in infant mental health, showing that this movement has already crossed several frontiers. Prepared by specialists in their own countries, they demonstrate the variety of approaches used to understand and help families who are dealing with problematic infants and young children, while taking into account culture-relevant elements involved in understanding and intervention.

Several theoretical currents are influential in infant mental health, but psychoanalysis, clinically and theoretically, holds a special place in our field. We may remember the importance that psychoanalysis has given to infancy in its theoretical development. Of course, for Freud, infancy meant the verbal child, and more specifically the 3- to 6-year-old during the Oedipal phase. Melanie Klein placed emphasis on earlier phases, though in doing so she attributed to the very young infant very destructive imaginary strivings and projections that she reconstructed from her treatment of older mostly psychotic children.

We know how much Bowlby questioned some of these psychoanalytic hypotheses. His observations of very young children in situations of separation, among other influences, led him to develop his theory of attachment, which has come to play a crucial role in research and clinical activities. With the contributions of Mary Ainsworth, Mary Main, and many others, attachment concepts have become central to research and clinical activities in many countries and have opened the way to a deeper understanding of both normal and psychopathological development. Infant mental health

is deeply influenced by the attachment paradigm.

We also have to note that family systems and family therapy are closely tied to attachment theory (Byng-Hall, 1990; Stevenson-Hinde, 1990); and thus also are very useful in infant mental health practice. Fundamental research done on the early father-mother-baby interactions (for instance in Lausanne, Corboz-Warnery, Fivaz-Depeursinge, Bettens, & Favez, 1993) is also bringing an interesting contribution to our practice.

It has almost become a postulate in our field that early intervention frequently leads to symptomatic and internal changes within the parent-child dyad or triad. More research is needed, but already significant results are available (Cramer et al., 1990; Landy et al., 1998; Robert-Tissot et al., 1996). Stern (1995) has developed the idea that early intervention for which there are many possible "ports of entry," has a good chance of mobilizing a system that has great mobility and offers true opportunities for change at this stage of life. This mobility has been well demonstrated all through this phase of life, from early pregnancy to age 2 to 3. We can now really talk of perinatality as a phase of life where an intervention, even of small proportions, can move the system in a durable manner (Gauthier, 1998).

There is an important corollary to this appreciation of the importance of early intervention: Several disciplines are involved in the care of infants, young children, and their families and must be aware that their role is essential. First-line workers, whatever their original discipline—nurse, midwife, child care worker, obstetrician, pediatrician, etc.—have to be trained in a truly systemic orientation. Examples of different types of training in this direction are reported in this handbook, opening the way to an essential transfer of knowledge between disciplines.

It also becomes clearer as we study infants and young families that parenting, mothering, and fathering do not start at birth, but are present as soon as a child is expected. Therefore, professionals have to become involved even during pregnancy, for there is evidence that even before birth the child becomes invested with affects and images that may influence development. Bydlowski (1997), Raphael-Leff (1993), and Molénat (1993), among others, have described well how this developmental phase is often marked by a "permeability of the unconscious" that often allows significant therapeutic work.

From a similar perspective, Fraiberg's clinical studies opened the way to the concept of intergenerational transmission, which finds interesting confirmation in recent research on transmission of attachment patterns (Benoit & Parker, 1994; Fonagy, Steele, Moran, Steele, & Higgitt, 1993). Important changes are being observed in the responsibilities that parents assume in the care of their children, just as greatly differing societies and cultures are developing new ways of socializing the infant and the young child. This handbook will bring us up to date on such issues.

Research on brain development shows the importance of the early years and the essential role of the environment in its development (Schore, 1994, 1996). Early intervention is essential for all, but particularly for high risk populations, since we now know that poverty and psychopathology are intricately connected, and that early intervention is essential to avoid repetitions and reach parents' desire for a new experience, one different from their own childhood, with their child. We also know that several situations constitute a risk for the coming child: Prematurity, substance abuse, depression, adolescent pregnancy, death of a previous child, and traumatized childhood are all conditions that call for early preventive intervention from professionals who are naturally in contact with mothers and fathers.

This handbook is an unusual sharing of knowledge from experts in several disciplines and all parts of the world, whose work focuses on infants and young families. It expresses the conviction, which has gradually come to all professionals working in this area of infant mental health, that early intervention is the best way to prevent the severe difficulties in the development of children and adults that often lead to psychopathology. Although such early intervention may be costly, it is certainly less so than later psychopathology is to societies. Let us hope that this major effort will be much read all over the world, so that it influences, in all parts of our global environment, the development of social policies that encourage and support an early involvement with infants and families.

References

Benoit, D., & Parker, K. C. H. (1994). Stability and transmission of attachment across three generations. *Child Development, 65*, 1444–1456.

Bretherton, I., & Waters, E. (Eds.). (1985). Growing points of attachment: Theory and research. *Monographs of the Society for Research in Child Development, 50* (1–2, Serial No. 209).

Bydlowski, M. (1997). *La dette de vie: Itinéraire psychanalytique de la maternité* (Le fil rouge). Paris: Presses Universitaires de France.

Byng-Hall, J. (1990). Attachment theory and family therapy: A clinical view. *Infant Mental Health Journal, 11*(3), 228–236.

Corboz-Warnery, A., Fivaz-Depeursinge, E., Bettens, C. G., & Favez, N. (1993). Systemic analysis of father-mother-baby interactions: The Lausanne triadic play. *Infant Mental Health Journal, 14*(4), 298–316.

Cramer, B., Robert-Tissot, C., Stern, D. N., Serpa-Rusconi, S., De Muralt, M., Besson, G., Palacio-Espasa, F., Bachmann, J. P., Knauer, D., Berney, C., & d'Arcis, U. (1990). Outcome evaluation in brief mother-infant psychotherapy: A preliminary report. *Infant Mental Health Journal, 11*(3), 278–300.

Fonagy, P., Steele, M., Moran, G., Steele, H., & Higgitt, A. (1993). Measuring the ghost in the nursery: An empirical study of the relation between parents' mental representations of childhood experiences and their infants' security of attachment. *Journal of the American Psychoanalytic Association, 41*, 957–989.

Gauthier, Y. (1998). Du projet d'enfant aux premières semaines de la vie: Perspectives psychanalytiques. In P. Mazet & S. Lebovici (Eds.), *Psychiatrie périnatale. Parents et bébés: Du projet d'enfant aux premiers mois de vie.* (Monographies de la psychiatrie de l'enfant). Paris: Presses Universitaires de France.

Landy, S., Peters, R.DeV., Arnold, R., Allen, B., Brookes, F., & Jewell, S. (1998). Evaluation of "Staying On Track": An early identification, tracking, and referral system. *Infant Mental Health Journal, 19*(1), 34–58.

Molénat, F. (1992). *Mères vulnérables.* Paris: Stock/Pernoud.

Raphael-Leff, J. (1993). *Pregnancy: The inside story.* Northvale, NJ, and London: Jason Aronson Inc.

Robert-Tissot, C., Cramer, B., Stern, D. N., Serpa, S. R., Bachmann, J. P., Palacio-Espasa, F., Knauer, D., De Muralt, M., Berney, C., & Mendiguren, G. (1996). Outcome evaluation in brief mother-infant psychotherapies: Report on 75 cases. *Infant Mental Health Journal, 17*(2), 97–114.

Schore, A. N. (1994). *Affect regulation and the origin of the self.* Hillsdale, NJ: Erlbaum.

Schore, A. N. (1996). The experience-dependent maturation of a regulatory system in the orbital prefrontal cortex and the origin of developmental psychopathology. *Development and Psychopathology, 8*, 59–87.

Stern, D. N. (1995). *The motherhood constellation: A unified view of parent-infant psychotherapy.* New York: Basic Books.

Stevenson-Hinde, J. (1990). Attachment within family systems: An overview. *Infant Mental Health Journal, 11*(3), 218–228.

Waters, E., Vaughn, B. E., Posada, G., & Kondo-lkemura, K. (Eds.). (1995). Caregiving, cultural and cognitive perspectives on secure-base behavior and working models: New growing points of attachment theory and research. *Monographs of the Society for Research in Child Development, 60*(2–3, Serial No. 244).

Preface

Joy D. Osofsky and Hiram E. Fitzgerald

In 1996, anticipating our 6th World Congress, we recognized with the Executive Committee of the World Association for Infant Mental Health (WAIMH) that our next World Congress planned for July 2000 would not only mark the beginning of the new millennium, but also, for WAIMH a celebration of our 20-year anniversary. Thus, the WAIMH Handbook of Infant Mental Health was "conceived" as a tribute to that occasion. We agreed to undertake the editing of a series of volumes that would present a comprehensive review and integration of work in the area of infant mental health from around the world. From the initial idea, with the help of our editors at John Wiley & Sons, we decided that four volumes were needed to truly represent the area covering the breadth of programs and approaches that would best describe the field including: I. Perspectives on Infant Mental Health; II. Early Intervention, Evaluation, and Assessment; III. Parenting and Child Care; IV. Infant Mental Health in Groups at High Risk. We were committed to making the book interdisciplinary and international to reflect the vision of WAIMH.

Many people have been very helpful and encouraging in bringing this major effort to an excellent conclusion. First, we want to thank the Executive Committee of WAIMH including Yvon Gauthier, Peter de Chateau, Tuula Tamminen, Elizabeth Tuters, Miguel Hoffmann, Antoine Guedeney, and Bob Emde who encouraged us from the outset. They thought it was an exciting and very worthwhile undertaking, and have been extremely helpful in assisting us in bringing many chapters to completion and editing others when we needed their help. Second, we are very appreciative of the vision and foresight of Kelly Franklin, first our editor and now publisher, who brought us to New York to discuss how Wiley could play a role in advancing the field of infant mental health. We hope that you will agree that her encouragement of us to develop the *WAIMH Handbook of Infant Mental Health* and her saying, "You can do four volumes!" was fortuitous.

We each have individual people to recognize and thank. I (JDO) want to thank my colleagues, especially Martin Drell, Head of the Division of Infant, Child and Adolescent Psychiatry at Louisiana State University Health Sciences Center who not only were available and supportive of this work, but offered inspiration as well. Through the Harris Center for Infant Mental Health that I direct at LSUHSC, I am constantly exposed to the excitement in our faculty and trainees as they learn more about and provide better interventions and treatment for infants and their families. In such an environment that values making a difference in the earliest years of life, the development of this publication has been encouraged and valued. My support staff for this book, including some who have moved on to complete their graduate education, have included Bridget Scott, Ana Linares, and Angela Black. I am appreciative of their careful record keeping and help with organizing this project. Of course my family, as always, has been very patient with me and encouraging as I spend endless hours in front of the computer writing and/or editing. Perhaps the best part of that support is seeing how my three growing and grown children have learned to value education, writing, and helping others. My husband, Howard, has always been there for me with encouragement and pride as such a major project has come to completion. I thank him for always providing a "secure base" and for his love and steadiness for all of us.

I (HEF) too have many individuals to thank, starting with my wife Dolores. Not only has she been a steadfast companion for the past 37 years, but she actually holds her own place in WAIMH's history (as Paul Harvey might say, see Volume 1, Chapter 1, page 20 "for the rest of the story!"). When writing and editing there is no more treasured commodity than time, and my colleagues at Michigan State University, Rachel Schiffman, Ellen Whipple, and Holly Brophy-Herb helped to release some of that by sharing responsibility for administering the interdisciplinary graduate programs in infant studies. I learned a great deal about infancy by participating in the rearing of three individuals each of whom has blossomed into a caring, compassionate adult who values education, children, and family life. Being a grandparent, however, provides insights into infant development and parent-infant relationships not afforded to parents as they play out the daily routine. So, thanks to Sean, Ryan, Mara, and Mallory for refreshing and renewing my opportunities to view again the truly wonderous early beginnings of human devleopment.

Finally, we want to thank the many infants, toddlers and families who have really "taught us all we know" about infant mental health. Without them, we would not only be less knowledgeable, but also, we would never have had the opportunity to appreciate the magic of human development. Combined we have probably directly sampled a small portion of the lifecourse of thousands of infants and their caregivers. The diversity of human development, the resilience to adverse outcome, and both the compassion and inhumanity of humankind, each, in its own way, challenges infant mental health specialists to hone their scientific and clinical skills, and to participate in advocating for policies that enhance the quality of life, especially during the early years.

These volumes are a beginning, not an end. They are intended to provoke discussion about the field of infant mental health and to frame a definition of that field. They unambiguously join scientific and clinical perspectives and boldly speak to public policy issues. We invite each of you to join this effort to help shape a perspective, one that will play out across disciplines, across national boundaries, and across the full spectrum of human development.

Joy D. Osofsky
New Orleans, Louisiana

Hiram E. Fitzgerald
East Lansing, Michigan

1

Toward a Theory of
Early Relationship-Based
Intervention

Robert N. Emde, Jon Korfmacher,
and Lorraine F. Kubicek

1

3

Introduction

This chapter offers a contribution toward a theory of intervention in infancy that is relationship-based. We begin with a set of assumptions about successful mental health interventions. We then discuss developmental motives in the context of the caregiving relationship and interventions, enhancing adaptive caregiving interactions, and the role of the interventionist in a network of relationships. Following this, we discuss a model for evaluating infant mental health programs. We conclude with thoughts for the practitioner of infant mental health.

Assumptions

Successful mental health interventions *throughout the life span* are characterized by four features. First, they are *experience-focused*. Successful interventions consider the meaning of interventions for the individual at both the psychological and interpersonal levels. From a humanistic perspective, individual meaning is taken into account not only to minimize suffering and self-destructive behavior, but also to make it possible for satisfying and productive adapta-

tions. Second, successful interventions are *developmentally-oriented.* They go beyond immediate symptom relief and are concerned with enabling individual adaptive developmental processes over time.

Third, successful mental health interventions throughout life are *relationship-based*. Interventions depend upon a sense of trust and availability as experienced over time with the intervener. Fourth, and less widely appreciated, successful interventions involve the *influence of relationships on other relationships*. Individual psychotherapies, for example, are based on therapist-client relationships. Such relationships are designed to influence two domains of other relationships: (1) problematic internalized (psychologically-represented) relationships that are conflictual or inadequate and (2) problematic interpersonal relationships outside the therapeutic encounter that deal with loving and other aspects of living. Other mental health interventions, such as family therapy, group psychotherapy, or casework, are often explicitly designed to make use of an interventionist relationship influencing a network of relationships in the family or in the workplace.

Successful mental health interventions *in early life* highlight special aspects of these four features. First, in these interventions, the *experience of both the child and the adult caregiver* is of central concern. Research has repeatedly targeted the individuality of the infant's experience, not only in terms of temperament (Chess & Thomas, 1986; Carey, 1970, 1972), but also in terms of interaction with caregivers and the infant's mastery of the environment (Bell, 1968; Osofsky & Danziger, 1974; Sameroff & Chandler, 1976). Even though the interventionist cannot access infant experience directly through language, it can be appreciated from emotional expressions and gestures that communicate needs and intentions. The experience of caregivers can be accessed through language, as well as behavioral observations. Such experience is often a target of mental health work, especially in the practice of parent-infant psychotherapy (see the special issue of the *Infant Mental Health Journal*, Summer 1998).

Second, the *developmental orientation* highlights a special emphasis of successful interventions in infancy: They are necessarily prevention-oriented. Because early developmental processes are rapid and involve the beginnings of pathways for adaptation and because early vulnerabilities hamper such pathways, the mental health interventionist is concerned with preventing future problems and strengthening future adaptations, in addition to dealing with current individual stresses and symptoms.

This brings us to the third feature, namely, the special aspects of the *relationship-based* nature of successful early interventions. Availability and trust of the intervener as experienced by the caregiver is a primary goal of intervention that, in turn, may enhance the relationship between caregiver and infant. Unlike adult psychotherapy, the client of an infant mental health intervention is not necessarily the adult caregiver but the caregiver-infant relationship itself. A focus on the early caregiving relationship is important because this experience for the infant is crucially different from subsequent life relationships. It is formative. All aspects of the infant's development are subsumed within it. Without the caregiver-infant relationship, there would be no infant (Tyson, Emde, Galenson, & Osofsky, 1985; Winnicott, 1960). Disturbances and problems in infancy are immersed in disturbances and problems of the caregiver-infant relationship (Sameroff & Emde, 1989a).

Thus, this chapter focuses on how the service provider may influence the caregiver-infant relationship by diminishing stresses and conflicts and by strengthening developmental processes in both partners and their interactions. In other words, this chapter places emphasis on the provider's relationship to the caregiving relationship. Such a focus is consistent with much of the emphasis of Fraiberg (1980) and of the practice of parent-infant psychotherapy and brings us to the fourth special quality of successful interventions in early mental health, namely, the *influence of relationships on relationships*. Not only must successful early intervention target the caregiver-infant relationship itself, but it also must be multifaceted, attending to a network of other social relationships that support the caregiver-infant relationship. Moreover, in addition to current relationships, the intervener also attends to parental influences represented from the past, influences of relationships that go across three or more generations. Fraiberg and colleagues (Fraiberg, Edelson, & Shapiro, 1975) drew attention to such psychodynamic influences in interventions in the classic essay entitled "Ghosts in the Nursery." Subsequently, such influences have been given added coherence from recent attachment theory and research (Fonagy, Steele, Moran, Steele, & Higgitt, 1993; Fonagy, Steele, & Steele, 1991; Main, 1993).

Developmental Motives, the Caregiving Relationship, and Intervention

Psychoanalytic contributions of the past 40 years have increasingly emphasized that the child's early motives are developmentally-based, preadapted for social interactions, and can, by implication, provide a framework for mental health interventions. The work of Spitz (1959, 1965), Bowlby (1969, 1973, 1980), Fraiberg (1980), and Mahler, Pine, and Bergman (1975) emphasized that early development is contained within caregiving relationships and that the child's developing autonomy occurs along with the young child's developing interconnectedness with others. Bowlby's ethnological considerations articulated that the human infant is born preadapted by evolution for social interactions and that attachment and exploration develop within the context of supportive and consistent caregiving interactions, points that were also enumerated in the theorizing of Spitz (Emde, 1983a). Fraiberg broadened con-

siderations of motivation important for the interventionists by bringing cognitive perspectives from Piaget. Fraiberg also pointed to the rapid development of the infant and founded approaches in infant-parent psychotherapy, wherein the infant was present during psychodynamic explorations with mother. Fraiberg's often quoted phrase "it's a little bit like having God on your side" (Fraiberg, Shapiro, & Cherniss, 1980, p. 53), considering the rapid development of the infant over the course of the early postnatal months, pointed to a positive developmental impetus that could be experienced, appreciated, and acknowledged as part of mother's caregiving. Such an impetus could be used by the therapists to help bolster the mother's self-esteem and, by implication, an empathic appreciation of this experience could add incentives to the mother's own development.

This leads us to consider some of the salient developmental processes in infancy that are made use of in intervention. Although these processes require nourishment from the caregiving environment, they represent potential and active strengths in each individual infant. In earlier publications, we summarized extensive multidisciplinary research regarding a set of basic motives of infancy (Emde, 1988a, 1988b; Emde & Robinson, in press). Such motives are inborn tendencies, manifest in earliest infancy, and fostered by caregivers who are emotionally available—that is, responsive to the infant's emotional signals of need, states, and interests. Since these basic motives continue throughout life, they can also be thought of as developmental motives (Emde, 1990). In other words, as

6

Fraiberg began to envision, these motives are aspects of developmental processes that become consolidated during the experiences of early caregiving and can also be mobilized in interventions.

Activity is a first basic motive. The infant is active, exploratory, and motivated to master the world and realize developmental agendas—given that there is a consistent caregiving environment (Emde, Biringen, Clyman, & Oppenheim, 1991). *Self-regulation,* a second basic motive, refers to the fact that there is an inborn propensity for regulation of behavior, as well as for physiology. Self-regulation of behavior is indicated by cycles of sleep, wakefulness, and attentiveness, as well as the longer term built-in propensity for the young individual to attain species-important developmental goals, such as self-awareness, representational thinking, and language, in spite of a variety of perturbations and variations. *Social-fittedness* is identified as a third basic motive. Infants are motivated and preadapted by evolution for initiating, maintaining, and terminating human interactions. Much research has documented the biological preparedness for the dynamic complexities of human interaction that exist in early infancy, providing there are caregiving experiences to foster its development (Papousek & Papousek, 1979; Stern, 1985).

Affective monitoring is identified as a fourth basic motive. There is a propensity from early infancy to monitor experience according to what is pleasurable or not pleasurable. The infant's affective expressions guide the caregiver to what is needed and when. One only needs to be reminded of the messages conveyed by an infant's cry, an interested alert expression, or a bright smile. During the middle of the first year, a major development takes place from the infant's point of view, that of social referencing. The infant begins to monitor emotional expressions of significant others in order to guide behavior when confronted by a situation of uncertainty. Accordingly, if a mother smiles, the infant is encouraged to approach a stranger or unfamiliar moving toy; if mother looks fearful or angry, there is reluctance or retreat (Emde, 1992).

Cognitive assimilation is designated as a fifth basic motive. From the beginning, an infant has a tendency to explore the environment, seeking what is new in order to make it familiar. Such a motive is related to that of activity but brings emphasis to a more directed tendency for the child to "get it right" about the environment. It makes use of what Piaget referred to as "cognitive assimilation" that in his cognitive theory was considered "a basic fact of life" (Piaget, 1952). This motive also incorporates the construct of mastery motivation, wherein the child experiences pleasure in performing newly-acquired behaviors and skills (Harmon & Murrow, 1995; MacTurk & Morgan, 1995).

Perhaps it is because the previously mentioned motives are universal features of normal development that they are generally assumed by developmental theories while not being specified as motivations. Still, when they are experienced by an infant with an emotionally available caregiving figure, we believe they become elaborated into important developmental structures prior to three years of age. Among these structures are what we consider early *moral motives*. We now believe important aspects of moral development occur earlier than previously thought, and they occur in a broader domain. Early moral inclinations can be observed prior to the preschooler's awareness of "Oedipal" urges and conflictual struggles within triangular family relationships (Emde, Johnson, & Easterbrooks, 1987). Most central to this chapter is our belief that developmental motives become early moral motives in infancy and in toddlerhood as a result of repeated everyday experiences within the caregiving relationship.

According to our theory, morality contains positive aspects (referred to as "do's" in early moral development) as well as negative aspects (referred to as "don'ts" in early moral development). The "do's" are prominent in the infant's early experience and seem to follow naturally from the basic motives described previously. For example, a propensity for social interaction, the basic motive of social-fittedness, involves reciprocity in exchanges. Inclinations of this sort result in rules being internalized for turn-taking. These rules are learned in the course of games and other social interactions with caregivers (Bruner, 1986; Kaye, 1982; Stern, 1985) and represent early forms of reciprocity that are included in all moral systems. Similarly, the basic motive of cognitive assimilation, of getting it right about the world, leads to the internalization of many rules which become accepted by the child in the course of everyday life.

Toddlers typically develop further moral inclinations during the second year.

When confronted by another's distress, a one and one-half-year-old may respond empathically—also experiencing distress and attempting to comfort, soothe, or share something with the distressed other (Zahn-Waxler, Radke-Yarrow, & King, 1979; Zahn-Waxler, Robinson, & Emde, 1992). Toward the end of the second year, children sometimes show anxiety when internal standards are violated. When faced with a familiar object that is changed, flawed, or dirty, the child may evidence distress, and there may be a tendency to repair or make it better (Kagan, 1981), another form of "getting it right."

The infant's sense of initiative takes on a new level with the onset of walking, which has further implications for early moral development. This was characterized by Erikson (1950) as a stage of "autonomy versus shame and doubt" in the toddler's experience. The internalization of prohibitions or "don'ts" occurs through repeated interactions with caregivers wherein rules of safety and family culture are imposed. Correspondingly, the toddler develops a sense of the semantic "no" (Spitz, 1957) and a developing sense of "good" and "bad" (Mahler et al., 1975; Sander, 1985). Such a process involves not only negative features but also aspects of the "do's" in terms of the toddler's wanting to get it right and in terms of processes of social referencing. The child, through repeated interactions, learns strategies of negotiation in the midst of emotional communications with caregivers, as well as the consequences of these strategies (Emde et al., 1987; Kochanska, Casey, & Fukamoto, 1995; Kochanska & Askan, 1995; Kuczynski & Kochanska,

1995). Dunn and Kendrick (1982) also documents the importance of interactions that include conflicts with caregivers and siblings, over such issues as possession, sharing, or destruction, for the internalization of expectations and rules about how to negotiate or cope with these situations. Much of what the child first learns in this area is "practicing knowledge" (Reiss, 1989), knowledge that is activated when particular people come together in family or group routines.

We have placed strong emphasis on these moral motives because they are extremely important aspects of successful social development. Many needy children, however, have not been provided the consistent caregiving routines and practices to support such early moral motives. We believe the assessment of the child's moral motives in the context of the family, for example, to reciprocate, repair, and follow rules, and the engagement of these motives within the family, in the context of mealtimes, bedtimes, play, and other daily routines, are an untapped resource for intervention. In the next section, we provide more detail regarding caregiving interactions and routines that may or may not engage these motives and implications for intervention.

Enhancing Adaptive Processes in Caregiving Interactions and Routines

The caregiver-infant relationship is founded, at least in part, on the recurring, day-to-day interactions in which infants and caregivers engage. An important aspect of these early social interactions is their organization or structure. Their structure leads to, and then comes to depend upon, expectations that infants and their caregivers share about their own and each others' behavior. We hope to show that intervention opportunities can occur at fine-grained levels of interaction. First, we consider the need for consistent, adaptive patterns of behavior which both promote coordination in interaction and facilitate interactive repair when miscoordination occurs. The importance of these processes for positive developmental outcomes is highlighted. Next, we consider the negative developmental consequences of inconsistent and/or maladaptive patterns of interactive behavior. Moving from fine-grained analysis of interaction, we additionally consider behavior patterns within the larger context of the family system and discuss the beneficial effects of family routines on family functioning and child outcomes.

Caregiving Interaction

Research on infant-caregiver interactions during the past 25 years has made it clear that, from the earliest days of life, the infant is capable of highly predictable behavioral responses to outside stimuli and is an active participant in social interactions with his caregivers (Lewis & Rosenblum, 1974; Schaffer, 1977; Stern, 1977; Tronick, 1982). This research has also made it clear that despite these often impressive abilities, the infant has much to learn before he can contribute, in a more equal and socially appropriate way, to the maintenance and regulation of his interactions with others.

Social interaction is a complex process which requires individuals to coordinate their separate actions into a joint, organized activity (Duncan & Fiske, 1977; Kendon, 1982; Lewis, 1969; Schaffer, 1984). The ability to achieve coordination in interaction is closely tied to the experience of consistency. When similar patterns of behavior are repeated over time, both infant and caregiver are likely to develop expectations and rules, that are largely unconscious, about what behaviors are expected of them and what behaviors they can expect from their partner. Once such a set of mutual, reciprocal expectations is established, it increases the likelihood that the pattern will be repeated when infant and caregiver are engaged in similar kinds of social exchanges (Bruner & Sherwood, 1977; Duncan, 1991; Duncan, 1997; Duncan & Farley, 1990; Kubicek, 1981; Kubicek, 1992; Schaffer, 1984; Stern, 1977). In this way, dyads begin to establish their own characteristic patterns of interacting over time.

The profound influence of the infant-caregiver relationship on the infant's learning about self and other is intimately tied to these characteristic patterns (Sameroff & Emde, 1989a; Stern, 1985; Tronick, 1989). What the infant learns about turn-taking, reciprocity, repair, emotional regulation, and social referencing will be strongly influenced by the nature of these formative patterns of interaction with the caregiver. Such patterns will not only affect the infant's expectations regarding interactions with the caregiver, but will likely generalize and influence the infant's expectations regarding interactions with others as well (Tronick, 1989).

Although characteristics of the infant clearly affect these interaction patterns from the start (an influence which increases with age), because of the infant's dependence, characteristics of the caregiver have a more predominant influence in the earliest years. Both research and clinical practice indicate that certain caregiver characteristics are likely to foster patterns that are beneficial to the infant's development, whereas others are likely to foster patterns that are harmful. We consider each of these situations in turn.

If a caregiver is sensitive, responsive, and consistent, the expectations an infant develops about self and others are likely to nurture development of the basic motives of infancy. That is, an infant who consistently experiences a nurturing caregiving environment is more likely to be motivated to explore the environment, develop adaptive means for self-regulation, develop social competence, be more aware and attuned to the emotions of significant others and rely on them as a guide for his or her own behavior, and take pleasure in mastering the environment.

Of course, this is not meant to imply that all infant-caregiver interactions will be synchronous, well-coordinated, or affectivity positive even if the caregiver is sensitive, responsive, and consistent. Although researchers have used these terms to describe the communicative "dance" that develops between a caregiver and an infant, we now know that these terms tend to apply only to the "best" exchanges between caregivers and infants (Tronick

& Gianino, 1986). Even among well-functioning dyads, everyday communication is likely to involve many missed cues and misunderstandings relating to the mistiming or misreading of signals and different goals (Biringen, Emde, & Pipp-Siegel, 1997; Tronick & Cohn, 1989; Kubicek, 1992; Golinkoff, 1983, 1986). The resulting mismatches or violations of expectations may create stress and generate negative emotions. The challenge for the dyad is to develop effective strategies to repair these mismatches or violations, through self-directed or other-directed regulatory behavior. Fortunately, caregivers and even very young children typically work together to repair their communicative errors, so that their exchanges can continue, especially when interactions are characterized by sensitivity, responsivity, and consistency.

To illustrate, consider the following sequence, videotaped during an evening home visit with a family (Kubicek, 1992). The family had finished dinner, and the father and toddler had gone into the living room, as they often did, to play with some puzzles. The father sat down in a large chair, and his son sat on the floor a few feet in front of him. The child initiated an exchange with an apparent request to the father to place a bunny puzzle piece in the puzzle board, a request that the father initially misunderstood. The turn exchanges that follow illustrate the kind of additional "interactive work" and cooperation that is required of both caregiver and child to maintain their exchange and eventually resolve their misunderstanding. Although this child was 15 months old at the time, he had relatively few words and relied heavily on nonlanguage behaviors to communicate. The following was observed:

> The child vocalizes to his father ("eh") as he bounces the bunny puzzle piece in the air. Father points to the bunny space in the puzzle board and sings, "Hippity hoppity hippity hoppity hippity hoppity back in his spot?" Next, the child holds the bunny piece out to Father, who responds, "Put him back in his spot?" The child frowns and repeats his initial vocalization ("eh"), but this time in a more fretful, insistent tone, and bounces the bunny piece in the air. Father repeats, "Hippity hoppity hippity hoppity." At this point, the child interrupts his father by getting up and walking over to his father's chair and placing the bunny piece on the arm of the chair. Father now seems to understand and replies, "Want me to do it?" The child smiles and immediately points to the space in the puzzle board. Father bounces the bunny piece in the air as he sings, "Hippity hoppity hippity hoppity hippity hoppity back in his spot!" Both smile and break into laughter.

This vignette helps to highlight an important finding regarding caregiver-child interactions. Even in well-functioning dyads, interactions frequently involve the expression of negative as well as positive emotions. What is important for healthy development, and illustrated here, is that both parent and child learn to regulate their emotions in response to one another and express them in adaptive ways (Sameroff & Emde, 1989a). For example, in this vignette, the child expresses some anger/frustration as he attempts for the third time to communicate what he wants his father to do. He frowns and vocalizes in a more fretful and insistent tone as he bounces the bunny piece in the air. Despite his distress, the child copes well and continues to engage his father, an adaptive response which was likely motivated by earlier successes in similar situations. For his part, the father does not become angry or impatient with the child but instead, calmly makes another attempt to understand what his son wants. Both are eventually rewarded with success and share a hearty laugh before going on to their next game.

When caregivers and their children are able to regulate their emotions adaptively and negotiate needed communication repairs successfully, such early exchanges can provide a foundation for positive development. Through repeated experience in these day-to-day interactions with sensitive caregivers, the child begins to learn important lessons about the world and about how interaction works. Specifically, he learns adaptive rules for turn-taking, social reciprocity, and emotion regulation, begins to develop expectations about behavioral regularities and interactive sequences, and learns to repair errors or misunderstandings in interaction which allow him to maintain engagement in the face of stress. These experiences also help the child to develop a positive affective core (Emde, 1983b) and to view the self as effective and the caregiver as reliable and trustworthy (Tronick, 1989).

Less adaptive exchanges, on the other hand, may have negative consequences for development. Problems can arise when caregiver characteristics such as immaturity or inexperience (Brooks-Gunn & Chase-Lansdale, 1995; Osofsky, Hann, & Peebles, 1993), depression (Field, 1995; Tronick & Field, 1986), drug use (Mayes, 1995; Zuckerman & Brown, 1993), or stress related to chronic poverty (Halpern, 1993; Norton, 1990) lead to insensitive, nonresponsive, and inconsistent care. Under such conditions there can be disorganization, with maladaptive expectations about self and others that are likely to undermine the development of the basic motives summarized earlier in the chapter.

Consider, for example, the following interaction sequence, also videotaped during an evening home visit, of a family participating in a recent longitudinal study. Following dinner, the mother and the father and their two-year-old son went into the living room to play with some toys the researcher had brought. The mother and father sat on the floor leaning against the couch, and their son sat a few feet in front with his back to them. The child was absorbed in playing with a shape sorter which required matching color-coded keys to doors in order to remove animal blocks from the sorter. For the first part of the vignette, father repeatedly tickles and gently pokes at the child, despite the child's repeated protests that escalate in intensity. Failing to stop his father, the child eventually gets up and moves across the room. Shortly after, the child invites his father to play. First the father ignores the child, then repeatedly asks what the child wants before helping him open the door. In contrast to the previous vignette, the turn exchanges that follow illustrate how disruptive it can be for a child when a caregiver is unable or unwilling to respond in a sensitive way to his requests and thwarts, passively and/or actively, his attempts to repair.

Father gently pokes at the back of the child's neck as he sits trying to open the sorter door. The child says, "No," and continues to play. Next, the father successively pokes the child in three different spots on his back and the child says, "No, no!" in a louder voice. The father persists, and the child turns and looks at his father and says, "No!" even more loudly and attempts to push his father's hand away. He then turns back to the sorter, and father resumes his teasing. The child turns to his father and screams "No!" in a high pitched voice and then moves to the other side of the room where he plays with another toy. A few minutes later, the child, with keys in hand, approaches Father and invites his help saying, "Daddy do it, Daddy do it." Father stares with a blank face. The child says, "Daddy do" and places the keys on his father's hand. When Father fails to respond, the child picks up Father's limp hand and tries to put the keys inside it, repeating, "Daddy do, Daddy do it," several times while looking at his father. The child slaps at Father's hand, then screams and pulls the keys while Father holds on. The child eventually gets the keys and again asks, "Daddy do it," then begins to cry as he tries to put the keys back in his father's hand. Finally, the father asks, "What do you want?" The child sighs, then says, "Daddy do it." There are several more turns in which Father repeats, "Do what?" each time the child says "Daddy do it." The child eventually points to the sorter door and says, "Daddy do." Father asks, "Do

you want me to open the door?" and the child says, "Yep." Father begins to explain how to open the door, and the child watches.

In this example, the father intentionally creates conflict/disruption by teasing his son and ignoring the child's request to stop, despite the child's increasing distress. Rather than helping the child regulate his emotion, the father contributes to dysregulation. After repeated attempts, the child's only recourse is to remove himself from the situation. After calming himself, the child returns to his father who ignores his attempts to repair, once again escalating the child's distress until he cries. Even then, the father persists in several question-answer exchanges before helping the child with the sorter. This leads to a brief period of joint play, but one that clearly lacks the shared joy evident in the previous example.

When child and caregiver are unable to regulate emotions adaptively and negotiate needed repairs successfully, the characteristic patterns of interaction they develop are likely to undermine, rather than support, positive development. Through repeated experiences in these kinds of day-to-day interactions, the child is more likely to see the world as insensitive and uninviting. As Tronick (1989) warns, this could lead to the establishment of a self-directed style of regulatory behavior to control negative emotions. The need to control negative emotions may take precedence over other developmental goals. Such experiences are likely to interfere with the development of a positive affective core (Emde, 1983b), and the child may begin to view the self as ineffective and the caregiver as unreliable (Tronick, 1989). Due to such destructive effects on the child's overall development, intervention is warranted.

The preceding discussion suggests that one appropriate entry point for intervention with the caregiver and infant is with their interactive behaviors. Several models of early intervention have followed such an approach. Interaction guidance (McDonough, 1991, 1992, 1995) is one such example. The interventionist guides the caregiver to strengthen healthy patterns of interactional behavior with her infant, often using reflective review of videotaped interaction. Intervention, in other words, takes place within the context of the caregiver-infant relationship, rather than focusing on problems in the infant or the caregiver themselves. Similarly, a major goal of the parent-infant mental health model developed by Kathryn Barnard and colleagues (Barnard et al., 1987) is to influence the caregiver-infant relationship through social interaction and communication as well. There is strong emphasis on enhancing caregiver-infant interaction by developing the caregiver's awareness of infant cues, encouraging the caregiver to vocalize, respond contingently, provide appropriate stimulation, and develop appropriate expectations about infant abilities. In addition, curricula such as the Partnership in Parenting Education (PIPE) (Dolezal, Butterfield, & Grimshaw, 1994; Butterfield, 1996) emphasize guiding parents in how to set the stage for positive interaction by helping them become more sensitive and emotionally available. Through demonstrations and interactive sessions, using the infant as "teacher" and talking through the infant, parent educators focus on emotional communication, mutual regulation between caregiver and infant, and relationship-building skills.

Routines

Another entry point for intervention may be in encouraging the development and maintenance of meaningful family routines. Family routines are patterned interactions that occur with predictable regularity in the course of everyday living. Routines help to organize family life, reinforce family identity, and provide members with a shared sense of belonging (Wolin & Bennett, 1984).

At least one reason why adherence to routines may be associated with these positive outcomes is that family routines can provide an ongoing context for strengthening the parent-child relationship by providing regular opportunities for parent and child to come together around a common goal and develop patterns of interaction that are adaptive and likely to enhance development. Through repeated participation in shared, meaningful activities such as greetings, mealtimes, bedtime routines, and social games, with sensitive and responsive caregivers, children begin to internalize basic procedures for emotional regulation and morality and learn the values and practices of their family and culture (Bossard & Boll, 1950; Fiese, Hooker, Kotary, & Schwagler, 1993; Reiss, 1981; Rogoff, Mistry, Goncu, & Mosier, 1993).

Routines are considered an almost universal attribute of family life that cuts across ethnic background and socioeconomic status (Bossard & Boll, 1950; Boyce, Jensen, James, & Peacock, 1983). Nevertheless, few details are known about the actual day-to-day practices of families with infants and young children, particularly those with low incomes. The scant literature that is available, however, suggests that the lives of many families living in poverty lack adequate structure and predictable routines (Aponte, 1976; Halpern, 1993). Norton (1990) has intensively studied the early experiences of a longitudinal sample of inner city, low-income children of adolescent mothers, noting deficits in caregiving routines and the structuring of experience through language, as well as consequent problems in the children's future-oriented sense of time. Similarly, Escalona (1987) has described a relative lack of structure in the daily lives of the poorest infants in her economically disadvantaged longitudinal sample of premature infants and has found an association between this relative lack of structure and impairments in cognitive development.

Two studies have highlighted the beneficial effects of family routines on child social and cognitive outcomes in low-income Head Start preschoolers. Keltner (1990) found that adherence to family routines was predictive of preschool social competence. Churchill and Stoneman (1997) found that for girls, family routines were associated with higher scores on standardized cognitive tasks and teacher ratings of peer interaction. Preliminary results from our own ongoing longitudinal study (Kubicek & Emde, 1998) of an ethnically diverse group of Early Head Start research

families suggest that there is meaningful variation in the number and kind of routines these families follow. We plan to explore the relation between differences in the practice of family routines in this low-income sample and a number of outcome assessments in the toddler and preschool periods.

These results suggest a promising area in need of more systematic research aimed at identifying strengths in existing routines as well as documenting areas of impoverishment and difficulty so that culturally appropriate interventions can be developed. Such an approach has been used therapeutically to help families cope with problems relating to transitions such as adolescence or remarriage as well as mental health issues such as children's fears or obsessions or parental alcoholism (Imber-Black, Roberts, & Whitney, 1988).

Emotional Availability and the Role of the Interventionist in a Network of Relationships

Overlaying structure and everyday routines in the early caregiving relationship is the construct of emotional availability. Regulation of the emotional communicative system is a central task facing parent and infant. Initially, the emotional availability of caregiver to child provides the main basis for regulation. Being emotionally available can be thought of as communicating an openness toward the other's feelings and expressed needs (Biringen & Robinson, 1991; Sroufe, 1995). Emotional availability reflects a quality of the developing relationship that is continuous, in that expectations include a responsiveness that will bring interest and pleasure, as well as relief from distress (Emde, 1980). Variations in emotional availability and caregiver sensitivity are extensive. Not only are there deficits that can be considered maladaptive, but there are excesses. Infants can become disorganized by too much excitement or distress and communicative signals can also become aversive for caregivers. Managing caregiver arousal to infant signals is, therefore, a challenge in sustaining availability to infants and may need support from interventionists.

It is relevant to our theory of intervention that, through repeated experiences with emotionally available caregivers, the child, especially during the second year, learns skills of self-control, emotional regulation, and negotiation, as well as empathy in helping others. Pride and shame typically develop during the child's second year, and the interventionists can enhance attunement to the child of the caregiver by highlighting a toddler's new skills and emotional reactions. As could be seen in the exchanges described in the previous section, the experience and expression of positive emotions are also vital aspects of communication and regulations that are adaptive. An intervention that focuses on interactions between caregiver and child must be attuned to the emotional tone of the interaction as well as the specific behaviors. Promoting positive engagement is, in fact, a focus of the approaches noted in the previous section (Barnard et al., 1987; Dolezal et al., 1994; Butterfield, 1996; McDonough,

1991, 1992, 1995). For some parents, intuitive bases for emotionally available engagement are not present, and they may need assistance in experiencing what "getting it right" feels like in interactions (Emde & Robinson, in press). An important principle of intervention in this area is that, once having experienced a positive response from the infant, parents experience inherent rewards that continue to motivate positive interactions (Emde, 1980).

A relationship-based theory of intervention also addresses the emotional availability of the interventionist. This involves broadening our focus, from the emotional availability seen within the caregiving dyad to the emotional availability between the interventionist and the caregiving dyad. The interventionist's emotional availability includes not only the ability to resonate with the emotions of the infant-caregiver relationship in a way that can facilitate relief of distress and encouragement of positive emotional communications and engagement, but it also refers to the openness to empathic communications in a broader sense. Communicating an understanding of painful past experiences and how they might motivate actions in the present can convey an open presence to caregiver that is appreciated. Equally important is a perspective over time. Maintaining a consistent supportive alliance encourages a hopefulness about the possibility of alternative positive outcomes both now and in the future. When an interventionist is able to help a parent view a child's developmental motives more clearly and see that "ghosts" from the past that distort perception need not be influential (Fraiberg et al., 1975), there are new opportunities for appreciation of the child's individual experience and growth.

The interventionist's emotional availability also extends to a larger network of relationships, including those in family, community, and staff of programs that work with the caregiver or child, such as Early Head Start or day care. Indeed, all interventions, from short-term to long-term and from crisis-focused to analytic, involve the influence of relationships on other relationships. This leads to at least two implications. First, if we acknowledge and assess these influences, we may further strengthen our interventions by discovering other supportive relationships and conflicting ones that can use attention. In the model described by Barnard and colleagues (1987), for example, intervention during pregnancy focuses on the caregiver's social skills and relationships with others in her life, with the assumption that the caregiver's ability to parent a child will be based, at least in part, on the caregiver's ability to maintain satisfying relationships with other adults. Second, our efforts may often be misplaced. That is to say, in our infancy work, we make use of our relationship to the mother, but what seems most important is the relation we have to the mother-infant relationship. Thus, our efforts may need to be concentrated on fostering that relationship instead of focusing on the mother or on the child.

When we think of interventions as the influence of relationships on relationships, we realize that there are different levels we may address within developing systems. It is often strategic to choose a level for working that offers maximum leverage, depending on the unique concerns and experiences of the family. For example, we may have long-term goals to influence the internalized relationships that are represented in the child, such as to improve "working models of attachments", or similar goals to influence the internalized relationships within the mother's representational world, an approach seen most commonly in parent-infant psychotherapy models (Fraiberg, 1980). Other targeted goals might include improving father-child and mother-father relationships within the family in the course of our interventions. Similarly, other goals might address enhancing other supportive relationships for the mother and, thereby, improve her relationship with her infant—goals that are often prioritized in family support programs. As noted previously, we may target a more direct and immediate level for our goal-setting that concentrates on bettering the repeated interactions between mother and infant in order to make such interactions more satisfying. In all instances, it seems clear that our intervention relationship is in relation to one or more other relationships which we hope to influence for the better.

We need more thinking to address these points. Family systems approaches currently come closest to addressing these matters, but with a few exceptions (Byng-Hall, 1995; Scharff & Scharff, 1987), they seldom consider relations to internalized representations of relationships and seldom consider development. What is needed is intervention theory which probes further in this area and can specify schemes for assessing leverage points in developing systems—one that can yield opportunities for influencing the effects of relationships on relationships and their consequences for intervention in particular circumstances.

Evaluation of Infant Mental Health Programs

A theory of mental health services for very young children and their families should also provide a guide for evaluation of the services. Obviously, a comprehensive overview of evaluation issues in infant mental health cannot be conducted here. In this remaining section, however, we will address four important and interrelated facets of evaluation that parallel points earlier addressed: (1) measuring the *experience* of families in intervention programs; (2) considering the *dynamic development* of the intervention; (3) examining the *relationships that interventionists form* with families; and (4) examining the *network of relationships* within a program, including the program's relationships to the evaluator. Each of these points lead to a general conclusion: Given the many different entry points into the caregiving system available to programs and interventionists, examining the processes by which interventionists achieve outcomes is just as important as examining the outcomes themselves.

Experience of Participants

A key to examination of intervention process is recognition that people, including infants, have unique and individual experiences with a program. Understanding the variable experiences that families have within the program and understanding the meaning that is attached to that experience is crucial. Although the need for this has been repeatedly addressed (Emde, 1988c), there are few empirical examinations of this issue. The simple outcome question "Does it work?" that is often asked in evaluation studies is overly reductionistic, denying the large range of experiences that families have in an infant mental health program. By being so focused on outcome, one may lose sight of the crucial question of "How does the intervention work for whom under what circumstances"?

Families enter a mental health intervention with different motivations and expectancies. We too readily assume that because families initially agree to be part of an intervention program, they will be knowledgeable consumers and enthusiastic participants, understanding fully what they are getting into and endorsing our attempts to help them. But it may be that caregivers agree to enter an intervention program because they were pressured by another family member or support agency to join or because they want to see changes in circumstances around them, without having to explore changes in themselves. Once in a program, families will have different experiences, based in part upon their differing motivations and expectations, but also according to variation in program factors, such as the relationship that forms with the interventionist (see following) and the critical events that occur during the course of treatment. In short, participant characteristics at the onset and their experiences within the program will influence the meaning that they attach to the treatment that they receive.

It is possible to study this experience, although it involves a more in-depth focus on participants than outcome studies typically provide. One may chart, for example, the quantity of contact that families have with their interventionist to examine the different "dosages" of treatment (Howard, Moras, Brill, Martinovich, & Lutz, 1996). Olds & Korfmacher (1998) demonstrated in a nurse home-visiting program for first-time mothers that mothers with lower feelings of self-control received more visits than mothers with stronger senses of control. Mothers, in a very basic way, had different experiences based upon this level of psychological resources, and this differential experience likely contributed to the low rates of child maltreatment seen at later time periods in the home-visited, lower-resource group when compared to mothers who did not receive home visits (Olds, Henderson, Chamberlin, & Tatelbaum, 1986).

Amount of contact, however, is most likely a proxy measure for more complicated aspects of "dosage." These other qualitative characteristics of the experience include how emotionally engaged family members are within sessions or the actual content of the intervention (e.g., topics discussed or use of specific techniques, such as videotape feedback). These characteristics can be examined quantitatively, using scales and checklists (Greenspan et al., 1987; McBride & Peterson, 1997).

Different studies, for example, have empirically demonstrated that parent's engagement in the intervention predicts program outcome (see Heinicke, 1993, for one review). The young child's experience as intervention participant is less well studied (Liaw, Meisels, & Brooks-Gunn, 1995, is an exception), although there is ample evidence from the child care literature (Howes & Smith, 1995) that child activities and relationships in a center-based setting can be reliably measured.

Qualitative methods are also important evaluation tools and may in fact be the best way to measure complex aspects of a patient's experience. Focus groups (Gilkerson & Stott, 1997) and narratives of case studies (Kitzman, Cole, Yoos, & Olds, 1997) provide detailed accounts of how both participants and helpers find value or struggle with challenges within interventions. Qualitative and quantitative methods can be used together in the search for important program elements. For example, a study using preliminary data from an evaluation of an Early Head Start program examined how children from low-income families responded to a structured and enriched Montessori environment, using both weekly rating scales filled out by teachers and ethnographic field notes from an anthropologist (Korfmacher, Spicer, & Emde, 1998). The combined data highlighted individual variation across children in their response to the classroom environment, changes in the child's response across time, and the importance of the period of transition from the infant to the toddler classroom. The study also highlighted to the investigators how study of a common theme is enriched by comparing and contrasting qualitative and quantitative data.

Development of the Intervention

As the previous example demonstrates, the experience participants have in an intervention is not static. Infant mental health programs deal with young children and families that are undergoing rapid developmental adaptation. In turn, we can assume that children and families will respond in different ways over the course of the intervention. They will have different levels of engagement, and they will focus on different issues. Psychotherapy research with adults, for example, shows that improvements in feelings of well-being are apt to occur earlier in the treatment cycle, followed by symptom relief and only later by changes in behavioral adaptation patterns (Howard et al., 1996).

The relationship family members have with their infant mental health provider and the relationship the provider has with the parent-infant relationship will change over time. Given this, infant mental health programs themselves should not be considered static entities. They too must change over time, altering themselves to fit to the individual needs of families as the families embark on different longitudinal pathways.

As families and the programs that serve them develop and change over time, so must evaluation and measurement of the program itself be able to adapt. Examining how the experience and meaning of treatment changes for families and how these changes affect outcome requires a means of collecting process data from multiple time periods and requires sophisticated approaches toward analyzing data. New methods of measuring individual differences in development (Howard et al., 1996; Speer & Greenbaum, 1995) provide opportunities for studying change in response to intervention. These techniques have not yet been used to study changes in experiential aspects of the intervention itself, such as the therapeutic relationship, although such an approach is certainly possible if programs collect such data at multiple time points.

A final point about the developmental orientation of program evaluations in infant mental health is crucial. Given that the goals of most programs are future-oriented, for example, to improve social emotional competence after early childhood and to enhance school readiness, longitudinal follow-up is essential. Long-term follow-up of interventions early in the life cycle have demonstrated important effects over a decade later for both children and their parents, such as promoting school achievement (Barnett, 1995), reducing child maltreatment (Olds et al., 1997), and reducing child and parent antisocial behavior (Olds et al., 1997, 1998).

Therapeutic Relationships

An important element of the individual experience in an intervention is the quality of the relationship formed with the therapist or service provider. Therapeutic or helping relationships are frequently shown to be strong predictors of positive adult psychotherapy outcomes (Orlinsky, Grawe, & Parks, 1994; Orlinsky & Howard, 1986), as well as early childhood intervention research (Osofsky, Culp, & Ware, 1988; Lieberman, Weston, & Pawl, 1991).

The concept of the helping relationship has been measured mostly in terms of contributions by the participating parent or caregiver, measuring, for example, program "taking" (Osofsky et al., 1988), achievement of treatment goals (Barnard et al., 1988), or commitment (Korfmacher, Adam, Ogawa, & Egeland, 1997). Such constructs are basic measures of the treatment alliance. It must be acknowledged that, although a premium is placed on the helping relationship in early childhood programs, as has been noted repeatedly in this chapter and elsewhere (Olds & Kitzman, 1993), this relationship is very difficult to measure. Individuals within the helping relationship—the client and the provider—construct psychological meanings of the relationship that are based on their own personal history and interpretation of events, and they will perceive the relationship in ways different from each other and from an outside observer (Orlinsky & Howard, 1986). There are also specific features of a given individual helping relationship. That is, the *match* between therapist and patient is frequently shown to be an important program element in adult psychotherapy (Beutler, Machado, & Neufeldt, 1994) and is assumed to be so in early childhood interventions as well (Korfmacher, 1998).

Additionally, since the relationship is dynamic, the quality of the match and the meanings individuals attach to the relationship will change over time. A productive and meaningful alliance comes from a therapist and a client finding a level where they work well together. Just as we have noted in the parent-child relationship, there are periods in the helping relationship of disruption and repair. How the service provider and the family member negotiate these times is an important and untapped area of study. For example, sequential analyses, as are used in psychotherapy research, are ways to examine the reactions of clients to interventionist actions (Lambert & Hill, 1994) within a session. The function of so-called "critical events" (Fraser & Haapala, 1987; Peterson & McBride, 1999), on which the quality of the intervention can shift, also plays a role here. For example, the Early Head Start study noted previously highlights how important transitions between classrooms are for young children in center-based programs (Korfmacher et al., 1998). The previously mentioned techniques have as yet had minimal application in infant mental health programs, but they are promising in allowing for the tracking of individual infants and families using services over time.

In summary, although there is converging evidence to support the importance of the helping relationship in infant mental health programs, we do not yet understand what are the critical dimensions of the helping relationship to study or how to examine them best. Although our theory and our practice highlight how crucial it is to attend to these relationships, in an evaluation context, the helping relationship is a moving target. This aspect of early childhood intervention research needs increased attention, with development of qualitative and quantitative measures better able to capture it and its complexity.

Evaluating a Network of Relationships

The problems of measuring helping relationships in early childhood intervention are compounded by a point made previously in this chapter. In early childhood interventions, the provider not only develops a relationship with the parent (the relationship most analogous to the adult psychotherapy alliance), but also develops a relationship with the infant and additionally hopes to influence the relationship between the parent and the infant. These different relationships, as well as relationships that the provider may develop with other family members in the context of assisting the parent-child dyad, are all being played out simultaneously and developmentally.

In most cases, these other relationships are not being measured. Although we know that the therapist's alliance with the parent may predict a positive outcome, how does one measure the therapist's relationship to the infant, and how does this intersect with the relationship developing with the parent? This topic is unexplored in early childhood intervention, although research on the relationships between parents and day care providers may offer a model of study (Elicker, Noppe, Noppe, & Fornter-Wood, 1997).

To add to the complexity noted previously, there is one more relationship to discuss—the relationship between the program and the researcher. Strict advocates of the scientific method may emphasize a need for evaluators to keep an objective distance from the program that they study. According to this view, researchers should act unobtrusively around the intervention, silently observing and measuring, interviewing families, and videotaping children, but not relating their impressions of measurements until well after the intervention is concluded. Attempts to provide feedback to programs are seen as "experimenter effects," threats to the study's internal validity, and, therefore, discouraged.

Although these concerns of losing objectivity and empirical rigor are valid in some evaluation contexts, there needs to be acknowledgment of the cost that this rigor can bring. Empirical research establishes artificial constraints to programs, setting boundaries and limitations that disrupt the natural flow of families into program and services. A randomized trial, for example, will alter the motivation of participants in joining a study/intervention, putting off some families who do not want the uncertainty of assignment but also encouraging others who have no interest in the study but the commonly-used financial incentives for taking part in the research.

Although program evaluations that are tightly experimentally-based (i.e., efficacy trials) by their nature do not allow for an active dialogue between the researcher and the clinician, such trials are but one evaluation tool. The model of continuous improvement analyses, for example, where evaluators feed back information to programs and providers during the course of the intervention in order to promote changes or improvements, is increasingly being promoted. It is but one example of "action research" methods (Lewin, 1947; Whyte, 1984) that assume a more dynamic and collaborative relationship between evaluator and program. These alternative assessment approaches should be seriously considered for interventions that are in their own period of growth and development or that exist in a community or context where a strict efficacy trial is not feasible. Such strategies fit well within the relationship-based framework of intervention that has been proposed in this chapter.

Conclusion: A Need for Theory in an Increasingly Active Field

We began the chapter with the viewpoint that a contemporary useful theory of mental health interventions in infancy has certain common features. Successful mental health interventions are experience-focused, developmentally-oriented, and relationship-based. Moreover, they involve the influence of relationships on other relationships. Interventions in infant mental health build on developmental motives within the context of the caregiving relationship. Such interventions enhance adaptive processes in caregiving interactions and routines so as to enhance the experience of both caregiver and child with positive expectations in everyday routines, as well as for development itself. Enhancing emotional availability in the caregiving relationship involves attention to emotional regulation, exchanges of signals, and consistency over time in interactions between infant and caregiver. Correspondingly, the interventionist also becomes emotionally available in relation to this relationship, with expressions of empathic concern and appreciative interest. Evaluation of infant mental health programs attends to each of these features of the relationship-based theory of intervention. Such evaluation also highlights the network of relationships involved in work that targets improved developmental outcomes for infants and toddlers.

We return to the concerns of the practitioner. A topic we have not yet addressed is diagnosis and assessment. A relationship-based model of intervention, however, has begun to influence thinking in this area. Diagnosis, in the practice of infant mental health, is regarded as an ongoing process. It is not a fixed designation, but it needs to be repeated over time because of dynamic influences of development and because of the changing contexts of different caregiving and other relationships. The process of diagnosis consists of two aspects: The assessment of individuals in context and the classification of disorders.

The assessment of individuals involves a variety of evaluations of an individual's functioning and symptoms within the context of a network of family relationships, as well as evaluations of culture and stresses that are both biological and environmental. In light of the multidisciplinary nature of early intervention activities, practitioners of early intervention are likely to be diverse and multiple paradigms and methods of assessment may be applied (Brazelton &

Cramer, 1990; Fraiberg, 1980; Gaensbauer & Harmon, 1981; Greenspan, 1981, 1997; Stern & Stern-Bruschweiler, 1987; Shonkoff & Meisels, in press)

The diagnostic process moves from assessment to considerations of classification. The classification of disorder involves linking to a system of ordering knowledge about symptom patterns and syndromes that can provide information about etiology, prognosis, and intervention outcomes. Such classification has a major function of allowing for communication among professionals, and it is important to bear in mind that we classify disorders, not individuals (Rutter & Gould, 1985).

No current classification exists for infancy and toddlerhood that has been shown to be reliable or valid. A recent advance has been the publication of *Diagnostic Classification: Zero to Three; Diagnostic classification of mental health and developmental disorders of infancy and early childhood* (DC: 0–3; Zero to Three, 1994), representing the work of a national task force of clinicians. The new system is intended to supplement DSM–IV (American Psychiatric Association, 1994), providing adequate coverage of early age. Relevant to our model, this diagnostic classification system recommends assessment prior to classification and incorporates a multiaxial system that not only allows for the features of assessment, but pays special attention to the evaluation of the caregiver relationship. A special axis exists in the DC: 0–3 system which deals with relationship disorder, following the recommended use of a parent-infant relationship global assessment scale which provides anchor points for clinical judgments.

In conclusion, recent research has provided a considerable amount of knowledge about developmental processes in infancy and their dependence on an emotionally available caregiving relationship experience. Recent clinical practice has provided an accumulated conviction that relationship-based assessments and interventions are what lead to successful outcomes. Additionally, attention is now being directed, both in program evaluation and in mental health interventions, to influences across a network of relationships. In the increasingly active field of mental health interventions, we are now aware that effects result from the influence of relationships on other relationships. Insights about this are more recent, and research is needed. Because of a lack of empirical knowledge, this chapter can only point to a framework rather than a theory in this area. It is our hope that future research on the topic of a theory of infant mental health intervention will build on forthcoming inquiry and investigation to develop a more specific model.

References

American Psychiatric Association. (1994). *Diagnostic and statistical manual of mental disorders* (4th ed). Washington, DC: Author.

Aponte, H. J. (1976). Underorganization in the poor family. In J. D. Guerin (Ed.), *Family therapy: Theory and practice* (pp. 432–448). New York: Gardner Press.

Barnard, K. E., Hammond, M. A., Sumner, G. A., Kang, R., Johnson-Crowley, N., Snyder, C., Spietz, A., Blackburn, S.,

Brandt, P., & Magyary, D. (1987). Helping parents with preterm infants: Field test of a protocol. *Early Child Development and Care, 27,* 256–290.

Barnard, K. E., Magyary, D., Sumner, G., Booth, C. L., Mitchell, S. K., & Spieker, S. (1988). Prevention of parenting alterations for women of low social support. *Psychiatry, 51,* 248–253.

Barnett, W. S. (1995). Long-term effects of early childhood programs on cognitive and school outcomes. *The Future of Children, 5*(3), 25–50.

Bell, R. Q. (1968). A reinterpretation of the direction of effects in studies of socialization. *Psychological Review, 75,* 81–95.

Beutler, L. E., Machado, P. P. P., & Neufeldt, S. A. (1994). Therapist variables. In A. E. Bergin & S. I. Garfield (Eds.), *Handbook of psychotherapy and behavior change* (pp. 229–269). New York: Wiley.

Biringen, Z., Emde, R. N., & Pipp-Siegel, S. (1997). Dyssynchrony, conflict, and resolution: Positive contributions to infant development. *American Journal of Orthopsychiatry, 67,* 4–19.

Biringen, Z., & Robinson, J. (1991). Emotional availability in mother child interactions: A reconceptualization for research. *American Journal of Orthopsychiatry, 61,* 258–271.

Bossard, J., & Boll, E. (1950). *Rituals in family living.* Philadelphia, PA: University of Pennsylvania Press.

Boyce, W. T., Jensen, E. W., James, S. A., & Peacock, J. L. (1983). The family routines inventory: Theoretical origins. *Social Science Medicine, 17,* 193–200.

Bowlby, J. (1969). *Attachment and Loss: Vol. I. Attachment.* New York: Basic Books.

Bowlby, J. (1973). *Attachment and Loss: Vol. II. Separation, Anxiety and Anger.* New York: Basic Books.

Bowlby, J. (1980). *Attachment and Loss: Vol. III. Loss, Sadness and Depression.* New York: Basic Books.

Brazelton, T. B., & Cramer, B. G. (1990). *The earliest relationship.* Reading, MA: Addison-Wesley.

Brooks-Gunn, J., & Chase-Lansdale, P. L. (1995). Adolescent parenthood. In M. H. Bornstein (Ed.), *Handbook of parenting, Vol. 3* (pp. 113–149). Mahwah, NJ: Erlbaum.

Bruner, J. S. (1986). *Actual minds, possible worlds.* Cambridge, MA: Harvard University Press.

Bruner, J. S., & Sherwood, V. (1977). Peekaboo and the learning of rule structures. In J. S. Bruner, A. Jolly, & K. Sylva (Eds.), *Play: Its role in development and evolution* (pp. 277–285). Harmondsworth, England: Penguin.

Butterfield, P. M. (1996). The Partners in Parenting Education Program: A new option in parent education. *Zero to Three, 17*(1), 3–10.

Byng-Hall, J. (1995). *Rewriting family scripts: Improvisation and systems change.* New York and London: Guilford.

Carey, W. B. (1970). A simplified method for measuring infant temperament. *Journal of Pediatrics, 77,* 188–194.

Carey, W. B. (1972). Clinical applications of infant temperament. *Journal of Pediatrics, 81,* 823–828.

Chess, S. & Thomas, A. (1986). *Temperament in clinical practice.* New York and London: Guilford.

Churchill, S. L., & Stoneman, Z. (1997, April). *Family routines and temperament as a predictor of child outcomes: Differences by sex of child.* Poster presented at the biennial meeting of the Society for Research in Child Development, Washington, DC.

Dolezal, S., Butterfield, P. M., Grimshaw, J.

(1994). *Listen, listen, listen.* Denver, CO: How to Read Your Baby.

Duncan, S. D., Jr. (1991). Convention and conflict in the child's interaction with others. *Developmental Review, 11,* 337–367.

Duncan, S. D., Jr. (1997). Early parent-child interaction grammar prior to language acquisition. *Language and Communication, 17*(2), 149–164.

Duncan, S. D., Jr., & Farley, A. M. (1990). Achieving parent-child coordination through convention: Fixed- and variable-sequence conventions. *Child Development, 61,* 742–753.

Duncan, S. D., Jr., & Fiske, D. W. (1977). *Face-to-face interaction: Research, methods, and theory.* Hillsdale, NJ: Erlbaum.

Dunn, J., & Kendrick, C. (1982). *Siblings.* Cambridge, MA: Harvard University Press.

Elicker, J., Noppe, I. C., Noppe, L. D., & Fornter-Wood, C. (1997). The parent-caregiver relationship scale: Rounding out the relationship system in infant child care. *Early Education & Development, 8,* 83–100.

Emde, R. N. (1980). Emotional availability: A reciprocal reward system for infants and parents with implications for prevention of psychosocial disorders. In P. M. Taylor (Ed.), *Parent-infant relationships* (pp. 87–115). Orlando, FL: Grune & Stratton.

Emde, R. N. (1983a). *Rene A. Spitz: Dialogues from infancy. Selected papers (with commentary).* New York: International Universities Press.

Emde, R. N. (1983b). The pre-representational self and its affective core. *The Psychoanalytic Study of the Child, 38,* 165–192.

Emde, R. N. (1988a). Development terminable and interminable I: Innate and motivational factors from infancy. *International Journal of Psycho-Analysis, 69,* 23–42.

Emde, R. N. (1988b). Development terminable and interminable II: Recent psychoanalytic theory and therapeutic considerations. *International Journal of Psycho-Analysis, 69,* 283–296.

Emde, R. N. (1988c). Risk, intervention, and meaning. *Psychiatry, 51,* 254–259.

Emde, R. N. (1990). Mobilizing fundamental modes of development—an essay on empathic availability and therapeutic action. *Journal of the American Psychoanalytic Association, 38,* 881–913.

Emde, R. N. (1992). Social referencing research: Uncertainty, self, and the search for meaning. In S. Feinman (Ed.), *Social referencing and the social construction of reality in infancy* (pp. 79–94). New York: Plenum.

Emde, R. N., Biringen, Z., Clyman, R. B., & Oppenheim, D. (1991). The moral self of infancy: Affective core and procedural knowledge. *Developmental Review, 11,* 251–270.

Emde, R. N., Johnson, W. F., & Easterbrooks, M. A. (1987). The do's and don'ts of early moral development: Psychoanalytic tradition and current research. In J. Kagan & S. Lamb (Eds.), *The emergence of morality* (pp. 245–276). Chicago: University of Chicago Press.

Emde, R. N., & Robinson, J. L. (in press). Guiding principles for a theory of early intervention: A developmental-psychoanalytic perspective. In J. P. Shonkoff & S. J. Meisels (Eds.), *Handbook of early childhood intervention.* New York: Cambridge University Press.

Erikson, E. (1950). *Childhood and society.* New York: Norton.

Escalona, S. (1987). *Critical issues in the*

early development of premature infants. New Haven, CT: Yale University Press.

Field, T. (1995). Psychologically depressed parents. In M. H. Bornstein (Ed.), *Handbook of parenting, Vol. 4* (pp. 85–100). Mahwah, NJ: Erlbaum.

Fiese, B. H., Hooker, K. A., Kotary, L., & Schwagler, J. (1993). Family rituals in the early stages of parenthood. *Journal of Marriage and the Family, 55,* 633–642.

Fonagy, P., Steele, M., Moran, G. S., Steele, H., & Higgitt, A. (1993). Measuring the ghost in the nursery: An empirical study of the relation between parents' mental representations of childhood experiences and their infants' security of attachment. *Journal of the American Psychoanalytic Association, 41,* 957–989.

Fonagy, P., Steele, M., Steele, H. (1991). Maternal representations of attachment during pregnancy predict the organization of infant-mother attachment at one year of age. *Child Development, 62,* 880–893.

Fraiberg, S. (1980). *Clinical studies in infant mental health: The first year of life.* New York: Basic Books.

Fraiberg, S., Adelson, E., & Shapiro, V. (1975). Ghosts in the nursery: A psychoanalytic approach to the problems of impaired infant-mother relationships. *Journal of American Academy of Child Psychiatry, 14,* 387–421.

Fraiberg, S., Shapiro, V., & Cherniss, D. S. (1980). Treatment Modalities. In S. Fraiberg (Ed.), *Clinical studies in infant mental health: The first year of life* (pp. 49–77). New York: Basic Books.

Fraser, M., & Haapala, D. (1987). Home-based family treatment: A quantitative-qualitative assessment. *Journal of Applied Social Sciences, 12,* 1–23.

Gaensbauer, T. J., & Harmon, R. J. (1981). Clinical assessment in infancy utilizing a structured playroom situation. *Journal of the American Academy of Child Psychiatry, 20*(2), 264–280.

Gilkerson, L., & Stott F. (1997). Listening to the voices of families: Learning through caregiving consensus groups. *Zero to Three, 18*(2), 9–16.

Golinkoff, R. M. (1983). The preverbal negotiation of failed messages: Insights into the transition period. In R. M. Golinkoff (Ed.), *The transition from prelinguistic to linguistic communication* (pp. 57–78). Hillsdale, NJ: Erlbaum.

Golinkoff, R. M. (1986). "I beg your pardon?": the preverbal negotiation of failed messages. *Journal of Child Language, 13,* 455–476.

Greenspan, S. I. (1981). *Psychopathology and Adaptation in Infancy and Early Childhood.* New York: International Universities Press.

Greenspan, S. I. (1997). *The growth of the mind.* Reading, MA: Addison-Wesley (with Beryl Lieff Benderly).

Greenspan, S., Wieder, S., Lieberman, A. F., Nover, R., Robinson, M., & Lourie, R. (Eds.). (1987). *Infants in multirisk families.* Madison, CT: International Universities Press.

Halpern, R. (1993). Poverty and infant development. In C. H. Zeanah, Jr. (Ed.), *Handbook of infant mental health.* New York: Guilford.

Harmon, R. J., & Murrow, N. S. (1995). The effects of prematurity and other perinatal factors on infants' mastery motivation. In R. H. MacTurk & G. A. Morgan (Eds.), *Advances in applied developmental psychology: Vol. 12. Mastery motivation: Origins, conceptualizations, and applications* (pp. 237–256). Norwood, NJ: Ablex.

Heinicke, C. M. (1993). Factors affecting the efficacy of early family intervention. In

N. J. Anastasiow, S. et al. (Eds.), *At-risk infants: Interventions, families, and research* (pp. 91–100). Baltimore, MD: Brookes.

Howard, K. I., Moras, K., Brill, P. L., Martinovich, Z., & Lutz, W. (1996). Evaluation of psychotherapy: efficacy, effectiveness, and patient progress. *American Psychologist, 51,* 1059–1064.

Howes, C., & Smith, E. W. (1995). Relations among child care quality, teacher behavior, children's play activities, emotional security, and cognitive play activity in child care. *Early Childhood Research Quarterly, 10,* 381–404.

Imber-Black, E., Roberts, J., & Wheling, R. A. (1988). *Rituals in families and family therapy.* New York: Norton.

Kagan, J. (1981). *The second year: The emergence of self-awareness.* Cambridge: MA Harvard University Press.

Kaye, K. (1982). *The mental and social life of babies: How parents create persons.* Chicago: University of Chicago Press.

Keltner, B. (1990). Family characteristics of preschool social competence among black children in a Head Start program. *Child Psychiatry and Human Development, 21*(2), 95–108.

Kendon, A. (1982). The organization of behavior in face-to-face interaction: Observations on the development of a methodology. In K. R. Scherer & P. Ekman (Eds.), *Handbook of methods in nonverbal behavior research* (pp. 441–505). Cambridge: Cambridge University Press.

Kitzman, H., Cole, R., Yoos, L., & Olds, D. (1997). Challenges Experienced by Home Visitors: A Qualitative Study of Program Implementation. *Journal of Community Psychology, 25,* 95–109.

Kochanska, G., & Aksan, N. (1995). Mother-child mutually positive affect, the quality of child compliance to requests and prohibitions, and maternal control as correlates of early internalization. *Child Development, 66,* 236–254.

Kochanska, G., Casey, R. J., & Fukamoto, A. (1995). Toddlers' sensitivity to standard violations. *Child Development, 66,* 643–656.

Korfmacher, J. (1998). Examining the service provider in early intervention. *Zero to Three, 18*(4), 17–22.

Korfmacher, J., Adam, E., Ogawa, J., & Egeland, B. (1997). Adult attachment: Implications for the therapeutic process in a home visitation intervention. *Applied Developmental Science, 1,* 43–52.

Korfmacher, J., Spicer, P., & Emde, R. (1998, July). *Examining the child's experience in an Early Head Start Program.* Poster presented at Head Start Fourth National Research Conference, Washington, DC.

Kubicek, L. F. (1981). Organization in two mother-infant interactions involving a normal infant and his fraternal twin brother who was later diagnosed as autistic. In T. Field, S. Goldberg, D. Stern, & A. Sostek (Eds.), *Interaction in high-risk infants and children* (pp. 99–110). New York: Academic.

Kubicek, L. F. (1992). *Organization of parent-child repair and non-repair sequences in routine interactions at 15 and 21 months.* Unpublished doctoral dissertation, University of Chicago.

Kubicek, L. F., & Emde, R. N. (1998, July). Similarities and differences in the family routines of an ethnically diverse group of Early Head Start research families. Head Start Fourth National Research Conference, Washington, DC.

Kuczynski, L., & Kochanska, G. (1995). Function and content of maternal demands: Developmental significance of early demands for competent action. *Child Development, 66,* 616–628.

Lambert, M. J., & Hill, C. E. (1994). Assessing psychotherapy outcomes and processes. In A. E. Bergin & S. L. Garfield (Eds.), *Handbook of psychotherapy and behavior change* (p. 72–113). New York: Wiley.

Lewin, K. (1947). Action research and minority problems. *Journal of Social Issues, 2,* 34–36.

Lewis, D. K. (1969). *Convention.* Cambridge, MA: Harvard University Press.

Lewis, M., & Rosenblum, L. A. (Eds.). (1974). *The effect of the infant on its caregiver.* New York: Wiley.

Liaw, F., Meisels, S. J., Brooks-Gunn, J. (1995). The effects of experience of early intervention on low birth weight, premature children: The Infant Health and Development Program. *Early Childhood Research Quarterly, 10,* 405–431.

Lieberman, A. F., Weston, D., & Pawl, J. H. (1991). Preventive intervention and outcome with anxiously attached dyads. *Child Development, 62,* 199–209.

MacTurk, R. H., & Morgan, G. A. (1995). *Advances in applied developmental psychology: Vol. 12. Mastery motivation: Origins, conceptualizations, and applications.* Norwood, NJ: Ablex.

Mahler, M. S., Pine, F., & Bergman, A. (1975). *The psychological birth of the human infant: Symbiosis and individuation.* New York: Basic Books.

Main, M. (1993). Discourse, prediction, and recent studies in attachment: Implications for psychoanalysis. In T. Shapiro & R. N. Emde (Eds.), *Research in psychoanalysis: Process, development, outcome* (pp. 209–244). Madison, CT: International Universities Press.

Mayes, L. C. (1995). Substance abuse and parenting. In M. H. Bornstein (Ed.), *Handbook of parenting, Vol. 4* (pp. 101–126). Mahwah, NJ: Erlbaum.

McBride, S. L., & Peterson, C. (1997). Home-based early intervention with families and children with disabilities. Who is doing what? *Topics in Early Childhood Special Education, 17,* 209–233.

McDonough, S. C. (1991). Interaction guidance: A technique for treating early relationship disturbances in parents and children. In J. Gomes-Pedro (Ed.), *Bebe XXI.* Lisbon, Portugal: Condor.

McDonough, S. C. (1992). Treating early relationship disturbances with interaction guidance. In G. Fava-Vizziello & D. N. Stern (Eds.), *Models and techniques of psychotherapeutic intervention in the first years of life.* Milan: Rabbaello Cortina Editore.

McDonough, S. C. (1995). Promoting positive early parent-infant relationships through interaction guidance. *Child & Adolescent Psychiatric Clinics of North America, 4*(3), 661–672.

Norton, D. (1990). Understanding the early experience of black children in high-risk environments: Culturally and ecologically relevant research in regard to support for families. *Zero to Three, 10*(4), 1–7.

Olds, D. L., Eckenrode, J., Henderson, C. R., Kitzman, H., Powers, J., Cole, R., Sidora, K., Morris, P., Pettitt, L. M., & Luckey, D. (1997). Long-term effects of home visitation on maternal life course and child abuse and neglect: Fifteen year follow-up of a randomized trial. *JAMA: Journal of the American Medical Association, 278,* 637–643.

Olds, D. L., Henderson, C. R., Chamberlin, R., & Tatelbaum, R. (1986). Preventing child abuse and neglect: A randomized trial of nurse home visitation. *Pediatrics, 78,* 65–78.

Olds, D. L., Henderson, C. R., Cole R., Eckenrode J., Kitzman H., Luckey D., Pettitt L., Sidora K., Morris P., & Powers J. (1998). Long-term effects of nurse home visitation on children's criminal and antisocial behavior: 15-year follow-up of a randomized controlled trial. *JAMA: Journal of the American Medical Association, 280,* 1238–1244.

Olds, D. L., & Kitzman, H. (1993). Review of research on home visiting programs for pregnant women and parents of young children. *The Future of Children, 3*(3), 53–92.

Olds, D. L., & Korfmacher, J. (1998). Maternal psychological characteristics as influences on home visitation contact. *Journal of Community Psychology, 26,* 23–36.

Orlinsky, D. E., Grawe, K., & Parks, B. K. (1994). Process and outcome in psychotherapy—noch einmal. In A. E. Bergin & S. L. Garfield (Eds.), *Handbook of psychotherapy and behavior change* (pp. 270–376). New York: Wiley.

Orlinsky, D. E., & Howard, K. I. (1986). Process and outcome in psychotherapy. In S. L. Garfield & A. E. Bergin (Eds.), *Handbook of psychotherapy and behavior change* (pp. 311–381). New York: Wiley.

Osofsky, J. D., Culp, A. M., & Ware, L. M. (1988). Intervention challenges with adolescent mothers and their infants. *Psychiatry, 51,* 236–241.

Osofsky, J. D., & Danziger, B. (1974). Relationship between neonatal character and mother-infant interaction. *Developmental Psychology, 10,* 124–130.

Osofsky, J. D., Hann, D. M., & Peebles, C. (1993). Adolescent parenthood: Risks and opportunities for parents and infants. In C. H. Zeanah, Jr. (Ed.), *Handbook of infant mental health* (pp. 106–119). New York: Guilford.

Papousek, H., & Papousek, M. (1979). Early ontogeny of human social interaction: Its biological roots and social dimensions. In K. Foppa, W. Lepenies & D. Ploog (Eds.), *Human ethology: claims and limits of a new discipline* (pp. 456–489). New York: Cambridge University Press.

Peterson, C. A., & McBride, S. L. (1999, April). *Home-visiting: Parent and provider perceptions of critical events.* Paper presented at the Biennial Meeting of the Society for Research in Child Development, Albuquerque, NM.

Piaget, J. (1952). *The origins of intelligence in children* (2nd ed.). New York: International Universities Press.

Reiss, D. (1981). *The family's construction of reality.* Cambridge, MA: Harvard University Press.

Reiss, D. (1989). The represented and practicing family: Contrasting visions of family continuity. In A. J. Sameroff & R. N. Emde (Eds.), *Relationship disturbances in early childhood—A developmental approach* (pp. 191–220). New York: Basic Books.

Rogoff, B., Mistry, J., Goncu, A., & Mosier, C. (1993). Guided participation in cultural activity by toddlers and caregivers. *Monographs of the Society for Research in Child Development, 58*(8, Serial No. 236).

Rutter, M., & Gould, M. (1985). Classification. In M. Rutter & L. Hersov (Eds.), *Child and adolescent psychiatry: Modern approaches* (pp. 304–321). London: Blackwell Scientific Publications.

Sameroff, A. J. & Chandler, M. (1976). Reproductive risk and the continuum of caretaking casualty. In F. D. Horowitz (Ed.), *Review of the child development research: Vol. 4* (pp. 187–244). Chicago: University of Chicago Press.

Sameroff, A. J., & Emde, R. N. (Eds.). (1989a). *Relationship disturbances in early child-*

hood: A developmental approach. New York: Basic Books.

Sameroff, A. J., & Emde, R. N. (1989b). Relationship disturbances in context. In A. J. Sameroff & R. N. Emde (Eds.), *Relationship disturbances in early childhood: A developmental approach* (pp. 221–238). New York: Basic Books.

Sander, L. (1985). Toward a logic of organization in psychobiological development. In K. Klar & L. Siever (Eds.), *Biologic response styles: Clinical implications.* Monograph Series of the American Psychiatric Press.

Schaffer, H. R. (Ed.). (1977). *Studies in mother-infant interaction.* New York: Academic.

Schaffer, H. R. (Ed.). (1984). *The child's entry into a social world.* New York: Academic.

Scharff, D. E., & Scharff, J. S. (1987). *Object relations family therapy.* New Jersey and London: Jason Aronson.

Shonkoff, J. P., & Meisels, S. J. (Eds.) (in press). *Handbook of early childhood intervention* (2nd ed.). New York: Cambridge University Press.

Speer, D. C., & Greenbaum, P. E. (1995). Five methods of computing significant individual client change and improvement rates: Support for an individual growth curve approach. *Journal of Consulting and Clinical Psychology, 63,* 1044–1048.

Spitz, R. A. (1957). *No and yes: On the genesis of human communication.* New York: International Universities Press.

Spitz, R. A. (1959). *A genetic field theory of ego formation.* New York: International Universities Press.

Spitz, R. A. (1965). *The first year of life.* New York: International Universities Press.

Sroufe, L. A. (1995). *Emotional development: The organization of emotional life in the early years.* Cambridge, England and New York: Cambridge University Press.

Stern, D. (1977). *The first relationship.* Cambridge, MA: Harvard University Press.

Stern, D. (1985). *The interpersonal world of the infant.* New York: Basic Books.

Stern, D., & Stern-Bruschweiler, N. (1987). *The mother's representation of her infant: Considerations of its nature.* Unpublished manuscript.

Tronick, E. Z. (1982). *Social interchange in infancy.* Baltimore, MD: University Park Press.

Tronick, E. Z. (1989). Emotions and emotional communication in infancy. *American Psychologist, 44,* 112–126.

Tronick, E. Z., & Cohn, J. F. (1989). Infant-mother face-to-face interaction: Age and gender differences in coordination and the occurrence of miscoordination. *Child Development, 60,* 85–92.

Tronick, E. Z., & Field, T. (1986). *Maternal depression and infant disturbance: Vol. 34. New directions for child development.* London: Jossey-Bass.

Tronick, E. Z., & Gianino, A. (1986). Interactive mismatch and repair: Challenges to the coping infant. *Zero to Three, 6*(3), 1–6.

Tyson, R. L., Emde, R. N., Galenson, E., & Osofsky, J. D. (1985). The origins and fates of psychopathology in infancy: a panel discussion. In J. D. Call, E. Galenson & R. L. Tyson (Eds.), *Frontiers of infant psychiatry: Vol. 2* (pp. 480–489). New York: Basic Books.

Whyte, W. F. (1984). *Learning from the field: A guide from experience.* London: Sage.

Winnicott, D. W. (1960). *Ego distortion in terms of true and false self: The maturational processes and the facilitating environment.* New York: International University Press.

Wolin, S. J., & Bennett, L. A. (1984). Family rituals. *Family Process, 23,* 401–420.

Zahn-Waxler, C., Radke-Yarrow, M., & King, R. A. (1979). Child rearing and children's prosocial initiations toward victims of distress. *Child Development, 50,* 319–330.

Zahn-Waxler, C., Robinson, J., & Emde, R. N. (1992). The development of empathy in twins. *Developmental Psychology, 28,* 1038–1047.

Zuckerman, B., & Brown, E. R. (1993). Maternal substance abuse and infant development. In C. H. Zeanah, Jr. (Ed.), *Handbook of infant mental health.* New York: Guilford.

Zero To Three. (1994). *Diagnostic classification: 0–3 Diagnostic classification of mental health and developmental disorders of infancy and early childhood.* Washington, DC: Author.

2

Relationships for Growth:
Cultivating Reflective Practice
in Infant, Toddler, and
Preschool Programs

Linda Gilkerson and Rebecca Shahmoon-Shanok

2

Introduction

An experience is something we assume that we should be able to take in all at once, yet we find ourselves asking questions of it in this hide-and-seek game. There are tender little touches that make us want to come up close and look. But then confidence wavers, and we have to step back and bring it into focus again. We may need to push to recognize new kinds of problems and complexities, to catch perception in our peripheral vision so that the images tighten up and become more stable. Indeed, peripheral experience can become the center of the work. We become aware of what it's like to gain glimpses of things, and to register information about

The authors wish to express appreciation to Zero to Three: The National Center for Infants, Toddlers and Families as the wellspring within which this work was refined, to David Wilson for his patience and skilled assistance with the manuscript, and to Bridget Scott for her help with references. We also thank each of the survey respondents who gave time from very packed days to reply to the questionnaires.

objects, even when we're not looking at them directly. It's a bit like seeing more than we can take in.°

Many programs serving young children such as Head Start and day care, have their roots in either an educational/school model, or in a medical model, such as programs serving young children with developmental disabilities. In the first instance, the zeitgeist inherited from the schools has home/school separation, classrooms, curriculum/cognitive learning, and year-to-year pacing at the center. In the second, the hindsight of burgeoning birth-to-three knowledge allows us to see that the emphasis on remediation of deficits often minimized attention to the child's social and emotional development. The relational and emotional needs of very young children which, in fact, have intrinsic roles in both cognitive growth and basic adaptation (Greenspan, 1997; Schore, 1994) are not at the center of practice in either model.

Recent blueprints for early care and education of infants, toddlers, and preschoolers stress the importance of a relationship-based approach to child and family development. The principles of Developmentally Appropriate Practice (DAP), articulated by the National Association for the Education of Young Children (NAEYC) (Bredecamp & Copple, 1997), propose that young children learn best when they feel safe and valued, when their physical needs are met, and when they are psychologically secure. DAP encourages a child-sensitive, interaction-centered approach to early learning. The principles of Early Head Start stress the continuity of relationships, the importance of the home culture, and the necessity for parent involvement and partnership at the highest level (Advisory Committee on Services for Families with Infants and Toddlers, 1994). These principles echo the primary value of the early intervention component (Part C) of the Individuals with Disabilities Education Act (IDEA): respect for the family. Within this framework, the nature of relationships is at the heart of the early childhood intervention process.

But while the *philosophy* of early care and education is shifting, *practice* in the range of infant, toddler, and preschool settings is much, much slower to change. In order for them to develop self-regulation, initiative, affective range, and eventually symbolic capacities (Greenspan, 1997; Schore, 1994), young children *need* an individualized, relational, Extended-Families Model (Axtmann, 1986; Shahmoon-Shanok, 1984, 1997b), where specific, affectively-lively relationships can flourish and adults can sustain attuned attention and mediate the experiential world for each individual child (Feuerstein, 1986; Vygotsky, 1978); where peer-based interaction stimulates, rather than overwhelms, each child's initiative, playfulness, learning, and prosocial capabilities (Axtmann, 1986; Shahmoon-Shanok, 2000; Shanok, Welton, & Lapidus, 1989); and where families can feel that they are heard, can hear, and where they can be and feel effective. Regardless of the degree of developmental resource or challenge, *all* infants, toddlers, and preschoolers have emotional and social needs and capacities; so, too, do their parents. Unless these developmental core processes are central to the mission and goals of an early childhood service, significant opportunities to strengthen children and families are lost. In order to promote relationally specific care, engagement, and the self-knowledge that makes this possible across the range of children and families, practitioners and programs must themselves develop and change: they must become reflective. It is reflection upon experience and knowledge that not only facilitates adult learning but also stretches the relational capacities of practitioners to include the evolving social/emotional dimension of each child and to work in authentic partnerships with the preciously various families they encounter.

Reflection is the mindful consideration of one's actions (Tremmel, 1993); a dialogue of thinking and doing through which one becomes more skillful (Schön, 1983); a process through which patterns of behavior become clear and insights dawn regarding the nature of our assumptions and motivations. Reflection, then, is both a means and an end. That is, reflection is a way of examining one's work, a way of approaching the work, and a way of preparing for the work: reflection-*on*-action, reflection-*in*-action, and reflection-*for*-action (Schön, 1983). Reflective practice integrates formal and informal knowledge, and embraces self-knowledge as a necessary professional competency (Bowman, 1989). Reflection serves as a tool for quality enhancement, increasing organizational effectiveness and strengthening practice (Gilkerson & Als, 1995).

Reflection is particularly essential when the focus is on early relationships. Fenichel notes that relationship-based work with

small children and families engages the emotions as fully as the intellect:

> Very young children stir powerful feelings in adults (the species is programmed that way). Moreover, parents and parent-child interaction evoke complex responses in professionals that are often difficult to sort out and respond to in ways that support the parent, the child, and the relationship between them. (Fenichel, 1992a, p. 10)

Flexible, enduring, and durable reflective capacities are "made," and only partially "born." While there are certain personality characteristics and skills, such as patience, empathy, emotional range, self-efficacy, and critical thinking, which lend themselves to reflective practice, in order for reflective qualities to become an intrinsic attribute of one's professional role—in order for them to be recognized, familiar and internalized rather than new and "tacked on" (Pine, 1985) to become a familiar, internalized, and central agent of the professional self—they must be exercised and guided in vivo, in an apprenticeship with more experienced, reflective partners. Yet, so far, few of the disciplines that work with young children and their families emphasize reflection upon how and what is communicated to specific children and their families with the goal of building relational and emotional development. Furthermore, few degree programs prepare their practitioners for work with very young children *and* their families (Klein & Gilkerson, in press) or for transdisciplinary team approaches, because most of the professions emphasize *either* the child, *or* the parent, *or* the disability.

It is a very, very wide range of families and children who present themselves in birth to six services. Why would anyone expect that any practitioner could do useful things with all of them, alone? Work with and within relationships virtually *requires* ongoing opportunities for reflection within the context of a supportive supervisory relationship. This means that time must be set aside on a regular basis, with an experienced and trusted colleague, to explore the "imperfect processes" (Belenkey, Clinchy, Goldberger, & Tarlue, 1986) of professional practice and one's own responses to the work. Reflection-*on*-and-*for*-action is undertaken "in tranquility, off-line" (Tremmel, 1993) to build the capacity for reflection-*in*-action: "processes of 'feeling,' 'seeing,' or 'noticing' what it is you are doing; then learning from what you feel, see, or notice; and finally, intelligently, even intuitively adjusting your practice" (Tremmel, 1993, p. 436).

Regular, dependable, ongoing in-service training is necessary to build the capacity of staff members to understand and relate to the emotional and social factors in both the child and his primary parenting figures and to build relationships within the team. Building on the work which we (Eggbeer, Fenichel, Pawl, Shanok, & Williamson, 1994; Gilkerson & Young-Holt, 1992; Shanok, 1992; Shanok, Eggbeer & Fenichel, 1994–1995; Shanok, Gilkerson, Eggbeer, & Fenichel, 1995b) and others (Fenichel & Eggbeer, 1991; Fenichel, 1992a; Pawl, 1995) have done through Zero to Three: The Na-

tional Center for Infants, Toddlers and Families, we propose that relationally attuned supervision is the heart of reflective practice, and that in order for programs to accomplish their missions, they must provide an ongoing staff development, in-service training program centered around the provision of regular, collaborative, reflective supervision for staff and for administrators.

We recognize this as a bold, even audacious, position to take in reference to programs and professions that do not have a tradition of reflective supervision. Moreover, we realize that many programs and providers, particularly those in Part C Early Intervention settings and those in the health care system, are under growing pressure to increase the amount of direct service billable time and, consequently, to decrease the amount of time available for any in-service education and team communication.

But to fulfill the trust that is literally in our arms anytime and anywhere services are delivered to our nation's youngest citizens and their families, programs and professionals must become relationally sensitive and emotionally alive. Five decades of research and clinical experience from diverse sources converge to make explicit the fact that early development is dependent upon the quality of relationships (c.f. Ainsworth, Blehar, Waters, & Wall, 1978; Bowlby, 1988; Fraiberg, Adelson, & Sharpio 1975; Greenspan, 1992; Mahler, Pine, & Bergman, 1975; Stern, 1985). Because our work is well described as the impact *of* relationships *upon* relationships (Emde, 1998), we must make available to frontline practitioners the resources needed to support relationship-based work.

> ... shared sense has emerged that the critical mental health challenge is not so much diagnosing problems or building specific skills, such as setting limits, but is in supporting the staff in caring for children, and helping them ensure that children's (and families') [parentheses added] emotional and social needs are being met. . . . (Yoshikawa & Knitzer, 1997, p. 31)

Yet, given the enormous pressures on programs as a consequence of severely limited financial resources, it is critical to think flexibly, creatively, and practically in order to achieve the establishment of ongoing opportunities for reflection in birth through five programs.

The purpose of this chapter is to describe the qualities of leadership, staff development, and supervision conducive and necessary to thoughtful, sensitive, intelligent, well-planned reflective practice with very young children and their families. In the spirit of beginning where programs/providers are, we first describe the perceptions of directors from a range of settings regarding the current status of supervision and consultation in their programs. Next, we present in greater depth the elements of reflective supervision. Finally, the current dilemma of availability is addressed by presenting workable models for the integration of *reflective process* and, eventually, *reflective supervision* into programs that have limited finances and with professionals who have not experienced it.

Voices from the Field

Early Impressions: 1991

In 1991, Zero to Three: The National Center for Infants, Toddlers and Families engaged in a series of activities—telephone interviews, leadership forums, and focus groups—to explore the perceptions of practitioners and administrators regarding supervision and mentorship in the infant/family field (Fenichel & Eggbeer, 1992b). Not surprisingly, they note that colleagues in programs closely associated with Zero to Three highly value supervision and mentorship. However, even these program leaders had difficulty in finding and protecting the necessary resources (time and money) to maintain regular supervision and reported that staff keenly felt the lack or loss of good supervision. Once staff have experienced supportive supervision, they do not want to be without it.

When asked to describe good supervisors, participants from all the groups listed the following qualities and experiences: sensitivity, good listening skills, someone who explains things, mutual respect, giving staff autonomy, constructive handling of conflict, someone who will work alongside you, and availability. For the infant/toddler childcare group, it is interesting to note that regularity in supervision did not seem as important as general availability. In these focus groups, supervisors and child care providers in public agencies less readily associated reflection with supervision. Rather, they most likely saw supervision as advice, performance appraisal, and staff evaluation.

Providers felt that supervision was particularly important in a "frontier" field, where so much learning comes through experience and where cultural and value differences can separate practitioner and family. The providers acknowledged that the consequences of inadequate supervision left them feeling "floundering" and "insecure" and at best resulted in not doing a good job, at worst, doing real harm. Yet when asked how they would spend a gift of $50,000 to their program, neither the practitioners nor the administrators were willing to spend the money on improving supervision. More direct services, more frontline personnel, and more training were priorities for the hypothetical resources. Supervision was seen as a luxury, rather than an essential component of professional practice and training, even for people who wanted it. The focus group designer concluded that convincing providers of the necessity of reflective supervision might require convincing them of their own importance in infant/family work. Indeed, she wrote,

> The most salient challenge to "selling" supervision is the lack of entitlement many of these practitioners feel. They see supervision as something for *them, rather than their clients, and [they feel that] they are not as important as the people that they serve* [italics added]. In order to really institutionalize good supervision and mentorship programs . . . education (will be needed) on how supervision translates into better care for their clients, so that practitioners feel entitled to ask for this help. (EDK Associates, 1991 as cited in Fenichel & Eggbeer, 1992b)

Update: 1998

Seven years later, we found that program directors report many of the same issues and concerns. Using a questionnaire format, one of the authors (LG) surveyed 20 directors of Part C early intervention programs and 18 directors of infant/toddler day care programs in Illinois and 8 directors/practitioners from a range of infant/toddler/preschool settings in the New York metropolitan area. First, we report the perceptions of the Part C Early Intervention Program Directors. Next, we compare their perspectives to those of center-based infant/toddler child care providers and, finally, we discuss the views of the New York group, who represent a range of community-based prevention and intervention programs.

PART C EARLY INTERVENTION DIRECTORS

Early intervention directors in Illinois reported that programs which offer individual supervision and organized group supervision are in the minority. Individual supervision is most frequently offered on an as needed basis. Only 10 percent of the programs offer individual supervision weekly, and another 15 percent offer monthly individual supervision. Organized group supervision occurs most frequently on an as needed basis.

The most common formats for supervision activity, available to nearly all early intervention providers, are team meetings/case reviews and informal peer support. Frequency of team meetings varied:

approximately one-half of the programs hold weekly team meetings while the other half meet biweekly, monthly, or as needed. One-half of the directors reported that informal peer support occurs on an as needed basis, while 40 percent report daily peer support.

Supervision to direct staff is primarily provided by the program directors, and to a much lesser extent, other senior staff members, administrators, and consultants share the supervisory responsibilities. The educational backgrounds of the directors are predominantly from the field of education: early childhood, early childhood special education or special education and, less frequently, from occupational therapy, speech-language therapy, and nursing. Only three of the supervisors had formal training in mental health. The most common issues that arise in supervision fall into four broad categories: child concerns, family concerns, team concerns, and systems/policy issues (see Table 2.1).

Perhaps what is most striking from this data is the relatively low percentage of directors who reported child issues as a focus for supervision, even though a great majority of them reported that the complexity of presenting problems among children en-

TABLE 2.1

Part C Programs: Issues Arising in Supervision[1]

Child Issues

- Complex social/emotional/behavior management challenges of children

Family Issues

- Boundary issues: What are appropriate family issues to address?
- Families' lack of participation/commitment in program
- When to call protective services
- Staff members stress/confusion about families

Team Issue

- Space, time, scheduling conflicts with other staff
- Interpersonal issues among staff
- Flow of communication among team members
- Staff insensitivity to families

Systems Issues

- Billing/funding issues
- Documentation of services; IFSP (Individual Family Service Plan)
- Lack of services to meet range of family need
- Understanding the new EI (Early Intervention) system and explaining it to parents

[1]Order of the issues as they are listed here does not imply frequency.

tering early intervention had increased. Specifically, directors noted that children present with more severe and multiple disabilities, with increasingly complex medical and/or social/emotional needs. Among those who did bring child concerns to supervision, behavior management was the focus. With greater numbers of children living in single family homes, in foster care, or with less extended family support than in prior generations, family issues appeared as the priority for supervisory support. Team issues centered primarily around conflictual interpersonal communication and attitudes among staff. Because of the recent change from a grant-funded program model to a fee-for-service systems approach to early intervention in Illinois, providers had many implementation issues regarding state and local policies and practices. When asked what kinds of issues directors themselves believed would be helpful for staff to address through supervision, most directors mentioned similar topics and added (a) problem-solving capability within the staff, (b) increased use of a less fragmented, discipline-specific approach to services, and (c) increased personal awareness.

Overall, fewer than half of the directors were satisfied with the current supervisory capacities within their agencies. Rather, directors would have liked to increase the amount of individual, personalized supervision and the amount of team time to discuss each child/family "at a [more] leisurely pace." The major barriers cited were lack of time and a dearth of money. Some directors were part-time. Others carried a sizeable caseload themselves. Thus, time for supervision was limited, eked out of overly scheduled and somewhat dizzying workdays. The most common barrier mentioned was the press for billable hours. One director wrote, "The staff are stretched to the limit and not allowed time to reflect and, in fact, to grow professionally and become more productive."

The lack of persons who could provide quality supervision was cited by only one program as a barrier to achieving an ideal supervisory plan. Yet, when the educational backgrounds of most directors/supervisors were factored in, it is likely that very few had any formal focus in their training on reflective processes, on analyzing self, or on the ideas of parallel process and shared power.

In terms of supervisory resources for the directors themselves, when they had it, program directors typically received supervision from an agency division director, vice president, or executive director. Yet, fully one-fourth of the directors reported that there was no one designated as their supervisor. Education was the most common background of those who supervised directors. The majority of directors who did report getting some supervision did not have a regularly scheduled time to meet with their own supervisors. When they did receive supervision, directors used it most frequently for (a) program planning and logistical concerns and (b) support around work with team members. When asked what kinds of concerns the directors bring to their own supervision, only one director mentioned discussion of child issues, and not one mentioned family issues.

Virtually all of the suggestions by respondents for improvement in director supervision related to increased regularity of supervisory contact: "It would be helpful to meet regularly, not just when there's something to do administratively." "Frequently, I access the supervisory process related to a crisis. I'd like to have the time to use a more proactive approach." Some directors expressed a desire for their supervisor to observe the program and meet with staff. The directors listed the following qualities as contributing most to their supervisor's effectiveness: knowledge of and experience in the field, interpersonal skills (supportive, positive, understanding listener, affirming), and effective problem-solving skills (brainstorming alternate solutions). Thus, it was notable that most respondent/directors had positive ideas about the supervisory process, whether they were the recipient or the provider and would like to see more opportunities for thoughtful, personalized supervision.

CHILD CARE DIRECTORS

As with early intervention programs, the most common form of supervisory activity in the infant/toddler programs surveyed were team meetings and informal peer support. Some opportunities for individual supervision were provided in 12 of the 18 centers. While more than one-half of the directors were satisfied with the supervision in place for providers, they also reported that, ideally, each staff member should receive individualized, hands-on supervision, including an ongoing relationship with a mentor or master teacher who does not have other classroom responsibilities. The directors wished for more time:

for direct observation; to videotape classrooms in order to offer providers a chance to observe themselves; and to monitor job performance and day-to-day interactions in the center. The directors also noted that more time was required for staff to discuss developmental goals and daily plans for the children and more funding was needed for training. They saw the primary barriers to supervision in child care centers as related to limits of time and money and to a lesser extent, their knowledge of supervisory models and the availability of persons able to provide good supervision. Neither lack of interest of staff nor lack of commitment from administrators was noted as major barriers to staff supervision.

The child care center directors received supervision from agency administrators, who typically had backgrounds in either education or in business/management. Most of the directors had a regular time to meet with their supervisors. Supervision focused on a range of topics including evaluation of their performance, support around work with families, staff, *and* children, and personal support. Tuition, salaries, and budget issues were also addressed. Several directors expressed the desire for their supervisor to be on-site more frequently in order for them to feel that the supervisor was backing the decisions they had made. The supervisors stressed a need for a hands-on supervisory model, for themselves as well as for their staff. That is, they believed that their program would be strengthened if their supervisors were present in the setting, gaining firsthand knowledge of the children, families, and staff and providing practical guidance. Further, they identified the need for a more organized support system with their own peers within the field.

Twelve of the 18 programs had access to consultation on an as needed or monthly basis. Child-related issues for consultation included developmental assessment, behavioral problems, and inclusion support. Family-related needs were primarily centered around inclusion and communication with families. Staff-related areas involved child-related concerns (e.g., observation and recording, curriculum development, classroom management), rather than issues of conflict resolution. The directors sought consultation regarding program development, staff supervision, and staff recruitment and retention. The professional backgrounds of the consultants related to the areas of need: early education/child development, nursing, social work, psychology, and special needs professionals—occupational therapy, speech therapy, and inclusion facilitation. Only one-half of the programs felt that the amount of contact with the consultant(s) was adequate. Directors of programs that did not have consultation saw the addition of this service as valuable. They saw their consultation needs as including communication with families, cultural diversity, working with families in crisis, child assessment, behavioral management, health and nutrition, teamwork, supervisory models, program development (environmental design, planning, continuity of care), and licensing.

NEW YORK PROGRAMS

The leaders from eight infant/toddler programs in New York echoed the perspectives of the Illinois directors: The supervision provided to frontline staff and program directors was not sufficient in frequency or in substance, given the increasing complexity of child and family needs. Ideally, programs would have liked to offer weekly individual or group supervision to supplement team meetings and informal peer support. Barriers included, in order of frequency, lack of time, lack of commitment from administrators, lack of qualified supervisors, lack of money, and lack of knowledge of supervisory models. Lack of interest of staff was mentioned by only one program. Five of eight directors reported regularly scheduled, weekly individual meetings with their own supervisors at work. In contrast to many Illinois directors, their own supervision at work focused primarily on work with children and families, and less so, on conflicts with team members or program planning and logistics.

However, all of the New York leaders surveyed were involved in advanced training in infant mental health[1] and, as part of their training program, received weekly, individual and group reflective supervision. Their own experience of respectful, responsive reflective supervision had, for several, been eye-opening at least and, for some, practice-changing.

Until this experience, I have had a negative view of supervision. Supervision I have had in the past (early on in my working in this field) can be described as destructive and/or painful. I felt the supervisors were not committed to intensive, constructive supervision. My current experience has been an extremely positive, helpful one and I see the great potential that such a constructive relationship can have.

The supervision I have received so far this year has been excellent and has made me realize how knowledgeable clinical supervision can stretch me, as well as help me provide better support and services to the folks I work with.

It was initially and still somewhat challenging to organize around supervision from a discipline different from my own. It has encouraged me to 'widen my lens.' I have benefited greatly from the weekly one-on-one supervision as well as group supervision.

It's made me a little more critical! At work, I've taken on more supervisees with a better sense of how to do it . . . being supervised on supervising has . . . intensified *'Doing unto others as I would have them do unto others.'*

Summary of Voices from the Field

Data from the three sets of programs revealed several common themes:

1. Most of what is referred to as "supervision" within service centers takes place in team meetings and informal peer support, circumstances in which supervision is not explicit and, most probably, not followed up either from the point of view of the staff member's own professional growth and development or, even in any fuller way, from the perspective of the situation discussed.

2. The individual supervision that does occur is often unscheduled and is typically provided by persons with an educational background whose own disciplinary training most likely did not include opportunities for or training about process-oriented and affectively-based reflective supervision.

3. While the respondents appear satisfied with the content (though not the duration or depth) of their supervisory contacts, the topics generated suggest that many significant areas for reflection are neglected or ignored.

4. Directors receive limited supervision, focused mostly on administrative or systems issues. Process concerns that were addressed related to team conflict and staff management. In child care programs per se, supervision and consultation addressed child-related and curriculum concerns. Children and families were rarely the focus of director supervision in early intervention, perhaps because of the roles and backgrounds of the directors' supervisors and the pressing issues related to the larger service delivery system. Clinical expertise, that is, knowledge of child and family work, then, must come from the director, program consultants, or the staff themselves.

5. Offering program directors (and other leaders) regularly-occurring reflective supervision may be one of the most potent ways to stimulate increased quality and perhaps even the quantity of supervision for direct service staff.

Thus, the survey indicated that a start toward the incorporation of supervision for purposes other than evaluation has been made, at least among directors and leaders interested enough in the topic to devote some of their precious, pressured time to respond to the questionnaire. Still, even among those programs/practitioners doing the most, there remained a profound gap between the state of the field and the state of the art. It is our hope that the following sections, that define, describe, and provide a vision of reflective supervision and practice and offer a potpourri of ideas about how to incorporate these practices—how to turn the vision into reality—will contribute toward moving the state of the field forward, even while the challenges inherent in integrating practices across disciplines continue to be uncovered, explored, and worked out.

Reflective supervision encourages you to actively look at the experience, to puzzle it out, notice the context, and abandon the fiction that the whole picture is available to you at once. Hunt for the appearance of the subtext, the emotional tone, and the narrative: Some aspects are more quickly recognized than others. °

Reflective Supervision

Essential Qualities

Intensive work with young children and their families routinely faces us with novel human challenges. No one of us alone is able to meet the whole range of those challenges. Just as we need to learn about how to take the next step in building relationally specific and constructive interactions with each child and his parent, so too, we must learn to generate constructive, specific relationships for professional learning within which there is trust and a sense of sufficient safety to expose and explore one's most painful or embarrassing practice questions or dilemmas.

Reflective supervision is a relationship for learning where "strengths are supported and vulnerabilities are partnered" (Shanok, 1992, p. 37). Attachments form within the context of safety and relational specificity generated by an engaged, contingent, resourceful, and more experienced colleague, in regularly occurring circumstances over a long period of time. It takes time to cultivate supervisory relationships on the part of the supervisee and the supervisor. That time needs to be made and kept as the precious resource and blessing it is, so that each knows she can count on such an oasis, a place that moves into slower motion, where trust can grow as details are replayed, sifted through, and looked at from many angles, and a plan for the very next step can be born, in a context of safety.

Given their own prior experience, supervisors know that there may be no solutions readily available and that an important role for a supervisor is to hold—to contain—the anxiety of the supervisee. This kind of supervision conveys the sense that long-term improvement and development are discovered by carrying out short-term plans. Observation and reflection upon what has just happened offers further information and the next step about which to reflect. So the work moves forward, step by thoughtful step.

REFLECTIVE SUPERVISION REQUIRES A TRUSTWORTHY, RESPONSIVE ENVIRONMENT THAT IS OPEN TO CHANGE

Laying bare one's performance for inspection implies vulnerability and openness— optimal states for learning. The stimulus for reflection is often rooted in a need to better understand areas where a practitioner feels incompetent and unsure—the very areas that most need to be addressed and which, in situations without supportive supervision, are most likely to be concealed. Thus, reflection requires a climate of trust. With a listening companion, isolation and stress diminish while optimism and resourcefulness increase.

To think reflectively is to actively pursue the possibility that existing practices or, perhaps, program policies themselves may need rethinking. Thus, reflective practice requires a responsive organizational culture that is open to change. This implies that in good reflective practice, communication—the important messages which cause people to imagine new possibilities—flows in several directions. The supervisor and *her* supervisor (often the director) should try to really hear the supervisee's ideas and make use of them. Indeed, leadership at all levels within programs serving young children and their families can actively promote creative shifts in program practice and policy, not only by utilizing good ideas, but also by using the criticisms, pattern of stress, and even the wishful thinking of supervisees as fodder with which to problem-solve.

Line staff become deeply engaged when they are heard—*respected*—and can be invited and helped to generate ideas for thoughtfully planned change. Thus it is that many shifts in practice and even in policy originate bottom up, not top-down, in wholesome organizations whose subunits enjoy respect, flexibility, and autonomy in key areas. Such decentralization is possible when the chain of command is not by-

passed and when unit and program leaders are themselves held in nonauthoritarian, respectful relationships which welcome and foster communication. To utilize the combined best of everyone's ideas and to work through differences, team members at all levels, beginning with the executive director of the organization, need to truly hear each other.

REFLECTIVE SUPERVISION MODELS
PARALLEL PROCESS: HOLDING SO
THAT OTHERS CAN HOLD

When supervisees are treated with enduring consideration and respect, they, by parallel process, are enabled to offer those qualities to the parents and children with whom they work. As Pawl (1995) put it, "Do unto others as you would have them do unto others." Patience, nurturance, and the respect inherent in a good listening ear, applied with sensitivity to developmentally appropriate relationships, tend to gather in and mobilize parallel qualities. Once we recognize the developmental-relational needs of small children and the deeply personal transitions and dilemmas faced by their parents, it becomes easier to recognize how critical this dimension is. For staff members to become able to discover the wide range of responsivity and individualized resourcefulness which various children and families need, they themselves need to be "held" in a supportive, relationally nuanced "space." That means that in all programs, even in relatively small programs such as Early Head Start or day care centers, each staff member, like every child and family, needs a primary, trustworthy, specific person of her own, someone who will be thoughtfully responsive to that staff member's needs.

REFLECTIVE SUPERVISION IS BASED ON SHARED POWER

Any supervisee recognizes her supervisor as someone with power over her. The greater the power, the greater the supervisee's anxiety. Yet, the supervisory relationship does *not* need to be about dominance or control. Acknowledging the asymmetry within the supervisory relationship, Shanok (1992, p. 39, drawing on Manis, 1979) describes how to tilt the balance of power that exists between supervisor and supervisee. That is, as much as possible, the locus of power needs to be transferred. In the relational model described here, the power is shared, which is a great relief not only to the supervisee but also the supervisor! The supervisor facilitates the articulation of a contract between the supervisee and herself, even as she helps the supervisee make explicit her contracts with families. Thus, the supervisee needs to have the right to:

- Join in the development of a set of shared understandings—a contract—defining reciprocal interactions
- Participate in developing the learning structure to which she is being exposed
- Take first responsibility in analyzing her own work,
- Contribute meaningfully to her own evaluation

Thus, while the supervisor/supervisee relationship *is* asymmetrical, it is still democratic. In sharing active responsibility for

these processes, the supervisee develops capacity for reflection, analysis, and planning. The supervisee becomes more responsible and is better able to think and contribute creatively to her own learning when she has a stake in developing the terrain to be covered, when the qualities of the learning specific to her are explicit, and when the supervisory relationship features openness. Figure 2.1 shows one possible Narrative Evaluation outline which can serve as a performance appraisal as well as a set of foci for the supervisee/supervisor's upcoming shared attention. The goal of both the supervisee *and* the supervisor is for the supervisee to gradually discover competence, power and a sense of control in the process. The views of the supervisor, both supportive and critical, when tactfully offered become interwoven with those of the supervisee, instead of being experienced as an opinion coming from the outside. Performance evaluation can be felt as caring support which guides a practitioner's own goals for development.

REFLECTIVE SUPERVISION BUILDS SHARED UNDERSTANDING OF PHILOSOPHY AND PRACTICE

Reflective supervision offers a way of conveying the values of the organization and of linking those values to everyday practice. The priorities of the organization and its beliefs about good practice are naturally woven into the discussions of the work and become its living philosophy. Sharing and further distinguishing the organization's philosophy become shared understanding in a oral tradition which is passed on, one person to the next, in context. In this kind

Name of Supervisee:

_____

Period Covered: **from** _____ **to** _____

Today's Date: _____

Name of Supervisor: _____

Background:

Strengths:

Areas for Growth:

Integrative Statement and Plans for Improvement:

_____

Signature of Supervisee/date   Signature of Supervisor/date

FIGURE 2.1

A sample outline for narrative evaluation
to be generated in ongoing, shared discussions between supervisee and supervisor.

of supervision which is so closely related to practice, the philosophy becomes conceptually and practically integrated with greater immediacy because it develops within meaningful and emotionally lively associations.

REFLECTIVE SUPERVISION DIMINISHES SCALE

Relational specificity and responsivity are undermined by ratios that overwhelm. These essential domains of reflective practice can more readily flourish in small organizations or in large ones organized into separate programs and subunits. Each program or unit needs senior personnel who function as responsive team leaders.

Many birth through five programs began small with a few staff members and a coordinator/director. The founding staff worked as a team characterized by flexible roles, a flat organizational model, and group consensus. Over the years, however, programs have grown, doubling and tripling in size. Many have not adjusted their structure to this growth and still attempt to function as a committee of the whole. In fact, the flat organizational models of the original founders can stand in the way of creating an organization with smaller, more effectively functioning teams. These teams or work groups, like the original model, function best with not more than six to eight members and with designated leaders who participate reflectively in a leaders' group with the director. Diminishing the scale in this way is usually a relief to directors and also offers some staff members the chance to take on increasing responsibility.

Reflective process in steady and enduring relationships within smaller, cohesive groups allows the scale of an overly large organization, such as a medical center or community-wide service agency, to come "down," encouraging enough safety to blossom so that it can hold the range of individual difference and of reactions and feelings (Shahmoon-Shanok, 1991, 2000). Every staff member must have access to their supervisor is and must feel that the supervisor will be responsive to concerns and questions. Correspondingly, every supervisor must know that she does not have so many supervisees and other responsibilities as to be unable to respond to such questions and concerns. Thus, even when one-on-one reflective supervision is not yet possible, each member of a reflective program staff needs and should have a primary, specific, responsive person of one's own. This can occur only when units or subunits are small, not more than six to eight members.

REFLECTIVE SUPERVISION SUPPORTS ETHICAL PRACTICE

Reflective supervision offers a system of checks and balances. It provides a way of helping the worker to decide how to behave in ethically charged or other anxiety-ridden dilemmas. Ethical reflection, a term used by Sokoly and Dokecki (1992), refers to the need to continually understand the discrepancies between theory and one's practice, between traditional treatment, top-down mindsets in which the professional is expert and families are recipients of that expertise, and newer models of shared responsibility, shared power, and mutual expertise. Sokoly and Dokecki (1992) propose that Lebacqz's (1985) ethical framework provides a structure for many questions in the infant/family field. This framework holds that:

> an adequate approach to ethical discernment, decision, and action requires (1) defining and interpreting the intervention situation in light of duty-based, morally relevant features and professional role expectations; (2) examining the character of the professional; and (3) analyzing the structures of power that influence interventions in actual situations of professional practice. (Sokoly & Dokecki, 1992, p. 26)

By virtue of having a pair of more experienced eyes present, eyes that accept fallibility and tension even while empathically delving into them and while they expect considered behavior, reflective supervision tilts the balance toward ethical practice and accountability. Within this relationship, professionals can explore situational demands and role expectations, their own capacities for considered, mutual decision-making, and the power balance inherent in their relationships with families. In reflective, ethical practice, professionals must have "not only expertise and knowledge about the other but also self-awareness that allows them to evaluate whether what they are doing helps or hinders the growth of the other" (Sokoly & Dokecki, 1992, p. 28). Further, ethical practice implies being aware of the other as a person, not as an object. This involves "being conscious of the other by grasping the other's meaning" (Winter, 1966, in Sokoly & Dokecki, 1992,

p. 29). Through reflective supervision, new and experienced practitioners can examine the nature of their relationships with families and with others, the degree of free, uncoerced communication which exists within these relationships, the dilemmas specific to a particular family and situation, and the extent to which the practitioner is an authentic, trustworthy, helpful partner to families.

Indeed, the very idea of *partnership with families* implies openness to a range of challenges since families themselves vary so widely in their strengths and vulnerabilities. The way one discovers to "partner" a teenage single mother, a dual career couple, or a mentally ill father requires much consideration, especially in a climate which tends to not formally allow for such differences (Shahmoon-Shanok, 1997a). This topic of what constitutes ethical practice is enormous when considered from the perspectives of differing professional traditions and lies well beyond the scope of this chapter. It needs further development as the birth-through-five field moves toward a robust generic practice base.

RECIPROCITY IN REFLECTIVE
SUPERVISION BEGETS INITIATIVE AND
EFFECTIVE, ENGAGED PRACTICE

Through reflective supervision, the worker experiences how it feels to be both *fully known and* respected. How engaging it is to be treated with respect and reciprocity by a teacher/mentor! This engagement begets initiative by helping people feel effective in their clinical work and within their team. When the program functions as a reflective organization, then supervisees experience the proactive sense that they are able to affect things programmatically and philosophically and touch not only their clients but their colleagues and leaders. This is the state most conducive to optimal, enthusiastic learning and to good morale.

REFLECTIVE SUPERVISION DEVELOPS THE ART OF REMEMBERING

Through the necessity of reporting in depth about cases to a supervisor, the supervisee is required to actively remember details of contacts with child and parent. This activity, *re-collecting* nuance of word, behavior, and feeling, becomes a facility which makes possible depth and breadth in the ability to organize and aggregate data. *Re-viewing* with a sympathetic and experienced person promotes reflection upon the data with an open, thoughtful, problem-solving attitude. Process recording notes are one vehicle from the social work tradition that work very well to develop these facilities. To perform this task, the practitioner writes down every detail of a contact he can recall, and the supervisor reads the notes to prepare for thoughtful discussion in the supervisory appointment. It is labor-intensive and time-consuming, but those investments made over time perhaps explain its effectiveness as a tool. Indeed, more seasoned practitioners report that when they are stuck, the discipline of process recording notes often reveals insight and generates next steps.

When reviewed and actively considered, videotape or audiotape can also be used as another aid to or form of remembering. The danger is that video or audio taping could be relied upon for recall, which would then actually undermine the growth of capacities for recall and reflection.

As you look longer, they change. Figures move in and out, and what seems solid at one moment isn't the next, similar in a sense to the complex and mysterious processes of seeing and remembering. . . . Reflection together invites the supervisee to become an active participant in producing the narrative, or meaning, of her experiences. °

Review promotes the ability to remember, organize, consider, and generate provisional hypotheses which guide immediate next steps.

Practitioners often have an initial self-critical reaction to seeing themselves work on videotape. Supervision can acknowledge this near universal response through gentle humor and introduction of the concept of *self*-empathy. This helps workers remember how they were feeling and thinking at the time. It also helps them consider what they believe about what the children, parent, or colleagues on videotape were aiming for and experiencing. For optimal training to occur, practitioners should have ongoing experiences with both approaches to remembering, process recording notes that draw on and exercise the capacity to recall, and videotape that allows a practitioner to see herself from the outside, while integrating what can be seen with her own recalled experience.

REFLECTIVE SUPERVISION CREATES AND HONES SELF-KNOWLEDGE

Practitioners "need time to reflect upon themselves with the same intensity and vigor that is given to the study of others" (Stott & Bowman, 1996, p. 179). Self-knowledge engenders the capacity for understanding one's own values and beliefs, gender-based perspectives, cultural practices, and professional biases; for developing an awareness of one's personal style, such as image, temperament, and coping style; and for learning to take responsibility for one's own reactions and interactions (Klein & Gilkerson, in press). Pawl (1995) points out that supervision in every discipline should, at a minimum, offer the individual the opportunity to discover her own beliefs, attitudes, and characteristic responses and to realize that he will be the recipient of the preformed—that is, the transferential, internal working model—ideas of others. The development of the capacity to observe one's self—the "observing self,"—is critical to the ability to track one's effect upon another and, as such, is a necessary professional competency (Bowman, 1989).

What is so significant is awareness of the subjectivity of vision, the possibility of a double, or even triple, reading of a scene, and the understanding that vision and memory cannot claim any kind of essential certainty. Rather we cultivate a profound sense of the nature of experience—an understanding of remembering as a process that extends over time and one that is dependent on the makeup of the observer. °

In the brief excerpt about reflective supervision with a home-based speech-language therapist that follows, Henderson (1997) offers a powerful example of gender-related countertransference, a topic often "not discussed either because [it is] not considered relevant or [because] the idea of exposing [such reactions] feels uncomfortable and/or unprofessional" (Henderson, 1997, p. 21, following Brown, 1984; Felton, 1986; Gabbard, 1994).

Jane started her supervisory session by saying she was concerned about the current treatment plan and wondered if she should offer the family a time when the mother could be more actively involved. She was worried that the mother would sense that the parent-child sessions were going better with the father and that the mother might feel rejected and pull her daughter out of treatment.

With some gentle prodding, Jane was able to connect to the real source of her anxiety. In the last session prior to supervision, father, daughter, and therapist were all sitting and interacting on the floor. At one point, the daughter did something really cute and Jane and the father made eye contact in a shared moment of pleasure. This moment of intimacy was extremely disconcerting for Jane. While she had grown in her ability to manage the intimacy with the mother, sharing an intimate moment with this father felt scary and wrong. She felt so threatened by her own reaction that she was ready to change the treatment plan.

Fortunately for all, she was able to share these feelings in supervision. While validating her fear and anxiety, I suggested that having a pleasurable feeling toward a father, even a pleasurable sexual feeling, was not wrong. It is possible to have such a feeling, take note of it, and not act upon it. I asked her if she could maintain her boundaries and she felt strongly that she could. She felt relieved that she could talk about the experience and also relieved to recognize the strength of her own boundaries, that is her ability to maintain a close but professional relationship with a man. (Henderson, 1997, pp. 21–22)

This example offers a glimpse into one type of complex practitioner feelings that can arise and, if unattended to, might undermine not only insight and connection but also, as in this case, the actual pattern of contacts. Thus, the entire range of practitioner feelings, including embarrassing ones, require shared attention within a reflective, thoughtful, ongoing context. Such attention yields the ability to effectively understand, manage, and even, at times, use emotional information to guide insightful, sensitive, and considered practice. The *way* that the supervisor probed and responded helped the supervisee nondefensively recognize her feelings and promoted her ability to use information contained in them.

As Foley put it so well in an article for birth through five supervisory staff (1994, February–March, p. 19):

Relationships are complicated. They are loaded with the "baggage" each party brings from his or her past experiences, as well as material arising from the present or "real" relationship. Thus *all* [italics added] relationships might be characterized as consisting of at least two important components: 1) the "real" relationships, which consist of themes that arise out of currently existing circumstances and undistorted interactions (Freud, 1954); and 2) the "illusory" relationship, or what some mental health professionals refer to as the transference and countertransference.

By transference, we mean the feelings, impulses and behaviors repeatedly experienced by the client in *relation to the psychotherapist, which arise not out of the "real" but out of recapitulations of earlier* [italics added] relationships (Freud, 1912; Sander, 1993). By countertransference, we mean the unconscious reactions that directed toward their clients in the present that are experienced by psychotherapists and which have their origins in the past. Both transference and countertransference can be thought of as "ghosts" from the past which haunt the present.

Reflective supervision hones the ability to maintain awareness of several levels of interaction at once, so that we "take in" both the manifest and the emotional, implied import of context, behavior, expression, and words. As practitioners become more self-aware, so, correspondingly, do the abilities to make such distinctions become stronger and more available.

REFLECTIVE SUPERVISION SUPPORTS CROSS-CULTURAL COMPETENCE

Along similar lines, a specific type of countertransferential material is each practitioner's long and deeply bred cultural vantage point. The matter is of great consequence in terms of sensitive practice in the helping professions, since aspects of it run so deep as to lie embedded somewhere below conscious recognition. Thus, fathoming one's own point of cultural perspective is critical. "Self-awareness is the first step on the journey toward cross-cultural competence" (Lynch & Hanson, 1992, p. 37). Through reflective supervision, we can attempt to bring to awareness the cultural beliefs, practices, and codes that subtly or grossly affect our perceptions of others and our responses to them. We can begin to become aware of our own blind spots and prejudices and expand our capacity to see from the other's perspective. It is not always possible to know another person's culture, but one can approach the other with the humbling knowledge that there will naturally be differences in fundamental areas of family life and child rearing, areas such as feeding and sleeping patterns, dependent behavior, discipline and the use of physical punishment, ways of showing feelings, and types of acceptable sources of help.

The goal is to avoid using our own culture, whatever it is, or the program's culture as *the* standard. Reflective supervision can help practitioners from all disciplines, which also may be understood as cultures themselves, to "understand and respond to areas of conflict and tension when we encounter individuals from unfamiliar cultures or experiences and learn to be more comfortable with being uncomfortable" (Rodriguez, 1995–1996, p. 12). With the help of each other, supervisor and supervisee may discover access to wider realms of experience, including that of cultural isolation and loneliness. The "not-knowing-how-things-are-done" of an immigrant family or a teenage parent coming to day care for the first time converge with their sense of not being known. Supervisory sharing can sensitize staff to these dimensions.

REFLECTIVE SUPERVISION AMPLIFIES CALM AND RESPONSIVITY

Individual development is generated in a supportive, attuned relational field, within a few relationships which amplify calm and responsivity. These relationships model best practice and, like wholesome adults with children, mediate experience so it does not overwhelm, but becomes an opportunity for growth. Just as the foundation of later development rests on the ability to achieve a state of calm alertness (Wolff, 1966; Greenspan, 1992), adults need time to revitalize—time to focus, organize, and reflect upon affectively lively and, not infrequently, anxiety-provoking situations and people. The physical and psychological environment needs to be thoughtfully and creatively conceived so that both supervisor and supervisee are freed from distractions and able to concentrate their energies in an unhurried atmosphere, an oasis in time and intensity.

REFLECTIVE SUPERVISION ENCOURAGES TRIAL ACTION AND CRITICAL THINKING

Freud said that "thinking is trial action." Such thinking is a discipline that requires both focus and consideration. It does not just happen but is, rather, a cultivated skill. Indeed, without pre-thinking what would "professional" practice be? When behavior and emotions are considered away from the actual event from a variety of angles, more nuanced and sensitive human contact is the likely result. Similarly, looking at behavior in context adds dimension and depth. For example, rather than demanding, "Stop the biting!" the reflective caregiver and her supervisor consider what led up to the behavior. Then, the supervisee can partner the child so that *his* strengths are cherished and *his* vulnerabilities are partnered. Often this kind of anticipatory consideration, *based on hindsight,* can make it possible to promote more mature functioning on the part of children and caregivers, wherein they are not reduced to frustration as in the biting incident.

Critical thinking requires the examination of our assumptions and acknowledgment of their presuppositions and limitations (Stott & Bowman, 1996). It requires reference to both formal knowledge and personal experience and to the affects generated from them. Thus, reflective supervision also serves as an optimal setting for the integration of theory and practice which becomes, over time and with guided experience, the ability to take in the perspectives of another, to see from varied and nuanced angles.

Play here with the idea that inconsistencies are always going to exist in the world, and that even if you look at something first with one eye, and then the other, there will be these slight differences . . . vision is binocular. We see with two eyes, and not one. The views of the world are not the same—there are complexities and inconsistencies in this—yet we have to work to reconcile them, based on deepening understanding, as all the while we tolerate the tension inherent.°

REFLECTIVE SUPERVISION IS ESSENTIAL FOR QUALITY IMPROVEMENT AND PROGRAM ACCOUNTABILITY

The aim of reflective supervision is to improve practice. It is worthwhile to the extent that it strengthens the capacities of workers and, therefore, of the program to provide quality services. "Just as an audit is an expected accountability element of the fiscal system of an organization, supervision must be an equally expected accountability element of direct services to children and families" (Gilkerson & Young-Holt, 1992, p. 113). Through careful examination of his own work, the teacher becomes accountable for the way he teaches, the home visitor, for the way he engages families and children, the director, for the way he leads. Individuals, then, are not persons who merely conduct a prescribed curriculum or predetermined strategies, but people who make rational choices and assume responsibility for those choices (Ross, 1987).

As supervisors, leaders share the responsibility for the clinical work and assume accountability themselves for the frequency and quality of the guidance provided for staff. Figure 2.2 is an outline written by a consultant for a specific director who was experiencing great difficulty supervising a dedicated but very intense senior supervisor on her staff, someone so heavy-handed in striving for program accountability that she was alienating both colleagues and supervisees.

Jeree Pawl (1995) has stated that "No one should make hard decisions alone." Reflective supervision provides a protected, professionally validated forum for sorting through difficult situations honestly and for arriving at the next step. Through this process, practitioners become responsible citizens not only of their programs, but also of their professions.

REFLECTIVE PRACTICE CONTRIBUTES TO PROFESSIONAL IDENTITY AND CAREER DEVELOPMENT

Every professional needs another who thinks with her about her professional

Evaluation

1. Set in motion a plan with her that 3 to 4 times a year you will make special appointments with her designated as feedback sessions about her and her work. These are sacrosanct, private, uninterruptable, and at least 1 hour, perhaps a little longer. Sometimes a second appointment to provide thinking or writing time in between is needed.

    a. While these sessions are mostly about her performance, process, work, and goals, the communication should be bidirectional. She should be free to also say how she is feeling and reacting to you as it is pertinent to the work.

2. In this context, she should be given first responsibility for her own evaluation and her own settings of objectives and goals. You then attach any additional idea(s) of yours to her own.

    a. Thus, let *her* talk about her strengths and weaknesses. Take notes so you can use her own words and let her write a draft of her own evaluation first.

    b. Then respond to what she has said beginning with her strengths. In that context, gently but clearly comment on the points of concern to you.

3. In between those evaluation/discussion sessions, if you are ever with her when you think she is heavy-handed, go over the incident with her as soon as possible afterwards. When you do, be very sympathetic and begin by asking her:

    a. What she was *feeling* when the instance occurred.

    b. What *she* thought about what had transpired.

    c. What *she* thought the result was for the other person.

    The goal is to get *her* to discover the pattern. That will not happen if *you* are heavy-handed with her.

4. *Whenever* you note her *strengths* tell her!

FIGURE 2.2

Guidance to a director who was supervising a key staff member who was alienating both her own colleagues and her supervisees by heavy-handed efforts at staff and program accountability.

goals and career directions. This kind of mentorship belongs at the heart of every supervisory relationship, even though it does not have to be focused upon very often. In some situations, this aspect of supervision can present a dilemma. When, for example, a supervisee is considering going back to graduate school and she works in a position that is very hard to fill, the supervisor may have mixed feelings addressing the issue. Further, the supervisee may hesitate to bring up her shifting aspirations. An-

other kind of dilemma may arise when a supervisee holds certain goals that the supervisor believes do not match the supervisee's capacities. The supervisor may need some support herself to expose and sort through her own reactions so that the difference is something that can be constructively spoken about between the two.

Becoming a professional inherently involves discomfort because it involves continually facing situations that are new: "unanticipated, uncontrollable, and contradictory" (Stott & Bowman, 1996, p. 177). Exploring one's capacity to deal with the anxiety intrinsic to giving up certain familiar views of self requires suspending autonomy to acquire competence (Grimmett, 1988). Shifts in personal identity flow from such explorations. Young professionals struggle with issues of identity and authority: Who am *I* to advise this experienced parent? Will the physician respect *my* recommendation? Mature women reentering the workforce after raising children seek to construct a professional identity when, for so many years, their primary role had been as mother or wife. Men in early childhood may feel invisible and isolated or too easily valued, placed on an unearned pedestal. Reflective supervision provides the setting to acknowledge these struggles and to take steps toward an enduring and integrated professional identity that embraces the past and present, an identity which conceives and spawns fresh ideas and deeply felt goals.

Stages of the Supervisory Interview

As your senses settle into the experience, you see some things very quickly. Other things come more slowly . . .°

Reflection is intimately intertwined with practice: during, after, and then prior to the actual work. All supervisory interviews have the following stages in common. Gilkerson (1995) and Shanok, Gilkerson, Eggbeer, and Fenichel (1995a & b) have described the process of the supervisory session: (1) Preparation, (2) Greeting/Reconnecting, (3) Opening the Dialogue/Finding the Agenda, (4) Information Gathering/Focus-ing on the Details, (5) Formulating Hypotheses, (6) Considering Next Steps, and (7) Closing. Shanok and colleagues (1995a) have prepared a teaching videotape with role play illustrating each phase of the supervisory process. Accompanying text describes the thought process of the supervisor and supervisee at critical points in the role play. This section expands that discussion to illuminate the rhythm and focus of each phase. These stages may be used as a means for supervisors to understand and to take to a deeper level some of what they may already be doing.

It is crucial to point out that ongoing supervisory sessions described take place within the boundaries of a supervisory contract, developed mutually by the supervisor and supervisee. The contract is usually formed in the first or second sessions and then shifts and deepens over time. It is an understanding between the parties, sometimes a written agreement, regarding the nature of the supervisory relationship, the role and responsibility of each member, the flow of the sessions, and the time commitment. Confidentiality regarding the people to be discussed, as well as that of the supervisee, is fleshed out as is the relationship of the supervisory sessions to the performance appraisal process or, if the supervisee is a student, to grading procedures. It is often helpful in the first session to talk about the supervisee's past experience with supervision and to explore her expectations, needs, and concerns.

PHASE 1: PREPARATION

In the first phase, preparation, the supervisor manages a "state transition" moving herself from her present tasks and preoccupations to a state of openness and empathic engagement. Whether it takes five minutes or five seconds, the supervisor resets her internal rhythm to ready herself to listen, to take in the state of another. By clearing her desk, as well as her mind, by putting her telephone on forward and the "Do Not Disturb" sign on the door, she creates a protected environment both for herself and for the supervisee. Even if the two were previously in another type of meeting together, the supervisor still takes a few moments to prepare: "I'm looking forward to our supervisory time together. Let's take a few moments, though, to shift gears and meet in my office or back here in a couple of minutes."

PHASE 2: GREETING/RECONNECTING

This portion of the session recognizes the need for a bit of social interchange that enables the supervisor and supervisee to reconnect as people and settle in. It is the time for regaining balance with each other through thoughtful, interested, yet brief semisocial contact. If the supervisor has not seen the supervisee for several days, she may notice her state of well-being: Is she relaxed and tanned, perhaps back from a short trip? Does she have a cast on her wrist? Does he look harried, tired, or have a bad cold? If the supervisor and supervisee have already been working together that day, the greeting and reconnecting helps to set the stage for this new joint activity. It may be as simple as noting: "It's good to have this quiet time together for supervision." These few moments of natural conversation are tactfully contained so that the time can shift to the supervisee's agenda.

PHASE 3: OPENING THE DIALOGUE/ FINDING THE AGENDA

To make the transition from the Greeting phase to Opening the Dialogue, the supervisor usually begins with a familiar open-ended question, such as: "How has this week been for you?" or "Let's begin." These ritual questions or opening phrases signal to the supervisee that the time is now focused on her and that she can take the lead. Over time, many supervisees themselves find tactful ways to move into the content. Toward the outset of the supervisory relationship, the supervisor has asked the supervisee to prepare for supervision by thinking about it during the period in between and coming with an agenda, a set of practice-related issues and questions in mind.

To create a safe environment for reflection, it is crucial that the supervisee have a significant degree of control. Setting the agenda provides tangible evidence to the supervisee of this and may be perceived as a message/metaphor about shared power. By following the guiding principle of social work, "Begin where the person is," the wise supervisor builds her own comments or concerns into the context set by the supervisee.

Sometimes a supervisee will have a specific topic, incident, or situation in mind. At other times, the supervisee may have many thoughts/needs or may simply be unfocused, and it is not clear to her where to begin. The supervisor could continue to listen, commenting that there seems to be a lot for the supervisee to share this week, or the supervisor might be more directive and inquire: "Where shall we focus our attention first?" or "You have a lot on your mind today. Where would you like to concentrate?" If the supervisee is conveying a jumble of material, the supervisor can simply move forward to the next phase of the session, focusing on the details.

PHASE 4: INFORMATION GATHERING/ FOCUSING ON THE DETAILS

When a topic has emerged and requires crystallization, the next phase is gathering the details, context, and nuance in order to respond to the needs of the supervisee vis-a-vis the practice problem. Without clear, rich information, there is no basis for the supervisor to provide guidance. The supervisor may ask questions to orient herself to the situation: "Tell me about this family," or "Remind me of how old the child is," or "You knocked on the door, the father opened it and walked away, and left you standing there? What happened next, and how did you feel?" During this phase the supervisor needs to create and sustain a climate in which the supervisee can begin to explore all sides of an interaction looking closely at her own contribution as well as at the contributions of others. The supervisor's most important role at this time is to listen: carefully, thoughtfully, and empathetically. Sometimes, though, she may need to probe and question in order to help the supervisee provide a full enough bridge so that she can vividly picture/feel the situation. She encourages the supervisee to convey a mix of summarized information as well as the nuance of detail. Videotape, audiotape, or process recording notes can provide supporting or contrasting vantage points (see preceding discussion about the art of remembering on page 54).

The very uncertainty of appearance of some of the elements slows down our perception of the image . . . and encourages us to take time over them; to become aware that some things are at that point of irresolution, which makes them difficult to identify, forcing us to keep scanning the surface to discover all sorts of incidents and nuances . . . The idea of a gaze that simply identifies or possesses an object is, in fact, undermined here.

A supervisee might present several separate, intensely connected topics. For example, she might want to discuss her difficulty in handling the behavior of a child and her disagreement with other team members about this child. It may be useful to distinguish between the two issues. Peeling back an interaction, looking closely at each behavior and feeling, can be very helpful. When it remains difficult for the supervisor to gather the sense of what occurred, it may be useful to engage in a role play so that the supervisor and supervisee can experience the emotional content and intensity of the interaction. When a supervisee presents an issue that is particularly difficult for her, she often begins in the middle of the story, where she is most confused or at the end, where she is most discouraged. Slowly reconstructing the interactions may help to reduce the anxiety and, therefore, increase the opportunity for insight, reflection, and resourcefulness.

PHASE 5: FORMULATING HYPOTHESES

As the details are uncovered, the supervisee and/or supervisor begin to formulate a hypothesis about underlying context or about a way to consider what has just occurred, usually in a shared way. This is a particularly fruitful time for the integration of theory and practice. "It sounds as if this mom is feeling so overwhelmed and hopeless, and that's affecting everyone in the family. It reminds me of that article we read on family systems, remember?" The supervisor might offer a hypothesis based on her experience and knowledge, or together they could explore alternative explanations. It is these formulations, based in large part on emotional information, which guide this process to the next stage.

PHASE 6: CONSIDERING NEXT STEPS

Given the hypotheses, the supervisee and supervisor can begin to consider possibilities for next steps. As in the initial phases, it may be helpful to have a phrase to mark this phase of the interview: "In the time we have remaining, let's consider what possibilities are available." This phase can include relatively concrete trial action, including brainstorming, role play, rehearsal, or materials development. One supervisee, for example, was struggling with her role on the assessment team. In exploring the issue, she began to realize that her frustration resulted not from the dynamics of the team but, rather, from a lack of focus within her own assessment observations. She used the remaining portion of the supervisory hour to develop a list of observation topic areas. This beginning tool increased her confidence and renewed her energy for the task at hand.

This phase may look very different for the supervisee who is helped to realize that her job is *not* to act. The supervisory sessions provide a safe place to sort out the feelings of urgency and to nourish the capacity to tolerate the tension inherent in guiding others toward developmental growth and change.

PHASE 7: CLOSING

The closing acknowledges the end of the session and validates the process that has just occurred. The supervisor might inquire about what lies ahead for the coming week. At this point of separation, the session usually ends by confirming the next appointment, a way of affirming ongoing partnership and assistance, part of the supervisory contract.

The foregoing steps work for other problem-solving conversations with the supervisee outside of the session. All the phases are there, but they are briefer. The process of focus, discovery, and next steps is similar, as is reassurance about future reconnection. The process also is helpful in guiding group supervision sessions, as described in the following section.

On the Way to Reflective Practice: Making It Happen

While we and others (Fenichel, 1992) advocate for individual supervision as an irreplaceable key to reflective practice in infant/family and preschool services, the unfortunate, present reality of the field is that precious few programs are able to offer staff the opportunity for regular, one-on-one supervision. In fact, individual supervision may be the final step rather than the first step, even for programs fully committed to reflective practice. We suggest a range of adaptive options for programs and for individual practitioners to consider as they move toward increasing opportunities for reflection within programs and/or with practitioners who have previously not experienced reflective supervision. These include adaptations of staff meetings and clinical meetings as well as the gradual establishment of opportunities for group supervision, individual supervision, and program consultation. While we are offering a range of valuable opportunities for generating reflective practice, individual supervision should remain a goal for all infant through preschool programs.

Prior to discussing these options for introducing and enhancing opportunities for reflective practice, it is essential to remember that their validity will be influenced by and will depend upon the larger context of the program. How each staff member experiences her job depends on her relationship with her immediate supervisor and on other intrinsic factors including the scale of the program, the current state of program stability, the characteristics of leadership, the support available to the leaders, and the nature of peer relationships. A review of these contextual contributors as background for the consideration of adaptations in program practices follows.

Context for Reflective Practice

It is helpful to realize that all programs cycle through periods of equilibrium and disequi-

librium, resulting from internal and/or external forces. Gilkerson (1993) identified four areas contributing to these cycles: financial stability, staff relationships (including staff/administatration relationships), staff changes (including new paradigms for practice), and critical program events (such as a move of the site to a new location or an eruption of community violence). In a program where the present leadership is characterized by unclear or punitive leadership styles, staff may be preoccupied with trying to figure out or cope with messages from the hierarchy. When external systems issues dominate, such as funding or policy shifts in early intervention programs, staff, even leadership, may be focused on program stability and job security. When, instead, the external and internal pressures are in relative balance and/or when leadership provides helpful structures and responsive support, staff can focus their energy on the work at hand. Informal relationships can provide mutual support. Conversation drifts naturally to the infants and families served.

When the leaders model one person helping another, peer interchange will more likely be supportive. In fact, the quality of peer relationships is a good indicator of the health of the organization and nature of the leadership style. Edna Adelson Fraiberg (in Gilkerson, 1992, p. 20) describes the essential role that collegial peer relationships played among the pioneering group of infant mental health practitioners:

It was a bit like a life raft mentality. We were all in there helping one another. When we'd be ready to dash out to a home visit, when the day had been particularly chaotic, there was someone to help you focus, to collect yourself. When you returned (to the office) and knew you couldn't do another thing until you talked it out, there was always someone with a cup of coffee to help you come back to earth. This work is just different from others. We left the book behind. We responded to families and let them lead us. . . . So much is subliminal; you're responding to signals you can't articulate without the eyes and ears of your colleagues. No one had the answer. We were all in there together. With all our goofs.

Wise administrators validate and protect such time for thoughtful, responsive, mutually generative staff relationships. Thoughtful leaders also ensure that they have a network for themselves—other leaders to support and reflect upon their own development and practice (see Bertacchi & Stott, 1991 for a model of a support group for directors). As each leader receives support, so she is able to support her staff. Reading and rereading, and discussing and rediscussing the characteristics of reflective supervision noted previously in this chapter in the context of the actual day-to-day life of the organization can transform each leader's practice. Only with nondefensive reflection upon her own practices can a leader make the shifts required to gradually shift her own understandings, emphases, and expectations at work. Each staff member needs to have a relationship of meaning and of openness, preferably with her superiors, in order for these changes to gradually germinate and take root, grow, and blossom.

Reflective Process in Group Meetings

This section discusses adaptations that can be made to existing group meetings, such as administrative or staff meetings and clinical meetings, and introduces the utility of group supervision. The potential of the group for self-reflection is also explored.

ADMINISTRATIVE MEETINGS

Reframing Meetings: A Community at Work

Fenichel and Eggbeer (1992b) point out that routine staff meetings can be a starting place for engendering reflection, particularly where isolation from birth-to-three colleagues is a "serious occupational hazard" (p. 23) such as for home visitors and child care teachers. Staff meetings represent shared time when the program community gathers to think together and, therefore, to do its communal work. It can be a time to share emotions, a "powerful antidote to the 'overwhelming nature of being alone'" (Doud, in Fenichel & Eggbeer, 1992b, p. 23). Viewed in this way, the vitality and depth of engagement during staff meetings is another marker for a wholesome, energized organization. Boredom, lack of animation, grumbling when a new meeting date is set, or a quiet dearth of ideas are signals that something significant is amiss.

The way communication is handled, individuals are treated, and the group is facilitated become, by parallel process, a working model for staff of the program philosophy. Indeed, how we are as a group conveys a great deal about what we believe about relationships. Who sets the agenda and by what process? What kinds of ideas are valued? Is a range of feelings encouraged? How are disagreements or new ideas handled? Are individual and group accomplishments celebrated?

Opportunities for Reflection within Existing Meetings

The operational question for each program becomes: In what ways can the program begin to use the meetings that already exist in new, more reflective ways? An excellent starting point is to explore with the group what their individual and collective experience is of the present meetings along the dimensions just mentioned and any others that staff members raise. What is the typical emotional tone/atmosphere of staff meetings? How are agendas determined? What about the purpose of these meetings? Do people agree on the purposes? Are the goals being achieved? Are meetings efficient, yet do they still offer opportunities for depth of discussion? What processes/structures keep the group focused? How do people feel after the meetings? How can staff meetings serve to promote professional growth and program responsiveness? What small, next steps could be taken to make the meetings more thoughtful, more constructive?

Fine-tuning opening rituals is one simple way to begin to shift the group process. One program decided to begin administrative meetings with a round-robin, offering each team member a few minutes to share what was new since they last had met. Another program decided to start in a lighter way, connecting as people first with "up close and personal" updates in addition to program news. Still a third began with time to "take the pulse," a few moments for each member to take stock, to give a reading on how each was doing during a particularly challenging period. These beginnings legitimize the importance of self-awareness as well as connection with others.

This reflective process begins to model the kind of thoughtful deliberation, considered planning, and mutual engagement we hope staff will bring to all aspects of their work. The capacity of leadership to hear staff concerns and ideas, to reflect upon them, to respond openly and nondefensively, and to follow through will make or break this initial step. Thus, the leaders, themselves, will need to process their reactions, feelings, and ideas about these directions. There is almost always a way to integrate the new and the old directions. If leadership decides against novel suggestions, it is essential that their rationale is explained to staff with opportunities for them to respond. We are talking about the building of honest interchange, which leads to mutual trust and respect.

In an open context, it is crucial to take time to build or tinker with an existing mission statement: What is the purpose of our program? What kinds of outcomes are expected? What do we believe about how to achieve our goals? People will be reassured when they experience the sense that *their* ideas count and become folded into the emerging whole.

Forming a "Committee on the Group"

To watch over the well-being of the group, the staff may want to form a committee to interact with the leader and help the leader think about the group and its needs. The committee and the leader then recommend to the group ways that it can grow and strengthen and solve problems. The committee represents the group by sorting through and integrating members' ideas and feelings and facilitating tactfully offered, but nevertheless, out-front messages in all directions. This process is an example of open communication. It is an efficient way to help the leader to know what people really feel and help the group to exercise constructive strategies for problem identification and resolution.

Providing Consistent Yet Flexible Leadership

In each type of meeting, there is designated, consistent leadership. Yet, in a democratically run organization, anyone can *actually* lead because everyone is heard. A new staff member may, for instance, volunteer a pivotal insight. Furthermore, individual members may chair certain portions of the meetings, take minutes, summarize and integrate important points, or organize a staff retreat. This is enabling to everyone and can be an enormous relief to designated leaders.

Group meetings provide a prime opportunity to model responsivity. It is a time when norms are reinforced and philosophy put into action. Leaders support cohesion by summarizing what has been said, thus drawing on what everyone has to contribute. The leader at such a meeting makes sense out of conflicting points of view by integrating and synthesizing. It is rare that there is not a kernel of worth in

what someone is saying. The key is to recognize that kernel and to bring it together with others. Generally, fine leaders see the value in what each person brings into the mix and make some use of it. Thus, real leaders become a force for integration, rather than for polarization. Leaders can deepen discussion on a topic by asking thoughtful questions or by offering their own insights and experience. Taking a topic to a deeper level encourages staff to stay with difficult issues. All this implies responsive, decentralized, nondefensive leadership—leadership open to thoughtful change.

Distinguishing Clinical Discussions from Administrative Management

A step which may be helpful to many programs is distinguishing (by labeling) administrative discussions from clinical/in-service discussions. Without making these distinctions, business/management topics too often tend to dominate the agenda of every meeting. Then administrative and clinical meetings can be held on separate days, one longer meeting can be divided into two parts, or administrative and clinical meetings can be held on alternate weeks. The program director with senior clerical staff might lead the management meetings, and senior clinical staff may lead the clinical review meetings. The meetings might have different formats, locations, and record-keeping procedures.

We advise that each program adopt a guideline regarding the percentage of group meeting time allocated to administrative/management issues and suggest that no more than 20 percent of time for group meetings be used for this purpose.

Making an explicit decision regarding the balance of administrative and clinical time requires that leadership and staff face the issue and asks that *both* take responsibility to address it. When possible, administrative items should be handled quickly. If they cannot be, then there are probably clinical implications that should be deferred to a clinical/in-service discussion or meeting. By recognizing these distinctions and placing such issues in the clinical context, concentration can then be appropriately placed on how it is that people *are* served vis-a-vis how they *should* be served or on larger programmatic issues that have significant implications for program design.

Incorporating Reflection into Management Meetings

Furthermore, it is also essential that business/management meetings always have a component that is reflective and/or engaging. No aspect of the work is unrelated to the program's philosophy and relational approach. A discussion of how fees are to be collected, for example, can be demoralizing or can lead staff to new ideas for more generative practice. To achieve quality in program practice, staff members need to continually remind themselves and each other that every procedure profoundly affects how families experience the program. In this time of increasing regulation of early childhood programs, we underscore the critical importance of generating and abiding by engaged, reflective, individualized practice when trying to fulfill requirements of funding and accrediting agencies. Given this, how can we use this new expectation to bolster and expand relationally and affec-

tively alive practice or how are we going to integrate this expectation with our philosophy of service, our knowledge of the families and communities we serve, and our current practices rather than how are we going to change to fulfill this external requirement?

Stepping Back to Move Forward: Coming Together to Appreciate and Understand One Another

When several times a year, one regular or extended staff meeting is devoted to the individuals who make up the staff, a sense of vitality and mutual appreciation ensues. We recommend that staff spend time exploring their stories of what brought them to the work. Who are they in the world? How do they define their role to others outside of the agency? What experiences in childhood and earlier in adulthood still keep them alive to the work? Staff can reflect upon their work with children and families over the past several months, taking stock of the mutual impact between themselves and the children and families they serve. Further, the group can consider its own evolution and developmental stage. How has this period been for the group as a whole? What challenges have they faced, and how did the group respond to these challenges? What were the low points? What were the high points? Ground rules such as the length of discussion time that each individual has to respond should be set in advance. There should be ample time for spontaneous discoveries of similarities and differences, for meandering and for depth of discussion.

Periodically, it is also helpful to conduct an oral history of the program: retelling its birth, remembering the founding members and their guiding principles, the populations served and the approach used, and, most importantly, how and why the program has changed over time (Gilkerson & Als, 1995). This activity is especially helpful when a significant number of new members join the group. As the history is told and retold, it is helpful to differentiate and name eras to mark time and thus, to create an opening for the next phase which will be shaped by the present team—new members included.

Creating Celebrations and Developing Rituals

In addition to creating regular opportunities for staff to reflect as a group on their own development, strong programs, like strong families, develop other rituals and celebrations, both to move through life cycle events and to honor the group, its good functioning, and all its hard work. All staff events mark important passages for the program and staff and create new opportunities for connection. Examples include birthday parties, Friday Lunch Bunch (staff order out from favorite restaurants and enjoy a group lunch), annual holiday celebrations, and anniversaries of years of service. To integrate the administration and multicultural staff of a large community agency, one program opted to hold a monthly potluck. All staff, including administrators who always attended, were required to come and to bring a dish to share. While much time was spent in informal, relaxed conversation, a compelling topic related to the work was also addressed in an interesting and engaging way, reinforcing their shared mission. These monthly

meetings offered personnel including secretaries, janitors, and drivers an opportunity to connect, to know one another and the agency at a deeper level and to feel and *know* that they were part of something bigger. What began as a requirement became so lively that people did not want to miss the chance to connect.

Celebrations for and with families are also an essential component of a caring and responsive program, such as children's birthdays, room picnics, reunions of "graduate families," and graduations or moving-on ceremonies for early childhood programs. When thoughtfully organized, these events celebrate both individuals and the group as a whole.

CLINICAL MEETINGS

The following sections offer a range of ideas. Each of them can be thought of as a cornerstone for in-service training. Indeed, the most important way to assist a staff to grow as individuals and as a program is to guide them to study and consider their practice together with regularity. Rather than spending precious dollars on brief "trainings," programs will improve over time only if they offer ongoing, regular, in-depth study of children and families they serve with leaders or consultants who know how to do so and to attach that study to a relevant conceptual, relationship-centered base, flowing from immersion in the in-depth knowledge of developmental factors.

Role of Parallel Process in Clinical Meetings

Clinical meetings are those where the actual work with children and families is discussed. These meetings may be called "staffings" or "case conferences," although the term "case" is being used less frequently in many infant/family settings out of respect for and sensitivity to families and children. The goal is always to join staff perceptions one to the other, deepening understandings of individual differences and of the child's and family's own perceptions and their developmental needs.

Discussions may center on particular children and families or on more generic issues in which staff discuss their work with children and families as examples of various concepts or strategies. The idea of "parallel process" suggests that meeting process can model reflective practice. It is essential that the clinical meetings be thoughtfully and responsively run.

Considering the Phases of Clinical Discussion

The same phases described for individual supervision also apply to the group process: time to prepare, greet and orient, honing in on the agenda, discussion of the work with patience and detail, taking one hour or longer to discuss a particular family in terms of each individual, the dyads and triads, and their systemic interrelationships or a child in terms of each aspect of his development, finding hypotheses, and considering next steps. These processes, which become familiar, encourage coherence, integration, and a sense of safety and openness. For many of the young children and their families, integration is among the most challenging aspect of their development. This reliable, consistent process is essential to reduce fragmentation and confusion within and among service providers. Thus, teamwork and role clarity is promoted.

Leadership of Clinical Meetings

Clinical discussions are best facilitated by one consistent person who is skilled in cultivating group process by creating a safe forum where everyone's ideas can be considered, cultivated, and integrated with others when appropriate. Knowledge of individual development and relational development across psychobiological, social-emotional dimensions is essential, as is depth of understanding about how to intervene using specific relational elements. This last factor will lead programs to move toward increasingly deep relationships of designated staff with particular children and families. Too many currently undermine their helping potential by being diffuse in their relational "offers." Everyone is pleasant to everyone, but richness of meaning and of exchange between people who come to engage deeply and developmentally together—the currency of growth promotion—suffers because no one person is designated and learns how to cultivate relationships for the purpose of growth.

Maintaining a Theme

To further enhance coherence in clinical discussions, it is helpful to focus upon a few continuous threads over time that emerge from practice-based challenges. Such themes could include what and how to communicate with parents or how to identify and meet complex developmental needs of an individual child. As the themes emerge and are made explicit, they can be explored during discussions and become the focus of in-service sessions and shared or assigned readings.

Following Affect

Emotions provide essential information about people and situations, yet professionals from disciplines other than mental health tend to use affect relatively unconsciously. In infant through school-age work, a goal of the field is to help workers become more aware of affects and their use, because experiencing and using emotions in the workplace is not only legitimate, it is necessary.

Through supervision and reflective discussion, emotions are honed and become an instrument that is virtually in constant use. Clinical meetings should model, cultivate, and teach this capacity (c.f. Copa et al., 1999). Occasional collaboration between supervisor and supervisee in an intervention session or other parts of the program is also an effective way to model, cultivate, and train staff to listen for both passion and subtle emotion. Discussion can then explore what staff members feel, understand, and finally, what choice of response might be made.

Videotaping is another way to offer staff members a chance to reflect upon how they felt in relation to how others perceive them. Watching a videotape alone and then sharing it with the team allows a staff member to see, feel, and identify with what the children and adults experienced, to consider what the experience might have been like for them. Further, what choices were made and why, what each participant was trying to accomplish, and for what self was he or she striving need to be actively considered. It can be surprising for professionals to note that there is a lack of synchrony between how they appeared and how they felt. For example, "I never knew that I look so stern when I'm asking questions," or "Wow . . . I looked so much calmer than I felt!"

CONSIDERING GROUP SUPERVISION

Group Process

Group supervision offers a more intensive, dynamically oriented process than is typically possible in larger clinical meetings. Yet, it is not as time or labor intensive as individual supervision. Group supervision involves a formal understanding with a relatively small number of staff (two to six) and an identified facilitator to meet regularly to discuss their work and their responses to the work. The minimum length should be one hour for a group of two and might last as long as two hours for a group as large as six. The facilitator should be an experienced, mature clinician with skill in group process. This is an excellent role for the mental health professional on the team or for a mental health consultant. The ground rules are set by the group facilitator. People say what they think and feel, but they must do their best to frame their messages tactfully to convey their reactions and ideas for group members' consideration.

This is good practice for clinical work: Framing important, even difficult messages in ways that another can hear them. When a member of the group is offended or upset by a comment, it becomes grist for the group's process. The person who made the comment learns how what occurred made the other(s) feel and to reflect upon or try out alternative ways to communicate. The person who was offended gets to practice self-protection, without blame or retaliation. For group supervision to fulfill its promise, the facilitator needs to be even-handed, attending to the protection of each individual as well as the safety and intactness of the group as a whole.

Typically, a group supervision session begins with time to take the pulse of the group by offering each person the opportunity to share briefly. The facilitator asks if anyone has a pressing issue to discuss. Several minutes are also set aside to follow up with the person who presented her work at the last meeting. Reviewing past discussions is vital to modeling coherent and *continuous* process, just what needs to be cultivated between staff and families and with families themselves. Generally, group members present their work and everyone participates in the discussion. The facilitator also actively participates but, typically, contributes after multiple perspectives have been shared. The facilitator may ask questions, draw parallels between the present work and that previously presented, or offer new insights and interpretations. Since the facilitator is selected for skill in group process *and* for clinical expertise, group supervision offers a wonderfully rich, situation-specific opportunity for teaching about clinical work. The facilitator teaches process by modeling an engaged, respectful, listening, reflective stance. Helping all members to aggregate and organize information and impressions, the facilitator helps the group to balance the needs of the supervisee with the needs of the family/child being discussed.

USING CONSULTANTS

Consultants may be employed as facilitators on a part-time basis. It is important that they come *to* the program and have time to get to know it and its cast of characters. Similarly, the consultant needs to become known and trusted. Programs may contract with a consultant from a local mental health clinic, college/university, or private practice to provide group supervision. Funds to hire a consultant can be built into the ongoing budget or, initially, can be secured through small foundation grants or other fundraising efforts. In some areas, members of the American Association for Marital and Family Therapy conduct group supervision pro bono for infant/parent programs, as a service to the community and as an opportunity to their members for professional growth. Similarly, in some locales, the local mental health agency supplies a staff member for several hours per week, or a graduate school of social work or clinical or counseling psychology might offer a field instructor to expand community/university connections. Group supervision sessions similar to those previously described are essential components of graduate education in two leading early childhood institutions: Bank Street College of Education and Erikson Institute. Increasingly, early childhood professional preparation programs are providing the foundation for reflective practice upon which ongoing professional development can build.

Reflective Process in Individual Supervision

Both 1991 and current survey results revealed that not only is individual supervision relatively rare, but also what is offered often falls short of minimum supervisory standards. To be considered individual supervision, meetings must occur on a regular rather than on an as-needed basis. Further, sessions should be held more than monthly, preferably weekly, and they should last for from 45 to 60 minutes each. The focus of supervision should be on the work with individual children and families, rather than on program planning, logistics, or coordination. Additionally, it should address the professional development needs of the supervisee, including exploring, as appropriate, issues of career development and professional identity. (See the section entitled Reflective Supervision Contributes to Professional Identity and Career Development earlier in this chapter.)

SUPERVISORY INTENSIVES

While ongoing individual supervision for each staff member is a standard practice in mental health settings and advanced training programs, it should become a long-term goal for infant through preschool programs. As programs move in this direction, we propose they implement the practice of "Supervisory Intensives," that is, time-limited periods where staff are guaranteed intensive, weekly supervision. In this model, every staff member receives a minimum of six continuous months of individual supervision every two to three years, depending upon the resources of the agency, and later begins or returns to group supervision. Supervisory Intensives would be provided by senior staff, program directors, or mental health staff or consultants. As noted previously, consultants can be hired from local

mental health clinics, colleges/universities, or therapists in private practice. Supervision can be paid for through existing program funds or through foundation or corporate grants. Every opportunity should be made to include individual supervision in grant-funded projects, such as Early Head Start or Healthy Families America. The message to policymakers is that individual reflective supervision is not a luxury, but a minimum standard for professional practice. The field must move toward becoming state of the art.

IN SITU SUPERVISION

When regularity, even in the limited form of Supervisory Intensives, is not possible, programs can provide staff with in situ opportunities for reflection with a mental health member of the team or a mental health consultant. This model, called Catching the Staff (Hefron, 1995) or Life-Space (Redl, 1966) Supervision, provides staff with easy access to a mental health professional for relatively brief discussions. For example, in the NICU (Neonatal Intensive Care Unit) at one hospital, the infant mental health specialist positions herself near the staff changing room when a change of shift occurs. Staff have come to expect and count on her presence, stopping to talk "as needed" about a difficult issue or simply to refuel for a moment before going home. The contacts in this model are staff-initiated. In another hospital setting, the consulting psychologist joins the nurses for Monday rounds, a time set aside to discuss staff/family relationships and emotional responses to the work. This session gives the psychologist a sense of the present issues and the needs of individual staff members. During the week, the psychologist visits the unit daily, making herself available to staff who seek contact, stopping by to talk with a nurse who appears to be having a difficult day, or reconnecting with a nurse who shared a troubling situation in Monday rounds. This consultation is very fluid, often brief, but carefully attuned to the immediate needs of the staff. It models the kind of "in the moment responsivity" required of staff in most community-based service delivery systems.

FORMALIZED PEER MENTORSHIP

Peer mentorship is another rich resource to support reflective practice and to expand limited resources for individual supervision. For example, a new staff member could be asked to keep a journal over the first months in the program and to meet periodically with an experienced team member to reflect upon the experiences, feelings, ideas, and concerns arising from this new role. This mentor relationship might continue formally throughout the first year in practice and then continue as a part of the natural network within the program.

Reflection with Families

As it is essential for professionals to step back and think through their work with colleagues, it is also essential to take time with families to think together about how the work is going. While families are unique and all suggestions must be considered only in light of the needs and capacities of each family and each provider, we recom- mend that programs extend the process of reflection from supervisory relationships into provider/family relationships. This can be as simple as taking a moment at the end of home visits to pause and ask: "How do you feel about what we did today? Did we cover what you hoped we would?" Another example is to have a ritual ending to parent groups where each member has a moment to comment on how the meeting was for them. As practitioners grow in their capacity to consider their own performance within a supportive supervisory relationship, they will be strengthened in their capacity to ask for, hear, and use feedback from parents. Periodic conversations with families to explore what is going well and what might be changed become a mainstay of professional practice.

Reflection can also be systematically built into the early intervention process. Carl Dunst and his colleagues (Dunst, Trivette, & Deal, 1994) designed the annual Individual Family Service Plan review process to include quiet time with the social worker, about two-thirds through the process, for the family to be encouraged to reflect upon and talk over what they have experienced and felt so far, and consider not only what still needs to be addressed, but also how they would prefer it to be addressed. This time to reflect lets the family decompress from the intensity of the interactions and gather their thoughts. It also offers time, if the family wishes, to talk about the feelings that have come up during the assessment and feedback sessions. Based on these reflections, the family has the opportunity to identify their unanswered questions and to set the direction for the remaining time with the assessment team. A family member might say, "I have heard all the numbers I can hear today. I only want to talk about what to do." In another situation, a family member might say, "I realize now that my major worry is my older child and how he is feeling about his little brother. I'd like to talk about that." In this approach, families also have time before the IFSP review day to consider what they want from the process and to develop specific questions for each professional they will see. Thus, "reflection for action" is incorporated as well as "reflection in action."

"Reflection on action" is illustrated in the Family Administered Neonatal Activities (Cardone & Gilkerson, 1988). The FANA is a three-phase process with new parents which begins with a family interview where families are encouraged to use the time to talk about how they are feeling, their labor and delivery, and what they already know about their baby. The next phase involves an active exploration of the newborn's capacities. The last phase is time to reflect—time to pause and consider what they have experienced. The facilitator asks questions such as: How do you feel about what we have just done together? What did you see that you expected to see? What did you see that surprised you?

Reflection is the continuing reconceptualization of what one is doing, observing, and feeling. This rich, generative process gets built into the very center of work *with* families and on behalf of families, when it flows from individuals who are also being supported by regular opportunities for shared reflection.

Conclusion

Reflective supervision and reflective practice provide an oasis in time, a place to breathe, remember, consider, and plan alongside an experienced, concerned, and dedicated professional. It minimizes loneliness and isolation and counteracts mediocrity.

In human services, there is no such thing as graduating from professional school knowing how to do the work. Preprofessional training and experience is simply the foundation. In fact, professional development is a lifelong process since one is constantly confronted with new challenges. No human situation is exactly the same. Reflection upon one's work is a central feature of professional growth and practice. Reflective practice can be achieved in many ways, but flourishes in a trustworthy environment, with responsive leadership and mutually supportive peer relationships. As James Baldwin wrote, "The moment we cease to hold each other, the moment we break faith with each other—the sea engulfs us and the light goes out."

To acquire the conceptual knowledge, the self-knowledge, and the experience needed to work effectively with young children and families and the capacity for relationally-specific, emotionally lively engagement, professionals must have multiple opportunities to experience respectful, responsive supervisory relationships over time. Workers, their supervisors, and their directors need sustained periods with intensive individual reflective supervision where the learning, knowing, doing, and being merge. Through this process, new affectively-lively knowledge and skills move from "the domain of new and 'tacked on,' to the familiar and indispensible" (Pine, 1985, p. 121), to an integral part of the professional self. With a parallel transformation, the agency or unit becomes a compelling and meaningful community in which to work and in which to grow, feel, and be effective.

Notes

*During the summer of 1998, while writing this chapter, one of us (RSS) viewed the paintings by Pierre Bonnard at the Museum of Modern Art in New York. Listening to the acoustiguide (by Glenn Loury, Director and John Elderfield, Curator), I was astonished to recognize the descriptions of the paintings as one metaphor after another for the internal experience of reflective practice. These quotations and ideas have been adapted from the narrative of the acoustiguide to illuminate the text which follows.

1. Respondents from New York all attended the Institute for Clinical Studies of Infants, Toddlers and Parents, part of the Jewish Board of Family and Children's Services.

References

Advisory Committee on Services for Families with Infants and Toddlers. (1994, September). *Statement of the advisory committee on services for infants and toddlers.* Washington, DC: Department of Health and Human Services.

Ainsworth, M. D. S., Blehar, M. C., Waters, E., & Wall S. (1978). *Patterns of attachment.* Hillsdale, NJ: Erlbaum.

Axtmann, A. (1984). The center for infants and parents at Teachers College, Columbia University: A setting for study and support. *Zero to Three, 4*(2), 3.

Axtmann, A., with Bluham, C. & Wolf, D. (1986). Friendship among infants? Yes, indeed! In *Beginnings.* Redmond, WA: Exchange.

Axtmann, A. (1998). Babies, Toddlers, Parents, Caregivers: Growing Together. Videotape available through Great Projects Film Company, Inc., New York, NY (212) 581-1700.

Belenkey, M. F., Clinchy, B. M., Goldberger, N. R., & Tarlue, J. M (1986). *Women's ways of knowing: The development of self, voice, and mind.* New York: Basic Books.

Bertacchi, J., & Stott, F. (1991). A seminar for supervisors in infant/family programs: Growing versus paying more for staying the same. *Zero to Three, 12,* 34–39.

Bowlby, J. (1988). *A secure base.* New York: Basic Books.

Bowman, B. (1989). Self-reflection as an element of professionalism. *Teachers College Record, 90*(3), 444–451.

Bredecamp, S., & Copple, C. (Eds.). (1997). *Developmentally appropriate practice in early childhood programs.* (Rev. ed.). Washington DC: National Association for the Education of Young Children.

Brown, F. (1984). Erotic and pseudoerotic elements in the treatment of male patients by female therapists. *Clinical Social Work Journal, 12*(3), 244–257.

Cardone, I., & Gilkerson, L. (1988). Family Administrated Neonatal Activities: an innovative component of family-centered care. *Zero to Three, 10*(1), 23–28.

Copa, A., Lucinski, L., Olsen, E., & Wollenburg, K. (1999, August–September). Promoting professional and organizational development. A reflective practice model. *Zero to Three, 20*(1), 3–9.

Dunst, C. J., Trivette, C. M., & Deal, A. G. (Eds.). (1994). *Supporting and strengthening families–Volume 1: Methods, strategies and practices.* Cambridge, MA: Brookline Books.

Eggbeer, L., Fenichel, E., Pawl, J. H., Shanok, R. S., & Williamson, D. E. (1994, October). Training the trainers: Innovative strategies for teaching relationship concepts and skills to infant/family professionals. *Infants and Young Children, 7*(2), 53–61.

Emde, R. (1998). *Verbal communication as Visiting Scholar to the Institute for Clinical Studies of Infants, Toddlers and Parents and the Early Childhood Group Therapy Program of Child Development Center.* New York: Jewish Board for Family and Children's Services.

Felton, J. R. (1986). Sex makes a difference—How gender affects the therapeutic relationship. *Clinical Social Work Journal, 14*(2), 127–138.

Fenichel, E. S., & Eggbeer, L. (1991). Preparing practitioners to work with infants, toddlers, and their families: Four essential elements of training. *Infants and Young Children, 4,* 56–62.

Fenichel, E. S., with NCCIP Work Group on Supervision and Mentorship. (1992a). In E. Fenichel (Ed.), *Learning through supervision and mentorship to support the development of infants, toddlers and their families.* (pp. 9–17). Arlington, VA: National Center for Clinical Infant Programs.

Fenichel, E. S., & Eggbeer, L., with NCCIP Work Group on Supervision and Mentorship. (1992b). Overcoming obstacles to reflective supervision and mentorship. In E. Fenichel (Ed.), *Learning through supervision and mentorship: A source book.* (pp. 18–26). Arlington, VA: Zero to Three.

Feuerstein, R. (1986). Learning to learn: Mediated learning experiences and instrumental enrichment. *Special Services in the Schools, 3*(1–2), 49–82.

Foley, G. (1994, February–March). Parent professional relationships: Finding an optimal distance. *Zero to Three, 14*(4), 19–22.

Fraiberg, S. H., Adelson, E., & Shapiro, V. (1975). Ghosts in the nursery: A psychoanalytic approach to the problem of impaired infant-mother relationships. *Journal of the American Academy of Child Psychiatry, 14,* 387–422.

Freud, A. (1954). The widening scope of indications for psychoanalysis: Discussion. In *The writings of Anna Freud* (Vol. 4, pp. 356–379). New York: International Universities Press.

Freud, S. (1912). The dynamics of transference. In *The standard edition of the complete psychological works of Sigmund Freud* (pp. 97–108). London: Hogarth.

Gabbard, G. O. (1994). Sexual excitement and countertransference love in the analyst. *Journal of the American Psychoanalytic Association, 42*(4), 1083–1106.

Gilkerson, L. (1992). Supports for the process of change in "program families." *Zero to Three, 12*(3), 19–21.

Gilkerson, L. (1993). *Taking the pulse: Understanding the dynamics of your unit.* Paper presented at the Contemporary Forums Developmental Interventions in Neonatal Care Conference, San Francisco, CA.

77

Gilkerson, L. (1995). Reflection on the process of supervision. In R. S. Shanok, L. Gilkerson, L. Eggbeer, & E. Fenichel (Eds.), *Reflective supervision: A relationship for learning. Discussion Guide* (pp. 41–49). Arlington, VA: Zero to Three.

Gilkerson, L., & Als, H. (1995). Role of reflective process in the implementation of developmentally supportive care in the newborn intensive care nursery. *Infants and Young Children, 7*(4), 20–28.

Gilkerson, L., & Young-Holt, C. L. (1992). Supervision and the management of programs serving infants, toddlers, and their families. In E. Fenichel (Ed.), *Learning through supervision and mentorship: A source book.* Arlington, VA: Zero to Three.

Greenspan, S. I. (1992). *Infancy and early childhood.* Madison, CT: International Universities Press.

Greenspan, S. I. (1997). *The growth of the mind and the endangered origins of intelligence.* Reading, MA: Addison Wesley.

Grimmett, P. P. (1988). The nature of reflection and Schon's conception in perspective. In P. P. Grimmett & G. L. Erickson (Eds.), *Reflection in teacher education* (pp. 147–176). New York: Teachers College Press.

Henderson, D. (1997). Women practitioners counseling men: Challenges and obstacles. *Zero to Three, 18*(1), 18–23.

Klein, N., & Gilkerson, L. (in press). Personnel preparation for early childhood intervention programs. In S. Meisels & J. P. Shonkoff (Eds.), *Handbook of early childhood intervention* (2nd ed.) Cambridge: Cambridge University Press.

Lynch, E. W., & Hanson, M. J. (1992). *Developing cross-cultural competence—A guide for working with young children and their families.* Baltimore: Brookes.

Mahler, M., Pine, F., & Bergman, A. (1975).

The psychological birth of the human infant: Symbiosis and individuation. New York: Basic Books.

Manis, F. (1979). *Openness in social work field instruction.* Goleta, CA: Kimberly Press.

Pawl, J. (1995). On supervision. In R. Shanok, L. Gilkerson, L. Eggbeer, & E. Fenichel (Eds.), *Reflective supervision: A relationship for learning. Discussion Guide* (pp. 41–49). Arlington, VA: Zero to Three.

Pine, F. (1985). *Developmental theory and clinical process.* New Haven: Yale University Press.

Redl, F. (1966). *When we deal with children.* New York: Free Press.

Rodriguez, B. M. (1995–1996, Fall–Winter). From self to other: Communication across cultures. *Family Resource Coalition Report, 4,* (3–4), 11–15.

Ross, D. D. (1987). *Teaching teacher effectiveness research to students: First steps in developing a reflective approach to teaching.* Paper presented at the Annual Meeting of the American Educational Research Association, Washington, DC.

Sander, A. M. (1993). An inquiry into the fate of transference in psychoanalysis. *Journal of the American Psychoanalytic Association, 41,* 627–651.

Schön, D. A. (1983). *The reflective practitioner: How professionals think in action.* New York: Basic Books.

Schore, A. N. (1994). *Affect regulation and the origin of the self: The neurobiology of emotional development.* Hillsdale, NJ: Erlbaum.

Shahmoon-Shanok, R. (1991). *Small Is Beautiful.* Opening Remarks at the Seventh Biennial Conference of Zero to Three: The National Center for Infants, Toddlers, and Families, Washington, DC.

Available from the author at ICS_ITP_ECGT@psinet.com or (212) 632–4741.

Shahmoon-Shanok, R. (1997a, April–May). Giving back future's promise: Working resourcefully with parents of children who have severe disorders of relating and communicating. *Zero to Three, 17*(5), 37–48.

Shahmoon-Shanok, R. (1997b). *Peer play groups: Enabling individual growth in very young children.* Remarks and chart presented as moderator at a Zero to Three National Training Institute session entitled Turning the Lens Toward Peer Relations in Groups of Children Under Three, with J. Bitetti and D. Wittmer, copresenters.

Shahmoon-Shanok, R. (2000). Infant mental health perspectives on peer play psychotherapy for symptomatic, at-risk and disordered young children. In J. Osofsky & H. Fitzgerald (Eds.), *WAIMH handbook of infant mental health: Vol. 4. Infant mental health in groups at high risk.* New York: Wiley.

Shanok, R. S. (1984). *Attachment and individuation: Implications for programming.* Invited address at First Northeastern Conference of the Center for Infants and Parents, Teachers College, Columbia University, New York. Available from the author at ICS_ITP_ECEGT@psinet.com or (212) 632–4741.

Shanok, R. S. (1992). The supervisory relationship: Integrator, resource and guide. In E. Fenichel (Ed.), *Learning through supervision and mentorship: A source book.* (pp. 113–119). Arlington, VA: Zero to Three.

Shanok, R. S., Gilkerson, L., Eggbeer, L., & Fenichel, E. (1995a). *Reflective supervision: A relationship for learning* [Videotape]. Washington, DC: Zero to Three.

Shanok, R. S., Gilkerson, L., Eggbeer, L. & Fenichel, E. (1995b). *Reflective supervision: A relationship for learning. A discussion guide.* Washington, DC: Zero to Three.

Shanok, R. S., with Eggbeer, L., & Fenichel, E. (1994–1995, December–January). Using relationship to teach relationship: The risky business of role playing. *Zero to Three, 15*(3), 46–52.

Shanok, R. S., Welton, S., & Lapidus, C. (1989). Group therapy for preschool children: A transdisciplinary school-based approach. *Child and Adolescent Social Work, 6*(1), 72–95.

Sokoly, M. M., & Dokecki, P. R. (1992). Ethical perspectives on family-centered early intervention. *Infants and Young Children: An Interdisciplinary Journal of Special Care Practices, 4*(4), 23–32.

Stern, D. (1985). *The interpersonal world of the infant: A view from psychoanalysis and developmental psychology.* New York: Basic Books.

Stott, F., & Bowman, B. (1996). Child development knowledge: A slippery base for practice. *Early Childhood Research Quarterly, 11,* 169–183.

Tremmel, R. (1993). Zen and the art of reflective practice in teacher education. *Harvard Education Review, 63*(4), 434–458.

Vygotsky, L. S. (1978). *Mind in society.* Cambridge, MA: Harvard University Press.

Wolff, P. (1966). *The causes, controls, and organization of behavior in the neonate. Psychological Issues #17.* New York: International Universities Press.

Yoshikawa, H., & Knitzer, J. (1997). *Lessons from the field: Head Start mental health strategies to meet changing needs.* New York: National Center for Children in Poverty, Columbia School for Public Health, and American Orthopsychiatric Association, Task Force on Head Start and Mental Health.

3

The Assessment of Infants and Toddlers with Medical Conditions and Their Families

Klaus Minde

3

Introduction

This chapter discusses ways to assess the emotional, social, and cognitive functioning of preschool children whose life has been compromised by a severe acute or chronic medical condition. As young children cannot be meaningfully evaluated in isolation, such an assessment will always include an evaluation of the child's family and wider social network and will focus both on the child's organizational abilities and affective and interpersonal experiences.

There is much in this process which is similar or even identical to an assessment of healthy noncompromised infants and toddlers. However, the burden of an illness or disability, with all the fantasies and conflicts such an event triggers in the parents and other family members, often requires additional skills and sensitivities in the clinician so that the assessment can help the family meet the reality of the "baby as is" (Brazelton & Cramer, 1990).

To deepen the reader's appreciation of the impact medical conditions can have on an infant's emotional, cognitive, and social development, three principles of early development are outlined. This is followed by reviewing the major developmental tasks of the first three years because the effects of medical illnesses are often translated into changes in the developmental trajectory of affected children.

The next section reviews key empirical studies which document the impact of illness early in life on later behavior and development. Special attention is given to studies which examine possible mediating variables, that is, look at what events or attitudes of caregivers bring about the translation of a medical illness at one or two years into a psychiatric condition, such as a somatoform disorder at age 10.

The chapter then outlines the assessment process as it should ideally take place. The framework used is that proposed by Greenspan (1991) and Lieberman and Slade (1997) who embrace the epigenetic premise that infants are able to organize experiences from birth onward and that this ability increases as the individual matures. Greenspan in this context talks about the phase-appropriateness, stability, and personal uniqueness of development. The second assumption of this framework is that each organizational level gives rise to specific affective experiences, well exemplified in the stranger anxiety of the 8-month-old infant. It is the interplay between these two phenomena and their modulation through an illness and the associated interpersonal caregiving experiences which need to be assessed by the infant mental health clinician.

The discussion of specific assessment procedures is based on empirical data as far as they are available and refers to the recently published "Practice Parameters for the Psychiatric Assessment of Infants and Toddlers" (Thomas et al., 1997) and the volume *New Visions for the Developmental Assessment of Infants and Young Children* edited by Meisels and Fenichel (1996) as major guidelines. Specific assessment practices are illustrated by providing the reader with clinical examples. Finally, those assessment procedures are highlighted which are considered to provide the most information in the shortest time

and for the least expense. This is done in an attempt to make the chapter practically relevant for the busy clinician.

General Principles of Early Development

Current thinking on early development tends to focus on the predictable unfolding of physical, cognitive, and social capabilities. While this is obviously correct, the first principle to remember is that these epigenetic changes are caused by multiple, interactive, and often nonobvious phenomena. This implies that it is incorrect to account for early development by only using the concept of neural maturation. While this process is important, it will not bring about development unless the neural structures are in interaction with people and events. In fact, it is psychological processes which organize individual experience, and it is social processes which regulate our relationships with others in the community. To be successful, for example, in walking, one needs to be able to have mastered the pattern of alternate leg movements (often a nonobvious phenomenon) and have the motivation to move forward (an interpersonal or psychological parameter).

The second principle of development states that periods of growth will be followed by instability and reorganization (Thelen & Smith, 1994). For example, if an infant can manipulate a toy in a specific way, the parents may then introduce the infant to a new toy which requires different ways of handling. Experience shows that infants will use these novel manipulative skills only occasionally in the beginning, falling back to their previously practiced modes of action at other times.

In addition to these perturbations and reorganizations, infants undergo some specific major qualitative changes in their cognitive development. For example, at approximately two months they become more attentive to qualitative features of the environment and can regulate their arousal level better (Emde et al., 1996). This has implications for their social development, as they now differentiate between a smiling face and a sad face and develop a social smile, and for sleep/wake regulations (they find it easier to get back to sleep on their own after a feeding at night). At eight to nine months, brought on by the ability to crawl, children become more aware of spatial relationships that in turn go together with their newly acquired dependence on distal emotional cues and stranger anxiety (Berthenthal & Campos, 1990). It is as if the onset of locomotion and the competence in making use of distant communication go together because the baby can now bridge the gap to the caretaker created by locomotion by using symbols (e.g., a look or encouraging sound by mother) to stay connected while taking off.

The third principle is that development occurs within a social context. Infants are surrounded by older people whose increased sophistication guides the development of the younger child (Rogoff, 1990). This also pertains to individual cultures which facilitates the development of cul-

ture specific abilities. For example, infants in New Guinea are able, with supervision, to handle knives and fire by the time they are able to walk, an event unthinkable in North America (Rogoff, 1990). Developmental achievements of the toddler, that is, increased representational capacity, shown in the use of symbols (e.g., play) and language or self-recognition and sexual curiosity about himself or herself and others follow the same three principles. A comprehensive evaluation, therefore, will need to take these principles into account and assess whether they have been affected by medical illnesses and the associated change of social context.

The Effects of Medical Illnesses on Development and Behavior

Epidemiology

The literature on the effects of medical illnesses on children's development is extensive but also difficult to interpret. There are various reasons for this. Foremost is the question whether only chronic but not acute medical conditions should be understood to impact on later development and behavior. Most authors seem to subscribe to this assumption although the definition of a chronic illness varies among them. For example, some authors define a chronic illness by its severity, others by its duration (Perrin et al., 1993). There is also a longstanding debate between those who claim that psychosocial concerns are specific to individual conditions such as asthma or diabetes (Lavigne & Faier-Routman, 1992) while others maintain that concerns are generalized and apply to all children and families coping with chronic conditions (Pless & Pinkerton, 1975). In addition, many studies of chronically ill children report on small, site-specific samples and rely on descriptive measures of behavioral or cognitive disturbances, generally obtained by only one rather than multiple observers. They also usually compare their samples to a chosen control group rather than test norms, a strategy known to decrease the risk comparison (Lavigne & Faier-Routman, 1992).

As mentioned earlier, the effects of acute illnesses on later development and behavior are rarely evaluated. The exception is the substantial literature on the impact of prematurity on infants and their families (Minde, 1993). In this chapter, the psychosocial and developmental risks of chronic health conditions as they have been defined by the Committee on Children with Disabilities and the Committee on Psychosocial Aspects of Child and Family Health of the American Academy of Pediatrics in 1993 are discussed.

Both committees defined a chronic condition as one that has lasted three months or longer. Severity is seen as the impact an illness has on a child's physical, intellectual, psychological, or social functioning (Stein et al., 1997). The impact may occur as a result of required treatments, persistent symptoms, limitations of activity or mobility, or interference with family activities. It is interesting that this definition does not include the impact a chronic condition can have on caretakers whose modified parenting style may then compromise their handicapped children's behavior and development.

The committee estimates that 10 to 20 million children and adolescents in the United States have some type of chronic health condition or impairment. If the number of individuals under age 25 in the United States is estimated to be about 72 million, this comes to about 20 percent of this population. The committee, furthermore, estimates that about 10 percent of children with chronic conditions, that is about 1.5 to 2 million children and adolescents, have a chronic illness severe enough to affect their daily life. If these figures are extrapolated to the infant and toddler age group, 250,000 infants are expected to have handicaps which impact on their day-to-day activities.

It should be emphasized that the number of chronically ill children who show psychological symptoms is 20 percent, that is, about twice as high as the number of children whose handicaps affect their daily lives (Cadman, Boyle, Szatmari, & Offord, 1987; Gortmaker, Walker, Weitzman, & Sobol, 1990). Such symptoms do not seem to be related to the severity of a chronic condition (Perrin, West, & Culley, 1989) but more to its duration (Hobbs et al., 1995). Nevertheless, these figures suggest that there are approximately one-half million infants and toddlers with chronic conditions and behavioral or developmental difficulties.

If the approximately 20 percent prematurely born children who show behavioral or developmental difficulties without being chronically ill are included, another 1 to 1.5 percent of the infant population is added to the symptomatic group, approximately 650,000 youngsters who require some form of mental health care during their first three years of life.

Symptoms and How They Come About

Symptoms which reflect the adjustment of infants and children to their physical disorders can vary widely and do not always imply the presence of "a problem." For example, a blind toddler may be hesitant in venturing away from his mother or display other behaviors usually classified as internalizing symptoms. Yet in the reality of this toddler, mistrusting nonfamiliar figures, showing unusual bouts of repetitive behaviors (e.g., engaging in self-stimulation), or displaying a low frustration tolerance may be a totally reasonable way of tackling the task of learning to live without vision. The toddler's family, in turn, may score as overly protective and even as controlling on well standardized Family Function Scales although the toddler in question clearly needs more direction and guidance than a visually competent toddler.

The first premise, therefore, is to emphasize that most measures of child psychopathology and family functioning used in pediatric settings were developed with normative samples of children or those referred or treated for mental health problems (LaGreca, 1994; McCubbin & McCubbin, 1988).

This is one reason why clinicians have tried to understand the problems of youngsters with a medical condition in more general terms. For example, researchers, besides recording internalizing and externalizing symptoms, have investigated the self-concept of such youngsters. Others have hypothesized that medically compromised children will more often show an insecure attachment and their clinical symptomatology will reflect this. Finally, authors have conceptualized a syndrome which is primarily seen in children with medical illnesses, naming it the Vulnerable Child Syndrome (Green & Solnit, 1964). What is the evidence for these various assertions?

There is indeed consistent evidence that children above age four with chronic medical conditions show about twice the number of externalizing and internalizing symptoms on child behavior checklists such as the CBCL developed by Achenbach (1991). This was best documented in a meta-analysis of 85 studies examining the behavior of children with chronic medical conditions by Lavigne and Faier-Routman (1992) that showed an overall increase in both internalizing and externalizing symptoms. However, some diseases seemed to produce more consistent difficulties than others. For example, chronic seizures, deafness, cardiac abnormalities, diabetes, and cystic fibrosis showed an effect size of at least .50 in five or more independent studies. Other conditions were not associated with an increase in behavior problems (e.g., rheumatoid arthritis, cerebral palsy, or chronic renal problems). However, they may not have qualified because there were too few well-controlled studies in each category for a proper analysis. These authors also documented that the self-concept of children with physical disorders was significantly lower than that of healthy children but that careful matching with norms (rather than the chosen control population) decreased the differences somewhat.

As the CBCL is of questionable validity for assessing children with chronic medical conditions, because its standardization is based on healthy youngsters, a shorter scale specifically designed for medically compromised populations was used in a population study examining 3,924 children and their families (Offord et al., 1987). These authors found very similar results to those described by Lavigne and Faier-Routman. Furthermore, Goldberg and her group in a series of studies examining the families and the development and behavior of infants with cystic fibrosis (CF) and congenital heart disease (CHD), as well as a control group from age six months onward, report that children with CHD in general show more demanding behaviors, a more negative mood, higher distractibility, and less acceptable behaviors as rated by both parents than both the control children and those affected by CF (Goldberg, Morris, Simmons, Fowler, & Levison, 1990). This suggests that precursors of the previously cited behavioral difficulties in children with medical conditions above age four can already be detected in infants and toddlers.

Similar findings pertain to the attachment patterns observed in the same children. Here again, among infants with cystic fibrosis, two-thirds were securely attached to their mothers (Fisher-Fay, Goldberg, Simmons, & Levison, 1988), as would be expected in normal populations. However, among infants with congenital heart disease, the proportion of securely attached infants was only 48 percent (Goldberg, Fischer-Fay, Simmons, Fowler, & Levison, 1989). This may suggest that a disease which presents within the context of an acute crisis like congenital heart disease has a more powerful effect on the parents than does a medical condition like cystic fibrosis which usually has a more insidious onset and requires no immediate surgical intervention.

Goldberg's work also touches on the important question of how a medical condition in an infant is transformed into problematic behavior and development. The work which has been done in this area has concentrated on creating models which could explain how the way parents perceive a medical condition may influence their interactions with their affected children. The model which best captures this complex process is the Vulnerable Child Syndrome, first described by Green and Solnit (1964). These authors reported on school-age children with severe behavioral and learning problems who had experienced a serious illness or accident earlier in childhood from which they had not been expected to recover. Although they had recovered fully, their parents continued to perceive them as highly susceptible to illness and even death. Green and Solnit who are highly esteemed psychoanalysts thought that such children may act to prove that death has not occurred by displacing the threat symbolically and to a limited part of their body (e.g., abdominal pain) or develop aggressive symptoms which in the end may serve to reinforce the parental perception of child vulnerability.

While the cases described by Green and Solnit almost certainly represent the extreme of a spectrum in which specific events can heighten parents' anxiety for many years, there are other reports which are consistent with an increased sense of vulnerability in some children and their caregivers. For example, Sigal and colleagues. (1973) reported on parents whose children had experienced a self-limiting severe croup or diarrheal illness (Sigal & Gagnon, 1975) and who showed heightened concerns for their welfare at least into later middle childhood. Minde and colleagues (1983) also showed how parents of very small premature infants (birthweight less than 1500 gr.) were affected by their children's medical complications in the neonatal nursery. When these complications lasted less than two weeks, the infant's recovery, documented by the baby's increasingly active behavior (e.g., more body movements, eye openings), was followed within a day by an increase in maternal activities (mothers touched or talked and smiled at their infants more). However, when complications lasted four weeks or longer, the recovering infants' increased activity level was not reciprocated by their mothers. It seemed as if the long and serious illness had closed off the parents' perception of their infants' actual state of health and they continued to perceive them and interact with them as if they had remained ill. A similar phenomenon was observed in the study of 65 very small premature twins where mothers within two weeks of the birth had delegated one of the twins to be a "problem baby" (Minde & Corter, 1984). This status remained constant in about 60 percent of the cases at least until age four and was primarily associated with health status at birth (the twin with the lower birth weight and higher perinatal problem score was usually designated the "problem child") and it had significant repercussions for the infants' behavioral development (Minde, Corter, Goldberg, & Jeffers, 1990).

Instruments That Assess Parental Perceptions of Medically Ill Children

Ten years ago, Forsyth and colleagues at Yale University began to design a Child Vulnerability Scale to measure parental perceptions of vulnerability and identify children who are perceived as vulnerable. After some preliminary clinical explorations with prematurely born children (Perrin et al., 1989) and children who had a history of feeding problems and much crying in early infancy (Forsyth & Canny, 1991), this group published psychometric data on their Child Vulnerability Scale, shown in Table 3.1, based on 1,095 mothers and their four- to eight-year-old children attending their pediatricians' offices (Forsyth, McCue, Horwitz, Leventhal, & Burger, 1996). The children were also rated on the CBCL (Achenbach, 1991), and visits to their pediatricians during the subsequent year were recorded. The eight-item Child Vulnerability Scale had a high internal consistency and 10.1 percent of all children were rated vulnerable by their mothers. Interestingly, 20 percent of the vulnerable children versus only 8 percent of the rest were given CBCL scores within the clinical range. Vulnerable children also visited their physicians more often during the subsequent year (5.9 vs. 3.9 visits). Of the subgroup who had at some time in their lives been diagnosed with a medical condition and whose mothers thought at some time that they might die, 50 percent scored within the vulnerable range.

TABLE 3.1

Parent Protection Scale

---

1. I blame myself when my child gets hurt.
2. I comfort my child immediately when he or she cries.
3. I encourage my child to depend on me.
4. I have difficulty separating from my child.
5. I trust my child on his or her own.
6. I let my child make his or her own decisions.
7. I have difficulty leaving my child with a baby-sitter.
8. I decide when my child eats.
9. I use baby words when I talk to my child.
10. I urge my child to try new things.
11. I determine with whom my child plays.
12. I keep a close watch on my child.
13. I feed my child even if he or she can do it alone.
14. I feel comfortable leaving my child with other people.
15. I protect my child from criticism.
16. I let my child choose what he or she wears.
17. I make my child go to sleep at a set time.
18. I go to my child if he or she cries during the night.
19. I encourage my child to play with other children.
20. I give my child extra attention.
21. I decide what my child eats.
22. I dress my child even if he or she can do it alone.
23. I decide when my child goes to the bathroom.
24. I know exactly what my child is doing.
25. I allow my child to do things on his or her own.

Source: Thomasgard , Metz, Edelbrock, and Shonkoff, "Parent-Child Relationship Disorders: Part 1. Parental Overprotection and the Development of the Parent Protection Scale." *Journal of Developmental and Behavioral Pediatrics, 16,* 244–250.

In a further development of this construct, Thomasgard and his colleagues (1995) developed a Parent Protection Scale based on their examination of 1,002 children ages 2–10 years, as shown in Table 3.2. The psychometric properties of this scale were satisfactory and all children above one standard deviation of the normative sample were identified as overprotected. It is of interest that overprotective mothers in this study in general were younger, nonmarried, from lower socio-economic backgrounds, and had only one child. History of the previous life threatening illness or injury for the child was not associated with maternal overprotection. This suggests that child vulnerability and overprotection are not identical or even associated phenomena and confirms retrospective studies which have associated child vulnerability with separation problems (Green & Solnit, 1964), overindulgent behaviors toward the child (Berger, 1977), school underachievement (Solnit &

TABLE 3.2

Child Vulnerability Scale

1. In general, my child seems less healthy than other children.
2. I often think about calling the doctor about my child.
3. When there is something going around, my child usually catches it.
4. I sometimes get concerned that my child does not look as healthy as he or she should.
5. I often have to keep my child indoors because of health reasons.
6. My child gets more colds than other children I know.
7. I get concerned about circles under my child's eyes.
8. I often check on my child at night to make sure he or she is okay.

Source: Forsyth, McCue, Horwitz, Leventhal, and Burger, "The Child Vulnerability Scale: An Instrument to Measure Parental Perceptions of Child Vulnerability." *Journal of Pediatric Psychology, 21,* 89–101.

Stark, 1959), and increased health care utilization (Levy, 1980; Thomasgard et al., 1993). In contrast, overprotection in children has been seen as a risk factor for adult dysthymia, anxiety disorders, and difficulties with close interpersonal relationships (Parker, 1983, 1993).

In a more recent study, Thomasgard and Metz (1996) reported on 114 children ages four to seven who were seen two years previously and rated on the Child Vulnerability Scale (CVS) by Forsyth and colleagues (1996) and the Parent Protection Scale (PPS) by Thomasgard and colleagues (1995). On follow-up, all children were also rated on the CBCL (Achenbach, 1991) by their mothers. Continuity over time was highest (93 percent) for children with low parental protection (–PPS) and low vulnerability (–CVS scores), medium for children with +PPS and –CVS (37 percent) or –PPS and +CVS (31 percent) scores, and lowest for children showing +PPS and +CVS (15 percent) scores. However, another 9 percent of the +PPS –CVS group and 10 percent of the –PPS +CVS group joined the +PPS +CVS group at follow-up. This means that only 31 percent of the vulnerable children and 37 percent of the overprotected children remained in their respective categories over a two-year period. Nevertheless, the 26 boys who had high perceived child vulnerability (+CVS) ratings during the initial evaluation showed significantly increased externalizing problems on the CBCL on follow-up, while the 16 +CVS girls showed increased internalizing problems. There were no behavioral correlates in the overprotected children, confirming that vulnerability and overprotection are different constructs and do not usually occur together.

There is other evidence which confirms the power parental representations have in predicting both parental mental health and child behavior. For example, Ireys and Silver (1996) showed that the perception 169 mothers had regarding the impact of their chronically ill children on family life was related to the mother's mental health after the child had been ill for a year but not initially. This suggests that an evaluation of family functioning and parental mental health after a diagnosis has been made may not always be able to accurately predict future family and child functioning. Meyer and colleagues (1995) in examining 142 mothers of premature infants also showed that maternal psychological distress was predicted by both maternal characteristics and infant variables.

On the other hand, there is also some evidence that certain aspects of family structure and beliefs can have a moderating or protecting effect on later developmental and psychological outcome. For example, Silver and colleagues (1996) in examining 352 families found that functional status of the children and their behavior was more strongly correlated in families with a single mother or a mother living with an unrelated partner than it was in two-parent families or those where mothers lived with a relative. The suggestion here is that more supportive family structures can successfully moderate the behavioral consequences of functional impairments. Likewise, Melnyk (1995) found that mothers who at the time of their child's hospitalization were given information about both their young children's expected behavior in the hospital and their own roles in dealing with it were more competent in handling their children and less influenced by their level of anxiety than when they did not receive this information. This suggests that the belief system of parents is an important mediating factor in children's development and that education is one way to bring about change.

In summary, there is persuasive evidence that caregivers' perception of a child's vulnerability is only weakly related to the severity of the actual illness of a child, but that it functions as a powerful mediator for later child psychopathology, family stress, and maternal emotional health. Firstborn children seem to be somewhat more at risk, but there is no relation with the child's sex. The actual problem behavior of children later on is thought to be related to the child's reaction to parental anxiety and can take the form of defiance and opposition or of joining the parents' anxiety and depression. In both cases, the child reinforces the parents' ongoing anxiety about the child's vulnerability.

The Socioemotional Assessment of Medically Compromised Infants and Their Families

Most frequently, infant mental health specialists express concerns about the medically ill infants' ability to develop normally and hope that the adverse effects of hospitalization or other aspects of the illness on behavior and development can be limited. Another goal of intervention is to optimize the relationship caregivers have with these "unusual" children and help them deal with behavior problems which may appear as a result of the child's medical condition. In infants, this may mean difficulties in feeding and sleeping or an apparent withdrawal from the world. In toddlers, one may observe aggression, defiance, overactivity, or developmental regression. In addition, children with chronic medical illnesses can show specific developmental delays and more or less subtle sensory-motor processing problems. Finally, infant mental health specialists are often asked to assist others in helping caregivers come to terms with an infant's chronic illness and prepare parents for a life with a "special" child.

It is obvious that, confronted with such a wide range of symptoms and questions, infant mental health specialists need to know a good deal about the impact and clinical course of various medical disorders and be cognizant of various formalized and clinical assessment procedures. These are discussed in some detail later.

There are a number of general principles which guide the evaluation and treatment of all infants and toddlers independent of their medical status. The most important of these is the need to understand and evaluate young children within the context of their family or primary caregiving unit. This means that clinicians must learn about a complex network of functions, each reflecting a mixture of biological, cognitive, and socioemotional endowments. They must be able to evaluate the significance of those functions within the child's milieu and culture and demonstrate them to his or her caretakers and other health care professionals. In addition, the clinician must be comfortable with talking about the inner life of these caretakers with them and assessing to what degree their subjective feelings or "internal representations" (Zeanah & Anders, 1987) influence their actual caretaking style. In summary, clinicians need to be experts in normal child development, knowledgeable about medical conditions and surgical procedures, and profoundly aware of the relationship life of adults.

Process of Assessment

The mental health assessment of a medically compromised infant or preschooler and his or her family consists of:

1. A clinical interview with one or more caregivers, which may include medical or rehabilitation personnel, to obtain an appropriate history of the presenting medical and psychological problems as well as a family and developmental history of both child and caretakers.
2. A clinical assessment of the infant or preschooler.
3. A more standardized assessment of the child, using appropriate and reliable testing procedures.
4. A parent-child relational assessment.
5. An assessment of the parenting skills of the primary caregivers.

The material obtained from this investigation should then be integrated in a dynamic fashion, so that it provides caretakers and health professionals with a coherent biopsychosocial narrative and an appropriate treatment plan.

The Clinical Interview with the Primary Caregivers

This interview is usually the first encounter between the clinician and the child's caretakers. Most parents of physically ill young children are anxious and concerned about meeting a mental health specialist because they may feel that "they cannot manage their child anymore" or their youngster "now in addition to physical problems also has a mental difficulty." They, therefore, frequently feel that they have failed as parents right from the start and may see this as a sign of their own inferiority or incompetence. The first aim of an evaluation, therefore, should be to establish a good working alliance between parents and the clinician. This will assure that the parents feel respected and allow the interview to become as much a mutual discovery of the past as it is active in the present (Hirshberg, 1993).

The format of the initial clinical interview will vary from clinician to clinician. Some find it useful to talk to the parents alone first. This allows parents to tell their stories without interruptions and gives them a sense of being important partners in the evaluation process. It also makes it easier for the clinician to probe gently in areas where parents may be defensive and may otherwise use their children's presence to avoid painful or embarrassing issues.

If the child in question is still hospitalized at the time of the referral, the initial contact of the mental health professional may be with the team of physicians and nurses looking after the infant or toddler because in many ways they may function as primary caretakers at that time. These individuals often have specific impressions or opinions about the strengths and difficulties of the child's parents and should be listened to carefully. Some of them may also have made valuable observations about the ill child, and their good will is often essential for helping the mental health clinician to create the psychosocially best possible treatment regime for a hospitalized or seriously ill child. If the child lives at home and

the parents bring the child along, one can begin assessing the parent-child relationship at that time. In practice, it is useful to tell the parents at the outset that they should do whatever they feel comfortable doing when caring for their child, and to facilitate this, for example, be careful not to continue the interview too quickly after the parents have interrupted the conversation to attend to their youngster. Such a practice allows the parents to alternate their attention between the interviewer and the child in a more relaxed way.

While the interviewing style will vary widely among individual clinicians, it always has to take into account the cultural traditions of the family. In fact, there is good evidence that different interviewing techniques will elicit similar information from the parents of young children. However, studies have also shown that factual historical data can best be obtained by direct questioning (Cox, Hopkinson, & Rutter, 1981). Feelings and opinions, in contrast, are elicited more easily by asking open questions such as "What does Marion do when you are occupied in the kitchen?" or using inferences or interpretations, for example, "This must have reminded you of your own hospitalization as a young girl" (Hopkinson, Cox, & Rutter, 1981). Such indirect emphasizing remarks are probably helpful because they suggest to parents that they have been understood, that the interviewer empathizes with their sentiments and can, therefore, be trusted.

Case Vignette 1
Marty, the oldest child of a Northern Aboriginal family, had been a healthy 13-month-

old boy until six days earlier when he had been admitted to a major pediatric teaching hospital's intensive care unit (ICU) after a 12-hour history of excessive vomiting which led to increasingly labored respiration. This began while his parents were traveling with him in a pickup truck from a northern village to a major city where his father was going to start a university-based training program. The child's cardiovascular functions seemed so precarious on admission that the question was posed whether he needed an immediate heart transplant or whether the illness was more systemic and required lengthy medical intervention. As it was recognized that these events had been very hard on Marty's family, a psychiatric consultation was requested.

At the time of the interview, Marty had been in the ICU for seven days and was totally anaesthetized to support his fragile respiratory and cardiac functions. In addition to his parents, a total of ten relatives had flown from his northern village to attend to him. Most of the relatives only spoke their native language, and two of them could often be found sitting at the foot of Marty's bed, silently looking up at the ceiling and speaking to no one. The medical team was unsure about how to deal with the family whom they perceived as matriarchically organized.

The infant psychiatrist initially read all the medical and nursing notes and spoke to various nurses and physicians about the baby. He also contacted a social worker who had already been involved with the family and spent some time watching the baby with his seemingly innumerable tubes and respirator-driven breathing patterns. He then met with the baby's parents and inquired about their perceptions of Marty's illness and their own past experiences with illness and hospitalization. Among other things, he

discovered that a 20-year-old paternal uncle had shot himself nine months ago after his girlfriend had died in a local house fire. He also learned that one maternal uncle had suddenly developed a "black throat," necessitating a helicopter transfer to a nearby hospital. However, the uncle had suffocated and died before the helicopter landed at the hospital. Another uncle had died as a three-year-old child of the complications of congenital heart disease. Finally, the father mentioned that he was wondering whether he might have inadvertently poisoned Marty by overlooking the possible leak of exhaust fumes from the truck into the cabin during their trip to the city.

This vignette touches on some of the special issues which can confront a clinician dealing with ill infants in the beginning of the assessment process. In the present case, cultural traditions had to be respected and taken into account, in particular when assessing the parents' feelings about the totally unexpected severe illness of their infant. We were also interested to learn how the family understood and managed the flood of questions which were directed at them by the medical specialists. Finally, it was unclear to what extent the unsettling fact of an unknown diagnosis and consequently uncertain prognosis for baby Marty was understood by his parents.

In more general terms, there has been some concern about the extent to which the retrospective nature of parents' reports on their childhood family environment is reliable and, therefore, valid. This can be a serious problem in a clinical interview which deals with both objective and subjective judgments about the parents' own past relationships. As parents early experiences are felt to be vital for understanding the transactional themes which determine the present child-parent relationship, the clinician needs to be aware of the possible limitations of the clinical interview as a means of obtaining valid information (Lyons-Ruth, Zoll, Connell, & Grunebaum, 1989).

On the other hand, work by Robins and her group (1985) indicates a 70 percent agreement on all factual background questions when two siblings were asked about them and a reported agreement ranging from 77 to 91 percent between childhood clinic records and adult responses regarding the family's stability. This suggests that the childhood events and feelings presented by parents of preschool children are reported with some accuracy. Furthermore, dynamic theory suggests that feelings and sentiments expressed by parents about their own upbringing are of relevance for their relationship with their child even if they cannot be fully confirmed as accurate (van IJzendoorn, 1985).

Vignette 1, Part 2
There were two additional issues which were of concern to the clinician. Marty's mother, age 20, was seven months pregnant and had never been away from the village in which she was born. Her English was also poorer than her husband's and made her dependent on his translation.

On the positive side, the father touched his wife during the interview on a number of occasions, something rarely found among these Northern people. There also seemed to be no violence between the couple, and both still had parents who lived with each other although some of their siblings had problems with alcohol or even committed

suicide. The parents were also obviously intelligent, the father having been chosen to pursue a university education.

Finally, in the five days of the infant's hospitalization, eight relatives of all ages had come to join Marty's parents, indicating substantial family support. The question remained, however, how we would explain the present status of this infant to the parents without destroying their sense of mastery and control over their infant's growth and development.

The content of the clinical interview of families with a medically compromised infant should be made up of factual information, encompassing data on the child (reason for referral, history of current difficulties) and the family (family history, including characteristics of other important caretakers such as grandparents, baby-sitters, or day care personnel). In this special population, the clinician should also gather information about the parents' own medical histories and their reactions to possible illness and injuries. This can be combined with an assessment of their past and present relationships with their own parents and important role models, their own parents' warmth and understanding of them, the type of punishment used in their homes, and possible family conflicts. Finally, the child's development should be assessed here. In this context, the medical history of the infant needs to be examined in detail. For example, note should be taken of the frequency and length of past hospitalizations, as well as the child's experience with painful procedures and reactions to them.

Vignette 1, Part 3

The concern expressed by Marty's father that he may have inadvertently poisoned his son during his long trip to the city and the presence of the relatives in the hospital provided an opportunity to have a meeting with all the members of the extended family and attempt to clarify Marty's medical problems in some detail. The psychiatrist first asked the group to select an interpreter and then slowly presented the facts about Marty's illness as they were known. He mentioned that a screen for any toxic substances in Marty's blood had found no evidence of any poison and then proceeded to explain the cardiovascular problems using the potential changes to a northern river, with which they were all familiar, in response to different types of pollution as an example for the possible etiology of Marty's cardiac failure. The group listened attentively although some continued looking at a magazine or even reading a book. At the end there were two questions, and then Marty's grandfather officially pronounced that he could see how we doctors had already begun to clean up some of the pollution and that they could now go home and tell the others about how brave and strong Marty was down in the big city.

The Clinical Assessment of the Child

This part of the assessment deals with the developmental status of the infant or toddler. Since medical conditions such as poorly controlled seizures of prematurity can be directly associated with developmental delays, the clinical assessment of the child is an important component of a comprehensive evaluation. Furthermore, medical illnesses in young children often affect their parents and cause them to de-velop inappropriate parenting strategies which, in turn, may lead to developmental abnormalities in the child. The models here are the Vulnerable Child Syndrome (Green & Solnit, 1964), discussed earlier, and transactional disturbances caused by other changes in the mother-child relationship, initially described by Sameroff and Chandler (1975). In short, these authors documented that there is always a dynamic interaction or transaction between a biological event (in this case an illness or handicap) and the environment (e.g., family or society). Furthermore, they showed that this interaction is dynamic, that is, the child influences the environment which, in turn, modifies the child's behavior.

This means that a developmental assessment may also highlight interactional difficulties, another reason to obtain the parents' collaborative participation. This also makes it easier for the parents to comfort and reassure their child and observe him perform the tasks given by the examiner.

The opportunity for this shared observation can be invaluable for several other reasons. To begin with, these young children are not challenged during an assessment by being separated from their familiar caretakers. Moreover, the examiner will demonstrate the strengths and/or weaknesses of the child's performance and so help the parents come to a more realistic perception of their infant's possibilities (Field, 1982). In addition, parents also witness and partake in a sensitive interchange between their youngster and another adult. Such an encounter can potentially teach them other ways to interact with young children and possibly introduce them to strategies that may modify or at least manage particular behavioral or cognitive deviations. Shared observations also facilitate later communication of the diagnostic formulation by the clinician.

Finally, the parents' presence in this situation allows the examiner to observe the parent-child interaction. Facets of this interaction may center around the parents' ability or wish to provide emotional support to the child, their possible intrusiveness in the testing situation, or their reactions to the displays of particular behaviors of the child toward the examiner (e.g., what do they do when their child smiles more at the examiner than at them during testing). This often also allows the clinician to combine the parent-child relational assessment with an overall developmental evaluation. However, for the purpose of clarity, the assessment of the young child's developmental skills and emerging capacities and the quality of the parent-child relationship are discussed separately.

The developmental assessment includes the following components:

1. Obtaining information about the child's past development.
2. Assessing the child's behavior during the formal testing procedure and observing his coping ability.
3. Possibly observing the child in different settings, such as the office, home, or day care environment.

The clinical assessment also includes a Mental Status Examination of the child. Such an examination is outlined in detail by Anne L. Benham in the recent "Practice Parameters for the Psychiatric Assessment of Infants and Toddlers" (Thomas et al., 1997) and includes, among others, an evaluation of the child's self-regulation, motor development, speech and language, thought, play, cognition, and relatedness. This includes the child's capacity for relating and showing interest in the examiner.

In children with acute illnesses like Marty, with families who live far away or are not easily engaged in extensive evaluations, it may be necessary to conduct the clinical assessment of both parents and infant in one interview. In such a situation, it is best to concentrate on the following aspects: Reason for referral, history of the parents' difficulties, the parents' past and present relationships with their parents and other members of their own families, the parents' present relationship with each other, their view of their child's personality and temperament since birth, and their vision of his future with his illness. Finally, the clinician should assess the degree to which the parents see themselves in a position to influence their child's future development.

Standardized Assessment Measures in Infancy

As discussed earlier, an important goal of every infant mental health professional is to help medically compromised infants and toddlers to avert a seemingly adverse outcome. This is a challenging proposition since evolving competence is dependent on context, both from within and without the child, and hence often cannot be reliably predicted at an early age. One way to help the clinician understand important risks and protective factors is the development of valid assessment instruments which can both identify problems early and monitor possible changes reliably. As Cicchetti and Wagner (1990, p. 248) state, "The standard definition of assessment is the measurement of the relative position of an individual in a larger defined population with respect to some psychological construct." This means that the assessment tool must have specific psychometric properties to monitor, for example, the effects of interventions. Unfortunately, traditional tests have been of little use here since even children with the same IQ do not necessarily have the same competencies in the same cognitive domains.

Driven by humanistic concerns for children with biological and social vulnerabilities (Shonkoff & Meisels, 1990), a wide range of daily intervention programs were, nevertheless, initiated during the past three decades (e.g., Head Start, Zero-to-Three, Project Care, and so on). Evaluations of these programs have shown that: (1) there is no linear relationship between early and later competencies and (2) social and family variables must be included to predict development (Sameroff & Fiese, 1990). Consequently, the most meaningful way to assess and predict future functioning is an assessment of a child's socioemotional development within the family context.

For a detailed review of the literature in this area refer to an excellent chapter by Stack and Poulin-Dubois (1998). Following are some assessment tools that show

sound psychometric properties and assess clinically meaningful details of child functioning.

Assessment of Socioemotional Competence

As discussed previously the socioemotional development of young children takes place within the context of the parent-child relationship and the milieu and culture in which they live. During the first years of life, children learn to communicate and regulate their emotions. They also learn to distinguish and respond appropriately to the emotional signals of others (Segal, Oster, Cohen, Caspi, Myers, & Brown, 1995).

The most widely accepted measures of the quality of a mother-child relationship and its socioemotional context is the face-to-face interaction. Specifically, researchers have studied factors that can interfere with an infant's capacity to regulate its emotions or modulate its signals as well as those which may compromise the ability of caregivers to provide the baby with sensitive and appropriate responses. Tiffany Field (1987) has written about this in detail and described various coding schemes (Field et al., 1980). The important task for the clinician is to observe how sensitively the caretaker is able to respond to the baby's cues and how the baby reacts to the caretaker's signals.

This is best done by seating mother and baby at eye level with each other and watching them during a series of brief interaction periods. Thus, the mother may talk to, smile at, touch, or engage in other aspects of interactions with the baby typical for her. The baby may join in, turn away if there is too much stimulation, or initiate a cueing game with the adult. The clinician can observe how the dialogue between the partners progresses, that is, if the mother stops stimulating the infant when the infant indicates that he or she has had enough, and so on.

There is another procedure called the Still-Face procedure developed by Tronick and colleagues (1978). This is a modification of the face-to-face procedures mentioned previously and is characterized by dividing the adult-child interaction into three periods. During periods one and three, the mother or another adult is asked to interact normally with the infant, that is, they can talk or touch the baby as seems appropriate. However, during period two, the adult is asked to suddenly stop his or her interactions and present the infant with a neutral nonresponsive "Still-Face" for 60 seconds. Infants will react to this unexpected situation by smiling or increased negative affect as if to say, "Come on mom, what happened to you?" If the mother persists with her "Still-Face," the baby will often look away in the end or fall asleep. The value of this particular paradigm is in the repeatedly documented observation that infants whose mothers are generally insensitive to their socioemotional needs will quickly turn away or fall asleep when their mother presents them with a "Still-Face." These children seem to have learned already at the age of three or six months that mother is not often available to them and that turning away is the best way to cope with this.

It appears that mothers or other caretakers who are consistently insensitive to their children's emotional needs or overtures have children who adapt by developing an expectation about the world which confirms the representations of their caretakers. Thus, infants who give up trying to get mother's attention back, for example, by making specific noises, as well-cared for children tend to do, behave as if they had learned already to expect little from their caretakers and try to contain their disappointment by looking away or falling asleep (Cohn, Campbell, & Ross, 1991).

Other measures which provide coding systems to evaluate the parent-child relationship during semistructured play are the Greenspan-Lieberman Observation System (GLOS; Greenspan & Lieberman, 1989) and the Emotional Availability Scales (EAS) developed by Biringen, Robinson, and Emde (1988).

A somewhat different paradigm for assessing children's socioemotional development is the "Strange Situation" developed by Aimsworth and her colleagues (1978). This test situation evaluates the caregiver-infant quality of attachment in a laboratory situation. It is, however, not a suitable test for clinicians as it requires a specially equipped laboratory and two assistants. Nevertheless, the differentiation between a secure and insecure attachment in children, that has resulted from the work of these authors as well as the work by Main and her colleagues (1985), can be a very useful guide for the practicing clinician, since it can be explored in clinical situations. For example, one can observe how a parent consoles a toddler who has hurt himself accidentally. If the mother responds to such an incident by telling the boy that he "should be more careful next time" and does so without picking him up or soothing him at the same time, it shows a lack of demonstrative understanding of his pain and discomfort. This may well indicate an overall pattern of "dismissive behavior" as defined by attachment theorists, that is, representing an interactive style where emotional issues are not taken seriously. Attachment patterns can also be evaluated by asking some specific questions. For example, while obtaining a developmental history from the parent one can ask how John or Mary used to accept being left for brief periods when they were 12 or 18 months old, that is, whether the parents were ever able to go to a movie or eat a meal outside the house. If this was impossible for them because of their ongoing concern for their baby, one might consider them to have an "overinvolved" or "enmeshed" relationship with their infant. This suggests that these parents have difficulties allowing their chronically ill child to individuate and are, thus, possibly compromising his developmental potential.

There are other assessment measures which try to conceptualize the caregiver-infant relationship in protocol-driven form. Roseanne Clark (1985) at the University of Wisconsin Medical School has developed the Parent-Child Early Relational Assessment (PCERA). Her paradigm asks parents to play with their children, have a snack with them, and then to get them to clean up the toys at the end of the session. Well-operationalized codes for distinct interactional variables are used to score these interactions. The PCERA has been used in intervention studies with toddlers (e.g., Minde et al., 1994), but requires a video camera and a specially equipped laboratory to provide valid data. Nevertheless, the categories used in assessing the parent-child interaction from the video screen can be helpful guides for the practicing clinician. Crowell and Feldman (1988) have also developed an assessment procedure which can be used with children ages 24–54 months. The procedure involves nine separate episodes of varying lengths of time designed to elicit behaviors indicative of different types of infant-caregiver relationships (e.g., free play, cleanup, bubble game, four teaching tasks, and a separation and reunion episode). It can be helpful in isolating various dimensions of the interactions of a dyad, and there are data which show a good correlation between the ratings on the Crowell procedure and specific attachment categories (Crowell & Feldman, 1991). One important advantage of Crowell's methodology is the comparative ease with which the interview can be scored.

Another way to investigate the caretaker-child relationship is by probing parental perception and attributions of their infant. Zeanah and Benoit (1995) have developed a semistructured interview, called the Working Model of the Child Interview (WMCI), to systematically examine and characterize this component of the relationship. The interview takes approximately one hour and should be videotaped for later review. The interviewer poses specific questions to the caregiver, that is, inquires about the child's personality, how the child is like or unlike his parents, and what the caretaker's anticipations are about the child's future development. The caregiver is also asked to select five adjectives which best describe the characteristics of the child. The interview is transcribed and coded following a specific coding scheme, allowing the parent-child relationship to be classified as balanced, disengaged, or distorted. The WMCI can be given during the later part of pregnancy and up to age 24 months. It has a high stability over time (89 percent for the balanced and 85 percent for the distorted category between pregnancy and 12 months of age) and also has a high concordance with Aimsworth's Strange Situation (overall match of 74 percent) (Benoit, Parker, & Zeanah, 1997). However, the scoring of the WMCI requires special training although the narrative of the interview can be clinically meaningful even for the untrained clinician.

Two easy paper and pencil tests which are useful in the assessment of medically compromised children are the Child Vulnerability Scale (Forsyth et al., 1996) and the Parent Protection Scale (Thomasgard et al., 1995) discussed in a previous section. Both questionnaires are brief, have good psychometric properties, and are scored using a four-step scale from 0 to 3 (see Tables 3.1 and 3.2). Some items are reverse coded (e.g., items 5, 6, 10, 14, 16, and 19 on the Parent Protection Scale). Both scales identify caretakers whose perceptions have been affected by the illness of their children and who as a consequence tend to model an unrealistic future to them. However, these scales should not be used in children under the age of two because they have not been validated in younger infants.

Finally, there may also be some value in obtaining an accurate assessment of an infant's temperament. Based on the pioneering work of Thomas, Chess, and Birch (1968), Fullard, McDevitt, and Carey (1984), and Simeonsson (1986) have developed reliable ways to label children either as "difficult," "easy," or "slow to warm up" (see Table 3.3).

What is important here is that some long-term studies found that temperament predicts later personality to some degree (Caspi & Silva, 1995) and membership in certain temperamental categories (such as "high withdrawal" and "slow adaptation") tends to be associated with certain affects and activity patterns later on, as in the description of the "inhibited child" by Kagan (1994). The scales developed by Fullard and Simeonsson are easy for caregivers to fill in and can be scored without specific training.

It should be recognized, however, that there is no evidence that children with acute or chronic medical illnesses are characterized by specific temperamental patterns. Nevertheless, I know that infants labeled as "difficult" tend to have more sleep problems and other behavior difficulties (Minde et al., 1993), especially if in addition they show an insecure attachment pattern. It is self-evident that the management of such infants will be even more difficult if parents also have to deal with an acute or chronic medical disorder. Table 3.4 provides a summary of standardized assessment measures in infancy which provide key references and an indication whether special training is

TABLE 3.3

Diagnostic Clusters of Temperament Traits

	High activity	Arrythmic	Withdrawal	Slow adaptation	Intense	Negative mood	Low persistence	Low distractibility	Low threshold
6		Difficult	Slow to warm up / Difficult	Slow to warm up / Difficult		Slow to warm up / Difficult			
5		Difficult			Difficult				
4									
3		Easy	Easy	Easy	Easy	Easy			
2	Slow to warm up				Slow to warm up				
1									
	Low activity	Rhythmic	Approach	Very adaptive	Mild	Positive mood	High persistence	High distractibility	High threshold

Source: Simeonsson, R. J. (1986). *Psychological and developmental assessment of special children*. Boston: Allyn & Bacon. Reprinted by permission.

TABLE 3.4
Standardized Assessment Measures

	Special Training	
Socioemotional Competence		
1. Still-Face Procedure	yes	Tronick et al., 1978 Cohen et al., 1991
2. Greenspan-Lieberman Observation System (GLOS)	yes	Greenspan & Lieberman, 1989
3. Emotional Availability Scales	yes	Biringen et al., 1988
4. Clinical Problem Solving Procedure	no	Crowell & Feldman, 1988 Crowell & Feldman, 1991
Parent-Child Relationship		
1. Parent-Child Early Relationship Assessment (PCERA)	yes	Clark, 1985 Minde et al., 1994
2. Child Vulnerability Scale	no	Forsyth et al., 1996
3. Parent Protection Scale	no	Thomas et al., 1995
4. Working Model of the Child Interview (WMCI)	yes	Zeanah & Benoit, 1995
Child Temperament		
1. Infant Temperament	no	Fullard et al., 1984
2. Infant and Toddler Temperament	no	Simeonsson, 1986

needed for the administration or scoring of the testing question.

Vignette 2

Genevieve B was seven months old when she was referred by her pediatrician for a consultation with an infant psychiatrist. The little girl had developed eczema on her arms and legs during the past three months causing much discomfort for her and anxiety for her parents, Martine and Pierre. Both of them had suffered from asthma since childhood, and while Pierre was much improved since graduation from college, Martine still used her puffer several times per week and had been on steroid medication for extensive periods during her life. The couple's older son George, age 6, had developed asthma at 24 months and was currently moderately affected. However, he had experienced four hospital admissions during the past three years for severe asthma attacks.

The main reason for the referral to the psychiatrist was the pediatrician's feeling that the B family seemed to handle Genevieve quite poorly. In particular, they did not seem to know when to give in to her demands for attention and how to contain her often angry demands for more holding, carrying around, and individual playtime with her mother. There were also conflicts between the parents about how to stop the girl from scratching the exposed parts of her eczema. This scratching or itching also affected her sleep, causing her to cry a lot and wake up her parents who tried to soothe their baby by moving her back and forth between their bed and her own crib, without much success. As a result, everybody's sleep was regularly disturbed.

The assessment consisted of an interview with both parents and a mother-child play session. During the session, the mother was extraordinarily solicitous toward Genevieve's apparent wishes. Any slight indication the girl made to play with a particular toy would be met by an overenthusiastic response by the mother. However, she would often quickly try to interest her infant in another toy or game, leaving no time for the development of a joyful reciprocal interchange between the two partners. In fact, two of the three play episodes ended in Genevieve crying and mother trying to soothe her in exasperation.

Treatment consisted of six sessions during which the mother and Genevieve came to play with a limited number of toys. The mother initially was instructed to let Genevieve lead the play and avoid suggesting novel activities to her for a 10-minute period. The girl was observed during the following months to become increasingly more imaginative in her play. She also looked more at her mother and developed longer play actions but still put great demands on her mother. The mother then was encouraged to set limits on Genevieve's most extreme demands (e.g., her wish to be in her lap at all times) in a calm fashion and was also asked to allow Genevieve to fall asleep in her own bed at night. The latter task was taken over by the father as the mother did not feel strong enough to carry it out. However, six weeks later Genevieve cried less, slept in her bed all night, and also scratched herself far less. Both parents then asked to come one more time to talk about their son George and learn how they might change their management of his asthma attacks.

This vignette shows the challenges temperamentally difficult children with a chronic medical condition can present to their families. The vignette also shows how rudimentary our tools for an empirically based socioemotional assessment are and how much all of us have to rely on our clinical expertise in developing intervention strategies. As far as the case of Genevieve is concerned, however, we know from the work of Mrazek and his group (1991) that an overinvolved parent-child relationship, observed within one month of the infant's birth, can predict the development of asthma if the child has the genetic predisposition for this illness. More importantly, Mrazek more recently documented that family-based interventions at that time can prevent the development of the clinical picture of asthma at least up to age four (Mrazek et al., 1998). The rationale seems to be that helping the parents modulate the children's affect and overall state control more effectively will give their children more control over their respiratory physiology.

In summary, there are few tools to reliably measure the socioemotional development of young children with medical problems. This necessarily compromises the ability to assess intervention programs for this population. Moreover, it will never be sufficient to merely evaluate the child since the difficulties may be related to the relationship the child has with his or her parents or to other physical stressors such as the physical pain he or she has experienced during the past few months. Therefore, guard against overvaluing "objective" measure paradigms and recognize the immense importance the setting (such as a hospital) and the parent-child relationship have on a child's behavior.

The Parent-Child Relational Assessment

The quality of the parent-child interaction is a critical factor in a young child's developmental functioning and, therefore, needs to be carefully assessed. Furthermore, directly observable interactive behaviors often reflect the presence and type of parental subjective experiences that may affect the child's overall development either positively or negatively. This means that the clinician should try to distinguish an observed interaction between a parent and a child that occurs only within a specific context (i.e., is a true interaction) from one that reflects a more persistent underlying parental attribution (i.e., a marker of the overall relationship between the parent-child dyad). Relationships tend to be less open to change and behaviors reflecting them are usually fairly enduring and consistent. Such behaviors are also often based on intergenerational continuities (Fonagy, Steele, & Steele, 1991).

How Can the Clinician Best Learn about the Parent-Child Relationship?

The setting where the interview takes place is of primary importance. While a medical ward or even the intensive care unit may at times be the site of a meeting with an infant and his family, it is useful to have a small room available that contains a few appropriate toys and is carpeted so that both adults and children can sit or move on the floor. Here the clinician can invite the parents to play or interact with the child as they see fit and observe the ensuing interactions for 15 to 25 minutes. Even if the initial meeting with the family takes place at the infant's bedside, it is advisable to conduct the formal intake assessment of the parents within the professional's office, away from the clinical ward. This will provide a "safe space" for the family members where they can share their thoughts and feelings in privacy and comparative comfort.

If the child is able to join the family for the parent-child relational assessment in the clinician's office, it may be useful to videotape the interactions. Such a videotape can then be used as a stimulus for later discussions and may open the door for treating possible infant-caregiver relationship disturbances (McDonough, 1993).

What Parameters Best Capture the Relationship between Parents and Their Medically Compromised Children?

Among the many parameters that can help the clinician in structuring his observations the six domains of functioning suggested by Emde (1989) appear the most relevant and inclusive. They are:

1. Attachment, including those aspects of behavior that deal with the child's and

caretaker's emotional or physical closeness and/or availability to each other, their ability to separate from each other, and/or the caretaker's support of the child's overall individuation.

2. Play, its style and symbolism.
3. Teaching and learning.
4. Vigilance and protection, reflecting behaviors of the caretakers that assure the physical safety of the child.
5. Power, control, and discipline.
6. Regulation of emotion or affect, including the expression and communication of emotion.

While the first three domains are equally relevant for physically healthy and ill children, the last three are especially meaningful for the medically ill youngster. For example, vigilance and protection of a handicapped child may have to be much more thoughtfully balanced because of the need such toddlers have to gain a developmentally appropriate sense of independence and autonomy. In assessing this aspect of the parent-child relationship one usually observes whether the parents appropriately intervene when the child gets into potential trouble. However, it is equally important to observe whether the toddler shows either excessive caution or undue recklessness in dealing with toys and equipment. Parents of medically ill children may be either overly anxious about their child's safety or careless and lacking in awareness as if to deny the special needs of this child.

Power, control, and discipline refer to the parents' regulation of their own and their children's behavior. The strategies parents use to control their children have long been seen as important predictors of the children's later social and intellectual competence (Maccoby & Martin, 1983). In addition, developmental researchers have identified a number of clearly demarcated styles of discipline which lead to a differential patterns of competence and adjustment in later life (Steinberg, Mounts, Lamborn, & Dornbush, 1991). In particular, there is now a professional consensus that parents can obtain control by imposing hostile, rejecting, authoritarian, harsh discipline using an authoritative parenting style, or using a generally permissive style. A harsh authoritarian type of discipline does not easily allow children to express their thoughts and feelings. As a result, in early childhood, such children may become passively hostile and, later, become aggressive adults. Children who are raised in a permissive fashion tend to be sensitive and caring later on, but are likely to have difficulties in organizing and disciplining themselves. For example, they may underachieve academically. In contrast, children who have grown up in families with an authoritative discipline style, that is characterized by clearly presented parental expectations, coupled with warmth and support, will do well academically and show sophisticated social skills (Steinberg et al., 1991).

Parents display these interactive patterns early in their children's life by the way they present themselves to the infant (e.g., as calm and in control vs. passive, overwhelmed, or tense and angry) and how they deal with routine parenting challenges. For example, a child who refuses to clean up at the end of a play session may demonstrate a caregiver's overall discipline style.

Here again, a medical illness often potentiates a parent's discipline patterns because many of these children do not find it easy to provide their parents with the feedback which may help them reassess their own control behavior. This may be due to the children's difficulties in expressing themselves (if they have neurological or other disorders affecting their cognition), their difficulties in modulating their behavior (causing them to be considered poor judges of their parents' behavior), or their lack of self-esteem and autonomy due to their excessive dependence on others. The latter difficulty often prevents them from even conceptualizing the inappropriateness of their parents' style of behavior control.

The regulation of emotion is a crucial area of relationship functioning, since the emotion or affect experienced in any interaction will determine its later psychological significance within the child's relationships. Early in life, children have limited self-regulatory capacities. Hence, the parents' ability to help them to organize their behavior at that time provides an important experience of tension release and some degree of mastery over their world. Responsive parents will facilitate their children's self-regulation by learning about their individual characteristics and building on their biological strengths to aid them in achieving a more harmonious way of relating to others.

Parents may find it more difficult to modulate the behavior of medically compromised children because their behavior is often harder to read (e.g., in premature infants) or their emotions are more difficult to regulate because of subtle Central Nervous System abnormalities. For those who communicate less well, the parents' task of soothing and regulating the infant's behavior may be more difficult but also more important for the infant's future development. In clinically assessing a regulatory pattern, it is useful to differentiate between caregivers who respond inappropriately because they do not see or experience the need of the child and those who perceive these needs but cannot act because of personal problems or limitations (e.g., depression or overwork). Some parents may also show a transient inability to perceive and/or respond to their children's needs because of fatigue or other environmental stressors. Others may follow cultural traditions in which emotions are shown in ways that are unfamiliar to most of us. Finally, it is important to recognize that the behavior of young children with the same person can vary and depend on the overall context. Thus, John may behave very differently toward his mother in the presence of his father or the clinician than in their absence.

Vignette 1, Part 4

As previously reported, baby Marty had been put on a respirator after his admission to the ICU and was fully anesthetized to minimize the demands on his heart. While he was on this regime, both his parents visited daily for one hour, sitting silently by his bed, often watching television. Two weeks later, Marty's sedation was gradually decreased and five days later the infant was awake for three hours per day. One week later, Marty was awake approximately eight hours per day, and his behavior changed dramatically. He now responded to the arrival of his parents with a huge smile and would spend much time during their visits touching their hands and drawing them into his games by pointing to specific objects and even taking a parent's hand to help him get a special toy. Marty also developed distinct preferences for special toys which were now kept in a special yellow bucket. He also insisted on watching "Barney" each day as he had done at home. He would cry profusely when his parents left in the evening but could be easily soothed by his two key nurses.

His parents, in turn, developed a personal interaction routine during their three-hour daily visits. One parent would sit next to Marty's bed and hold his hand or watch television with him while the other parent sat on a chair behind the television, peeking at the boy only once in a while. Every 15 to 20 minutes, the parents would exchange places and take on the other's respective role. They both rarely talked to Marty directly although there was a constant smile, especially on the father's face when he had his turn with him. Marty did not seem to mind the lack of conversation with his parents but instead repeatedly showed them his favorite toys and play activities.

The ICU staff was delighted with Marty's progress as he "seemed to have been resurrected from the dead" (there was still no definite diagnosis). The psychiatrist in turn was delighted with the boy's strong attachment behaviors. They had obviously survived his 3½-week anesthesia and also suggested good cerebral functioning. This was especially gratifying as the parents showed none of the exuberance or direct emotional responsiveness seen in securely attached dyads, demonstrating the power which an attentive though comparatively silent presence of the caretaker can have on such a sick child's attachment patterns.

Assessment of Parenting Skills

Much of the information obtained during the assessment process described in the previous sections of this chapter relates to the primary caretakers' ability to meet the young child's developmental needs. Yet, the overall assessment of this ability remains a difficult task. It ranges from providing basic shelter, food, and warmth to recognizing that John and Mary are not merely small adults but developing individuals. Further complexities in measuring parenting abilities arise because mother's care may be "good enough" to use a phrase by Winnicott (1960) during the first six months of a child's life because she enjoys the seemingly unlimited giving of comfort to the young infant. However, this same mother may resent the infant's increasing demands for separation and individuation later.

Children are also differently equipped to cope with a marginal environment. Some may "make do," while others wither helplessly. The phenomenon of discontinuity in development can also work for or against a given child. For example, by becoming mobile and acquiring language, an older toddler may find substitute sources of stimulation and aids to cognitive growth that were not accessible to him before (Minde & Minde, 1986). It is in this area that a medical condition can significantly change the developmental trajectory of a child since being blind or motorically handicapped may not allow this toddler to actively contribute to the modification of his environment.

A child with a medical condition may also require special handling techniques which are not usually part of a mother's repertoire of caretaking practices. Here a failure to provide developmentally appropriate caretaking may reflect the parents' ignorance of the "right way" of handling their child rather than particular psychological or psychosocial limitations. For example, early on, prematurely born children usually need a more directive handling style as they often have difficulties in overall CNS organization (Minde, Marton, Manning, & Hines, 1980). Such a situation may present a purely interactive difficulty and not a relationship problem.

What then should you look for in parents of young children whose parenting competence you seek to assess? I suggest that parents be rated on five general and relatively stable dimensions that contribute to their interpersonal interactions regardless of the child's developmental stage (Minde & Minde, 1986). These are:

1. General emotional and physical health
2. Self-esteem
3. General coping and adaptation skills
4. Child rearing attitudes
5. Willingness and/or ability to provide developmental encouragement

Assessment of the parents' past and present emotional and physical health may be helped by using a standardized assessment device such as the SCL90–R Checklist (Derogatis, 1987). This scale is a useful tool in assessing physical and mental stages of parental anxiety, depression, and other abnormal thought processes.

Self-esteem can best be estimated from incidental statements of the parents. For example, mother may say, "Michael never listens to me nor does anyone else in the family." Father may remark, "Marilyn does not want to walk at all anymore. Obviously have not been successful in making her want to try." Both of these statements may be a reflection of low self-esteem and should alert the clinician to search for other signs of self-deprecation.

General coping and adaptation skills can be assessed by inquiring how previous stresses have been managed. When asked directly, parents will often report such data quite accurately. It should, nevertheless, be remembered that there are many ways of coping with difficulties, ranging from complete denial to active working through. The final rating of coping skills will be based on the effectiveness of these strategies rather than on the type of defense or coping mechanism used.

Authoritarian or democratic attitudes toward parenting can be assessed by evaluating the decision-making process in a family. This can be done by asking how other children in the family behave and are managed. If there is a history of placement of a sibling or of family conflicts with other children, one may want to explore how, by whom, and about what are decisions made in a family and how they are accepted by the children. As was discussed previously, families may function in a primarily authoritarian or indulgent way. However, few families subscribe totally to one mode of disciplining. It is also important to establish how well a specific interaction pattern seems to work. For example, in the interaction between handicapped and developmentally delayed children and their caregivers, more directive management patterns are likely to be found (Kogan, 1980; Minde et al., 1980). Moreover, it appears that for such children, more direct guidance and a less democratic management style may be developmentally appropriate.

The willingness of parents to provide developmental encouragement does not refer only to their ability to "stimulate" an infant. In fact, parents who are withdrawn and unavailable to their children can also be intrusive and hyperstimulating or can shift between the two modalities. Both extremes tend to be maladaptive and may undermine the expression of the child's present and expected capacities.

In addition to these general ratings, it useful to inquire about the routines of an average day of a young child and his family. This can provide the examiner with a sense of the stresses the family faces and simultaneously afford the possibility of assessing the family's support system and child rearing attitudes. Also make note of the caretakers' response to the clinicians as professionals or people, noting their predominant mood and thinking style. Such observations can help to predict the caregiver's readiness and/or ability to engage in a therapeutic relationship and may forecast the likelihood that the parent-child relationship can be influenced.

Conclusion

In this chapter, the impact illness early on in life can have on later behavior and development has been examined and ways have been outlined that permit a mental health professional to assess the psychosocial functioning of medically compromised infants and toddlers and their families.

The assessment strategies have been based on empirical evidence as far as it is available but recognize that much of our day-to-day work in this area is still based on clinical intuition and experience. Nevertheless, there is a rapidly increasing scientific literature emerging from the field which makes the assessment and treatment of medically compromised high-risk infants an ever more exciting and rewarding part of clinical activities.

References

Achenbach, T. M. (1991). *Manual for the child behavior checklist and revised child behavior profile.* Burlington: University of Vermont, Department of Psychiatry.

Ainsworth, M. H., Blehar, M. C., Waters, E., & Wall, S. (1978). *Patterns of attachment: A psychological study of the strange situation.* Hillsdale, NJ: Erlbaum.

Benoit, D., Parker, K. C. H., & Zeanah, C. H. (1997). Mothers' representations of their infants assessed prenatally: Stability and association with infants attachment classifications. *Journal of Child Psychology and Psychiatry, 3,* 307–313.

Berger, E. (1977). Parental overprotection and rejection: Implications for the epileptic child. *Maryland Medical Journal, 26,* 63–67.

Bertenthal, B. I., & Campos, J. J. (1990). A system approach to the organizing effect of self-produced locomotion during infancy. In C. Rovee-Collier & L. P. Lipsitt

(Eds.), *Advance in infancy research* (Vol. 6, pp. 1–60). Norwood NJ: Ablex.

Biringen, Z., Robinson, J. L., & Emde, R. N. (1988). *The emotional availability scales.* Unpublished manuscript, University of Colorado Sciences Center, Denver.

Brazelton, T. B., & Cramer, B. G. (1990). *The earliest relationship.* Reading, MA: Addison-Wesley.

Cadman, D., Boyle, M., Szatmari, P., & Offord, D. R. (1987). Chronic illness, disability, and mental and social well being: Findings of the Ontario Child Health Study. *Pediatrics, 79,* 805–813.

Caspi, A., & Silva, P. A. (1995). Temperamental qualities at age three predict personality traits in young adulthood: Longitudinal evidence from a birth cohort. *Child Development, 66,* 486–498.

Cicchetti, D., & Wagner, S. (1990). Alternative assessment strategies for the evaluation of infants and toddlers: An organizational perspective. In S. J. Meisels & J. P. Shonkoff (Eds.), *Handbook of early childhood intervention.* New York: Cambridge University Press.

Clark, R. (1985). *The parent-child early relational assessment.* Unpublished manuscript, University of Wisconsin Medical School, Madison, Department of Psychiatry.

Cohn, J. F., Campbell, S. B., & Ross, S. (1991). Infant response to the still-face paradigm at 6 months predicts avoidant and secure attachment at 12 months. *Development and Psychopathology, 3,* 367–376.

Committee on Children with Disabilities and Committee on Psychosocial Aspects of Child and Family Health. (1993). Psychosocial risks of chronic health conditions in childhood and adolescence. *Pediatrics, 92,* 876–878.

Corter, C., & Minde, K. (1987). The impact of infant prematurity on family systems. In M. Wolraich & D. Routh (Eds.), *Advances in developmental and behavioural pediatrics* (Vol. 8, pp. 1–48). Greenwich, CT: JAI Press.

Cox, A., Hopkinson K., & Rutter, M. (1981). Psychiatric interviewing techniques II. Naturalistic study: Eliciting factual information. *British Journal of Psychiatry, 138,* 283–291.

Crowell, J., & Feldman, S. (1988). The effects of mothers' internal working models of relationships and children's behavioral and developmental status on mother-child interaction. *Child Development, 59,* 1273–1285.

Crowell, J., & Feldman, S. (1991). Mother's working models of attachment relationships and mother and child behavior during separation and reunion. *Developmental Psychology, 27,* 597–605.

Derogatis, L. (1987). *SCL–90–R: Administration, scoring and procedures.* Baltimore: Clinical Psychometric Research.

Emde, R. N. (1989). The infant's relationship experience: Developmental and affective aspects. In A. J. Sameroff & R. N. Emde (Eds.), *Relationship disturbances in early childhood* (pp. 33–51). New York: Basic Books.

Emde, R. N., Gaensbauer, T. G., & Harmon, R. J. (Eds.). (1996). Emotional expression in infancy: A biobehavioral study. *Psychological Issues Monograph series, 10* (37).

Field, T. (1982). Interactions of preterm and term infants with their lower-and middle-class teenage and adult mothers. In T. Field, S. Goldberg, D. Stern & A. Sostek (Eds.), *High-risk infants and children: Adults and peer interactions* (pp. 113–132). New York: Academic Press.

Field, T. (1987). Affective and interactive disturbances in infants. In J. D. Osofsky (Ed.), *Handbook of infant development* (pp. 972–1005). New York: Wiley.

Fischer-Fay, A., Goldberg, S., Simmons, R. J., & Levison, H. (1988). Chronic illness and infant-mother attachment. *Journal of Developmental and Behavioral Pediatrics, 9,* 266–270.

Fonagy, P., Steele, H., & Steele, M. (1991). Maternal representations of attachment during pregnancy predict the organization of infant-mother attachment at one year of age. *Child Development, 62,* 891–905.

Forsyth, B. W. C., & Canny, P. F. (1991). Perceptions of vulnerability 3½ years after problems of feeding and crying behavior in early infancy. *Pediatrics, 88,* 757–763.

Forsyth, B. W. C., McCue, S., Horwitz, S., Leventhal, J. M., & Burger, J. (1996). The child vulnerability scale: An instrument to measure parental perceptions of child vulnerability. *Journal of Pediatric Psychology, 21,* 89–101.

Fullard, W., McDevitt, S., & Carey, W. B. (1984). Assessing temperament in one- to three-year-old children. *Journal of Pediatric Psychology, 9,* 205–217.

Goldberg, S., Fischer-Fay, A., Simmons, R. J., Fowler, R. S., & Levison, H. (1989, April). *Effects of chronic illness on infant mother attachment.* Paper presented at the Society for Research in Child Development, Kansas City, MO.

Goldberg, S., Morris, P., Simmons, R. J., Fowler, R. S., & Levison, H. (1990). Chronic illness in infancy and parenting stress: A comparison of three groups of parents. *Journal of Pediatric Psychology, 15,* 347–358.

Gortmaker, S. L., Walker, D. K., Weitzman, M., & Sobol, A. M. (1990). Chronic conditions, socioeconomic risks, and behavioral problems in children and adolescents. *Pediatrics, 85,* 267–276.

Green, M., & Solnit, A. J. (1964). Reactions to the threatened loss of a child: A vulnerable child syndrome. *Pediatrics, 34,* 58–66.

Greenspan, S., & Lieberman, A. F. (1989). Infants, mothers and their interaction: A quantitative clinical approach to developmental assessment. In S. I. Greenspan & G. H. Pollock (Eds.), *The course of life: Vol. 1. Infancy* (pp. 503–560). Madison, CT: International Universities Press.

Greenspan, S. I. (1991). *Psychopathology and adaptation in infancy and early childhood: Principles of clinical diagnosis and preventive intervention.* New York: International Universities Press.

Hirshberg, L. M. (1993). Clinical interviews with infants and their families. In C. H. Zeanah (Ed.), *Handbook of infant mental health* (pp. 173–190). New York: Guilford.

Hopkinson, K., Cox, A., & Rutter, M. (1981). Psychiatric interviewing techniques III. Naturalistic study: Eliciting feelings. *British Journal of Psychiatry, 138,* 406–415.

Ireys, H. T., & Silver, E. J. (1996). Perception of the impact of a child's chronic illness: Does it predict maternal mental health? *Journal of Developmental and Behavioral Pediatrics, 17,* 77–83.

Johnson, E., Silver, E., Stein, R. E. K., & Dadds, M. R. (1996). Moderating effects of family structure on the relationship between physical and mental health in urban children with chronic illness. *Journal of Pediatric Psychology, 21,* 43–56.

Kagan, J. (1994). *Galen's prophecy: Temperament in human nature.* New York: Basic Books.

Kogan, K. L. (1980). Interaction systems between preschool handicapped or developmentally delayed children and their parents. In T. Field (Ed.), *High-risk infants* and children: Adult and peer interaction (pp. 227–247). New York: Academic.

LaGreca, A. M. (1994). Editorial: Assessment in pediatric psychology: What's a researcher to do? *Journal of Pediatric Psychology, 19,* 283–290.

Lavigne, J. V., & Faier-Routman, J. (1992). Psychological adjustment to pediatric physical disorders: A meta-analytic review. *Journal of Pediatric Psychology, 17,* 133–157.

Levy, J. (1980). Vulnerable children: Parents' perspectives and the use of medical care. *Pediatrics, 65,* 956–963.

Lieberman, A. F., & Slade, A. (1997). The first year of life. In J. D. Noshpitz (Ed.), *Handbook of child and adolescent psychiatry* (Vol. 1, pp. 3–11). New York: Wiley.

Lyons-Ruth, K., Zoll, D., Connell, D., & Grunebaum, H. (1989). Family deviance and family disruption in childhood: Associations with maternal behavior and infant maltreatment during the first two years of life. *Development and Psychopathology, 1,* 219–236.

Maccoby, E., & Martin, J. (1983). Socialization in the context of the family: Parent-child interaction. In E. M. Hetherington (Ed.) & P. H. Mussen (Series Ed.), *Handbook of child psychology: Vol. 4. Socialization, personality and social development* (pp. 1–101). New York: Wiley.

Main, M., Kaplan, N., & Cassidy, J. (1985). Security in infancy, childhood and adulthood: A move to the level of representation. In I. Bretherton & E. Waters (Eds.), *Growing points of attachment theory and research* (50, pp. 66–104). SRCD Monographs.

McCubbin, M. A., & McCubbin, H. I. (1988). Family systems assessment. In P. Karoly (Ed.), *Handbook of child health assessment* (pp. 227–264). New York: Wiley.

McDonough, S. (1993). Interaction guidance: Understanding and treating early infant-caregiver relationship disturbances. In C. H. Zeanah (Ed.), *Handbook of infant mental health* (pp. 414–426). New York: Guilford.

Meisels, S. J., & Fenichel, E. (Eds.). (1996). *New visions for the developmental assessment of infants and young children.* Landover, MD: Corporate Press.

Melnyk, B. M. (1995). Coping with unplanned childhood hospitalization: The mediating functions of parental beliefs. *Journal of Pediatric Psychology, 20,* 299–311.

Meyer, E. C., Garcia-Coll, C. T., Seifer, R., Ramos, A., Kilis, E., & Oh, W. (1995). Psychological distress in mothers of preterm infants. *Journal of Developmental and Behavioral Pediatrics, 16,* 412–417.

Minde, K. (1994). The social and emotional development of low-birthweight infants and their families up to age 4. In S. L. Friedman & M. D. Sigman (Eds.), *The psychological development of low birth weight children: Advances in applied developmental psychology* (pp. 157–185). Norwood, NJ: Ablex.

Minde, K., & Corter, C. (1984). The contribution of twinship and health to early interaction and attachment between premature infants and their mothers. In J. D. Call, E. Galenson, & R. L. Tyson (Eds.), *Frontiers of infant psychiatry II* (pp. 160–175). New York: Basic Books.

Minde, K., Corter, C., Goldberg, S., & Jeffers, D. (1990). Maternal preference between premature twins up to age four. *Journal of the American Academy of Child and Adolescent Psychiatry, 29,* 367–374.

Minde, K., Marton, P., Manning, D., & Hines, B. (1980). Some determinants of mother-infant interaction in the premature nursery. *Journal of the American*

Academy of Child and Adolescent Psychiatry, 19, 1–21.

Minde, K., & Minde, R. (1986). *Infant psychiatry: An introductory textbook.* Beverly Hills: Sage.

Minde, K., Whitelaw, A., Brown, J., & Fitzhardinge, P. (1983). The effect of neonatal complications in premature infants on early parent-infant interactions. *Developmental Medicine and Child Neurology, 25,* 763–777.

Mrazek, D. A., & Klinnert, M. D. (1998). Preventing asthma through modification of parent-child interactions. In preparation.

Mrazek, D. A., Klinnert, M. D., Mrazek, P., & Macey, T. (1991). Early asthma onset: Consideration of parenting issues. *Journal of the American Academy of Child and Adolescent Psychiatry, 30,* 277–282.

Offord, D., Boyle, M. H., Szatmari, P., Rae-Grant, N., Links, P., Cadman, D. T., Byles, J. A., Crawford, J. W., Monroe-Blum, H., Bynne, C., Thomas, H., & Woodward, C. A. (1987). The Ontario child health study: Prevalence of disorder and rates of service utilization. *Archives of General Psychiatry, 44,* 832–836.

Parker, G. (1983). *Parental overprotection: A risk factor in psychosocial development.* New York: Grune & Stratton.

Parker, G. (1993). Parental rearing style: Examining for links with personality vulnerability factors for depression. *Social Psychiatry and Psychiatric Epidemiology, 28,* 97–100.

Perrin, E. C., Ayoub, C. C., Willet, J. B. (1993). In the eyes of the beholder: Family and maternal influences on perceptions of adjustment of children with chronic illness. *Journal of Developmental and Behavioral Pediatrics, 14,* 94–105.

Perrin, E. C., West, P. D., & Culley, B. S. (1989). Is my child normal yet? Correlates of vulnerability. *Pediatrics, 83,* 355–363.

Perrin, J. M., Maclean, W. E., & Perrin, E. C. (1989). Parental perceptions of health status and psychologic adjustment of children with asthma. *Pediatrics, 83,* 26–30.

Pless, I. B., & Pinkerton, P. (1975). *Chronic childhood disorder: Promoting patterns of adjustment.* London, England: Kimpton.

Robins, L. N., Schoenberg, S., Holmes, S., Ratcliff, K., Benham, A., & Works, J. (1985). Early home environment and retrospective recall: A test for concordance between siblings with and without psychiatric disorders. *American Journal of Orthopsychiatry, 55,* 27–41.

Rogoff, B. (1990). *Apprenticeship in thinking.* New York: Oxford University Press.

Sameroff, A., & Chandler, M. (1975). Reproductive risk and the continuum of caretaking casualty. In F. D. Horowitz (Ed.), *Review of child development research* (Vol. 4, pp. 187–244). Chicago: University of Chicago Press.

Sameroff, A. J., & Fiese, B. H. (1990). Transactional regulation and early intervention. In S. J. Meisels & J. P. Shonkoff (Eds.), *Handbook of early childhood intervention* (119–149). New York: Cambridge University Press.

Segal, L. B., Oster, H., Cohen, M., Caspi, B., Myers, M., & Brown, D. (1995). Smiling and fussing in seven-month-old preterm and full-term black infants in the still-face situation. *Child Development, 66,* 1829–1843.

Shonkoff, J. P., & Meisels, P. C. (1990). Early childhood intervention: The evolution of a concept. In S. J. Meisels & J. P. Shonkoff (Eds.), *Handbook of early childhood intervention* (3–31). New York: Cambridge University Press.

Sigal, J., Chagoya, L., Villeneuve, C., & Mayerovitch, J. (1973). Later psychological sequelae of early childhood illness (severe croup). *American Journal of Psychiatry, 103,* 786–789.

Sigal, J., & Gagnon, P. (1975). Effects of parents' and pediatricians' worry concerning severe gastroenteritis in early childhood on later disturbances in the child's behavior. *Journal of Pediatrics, 87,* 809–814.

Simeonsson, R. J. (1986). *Psychological and developmental assessment of special children.* Boston: Allyn & Bacon.

Solnit, A. J., & Stark, M. H. (1959). Pediatric management of school learning problems of underachievement. *New England Journal of Medicine, 261,* 988–993.

Stack, D. M., & Poulin-Dubois, D. (1998). Socioemotional and cognitive competence in infancy. In D. Pushkar, W. M. Bukowski, A. E. Schwartzman, D. M. Stack, & D. R. White (Eds.), *Improving competence across the lifespan* (pp. 37–57). New York: Plenum.

Stein, R. E., Gortmaker, S. L., Perrin, E. C., Perrin, J. M., Pless, I. B., Walker, D. K., & Weitzmann, M. (1997). Severity of illness: Concepts and measurements. *Lancet, 2,* 1506–1509.

Steinberg, L., Mounts, N., Lamborn, S., & Dornbush, S. (1991). Authoritative parenting and adolescent adjustment across various ecological niches. *Journal of Research on Adolescents, 1,* 19–36.

Thelen, E., & Smith, L. B. (1994). *A dynamic systems approach in development of cognition and action.* Cambridge, MA: MIT Press.

Thomas, A., Chess, S., & Birch, H. (1968). *Temperament and behavior disorders in children.* New York: New York University Press.

Thomas, J. M., Benham, A. L., Gean, M., Luby, J., Minde, K., Turner, S., & Wright, S. S. (1997). Practice parameters for the psychiatric assessment of infants and toddlers (0–36 months). *Journal of the American Academy of Child and Adolescent Psychiatry, 36,* 21S–36S.

Thomasgard, M., & Metz, W. P. (1996). The 2-year stability of parental perceptions of child vulnerability and parental overprotection. *Journal of Developmental and Behavioral Pediatrics, 17,* 222–228.

Thomasgard, M., Metz, P., Edelbrock, C., & Shonkoff, J. (1995). Parent-child relationship disorders: Part 1. Parental overprotection and the development of the parent protection scale. *Journal of Developmental and Behavioral Pediatrics, 16,* 244–250.

Tronick, E. Z., Als, H., Adamson, L., Wise, S., & Brazelton, T. B. (1978). The infant's response to entrapment between contradictory messages in face-to-face interaction. *Journal of the American Academy of Child Psychiatry, 17,* 1–13.

van IJzendoorn, M. H. (1995). Adult attachment representations, parental responsiveness, and infant attachment: A meta-analysis on the predictive validity of the adult attachment interview. *Psychological Bulletin, 117,* 387–S403.

Zeanah, C. H., & Anders, T. F. (1987). Subjectivity in parent-infant relationships: A discussion of internal working models. *Infant Mental Health Journal, 8,* 237–250.

Zeanah, C. H., & Benoit, D. (1995). Clinical applications of a parent perception interview. In K. Minde (Ed.), *Infants psychiatry, child psychiatric clinics of North America* (pp. 539–554). Philadelphia: W. B. Saunders.

4

Infant Mental Health Assessment through Careful Observation and Listening: Unique Training Approaches

Deborah J. Weatherston

4

Introduction

Training requirements for infant and family practitioners from multiple disciplines are complex. First, practitioners need to construct *a knowledge base* from which to observe an infant or toddler, think about a parent, and wonder about the complexity of early development within the context of caregiver-child relationships. Second, they need opportunities to develop and refine *assessment and treatment skills through direct service experiences* with children under three and families whose strengths and capacities vary. Third, they need *a context* in which to discuss the details of what they see and hear, a place in which to ask questions about infancy and early parenthood, relationship risks, disorders of development, and strategies for effective work. Fourth, they need individual guidance and opportunities for reflection with *a training supervisor* who is knowledgeable about early development and relationships and able to sustain them in their work. These four training elements—a knowledge base, skill development through direct service experiences, a context in which to question, and reflective supervision—are consistent with the training experiences first proposed by Selma Fraiberg and her colleagues in the Child Development Project in Ann Arbor, Michigan in the 1970s (Fraiberg, 1980). They reflect the early training guidelines recommended by the Michigan Association for Infant Mental Health (1983) to influence the design of university and community-based programs in the preparation of infant

mental health trainees and strengthen the practice of infant mental health. They mirror the training principles proposed by staff who are affiliated with the National Center for Infants, Toddlers and Families in Washington, D.C. and are highly regarded for their leadership in preparing infant and family practitioners (Fenich & Eggbeer, 1990). They also reflect current thinking among those who are preparing practitioners from multiple disciplines to assess and treat young children with respect to the social and emotional context in which they are raised (Meisels & Fenichel, 1996; Harmon & Frankel, 1997; Lieberman, Van Horn, Grandison, & Pekarsky, 1997; Weatherston & Tableman, 1989; Trout, 1987; Fisher & Osofsky, 1997; Bernstein, Pekarsky, & Wechsler, 1996).

The preparation of students and professionals from multiple disciplines and perspectives to provide services that enhance the lives of infants, toddlers, and their families clearly presents a significant challenge to educators, health care professionals, mental health practitioners, and policymakers at state and federal levels. What is it that early development practitioners need to know in order to work successfully with children zero to three years of age and their families? How will they translate their knowledge about infancy, development, and early parenthood into skillful practice with young children and families? How will their understanding of what is "best" for children and families affect the assessment process and treatment services that they provide? What will they need to support and sustain their continuing development as early intervention professionals? There is not one design suitable for all students or professionals interested in early identification and services for children under three and their families. However, there are approaches that offer guidelines for meaningful growth in the areas of infant and family assessment and support with attention to social and emotional development within the context of relationship and daily care.

What follows is a discussion of several training approaches that have been designed to teach and support graduate students and professionals in providing assessment and treatment services to infants, toddlers, and their families. The organizing principle that is evident in each of these models is the belief that optimal development occurs within the context of relationship. The programs differ in many ways, for example, size, composition, format, frequency of meetings, and length of time. However, each approach illustrates that it is possible to strengthen the knowledge base and clinical practice skills of practitioners from multiple disciplines who are interested in working with children under three and their families.

In this discussion, we continuously examine what practitioners need to understand in order to work effectively with children under three and their parents. What clinical skills are essential to accomplish the dual and delicate tasks of assessing and treating young children and families with sensitivity to relationship growth? How will they learn to observe carefully and respectfully, identify competencies, and understand risks within the context of each parent-child relationship? What experi-

ences nurture the art of clinical questioning, careful listening, and empathic response? These are questions that stakeholders need to ask when considering the design of training experiences and programs to prepare practitioners to work with very young children and their families.

A Training Legacy: Selma Fraiberg

Overview of Services

The legacy that Selma Fraiberg and her colleagues left us includes a powerful model for the practice of infant mental health (Fraiberg, 1980), as well as a strong design for training. Unique in the treatment of very young children and their families, Selma Fraiberg's model embraced early developing relationships, working with parent(s) and infant together most frequently in the intimacy of their own homes and offering a context for shared observations, careful listening, and empathic response. Infant mental health services, as designed by Fraiberg, offered an array of strategies for assessment and intervention: Emotional and concrete service support, developmental guidance, and parent-infant psychotherapy. Each strategy helped parents and practitioners to understand early development and to nurture relationships through a careful assessment and treatment process.

INFANT MENTAL HEALTH STRATEGIES
Included here is a brief description of infant mental health strategies that are inte-

gral to the early practice of infant mental health (Fraiberg, 1980; Weatherston, 1997). *Emotional support* is defined as compassion offered to a parent who faces a crisis in caring for a new baby or toddler. Alone or without emotional reinforcement a parent must have someone who is emotionally available, listens carefully, and holds the many feelings that threaten to overwhelm or confuse. *Concrete resource assistance* refers to the meeting of basic needs for food, clothing, medical care, shelter, and protection. The practitioner who feeds, clothes, or takes a family to the clinic assures parents and young children that he or she cares about them and will work to ease their burdens of care. *Developmental guidance* is the shared understanding about the baby's development and specific needs for care. The practitioner and parent carefully identify emerging strengths and concerns, reaching an understanding of the uniqueness of each baby through careful observation and words. *Infant-parent psychotherapy* offers a parent the opportunity to explore thoughts and feelings awakened in the presence of a baby. In the intimacy of the home visit, a parent may share stories of past experiences and significant relationships, major fears, disappointments, and unresolved losses as they affect the care of a baby and the early developing relationship between parent and child.

THE WORKING RELATIONSHIP

Crucial to the effectiveness of these strategies is the working relationship that develops between each infant mental health practitioner and parent (Fraiberg, 1980; Lieberman & Pawl, 1993). Respectful and consistent, the practitioner remains attentive to each parent's strengths and needs. Within the safety of this relationship, parents feel well cared for and secure, held by the therapist's words and in her mind (Pawl, 1995). The practitioner listens carefully, follows the parent's lead, remains attuned, sets limits, and responds with empathy. Well held, the parent experiences possibilities for growth and change through the relationship with her own infant.

The practice of infant mental health as defined by Selma Fraiberg and her colleagues is as relevant today as it was 25 years ago. Principles inherent in the original model guide assessment and treatment services for infants and parents in community mental health programs (Weatherston & Tableman, 1989; Lieberman & Pawl, 1993), specialized community-based projects (Fisher & Osofsky, 1997), early development services (Thomas, Guskin, & Klass, 1997), child psychiatry settings (Harmon, 1994/1995), and child and family diagnostic centers (Hirschberg, 1993; Zeanah et al., 1997).

"What About the Baby?" An Extraordinary Training Plan

Unique in its focus on children under three, parents, and relationships, the practice of infant mental health, as developed by students and staff under Selma Fraiberg's direction in the early 1970s called for a dramatic shift in thinking and practice. Graduate students, interns, and professionals from many disciplines required intensive and continuous training as they learned to identify clinical and developmental risks in infancy and structure relationship-based interventions through the very new practice of infant mental health. "What about the baby?" Fraiberg asked, with passion and determination. Efforts to answer that question left an indelible mark on the training experiences that included clinical work with children under three and their families, regularly scheduled clinical supervision to discuss that work, and lectures and group seminars, as well as opportunities for research (Fraiberg, 1980; Schafer, 1988). What follows is a discussion of that remarkable training model that gives us a framework for considering an approach to learning that is relevant today.

SEMINARS

Developmental and clinical seminars provided a context for group study. Early discussions centered on the contributions of infants and caregivers to each relationship, the identification of risks, and the needs of infants and families for concrete and emotional support, developmental guidance, and/or intensive, infant-parent psychotherapy. Each staff member and student intern presented clinical experiences to the group throughout the training year. Senior staff struggled beside student trainees. They discussed what they observed and learned to speak openly about their clinical experiences, in home, with infants and families, refining their own understanding of principles and techniques vital to infant mental health assessment and treatment services. Senior staff and student trainees presented videotaped segments of home visits as well as carefully prepared and detailed process notes from home visiting and the occasional office sessions. The intent of

the group experience was to inform and support clinical questioning and developmental competence among all participants within the Child Development Project (Fraiberg, 1980; Schafer, 1988).

INDIVIDUALIZED LEARNING

Because senior staff and clinical trainees came from very diverse backgrounds, some of the preparation for early assessment and treatment services had to be individualized. Knowledge of infancy, early relationship development, and assessment practices were fundamental. Selma Fraiberg took great care to assure that each staff person and trainee had an adequate understanding in these areas through tutorials, supervisory sessions, written materials, and study within small groups. Fraiberg recognized the individual skills that each professional and student had and designed experiences to enhance them.

CLINICAL EXPERIENCES

Clinical interns and staff responded to requests that were quite urgent, for example, infants who were failing-to-thrive and toddlers at risk of removal due to abuse and neglect. In the process of responding, interns and staff developed an array of strategies, described previously, as they followed children and families into their homes. Students and staff, including social workers, psychologists, nurses, and pediatricians, returned to "the kitchen" as the source for understanding the complexities of early infancy and parenthood, the risks of developmental failure, and the joys.

The early practitioners expected to see a family four to six times for the purpose of gathering information about the baby and the family, as well as building a relationship in which the family could begin to feel safe. They integrated informal assessment approaches with more formal measures of the infant's development and a parent's concerns, to determine ways that they might be helpful to a family and the family's capacity to accept them. Elegant case studies (Fraiberg, 1980; Fraiberg & Adelson, 1977; Fraiberg, Shapiro, & Adelson, 1976) describe the construction of infant mental health services, offered weekly or more frequently, beginning with the assessment and extending treatment through each infant's first or second year.

CLINICAL SUPERVISION

The model for supervision was extraordinary. All interns and staff met regularly and frequently for supervision, receiving one hour of supervision for every hour of service to a family. Fraiberg was clear in her belief that individual supervision was fundamental to clinical training and growth. Supervision provided a context for individualized guidance and support. A trainee could bring the details of his or her work to a trusted supervisor for careful review. Hour after hour, each training supervisor gave time and attention to a trainee, offering the experience of consistency, respectful listening, and guided support. Supervision provided a relationship for learning about infants and their families, a place for clinical questioning and individual growth.

A SUCCESSFUL APPROACH TO TRAINING

This was clearly an extraordinarily successful training approach. Many of the staff and trainees involved in the Child Development Project, over 25 years ago, are leaders in the field of infant mental health today, for example, Jeree Pawl and Alicia Lieberman in California and William Schafer in Michigan. They have continued to train others in the traditions established by Selma Fraiberg, modifying their approaches to accommodate new understanding about infancy and early parenthood, as we better understand the interplay between individuals and their environments that offers continuous opportunity for clinical growth and change (Emde, 1997).

Beyond the University's Borders: A Community Training Plan

In 1973, the Child Development Project reached out beyond the borders of the University of Michigan to reach front-line clinicians within Michigan's Department of Community Mental Health (Shapiro, Adelson, & Tableman, 1982). Betty Tableman, Director of Prevention Services for Michigan's Department of Mental Health, worked with Selma Fraiberg and Child Development Project staff, Vivian Shapiro and Edna Adelson, to design and carry out a community-based training program. This collaborative partnership led to the training of a cadre of community mental health practitioners (12 persons trained in two separate groups) who would incorporate what they learned about assessment and treatment services to children under three and their families into prevention programs across the state. Those who participated in the intensive, yearlong, community-based infant mental health training project made up the next generation of skilled, infant mental health practitioners in Michigan. It is truly remarkable that many of these "pioneers" have stayed in the field to influence the development of infants, families, and practitioners for more than 20 years.

A Modified Training Plan

Knowledge about infancy and early parenthood, theories vital to early relationship development and emotional health, assessment through observation and inquiry, and intervention strategies unique to the practice of infant mental health remained essential to the community mental health training plan. The training format changed to meet the needs of practitioners who lived far away from the Child Development Project (CDP). Twelve trainees met for one day of training at the CDP every other week for one year. Each trainee carried a "study" case, for example, a family at no or low risk for the purpose of training in infant and family observation, as well as clinical cases from their own communities, for example, infants and families at serious and early developmental and relationship risk. They shared the details of their observations and clinical experiences with seasoned supervisors at the CDP. They also discussed clinical hypotheses and strategies within the full training group.

The training experience required energy, commitment, constancy, and courage. In the process, each community mental health trainee learned to think about the baby within the context of the family, identify risks, and support strengths. Trainees

moved their clinical practice out of the office and into infants' homes where they worked with infants and parents together, on behalf of optimal development and to reduce relationship risks. They learned the importance of their own relationships to the developing relationships between parents and children. They learned to keep their eyes on each baby, nurture new parents, invite and listen intently to stories offered by parents, and respond with empathy to the stories told. They learned to watch infants in interaction with their parents and respect the courage each family displayed. They watched for developmental milestones and spoke about emerging capabilities and needs. They learned to hold parental disappointments, failures, grief, and unresolved losses. They experienced parental ambivalence, rejection, and despair. They learned to speak for those who could not—parent and child. They learned to move between the parent's past and present realities, address painful experiences as they threatened to make the care of a baby difficult, and offer hopefulness for change within each newly developing relationship between parent and child (Schafer, 1988; Tableman, 1982).

How Did They Learn These Things?

CLINICAL QUESTIONING

In addition to lectures in which senior staff presented information related to clinical and developmental theory and meetings with clinical supervisors, trainees asked each other questions and questioned clinical staff. What factors protect infants in the first months of life? What makes caregiving difficult, leading to abandonment, abuse, or neglect? What makes holding or feeding the baby almost impossible for a parent? What explains the disturbance in the development of a relationship between parent and child? What enables the infant or parent to progress? Senior staff and trainees wrestled with these questions and similar questions in supervision and within specialized discussion groups.

Of additional importance, clinical trainees studied videotaped interactions of infants and families with whom they worked. Videotaped sequences of infants and parents together, in interaction with one another, provided opportunities for trainees and staff to discuss what they saw, raise questions, and consider infancy and early development from many perspectives, assessing capacities and risks. In the course of one year, the infant mental health trainees learned how to observe infants and families, assess their strengths and needs, offer support and guidance as appropriate to each infant and family referred, and reflect on what they experienced with infants and families in their homes (Fraiberg, 1980; Schafer, 1992).

INFANT-PARENT PSYCHOTHERAPY

The teaching of infant-parent psychotherapy was more complex. This strategy was reserved for those families at highest risk, where parental issues of unresolved loss, abuse, or neglect placed infants at grave developmental and emotional risk. Infant-parent psychotherapy required extraordinary sensitivity to the baby, attention to the relationship, and responsiveness to the parent's own relationship history and in-

tense longing for consistent care (Wright, 1986). Selma Fraiberg believed that infant-parent psychotherapy could be most successfully taught and explored within the supervisory relationship between a senior staff person and individual trainee (Fraiberg, 1980). She placed great emphasis on the importance of this relationship to the training of competent infant mental health trainees and staff. Her unwavering belief that relationships affect relationships influenced the training model that she and her staff developed to guide and support new community mental health trainees. It is this model that has influenced very profoundly the next "generations" of infant mental health training models, trainers, and trainees.

The Graduate Certificate Program in Infant Mental Health, Merrill-Palmer Institute, Wayne State University, Detroit, Michigan

Many training approaches reflect the principles in which Selma Fraiberg believed. One training program that reflects Fraiberg's commitment to infant mental health theory and supervised clinical practice is the Graduate Certificate Program in Infant Mental Health at the Merrill-Palmer Institute, Wayne State University, Detroit, Michigan. The program offers graduate students and professionals from multiple disciplines opportunities to study infancy and early parenthood, family relationship development, approaches to assessment, developmental risks and jeopardized relationships, and strategies for effective, home-based intervention.

The training program provides a context for master's and post-master's students and professionals from the fields of social work, psychology, early childhood, special education, and nursing to study theories about development and early intervention and develop new skills in the practice of infant mental health. In addition to the academic coursework, graduate students enroll in a yearlong clinical practicum that encourages the application of theories through supervised observation, assessment, and clinical experiences. The clinical practicum is the cornerstone of the graduate certificate program. Observation and clinical casework, individual supervision, group discussion within a biweekly clinical seminar, and supportive relationships with new colleagues and peers are of fundamental importance to each trainee's development within the clinical training year. Training experiences within the Graduate Certificate Program at Wayne State University are described in greater detail following.

Assessment through Observation

Observation is fundamental to the assessment process. How one observes an infant and family affects the quality of the entire assessment. For the purpose of this chapter, we examine principles that support the process.

Basic Principles

Early assessment principles, stated eloquently by Fraiberg (1980) and restated by Hirshberg (1993), Lieberman and Pawl (1993), Lieberman and colleagues (1997), Meisels and Fenichel (1996), Meisels and Provence (1989), Trout (1987), and Weatherston and Tableman, (1989) are integral to infant mental health practice and early development services. They shape the ways in which practitioners approach infants and families and influence the ways in which infants and families may be understood. Trainees who are new to the field of early intervention or infant mental health will use these principles to guide them in their work. For some, the "rules" will seem odd or inconsistent with previous training. They may struggle to integrate a relationship-guided assessment approach with one that focuses more individually on an infant or the parent of a child. Over time and within the context of supportive training relationships, infant mental health practitioners and trainees from very diverse fields learn to provide relationship-based assessments with these important tenets in mind.

INFANT AND PARENT TOGETHER
First, the trainee watches the baby in the context of a relationship in order to understand who that baby is, what the baby brings to the relationship, what the caregiver provides, and the nature of their relationship with one another. Looking at one or the other alone will yield half of the story. As Donald Winnicott (1965) so beautifully reminds us, "There is no such thing as an infant." By this he meant that there is always a baby and a caregiver. This powerful concept directs the infant mental health practitioner to consider both infant and

parent together, not one in isolation from the other.

FAMILIAR SETTING

Second, the assessment occurs in a setting familiar to the baby and the family, most ideally, the home. The practitioner or trainee observes the surroundings in which a young child is raised in order to understand what life is like for the baby and the parent, what is going well, and basic wants or needs. Another argument, eloquently stated by Selma Fraiberg (1980) is the fact that a parent caring for a new baby and being overwhelmed by the baby's care may find it difficult to get out of the home. Lack of reliable transportation for many families makes this more problematic. Some parents and infants may need the trainee to reach out, knock on the door, and enter their home. In addition to better assuring that the infant and family will be seen for an assessment, visits where the family lives may be more comfortable and less threatening. Of additional importance, home visiting may strengthen the working relationship between the practitioner and family, reinforcing the practitioner's interest and offering a basis for greater trust.

TIME

A third important principle involves the number of visits needed to appreciate the problem with the baby or reason that the infant and family were referred. Selma Fraiberg (1980) advised her staff many years ago that an assessment might occur over four to six visits, including the use of informal and formal strategies. Others suggest four to eight visits (Lieberman

et al., 1997). Important to understand is that a thoughtful, systematic assessment takes time. The process requires attention to the concerns that parents have, the opportunity for a relationship to develop with the infant or toddler's parent(s), structured and unstructured observations, details of the child's development, and family stories, past and present (Greenspan & Meisels, 1996). The practitioner or trainee needs time to observe, listen, and begin to understand what is going well in a particular family, what worries exist and ways to be helpful.

WORKING RELATIONSHIPS

Finally, but of singular importance, is the fact that parents must be considered partners throughout the assessment process (Hirshberg, 1996). The working relationship between each parent and infant mental health trainee is vital to the success of the assessment (Davies, 1992). A parent or caregiver is present, allows the practitioner to be involved, and understands why the infant has been referred. One significant challenge that the new practitioner or trainee faces is to earn the parent's trust. Without trust, very little can happen. In relationship-focused service, a working alliance with each parent or caregiver on behalf of a young child is a requirement for best practice (Lieberman, 1998).

Translating Principles into Practice

With these ground rules for assessment in place, how do trainers or supervisors help trainees or practitioners reach an understanding of the infants and families referred to them for services? What tools do they need to guide them through the process? What training techniques encourage clinical growth? An infant mental health trainee or practitioner learns to observe and listen carefully to a family referred for assessment and/or treatment services. The coursework mentioned in the preceding section, as well as observation experiences with a low to no risk infant and family, prepares a practitioner/trainee to assess strengths and risks when a young child or family, believed to be in jeopardy, is referred for assessment and/or treatment. In instances where there is no formal training program or where it is not possible to observe a family at "low or no risk," the training supervisor has a particularly important role. Experienced in providing relationship-based assessments and treatment services, the training supervisor will have to guide practitioners in the art of careful observation, listening, and relationship-focused practice.

Infant and Family Observation: Historical Significance

The training of clinicians through the observation of infants and relationships has a distinguished history. An approach attributed to Esther Bick (1964), infant observation was instituted at the Tavistock Clinic by John Bowlby and has continued there as a method of training (Reid, 1997), as well as at the Anna Freud Centre in England (Freud, 1975). As discussed in some detail earlier in this chapter, Selma Fraiberg assigned healthy infants and families to trainees for the purpose of learning about

development (Fraiberg, 1980). Similarly, Elizabeth Tuters offered training to mental health professionals through Infant Observation Seminars at the Hinckes Institute in Toronto. Reported to be important for the understanding of infant development, the observation experience also invites discussion about the emotions aroused in the presence of a particular infant and expressed within the developing parent-infant relationship (Tuters, 1988). Miller, Rustin, Rustin, and Shuttleworth (1989) and Reid (1997) relate in detail the meaning of infant observation to interdisciplinary groups of trainees at the Tavistock Clinic today.

Of additional significance, infant and family observation offers opportunities to understand variations in parenting styles, adjustments to newly developing relationships, and transitions to early parenthood (Weatherston & Baltman, 1992). The observation of an infant within the context of his or her family provides a trainee or practitioner with a remarkable opportunity to study early infancy, relationship development, and a family's unique adjustment to a baby's care (Fraiberg, 1980; Baltman, 1994; Tuters, 1988; Reid, 1997; Miller et al., 1989). A most thorough discussion of infant observation and its application to clinical training and research appears in *Developments in Infant Observation: The Tavistock Model* (Reid, 1997). In summary, observation is a compelling experience that extends knowledge about infancy and early developing relationships, while at the same time preparing practitioners, who wish to work or who are working with children under three, for work with and within family relationships.

One Training Experience in Infant and Family Observation

OVERVIEW

What follows is a detailed discussion of the Infant and Family Observation experience that is a significant part of the clinical training component of the Graduate Certificate Program in Infant Mental Health at Wayne State University, Detroit, Michigan (Weatherston & Baltman, 1992; Baltman, 1993). Clinical staff designed the infant and family observation experience to complement work with higher risk infants and their families. The observation experience offers clinical trainees the opportunity to learn from infants and families who are at no identified risk, often beginning during the pregnancy and continuing through the baby's first year. The study includes infant behavior and development, as well as caregiving experiences and adjustments necessary as the baby and parent(s) enter into relationships with each other and accomplish the major task of attachment. Clinical supervisors and trainees agree that the opportunity to learn from an infant and family, under the guidance of a clinical supervisor, is remarkable. The experience prepares them to observe and listen carefully, notice the details of development, interaction, and relationship, and reflect on what they see and hear.

PREPARING FOR THE OBSERVER ROLE

How does a clinical trainee or practitioner new to the field of early intervention or infant mental health prepare to observe new parents caring for their baby? It is helpful for the trainee to have an intellectual appreciation of infant development within the context of the parent-child relationship, with awareness of the caregiving environment that surrounds them all. Coursework or readings specific to infancy, attachment theory, family dynamics and development, and techniques of assessment help to prepare trainees for the intellectual and emotional challenge of the infant and family observation experience. Table 4.1 offers a synopsis of observation guidelines for trainees.

The family's willingness to enter into a relationship with a trainee at a time when they are beginning their own relationship with the baby offers the trainee an exquisite opportunity to observe the complexities of early development in the family's first year. The trainee looks closely at the infant, noting weight, size, degree of activity, and responsiveness to face and voice. He or she notices if the baby is quiet, easy to comfort, feed, and hold. The trainee may notice that the baby is active, awake for many hours, and eager for stimulation, sometimes difficult to soothe or console. Trainees note the ways that a parent attends to the baby, cradling, picking up, or setting down. They watch the parent(s) and eagerly note their interest in the baby, "the dance," and, not so eagerly, recognize the parent's fatigue, ambivalence, and uncertainty about what might happen next or how to respond.

ARRANGEMENTS

Each visit lasts for about one hour. The trainee schedules appointments when it is most convenient for the family and when the baby is most likely to be awake. The trainee

TABLE 4.1
Observation Guidelines for Attention to a Nonclinical Infant and Family

The following guidelines help trainees to organize what they see during each visit to the family's home. The topics are not all inclusive, but meant to stimulate their thinking about the hour and to record in some detail what they observed (Weatherston, 1990).

Infant: Physical description (unique characteristics); emerging developmental capabilities in multiple domains; interest in people and playthings; developing abilities to engage, interact, and respond.

Parent: Developing interest in, attention, investment, and responsiveness to the baby; changing ability to organize around the baby's wants or needs; adjustment to infant's care; new roles and relationships.

Interactions: Infant's and parent's abilities to attend, listen, smile, vocalize/speak, engage, reach, hold, and follow; exchange during a feeding or at playtime, diapering, or bathing, mutuality of interests, pleasures, and capacities for affectionate response.

Quality of the Developing Relationship: Attentive, responsive; expressive, adaptive; comfortable and comforting; mutually satisfying, rewarding and appropriate; baby's use of parent(s) as source of comfort and security; response to separations and reunions; baby's use of parent(s) as a safe haven or secure base; parent's capacity to keep safe and secure; set limits.

Caregiving Environment: Parents, grandparents, siblings, and day care providers important to the baby's daily care; level of activity and stimulation in the home (or child care setting); description of home setting; degree of organization; toys available for the baby to play with; caregiving routines.

Infant history: Pregnancy; preparations for birth; labor and delivery; hospital stay; father's presence; the homecoming; experience of early care; special circumstances; illnesses or hospitalizations; concerns as expressed by parent; significant separations; arrangements for child care.

Network of Support: Family relationships significant to the parent's ability to care for the baby; quality and availability of family's support, network of friends surrounding parent(s) and infant, and parent's ability to use the support.

There are other observations to make in the course of the year's observation of a nonclinical family. Each is important to the trainee's clinical growth and personal development.

Emotional Response: The infant's response to each parent; each parent's response to the infant; the emotions contained and expressed within their relationships; the meaning of each relationship to the baby and to each parent.

Personal Responses: Feelings that the trainee is aware of as he or she meets with the infant and parent(s); identification with either the baby or the parent; memories or events recalled; the developing relationship between trainee and each member of the family and feelings surrounding that relationship.

videotapes the family for five to ten minutes once per month, capturing an early feeding sequence, playtime, the introduction of a new toy, diapering, bathing, or "being with the baby." Each videotaped sequence provides a powerful record of one baby's development within the context of the family.

EACH TRAINEE PREPARES A WRITTEN SUMMARY FOLLOWING EACH OBSERVATION

In this way, the trainee records changes in the baby's development, the early relationship and parental response over the course of one year, sharing the details of those observations in supervision or within the clinical training group. This strengthens the trainee's understanding of development in multiple domains and assures attention to individual differences in relationship development, security of attachment, and the subjective experience of one to the other.

VIDEOTAPED SEGMENTS

Videotape provides trainees with many opportunities for shared observation and discussion with his or her training supervisor and with other trainees. The material offers compelling examples of infants and parents in interaction with each other, for example, at play, during bath time, or during a feeding. This leads to thoughtful comments, in supervision or within the training seminar, about the observed experience as well as attention to the practitioner's emotional response.

THE LEARNING EXPERIENCE

Within the course of the year, each trainee concentrates on the baby's many and emerging adaptive capacities, milestones

reached, and relationship domains. Each trainee observes the parent's responsiveness to the baby and watches carefully for signs of an early developing relationship, negotiation of crises, and individual resolutions within that first year. Growing more skilled at observing and listening, the trainee learns to hold the uncertainties such as the wonder, questions, and concerns about feeding and sleep routines, a father's loneliness, early separations, and the mother's return to work. The trainee works hard to contain what he or she encounters: The stresses, frustrations, and delights. In the process of recording observations and bringing them to supervision, the trainee finds his or her "voice." He or she begins to clarify what has been observed and speak about the infant and parent's behavior and development within the context of their emerging relationship.

SELF-REFLECTION IS SIGNIFICANT TO THE OBSERVATION EXPERIENCE

Supervising faculty at the Wayne State University program note that it is in the discussion of the observation family that a trainee begins to reflect on his or her own values about infancy and early parenthood (Weatherston, 1998). There is time to consider more personal experiences, as a parent or child within a family, recently or many years ago. "The baby is so quiet. I'm wondering what it is like for his mom to try so hard to get his attention and get so little in return?" Then, "My baby was like that, too. I remember being somewhat disappointed because I expected him to be more playful. It was a long time before I understood that he was just different from me. I haven't thought about Jamie as a baby in a very long time." In the presence of an observation family, many thoughts and feelings, some of them sobering, some of them not, are aroused. A trainee may bring these thoughts to supervision for further reflection where they may be shared and safely explored. For many trainees, this is the first and only opportunity they have had to talk deeply about infancy, parenthood, and early development or to consider their more personal responses to families, relationship development, and early infant care.

SUMMARY

Trainees discover many unexpected rewards as they sit quietly and follow the parent and infant's lead. They learn to listen more carefully and begin to really hear what a parent has to say. They learn to watch the details of infant and relationship development that may have been overlooked. They learn about the baby's contribution to a relationship and the importance of each parent's emotional response. They experience the regulation of each unique relationship in the course of the training year. They also grow aware of their own thoughts and feelings in the process of playing a more passive role. At the same time, trainees discover the wisdom of "sitting on one's hands" in the presence of infant and parent(s) (Baltman, 1993), wondering about early development and relationship change.

Learning to Look: The Use of Videotaped Materials as Observational Tools

DEVELOPMENTAL OBSERVATIONS

Some training programs use videotaped materials of parents and infants in interaction with one another as a focal point for developmental observations and discussions. Bernstein and colleagues (1996) describe a unique training and support program for home-visiting staff, supervisors, and parent group facilitators that uses videotapes to generate discussion. Staff study videotaped interactions of infants and families who are not enrolled in their program. They share their observations with each other, identifying developmental strengths and noticing when parents provide appropriate care. Monthly meetings offer multiple opportunities for reflection and new understanding as they enhance developmental observational skills.

WATCHFUL EYES

Other programs describe the use of videotaped materials to sharpen clinical observations of practitioners who are working with infants and families who are at risk and have been referred for assessment and treatment services (Weatherston & Tableman, 1989). Under the watchful eyes of a trusted supervisor or with others in a discussion group, the practitioner uses videotaped sequences to observe a baby, alone or in interaction with someone, and wonders about both. The supervisor or trainer might first ask, "What about the baby?" "Describe in some detail what you see." The practitioner in training is invited to pay attention to details: The baby's age and size, level of activity, interest in his or her mother's face or voice, the way in which he or she approaches her, and his or her steady gaze, engaging smile, or mournful cry. Other questions follow. What does the baby bring to the newly developing relationship? What kind of care does he require? Questions like these encourage each training participant to look at the baby and wonder about his or her development within the context of a particular relationship. For many, this is the first opportunity they have to watch a baby so carefully and think about what they see. It takes an enormous amount of courage and practice to do this. The supervisor or trainer proceeds quite carefully, following the practitioner's lead and listening to the observations each makes with great care.

Because the baby exists in a partnership, never alone, the trainee also looks at the mother or father or caregiver. The supervisor or trainer might ask next, "What about the parent?" "How old does she appear to be? What does the parent bring to the baby in this brief videotape clip? How interested in or responsive does she seem to be to the baby? How able is he to attend to the baby's immediate needs?" Questions like these ask the trainee to study the parent's appearance and behavior and to wonder about both. The training supervisor may also ask, "What do you think it is like to be this parent caring for this baby day after day?" With questions like these, the trainee may be drawn into the infant and parent's worlds, but the observation does not stop there.

ENHANCING THE STUDY
OF RELATIONSHIPS

Videotape makes it possible to study early interactions and relationship, what happens in the space between parent and child. By examining moments on videotape, pleasurable or painful, the trainee has

time to think about the intricacies of relationship and the uniqueness of a particular infant-parent pair. The supervisor or trainer may ask, "How do they interact with one another? How satisfying does their relationship seem to be? What emotions are contained within the interaction, expressed or silently shared?"

REFLECTION

The observation of videotaped materials lends itself to personal reflection. Training consultants may ask practitioners questions that encourage thoughtful responses (Schafer, 1995; Goldberg, 1998; Foulds, 1997). What do you find yourself thinking about as you watch this mother-baby pair? Some have never been asked this question before and may not know quite what to say. Many respond with a thought about the baby's development or the mother's health. "I wonder if the baby has a delay. He doesn't babble or make the sounds other babies his age make." "I wonder if she is using again. She's so agitated." Others may offer a story about a family with whom they are currently working that relates to the family under close observation in a similar way. "I was reminded of the Smith family as I watched this mother-baby pair." Still others may be more introspective, remembering the care they gave to their own infants many years ago. "I can't help but think about my own baby when he was one year old and the fun we had. I loved taking care of him. That was a long time ago." They may remember aspects of their own early experiences with a mother or father or grandmother. "I wondered about my own mother and how alone she must have been when I was born." Many thoughts and feelings may wash over trainees as they begin to reflect, perhaps for the first time, on what they see or the meaning of relationship development to them and the importance of early infant care.

Over time and within the context of a thoughtful supervisory or training relationship, most trainees/practitioners find words to describe what they see and feel as they study videotaped sequences of parents and infants together. Many grow increasingly skillful in assessing the details of development in infancy and early parenthood, emerging capacities and developmental as well as caregiving risks. These observations fuel their understanding of infants and relationships and help them to develop, in partnership with caregivers, more careful assessment and treatment plans.

EMOTIONS EXPRESSED

It is important to note that as most trainees begin to observe and assess more carefully, they become more sensitive to a range of risks (Wright, 1986). They may feel increasingly uncomfortable, frustrated, angry, or tense as they review a particular videotape. They may feel lonely or deeply sad in response to a baby they see. Some protect themselves by detaching from the experience, shutting down, or turning away. Others may deny that they feel anything at all. Still others may express some ambivalence about the observation experience, the field of infant mental health, or grow increasingly active in their attempts to solve "the problem" or develop a working plan. It is important for the supervisor or trainer to allow these feelings to be experienced, hold them respectfully, and establish a place within the training relationship or the group where it feels safe for each practitioner to speak (Schafer, 1995).

A SAFE PLACE

Practitioners, newly developing and experienced, need many opportunities to talk as they observe infants and families in the course of training. The supervisory relationship or training group provides the place where it is safe to do this. The trainer remains attentive to the practitioner's sad, angry, or still face and gives permission to talk by asking, "Is this something you would like to talk more about?" The question carefully acknowledges the trainee/practitioner's need to be heard right then and the trainer's ability to listen. This allows the trainee to connect with what she is feeling and puts the power back into her hands. It also helps to restore the possibility of becoming the kind of practitioner she hopes to be (Schafer, 1995). In addition to supporting the trainee, this approach serves as a template for the practitioner's careful response to parents when with them in the clinic setting or at home.

In summary, these experiences in the use of videotape for observation encourage practitioners from many disciplines to watch each infant or toddler with care, keep their eyes on the interaction, wonder about the uniqueness of each developing relationship, and listen closely to what parents have to say. Immersed in the details of interaction and development through the study of many infants and families, trainees grow more confident in responding to requests for assessment when there are significant risks, suspected delays, or heightened caregiving concerns.

Learning to Look: Observing within the Context

DEFINING THE RELATIONSHIP

In all instances, the practitioner/trainee must be able to define the relationship (Schafer, 1995; Zeanah, 1997). This means that the practitioner/trainee will try to observe and understand the infant and parent within the context of their relationship with one another, appreciate the dynamics of interaction moment to moment, and contain the feelings expressed or aroused. In order to do this, the trainee observes the infant and parent(s) together. For many, this is a unique requirement. Students and professionals are customarily trained to work with children or with adults. In relationship work, the presence of the parent is vital to understanding the infant (Hirschberg, 1993; Meisels & Fenichel, 1996; Winnicott, 1965). The presence of the infant is a powerful contributor to understanding the dynamics of relationship within families and caregiving responses, both nurturing and problematic (Fraiberg, 1980).

PARAMETERS

Training programs/supervisors set clear parameters for early development practitioners or trainees. Practitioners within the field of infant mental health are taught to work with the infant and parent together (Fraiberg, 1980; Weatherston & Tableman, 1989; Wright, 1986; Trout, 1982; Lieberman & Pawl, 1993). Trainees make appointments when both parent(s) and infant are able to be present and at a time that is convenient for the family. If possible, trainees may make arrangements to visit parent(s) and infant in the home, limiting the observation or assessment to 1 to 1½ hours, for four to eight visits. In instances where home visiting is not possible, trainees work with parent(s) and infant in an office or playroom or center-based program. Regardless of the place, trainees are taught to approach families with kindness and respect, keeping in mind the centrality of the therapeutic relationship to the success of assessment and treatment.

These expectations are consistent with infant mental health practices as described by Selma Fraiberg (Fraiberg, 1980), Lieberman and Pawl (1993), Wright (1986), Weatherston and Tableman (1989), and Trout (1987). They are most important when a parent expresses concern about the development of an infant, a professional is worried about the caregiving capacity of a parent, or an agency suspects a relationship disturbance or disorder, due to serious neglect, abuse, or placement in foster care.

The Use of Formal Assessment Instruments to Enhance the Observation Process

INFANT OR TODDLER DEVELOPMENT

Assessment within the fields of infant mental health and early intervention is a complex process (Trout, 1987; Greenspan & Meisels, 1996), involving informal methods of observation and questioning (Weatherston & Tableman, 1989), as well as the use of formal tools. The training of practitioners to use specific assessment tools is beyond the scope of this chapter. What is important to note is that there are many instruments available to help professionals and parents consider the uniqueness of an infant or toddler's development and answer particular developmental questions. Most familiar are the Brazelton Neonatal Assessment Scales (Brazelton, 1973), the Bayley Scales (Bayley, 1969, 1993), and the Washington Guide (Barnard & Erickson, 1976). These formal infant assessment instruments guide practitioners and parents to focus on the infant's adaptive and developing capabilities, celebrate emerging strengths, and describe observed behaviors and/or delays. In summary, formal tools provide a structure for observation and questioning about a baby's progress and concerns that parents may have related to development, emerging capacities, and risks.

A well-trained practitioner is familiar with developmental assessment instruments in order to observe infants or toddlers carefully and respond with knowledge and sensitivity to parental questions and concerns. There is no substitute in the preparation of practitioners for training for the use of specific assessment measures. Each instrument has its own training guidelines. Practice in the use of a particular infant scale, under the guidance of a professional individually or in a group, is a requirement for proficiency.

INFANT-PARENT/ CAREGIVER INTERACTION

As mentioned previously, infants develop within a context of caregiving relationships, at least one. In assessing any infant, formally or informally, the practitioner learns to look at that infant with an eye on interaction and relationship development. There are many formal scales that invite the study of infants or toddlers in interaction with parents or caregivers. Two are of particular interest here: The Feeding and Teaching Scales from the Nursing Child Assessment Satellite Training (NCAST) Project (Barnard, 1976) and the Massie-Campbell Scale of Mother-Infant Attachment During Stress (ADS) (Massie & Campbell, 1983).

The NCAST captures the essence of interaction and relationship by teaching practitioners to focus on the infant's ability to signal wants or needs clearly, as well as the mother's sensitivity and responsivity to her baby's cues. The ADS assesses the infant's use of the parent-child relationship when under stress and the parent's ability to comfort or respond. These instruments guide the practitioner in training to look at the infant or toddler within a particular relationship. In a field that prides itself on relationship-based practice, these instruments are particularly useful. Once trained in the use of these measures, the practitioner is better prepared to examine what the infant and the parent each contribute to the relationship and their developing capacity to signal and respond. In actuality, the practitioner may use these measures as frames of reference when thinking about the child and family. The observation skills that each trainee develops when learning to use these tools are fundamental to careful infant mental health practice.

THE CAREGIVING CONTEXT

The context in which an infant or toddler and parent develops may also be measured. The Home Observation for Measurement of the Environment Inventory (HOME) (Caldwell, 1978) contains 45 items collected by observation and interview. The HOME teaches trainees and practitioners to consider the emotional and verbal responsiveness of the parent, the organization of the baby's world, opportunities for play, and caregiving routines. Training in the use of the HOME strengthens the practitioner's skillfulness in observing details of the environment that affect a small child's development and can easily be incorporated into strategies for relationship-based assessment and continuing intervention. Considering the importance of the environment to understanding parent(s) and infant(s) and the course of later development, the HOME is a critical observation tool for infant mental health and early intervention practice.

The Art of Questioning and Listening: Continuing the Assessment Process

Careful Questioning as Essential to the Assessment Process

THE INFANT OR TODDLER

Careful questioning enriches the assessment process. In addition to the formal assessment inventories or scales that are mentioned previously, the practitioner considers questions that will guide his or her thinking about a particular baby or parent, the dynamics of their relationship, and the caregiving environment. Some initial questions may include the following: Who is the baby in need in this family? How old is he or she at the time of your visit? What are some of the unique characteristics of the baby? Does the baby smile in response to a face or a voice? Is the baby able to communicate wants or needs clearly? Is the baby active, responsive, engaging, or not? Is the baby aware of or interested in people or activities? Is the baby responsive to caregivers? Does the baby brighten, gurgle, vocalize, or talk? Can the baby be comforted? What happens when the parent holds, touches, or amuses the baby?

The questions will vary according to the baby's age and ability. The practitioner learns to keep the questions in mind in order to keep the focus on the baby and to continuously record or note the changing developmental capacities or risks.

THE PARENT

The practitioner in training also wonders about the parent. The following questions may guide the practitioner in thinking deeply about the parent alone and in relationship to the infant: How old is the parent? How does he or she interact with or respond to you? Is he or she able to hold, stroke, comfort, feed, or attend to the baby's needs? Does he or she appear agitated, depressed, tearful, angry, or lonely? Is the mother or father's health or mental health a concern? Is he or she able to recognize the baby's cues and respond appropriately? Is he or she able to differentiate cries and cues? Is he or she consistent in offering care, emotionally responsive, understanding of wants and needs, and able to set limits that are appropriate to the infant's age? Is he or she able to follow the baby's lead?

THE RELATIONSHIP

When observing the infant and the parent together, the practitioner also learns to consider the developing relationship: Are the interactions synchronous, smooth, and carefully tuned? Do parent and infant follow each other's lead, smiling, talking, reaching, or touching? Is there a sense of pleasure shared in the games they play? How would you describe the relationship that is developing between them? Does the infant appear safe with the parent, protected and secure?

These and similar questions invite trainees or practitioners new to the field to think deeply about the details of early development as they are observed within a relationship context and incorporate those details into the assessment (Weatherston & Tableman, 1989; Hirshberg, 1993, 1996). Table 4.2 summarizes basic competencies for building a relationship with the parents and the infant.

THE CONTEXT FOR DEVELOPMENT

Finally, the practitioner also organizes his or her observations about the environment in which an infant and parent live. What is life like for this baby and this parent every day? Questions may include: Where does the baby reside (home, hospital, or foster care)? Who provides for the baby's daily care? Who else lives there? How safe does the baby appear to be? What is the level of activity in the home? Where does the baby sleep? Are basic needs for food, clothing, and protection met? Are there family members or friends to offer guidance and support?

Answers to these questions may come slowly. They are most important as guides throughout the assessment process.

Listening

A SAFE BASE

The practitioner learns to create a context in which families feel safe enough to talk. Attentive, respectful, and genuinely concerned, the practitioner or trainee follows the parent's lead and listens without interruption, approaches with consideration and warmth, and is nonjudgmental. Sensitive to each parent's successes and to each infant's strengths, the practitioner learns to identify what is going well. The practitioner is also attentive to the vulnerabilities, learns to clarify a parent's wants and needs, and permits the expression of worry or despair. Able to use the relationship with the practitioner as a safe base, parents begin to share their own observations about the baby, their adjustments, developmental questions, and, as appropriate, the details of the pregnancy and the baby's early care.

QUESTIONS

The practitioner or trainee is prepared with an array of questions: When did you first know that you were pregnant? What was your reaction to the news? How did you feel during your pregnancy? Did you expect a baby girl or baby boy? Was someone with you during the baby's birth? Did your labor and delivery go as you expected? Were there any complications or changes in your plans? Did the baby leave the hospital with you? What were the first weeks at home like? How did the early feedings go?

Did you have any help from your family? Was the baby's father able to be around? Does he share in the baby's care?

These and similar questions lead to a shared understanding of the baby's early development and relationship history and the family's needs for support and continuing care (Trout, 1987). Practitioners and trainees learn to ask these questions directly or indirectly, inviting parents to talk about the baby and demonstrating a willingness to listen. The practitioner in training moves slowly, allows parents to set the pace, and proceeds carefully.

PARENTAL HISTORIES

Finally, parental histories may also explain caregiving difficulties and relationship risks. Trainees learn about the importance of personal history as it affects caregiving capacity and parental response. The understanding of dynamics related to family relationships and early child care are vital to the assessment process. Questions that trainees wonder about are those related to abandonment, abrupt and extended separations from parents who provided primary care, histories of physical abuse or neglect, interruptions in relationships, removal to foster care, sexual abuse, exposure to trauma, and unresolved losses. The practitioner gathers historical information carefully and slowly, within the context of a working alliance that is comfortable. This is fundamental to a respectful and skillful assessment process.

Clinical Skillfulness

The infant mental health trainee often visits families in their homes. Close to the source, he or she has an endless number of

---

TABLE 4.2

Basic Competencies for Relationship Building

Use of gestures and expressions that communicate attention and interest in both parent and child.

Communication of sensitivity to parent's and infant's strengths and successes.

Demonstration of a willingness to listen to what each parent has to say.

Acceptance of parent's vulnerabilities, worries, or fears.

Expression of empathy in response to parent's present feelings and concerns for the baby.

Clarification of parent's wants and needs related to the infant.

Offering of patient and consistent support throughout the observation/interview process.

Acknowledgment of parent's wishes to take good care of the baby.

Staying alert to parent's experience of the clinical interview/process.

Wondering about a parent's reluctance or resistance, considering the question (silently), "What is making it difficult for this parent to relate to the baby or to accept my offer of help?"

---

opportunities to watch the infant and parent(s) together, listen, support their interactions, and offer help within the context of the therapeutic relationship. A visitor, the trainee enters thoughtfully and makes the family comfortable in her presence. He or she is sensitive to the parent who is vulnerable: The mother who finds it difficult to hold and feed her baby, the father whose baby has multiple disabilities and delays, or the foster mother who is caring for two toddlers who were removed from their mother's care. Carefully following the parent's lead, the practitioner observes who is there and what is happening, asks careful questions, listens, and responds respectfully. A guest, the trainee does not overwhelm, intrude, or offer judgments prematurely. He or she is there to learn from the family about their baby and how it is he or she might be able to help them (Weatherston, 1997).

In preparing trainees or new practitioners to gather information about the infant or toddler, the parent(s), the nature of their relationship(s), and the caregiving environment, trainers and/or supervisors invite trainees to wonder about many things. The questions raised in the previous section guide trainees in their efforts to learn what is important when assessing the capacities and the risks of each child and family referred for infant mental health or early developmental services. The questions are meant to encourage reflection. They may or may not be asked directly. The trainee is advised to approach each family individually and to take great care when interviewing for clinical concerns (Hirshberg, 1996; Trout, 1987; Weatherston & Tableman, 1989).

Building an Alliance

As noted earlier in this discussion, the assessment of children under three and their families requires a commitment to working relationships. The development of a trusting relationship between each parent/caregiver and trainee/practitioner is essential to the assessment process. As trainees and practitioners new to the field of infant and family practice build relationships with families, they experience how vital relationships are to the assessment process.

Incorporation of these experiences into a training program helps trainees to learn how to establish a context for relationship with a parent, understanding the importance of what occurs within it (Hirshberg, 1993). This is fundamental to effective practice.

Identification of Risks

Indications of Risk

The identification of risk in infancy and early parenthood is essential to the assessment process. Most generally, the indications of risk and need for supportive intervention lie within the infant or toddler, the parent or mothering figure, their developing relationship, and/or the context in which the infant and parent(s) live. In some instances, the risks are constitutional and rest mainly with the infant or toddler. In other instances, the risks cluster around the parent as primary caregiver, often the mother. In many cases, there are worries about both child and parent, including constitutional and maturational factors, psychosocial indicators, and the context of relationship care (Emde, 1989).

A trainee or practitioner new to the practice of infant mental health becomes familiar with many risk indicators, so he or she can observe or inquire about them, listen carefully to the parent's concerns, and relate them all, in partnership with parents, to a meaningful service plan. At the same time, he or she keeps in mind the infant or toddler's strengths, parental capacities to provide adequate care, and aspects that offer hopefulness for development and change. The last is often a challenging requirement, but extremely important to the early identification of strengths and risks and the possibility for intervention through a trusting relationship with each family referred.

Early Indicators of Risk:
The Infant or Toddler

Trainees and beginning practitioners learn to appreciate the variety of risks that encompass early development programs. The infants referred may be constitutionally vulnerable babies who cannot wait beyond the first weeks or months of life for prevention or early intervention support. They may be premature babies, underweight, irritable, difficult to comfort, or difficult to feed. Slow-to-gain or failing-to-thrive, they are at high risk for significant disabilities or developmental delays. Others may be difficult to engage, inattentive, unresponsive, or withdrawn. Still others may be highly active and hypersensitive, disorganized in their approaches to people or playthings, and unable to send clear signals to tell their caregiving parents what

they want or need. They may be unrewarding babies to take care of and at high risk for problematic care.

Other babies may be referred because of maturational concerns. A health care provider may suspect a delay in one or several developmental domains, for example, slow to sit or crawl, slow to smile or respond, or unable to separate. A parent may worry about a disturbance in development, a regression or developmental arrest. Still other referrals may be made because of a toddler's behavior, for example, biting, head banging, aggression that is out of control, significant withdrawal, or emotional retreat. Infant mental health trainees learn to observe a range of conditions in early infancy in order to be familiar with a range of developmental risks and delays.

Early Indicators of Risk:
The Parent(s)

In a substantial number of cases, a referral may be made during pregnancy or immediately following a baby's birth. The pregnancy may be healthy, and the infant may be constitutionally robust at delivery, with capacities to adapt and interact from the moment he or she opens his or her eyes. The referral is made because someone is worried about the parent(s). Will he or she be able to take care of the baby without clinical support? What factors may concern practitioners? If pregnant, a parent may express strong ambivalence or hostility about the birth of another child. A woman may have considered abortion or adoption up until the delivery of her baby. She may have lost previous pregnancies or delivered a still-born child. All of these factors raise "red flags" and suggest that the supportive presence of an infant and family specialist may reduce the risk of rejection of the baby, a jeopardized attachment relationship, neglect, abuse, or developmental delay.

Other conditions place infants and relationships at risk. The primary caregiver, usually the mother, may appear unprepared for the care of a baby, overburdened, or seriously depressed. She may be inattentive to the baby's needs, unable to be emotionally present. She may not be able to hold, feed, or provide routine care. She may not be able to enter into a loving relationship, provide developmental encouragement, or keep the baby safe. Of additional concern, a parent may have a history of early and unresolved losses that makes the care of this baby troublesome, for example, extended separations in early childhood, maternal rejection, neglectful care, or placement in foster care. Another parent may be too young, alone in the care of her baby, impulsive, or unrealistic in her expectations. Of additional concern is a parent who has a serious mental illness or developmental delay and, when faced with the responsibilities of parenthood, is not able to provide consistent or contingent care. All of these factors place an infant or toddler and parent at risk. Early referral for assessment and treatment may reduce the likelihood of developmental failure, abuse, or parental neglect.

Early Indicators of Risk: The Caregiving Environment

Of equal concern is the context in which an infant is raised. Homelessness, hunger, joblessness, poverty, alcoholism, and drug use place enormous burdens on families. These factors exacerbate the risks that parents face in taking care of their children, in responding to their needs to be fed when they are hungry, clothed, sheltered, comforted, and safe. Any of these conditions place infants and families in jeopardy, at risk for developmental failures. In combination, they alert infant mental health trainees to the need for immediate outreach, observation and inquiry, careful listening, early nurturing, and relationship-focused response.

The stakes are high. Babies and families in crisis cannot wait. Trainees and practitioners new to the field learn about infancy, early parenthood, relationship development, family functioning, capacities, and risks. Trainees identify the realities of young children's lives within the context of caregiving and family relationships.

Effective practitioners observe infants and parents together and wonder about the nature of early interactions and relationships. Families need practitioners who are able to listen carefully, ask questions that are thoughtful, gather information about the baby and early caregiving, and use formal developmental guides or diagnostic criteria, as appropriate. Above all, infants and families need practitioners who are able to invite parental participation throughout the assessment process, make an effort to establish warm and trusting relationships with the family, and consider parents' feelings in response to the observations and interviews. Knowledgeable and skillful, practitioners learn to organize their understanding in a meaningful and practical way, communicate carefully, and invite a supportive partnership with parents. Finally, all screenings and assessments should be carried out within the context of a team or supervisory relationship where observations may be discussed, questions raised, and the process explored (Meisels & Provence, 1989).

Clearly, the issues surrounding the preparation of professionals to assess young children and families are complex. They require attention to development (Meisels & Provence, 1989; Greenspan & Meisels, 1996), the environment (Sameroff & Fiese, 1990), context (Messick, 1983), and process (Meisels, 1996). University-based academic programs or in-service programs that are part of a personnel development plan must be designed to address these issues. At the least, training programs must offer opportunities for students and practitioners to use screening and assessment approaches appropriate for infants and toddlers and understand and relate to families.

Assessment within the Context of Careful Supervision

Supervision: The Learning Relationship

Careful observation of the infant and parent(s) together, the use of formal or informal scales or tools, gentle questioning, and thoughtful listening are requirements for a successful assessment. The practitioner in training learns to organize an abundance of information about a baby, the family, devel-

oping relationships, and the caregiving environment. In the best of circumstances, the trainee brings the details of his or her visits into individual meetings with a training supervisor. Together, they will consider the infant's developing competencies, contributions to the parent-infant relationship, disturbances, and risks. They will think about the parent(s), their capacities to nurture and respond to the infant, their worries, and their hopes. Supervisor and trainee will review the details of developmental observations and clinical interviews. They will wonder what might explain disturbances, delays, or an inappropriate caregiving response. Later, as their trust in one another grows, supervisor and trainee will look more closely at the feelings awakened in the presence of a particular parent and infant as they relate to the assessment process and to the trainee. At its best, the relationship between supervisor and trainee is a learning relationship (Bertacchi & Coplon, 1991; Shanok, 1992), offering a place for questioning, shared understanding, guidance, and support.

With time and attention, the supervisory relationship will develop. Many programs offer training and supervision for one year. The training supervisor has many responsibilities. He or she needs to be reliable, consistent, and emotionally available to the trainee. He or she establishes a routine, agreeing to meet regularly at a certain time and in a certain place. There should be no interruptions so that the supervisor is able to watch and listen carefully. Attentive throughout the hour, the supervisor sends a powerful message to each trainee. "You are most important right now. You will get all of my attention." Emotionally present, the supervisor creates a context in which each trainee feels protected and safe. He or she follows the trainee's lead, attending to verbal and nonverbal cues, observing carefully, and offering guidance or an empathic response. Devoted and invested, the supervisor serves as a continuing source of knowledge and support. He or she offers reassurance and praise as appropriate, building the trainee's confidence in observing and assessing infants and families referred for early services and providing continuing services.

As relationship-based services to infants and families have increased, practitioners and supervisors have written about the importance of the supervisory relationship to effective service designs. Rebecca Shamoon Shanok (1992, p. 37) writes, "When it is going well, supervision is a holding environment, a place to feel secure enough to expose insecurities, mistakes, questions and differences." Within the supervisory relationship, so much growth is possible for a trainee. Safely held, the trainee grows more resourceful and confident, informed about the observations he or she makes, and more emotionally available to the families he or she serves. At the same time, he or she may begin to consider personal responses to the clinical relationships he or she has entered (Bertacchi & Coplon, 1991; Schafer, 1996). The trainee flourishes within this encouraging and trusting teaching relationship.

As in the work itself, each training relationship is unique. The supervisor establishes the parameters and offers a context in which each trainee may discuss and explore assessments and continuing services to infants and families. The depth and intensity of the relationship varies according to the individual experiences and needs of each trainee. Important to Selma Fraiberg's original training model, the supervisory relationship continues today to be most significant to the trainee's learning process (Fenichel & Eggbeer, 1990; Schafer, 1996).

Assessment through Observation: A Clinical Example

What follows are details from a trainee's first visit to a family referred for assessment services. The summary illustrates the complexity of the assessment process and many challenges that a practitioner or trainee faces when asked to integrate theories, principles, and practices into real work with children under three and the family.

Come with me into the kitchen. It is approximately 10 o'clock in the morning. Dishes are piled high in the sink, and food from last night's dinner sits on the counter. The room is hot. The windows are shut, and although the sun shines high in the sky outside, the shades are drawn as if to protect against the intrusion of light. The 26-month-old toddler protests. He wants to get out of his high chair. His mother ignores him until he shrieks. She sets him free. The baby, 6-months-old, restrained in her infant seat, cries in the next room. The toddler brings me toys and wants to climb up on my lap, me, the strange home visitor. The toddler's face is smudged with traces of breakfast. He uses no words, just tugs at my sleeve to invite my interest. I respond, but very carefully, knowing that his mother, distracted and anxious, also needs my attention.

A visiting nurse had made the referral of this family several weeks ago. She was concerned about the baby's poor weight gain, the toddler's development, and the mother's depression. When I had called to inquire about the mother's interest in the Infant-Parent Program, she agreed, somewhat reluctantly, to let me come. "I'll be here, but I don't know what you can do."

As I sit at the table, I see that she is overwhelmed by the care of two small children. She does not seem to hear the baby's cries and grows impatient with the 26-month-old, who continues to bang a toy on the floor. She reaches to take the toy from his hand, but he moves quickly and darts away, ignoring her and now out of reach. She shouts, "Come here!" He says nothing. New at this job, I watch and listen ever so carefully, trying to make sense of what they are showing me, but uncertain about what to say. I wonder how often one of them has reached out only to have the other turn or move away. I wonder what explains the struggle between them. I comment quietly, "He moves so quickly. How do you keep up with him and the baby, too?" She smiles, "He is quick. Gets away from me now." I continue to describe what I see—a toddler who is pretty coordinated and likes to run and is curious. I also ask her if there is something she and he like especially to do. "Well, we used to have fun together, just him and me, until the baby came and was so sick and everything." I invite her to tell me more about this. As if no one has asked or listened to this story before, she begins to tell me. "The baby came too early. They had to take her from me. She was very small and blue. They held her up for me to

see her, but then they took her away in a hurry. I couldn't hold her or see her for almost a day. It was really scary and for a while I didn't think that she was going to live." The story is a difficult and painful one, but I try to remain attentive and respond by saying, "How very frightened you must have been! That was a very difficult beginning for you and for your baby."

She tells me a little more, and I notice some relief. She glances again at the toddler who has moved closer to her feet. She reaches out to him, and this time he allows her to pull him onto her lap. I notice that it is almost time for me to leave and tell them, "Our time is almost up. What has happened is very difficult and important for you to talk about. I could come back next week if you would like." The young mother agrees, and before she lets me out, she sets the toddler down on the chair and goes to get the baby. "She was crying real hard. Maybe she's hungry. Hold her while I get her bottle filled," she demands and thrusts the baby into my arms. I notice that the baby has a few curls and staring eyes. Her arms thrash about making it difficult for me to hold her easily. She continues to cry, and I call out to her mother, "She's not very content with me. She seems to be looking for you!" Janna returns with a warm bottle of milk, takes the baby, and begins to feed her. They both settle down. I say quietly, "That's just what she wanted, her mom and her bottle!" I am distracted by the toddler who now lies quietly on the floor, slightly withdrawn, rocking side to side, and sucking his thumb. I would like to stay, but need to go. "Bye-bye, see you next week," I tell him. "I'll come next Tuesday at 1 o'clock in the afternoon," I remind Janna.

I leave, feeling overwhelmed, emotionally exhausted, and ambivalent about going back. I'm hungry. I drive away as quickly as I can to the nearest fast-food line. Once fed, I settle down and wonder about the hour's home visit. "What about the baby?" I hardly got a glimpse. She looked so tiny and distressed. "What about the toddler?" He was fussy, lively, and then so quiet. I wonder if he has some significant delays or if he, too, might be depressed. "What about Janna? Does she have family or friends around to help her? Is she caring for these children by herself? Where is the baby's father?" Many questions dance around in my head. "Will I be able to really connect with Janna, so she can more consistently hold and feed and take pleasure in the care of her children? Will I be able to listen to all she needs to tell me about her babies, her role as a new mother, and relationships, past and present? Will I be able to find and speak about competencies in the midst of all this? Will I be able to understand the risks and do something about them, too?"

The young trainee will bring the details of her initial visit to her supervisor for guidance and support as they reflect on the details of the observation and their meaning to the assessment process.

Assessment within the Context of Supervision: An Example

Supervision is vital for clinical growth. Regularly scheduled meetings with a trusted supervisor create opportunities for the trainee to think deeply about babies and families. Together, they will explore the importance of relationships for early development and health and consider strategies for effective assessment and intervention. As the trainee finds words to describe what he or she has seen and experienced in the presence of a particular family, the training supervisor follows the trainee's lead carefully. The following example illustrates the supervisory meeting following the trainee's visit to Janna and her two young children. The trainee, a master's prepared social worker, is new to the practice of infant mental health and has been enrolled in the training program for three months. She expresses considerable alarm following her visit to this young family.

"The baby looked so lonely. She was strapped into her infant seat almost the whole time I was there. Janna didn't pick her up, until the very end. She didn't seem to notice how uncomfortable the baby was." The supervisor listens to the trainee's poignant description and acknowledges that it takes a great deal of courage to observe a baby so closely and to feel her distress. The trainee continues to offer details about the hour's visit. She describes the mother as "Young, alone, and fearful. She could hardly look at me when she talked." The supervisor again acknowledges how strong one has to be to experience the neediness of a mother who appears lonely and afraid. The trainee wonders how she can really help them. "They need so much, and I am so new." Her own uncertainty is clear. The supervisor offers supportive comments. "You learned so much in this first visit that will be helpful in understanding what the baby and her brother and mother might need. You are quite a careful observer and listener."

The supervisor continues by inquiring about what the trainee thinks the baby needs right now. "I guess she needs someone to notice that she is there, hold or comfort her when she cries, and offer her something to eat when she is hungry," the trainee says. The supervisor agrees and wonders if those same things might guide the trainee in planning for the next visit. "Continue to notice what each is doing. Stay very attentive and follow their lead. This might begin to feel difficult. You may want to be more active. You may want to pick the baby up out of that seat or be more directive with the toddler! Instead, hold them with your presence and also with your words. Invite the mother to tell you more about the baby since she seemed to respond to that. You might be the first person to have asked this. Respond with as much empathy as you can. She is young and new at this and seems pretty overwhelmed! If her eyes wander to the toddler, ask her a little more about him—what kind of a child he is, what he likes to do now. Reassure them that you will come back again."

The trainee looks more confident. The color returns to her face. Before the hour ends, the supervisor confirms the time of their next meeting and invites the trainee to call her before that if she has any questions at all. As the session ends, the supervisor says, "They are so lucky to have you take an interest in the baby's development and in the toddler's care. I imagine no one else has watched or listened so intently. I'll be thinking of you." At its best, supervision offers trainees a place for reflection about one's observations and the development of one's professional growth (Bertacchi & Coplon, 1993).

Conclusion

In conclusion, the training of infant mental health practitioners to assess infants, tod-dlers, and their families requires knowledge about infancy and early parenthood, opportunities to observe and listen, a place in which to think and ask questions, and learning relationships with trusted supervisors and peers. These are the cornerstones of reflective and effective infant mental health practice.

References

Baltman, K. (1993, October–December). Training professionals to look into space. *The Infant Crier,* no. 62, p. 4.

Barnard, K., & Erickson, M. (1976). *Teaching children with developmental problems: A family care approach.* St. Louis: Mosby.

Bayley, N. (1993). *Bayley Scales of Infant Development II* (2nd ed.). San Antonio: The Psychological Corporation.

Bernstein, V., Pekarsky J., & Weschler, N. (1996). Strengthening families through strengthening relationships: The ounce of prevention fund developmental training and support program. In M. Roberts (Ed.), *Model programs in child and family mental health.* Chicago: Earlbaum.

Bertacci, J., & Coplon, (1991). The professional use of self in prevention. In E. Fenichel (Ed.), *Learning through supervision and mentorship* (pp. 84–90). Zero to Three. Washington, DC.

Bick, E. (1964). Notes on infant observation in psychoanalytic training. *International Journal of Psychoanalysis, 45,* 558–566.

Brazelton, T. B. (1973). *Neonatal Behavioral Assessment Scale.* Philadelphia: Lippincott.

Caldwell, B. (1978). *HOME Scale.* Center

for Research on Teaching and Learning. Little Rock: University of Arkansas.

Davies, D. (1992, April). *Beginning an infant mental health case.* Paper presented at the Michigan Association for Infant Mental Health Conference, Ann Arbor, MI.

Emde, R. (1989). The infant's relationship experience: Developmental and clinical aspects. In A. J. Sameroff & R. N. Emde (Eds.), *Relationship disturbances in early childhood* (pp. 33–51). New York: Basic Books.

Fenichel, E., & Eggbeer, L. (1990). *Preparing practitioners to work with infants, toddlers and their families.* National Center for Clinical Infant Programs, Washington, DC.

Fisher, C. & Osofsky, J. (1997). Training the applied developmental scientist for prevention and practice: Two current examples. *Social Policy Report, 11*(2) 6–18.

Foulds, B. (1997). Personal training materials, Detroit, Wayne State University, MI.

Fraiberg, S. (Ed.). (1980). *Clinical studies in infant mental health.* New York: Basic Books.

Fraiberg, S., & Adelson, E. (1977). An abandoned mother, an abandoned baby. *Bulletin Menninger Clinic, 41,* 162–180.

Fraiberg, S., Shapiro, V., & Adelson, E. (1976). Infant-parent psychotherapy on behalf of child in a critical nutritional state. *Psychoanalytic Study of the Child, 31,* 461–491.

Freud, W. E. (1975). Well-baby profile. *Psychoanalytic Study of the Child*

Goldberg, S. (1998). Personal training materials. Detroit, MI: Wayne State University.

Greenspan, S., & Meisels, S. (1996). Toward a new vision for the developmental assessment of infants and young children. In S. Meisels & E. Fenichel (Eds.), *New visions for the developmental assessment*

of infants and young children (pp. 11–26). Washington, DC: Zero to Three.

Harmon, R. (1994/1995). Diagnostic thinking about mental health and developmental disorders in infancy and early childhood: A core skill for infant/family professionals. *Bulletin for Zero to Three, 15*(3), 11–15.

Harmon, R., & Frankel, K. (1997). The growth and development of an infant mental health program: An integrated perspective. *Infant Mental Health Journal, 18,* 126–134.

Hirshberg, L. (1993). Clinical interviews with infants and their families. In C. Zeanah (Ed.), *Handbook of infant mental health* (pp. 173–90). New York: Guilford Press.

Hirshberg, L. (1996). History-making, not history-taking. In S. Meisels & E. Fenichel (Eds.), *New visions for the developmental assessment of infants and young children* (pp. 85–124) Washington, DC: Zero to Three.

Lieberman, A. (1998). An infant mental health perspective. *Bulletin for Zero to Three, 18*(3), 3–5.

Lieberman, A., & Pawl, J. (1993). Infant-parent psychotherapy. In C. Zeanah (Ed.), *Handbook of infant mental health* (pp. 427–42). New York: Guilford Press.

Lieberman, A., Van Horn, P., Grandison, C., & Pekarsky, J. (1997). Mental health assessment of infants, toddlers, and preschoolers in a service program and a treatment outcome research program. *Infant Mental Health Journal, 18,* 158–170.

Massie, H., & Campbell, B. K. (1983). *Attachment during stress.* San Francisco: Children's Hospital and Medical Center.

Meisels, S. (1996). Charting the continuum of assessment and intervention. In S. Meisels & E. Fenichel (Eds.), *New visions for the developmental assessment of infants and young children* (pp. 27–52). Washington, DC: Zero to Three.

Meisels, S., & Fenichel, E. (Eds.). (1996). *New visions for the developmental assessment of infants and young children.* Washington, DC: Zero to Three.

Meisels, S., & Provence, S. (1989). *Screening and assessment: Guidelines for identifying young disabled and developmentally vulnerable children and their families.* Arlington, VA: Zero to Three.

Messick, S. (1983). Assessment of children. In W. Kessen (Ed.), *Handbook of child psychology: Vol. 1* (pp. 477–526). New York: Wiley.

Michigan Association for Infant Mental Health. (1983). *Training for infant mental health specialists: Suggested guidelines for teaching institutions.* Lansing, MI: Author.

Miller, L., Rustin, M., Rustin, M., & Shuttleworth, J. (Eds.). (1991). *Closely observed infants.* London: Duckworth & Co.

Pawl, J. (1995). On supervision. In L. Eggbeer & E. Fenichel (Eds.), *Educating and supporting the infant/family work force: Models, methods and materials* (pp. 21–29) Arlington, VA: Zero to Three.

Reid, S. (Ed.). (1997). *Developments in infant observation: The Tavistock model.* London: Routledge.

Sameroff, A. J., & Fiese, B. H. (1990). Transactional regulation and early intervention. In S. J. Meisels & J. P. Shonkoff (Eds.), *Handbook of early childhood intervention* (pp. 119–149). New York: Cambridge University Press.

Schafer, W. (1992). The professionalization of early motherhood. In E. Fenichel (Ed.), *Learning through supervision and mentorship* (pp. 67–75). Arlington, VA: Zero to Three.

Schafer, W. (1995). Clinical training seminar. Detroit, MI: Wayne State University.

Schafer, W. (October–December 1996). Clinical supervision is a necessity for infant specialists. *The Infant Crier,* No. 77, p. 6.

Shanok, R. (1992). The supervisory relationship: Integrator, resource and guide. In E. Fenichel (Ed.), *Learning through supervision and mentorship* (pp. 37–41). Arlington, VA: Zero to Three.

Shapiro, V., Adelson, E., & Tableman, B. (Eds.). (1982). The introduction of infant mental health services in Michigan. *Infant Mental Health Journal, 3,* 69–141.

Tableman, B. (1982). Infant mental health: A new frontier. *Infant Mental Health Journal, 3,* 72–76.

Thomas, J., Guskin, K., & Klass, C. (1997). Early development program: Collaborative structures and processes. *Infant Mental Health Journal, 18*(2), 198–208.

Trout, M. (1982). The language of parent-infant interaction. In J. Stack (Ed.), *The Special Infant* (pp. 265–82). New York: Human Sciences Press.

Trout, M. (1987). *Working papers on process in infant mental health assessment and intervention.* Champaign, IL: The Infant-Parent Institute.

Tuters, E. (1988). The relevance of infant observation to clinical training and practice: An interpretation. *Infant Mental Health Journal, 9*(1), 93–104.

Weatherston, D. (1998). Personal clinical training seminar materials. Detroit, MI: Wayne State University.

Weatherston, D. (1997). She needed to talk and I needed to listen. *Bulletin for Zero to Three, 18*(3), 6–12.

Weatherston, D., & Baltman, K. (1992, September). *The training of infant mental health practitioners.* Paper presented at the World Association for Infant Mental Health Conference, Chicago, IL.

Weatherston, D., & Tableman, B. (1989). *In-*

fant mental health services: Supporting competencies/reducing risks. Lansing, MI: Michigan Department of Mental Health.

Winnicott, D. (1965). *The maturational processes and the facilitating environment.* Madison, WI: International Universities Press.

Wright, B. (1986). An approach to infant-parent psychotherapy. *Infant Mental Health Journal, 7*(4), 247–263.

Zeanah, C., Boris, N., Heller, S., Hinshaw-Fuselier, S. L., Larrieu, J., Lewis, M., Palomino, R., Rovaris, M., & Valliere, J. (1997). Relationship assessment in infant mental health. *Infant Mental Health Journal, 18,* 182–197.

5

—

Preventive Infant Mental Health: Uses of the Brazelton Scale

J. Kevin Nugent and T. Berry Brazelton

5

Introduction

The Brazelton Neonatal Behavioral Assessment Scale (BNBAS) has been in use for over 25 years in research and clinical settings across the world, and as such, it can be said that it has played a major role in expanding our understanding of the phenomenology of newborn behavior. The Brazelton Scale is a neurobehavioral assessment scale and was designed to describe the newborn's responses to his or her new extrauterine environment and document the contribution of the newborn infant to the development of the emerging parent-child relationship (Brazelton, 1973, 1985; Brazelton & Nugent, 1995). It has also enriched our understanding of the competencies and complexities of newborn behavior and helped us identify the multiplicity of variables which influence newborn behavior and development. It has, therefore, added to our understanding of what can be considered normal or typical and has broadened our appreciation of the range of variability of newborn behavior and the relationship between prenatal influences and newborn behavior and the relationship between newborn behavior and later development. The research generated by the Brazelton Scale has also contributed to the clinician's understanding of the *process* of neonatal adaptation and the development of the emerging parent-child relationship.

While the Brazelton Scale has been used in hundreds of research studies as an outcome measure and continues to be used as a means of assessing the effects of a wide range of pre- and perinatal influences on newborn behavior, there has been a gradual shift toward its use as an educational tool with parents in clinical settings. Today,

The authors would like to thank Beth Higley for her critical comments and Sinead O'Connor and Allison Clapp for their assistance in preparing this chapter.

it is being used by many mental health clinicians as a means of supporting parents in their efforts to meet the needs of their new baby and as a means of forming a relationship with or developing a therapeutic alliance with parents (Bruschwieler-Stern, 1997; Candilis-Huisman, 1997; Cardone & Gilkerson, 1990; Keefer, 1995; Nugent, 1985; Nugent & Brazelton, 1989; Stern, 1995). The BNBAS is unique in that it can be used by the clinician to gather objective data about the infant's behavior. In the context of conducting a clinical session with parents, these data yield a comprehensive profile of behavior that is at the core of the treatment and is used to organize the experience of the family around the new infant. In practice, the value of the BNBAS for the mental health clinician is that the scale provides an assessment of the infant's current level of functioning across behavioral domains, describing both strengths and weaknesses while at the same time providing a blueprint to help parents better understand their infant and, thereby, support them in developing a positive and productive relationship with their infant.

Newborn Behavior and Development

Over the past 10 years, an ever-expanding canon of research confirms that the neonate's behavior can no longer be assumed to be biologically determined (Sameroff, 1993). Infant behavior at birth is phenotypic, not genotypic, so that intrauterine nutrition, infection (Lester & Brazelton, 1982;

Oyemade et al., 1994), and drugs (Fried & Makin, 1986; Coles, Platzman, Smith, James, & Falek, 1992; Beeghly & Tronick, 1994; Chasnoff, Griffith, MacGregor, Dirkes, & Burns, 1989; Dreher, Nugent, & Hudgins, 1994; Eyler, Behnke, Conlon, Woods, & Wobie, 1997) are affecting the fetus throughout pregnancy, interacting with genetic endowment to shape newborn behavior. There is rapidly accumulating evidence that the newborn infant is powerfully shaped before delivery, and routine perinatal events, such as maternal medication and anesthesia and episodes of hypoxia, further influence his or her reactions (Sepkoski, Lester, Ostheimer, & Brazelton, 1992). Research shows that extrauterine stimulation which involves the pregnant mother may also be shaping the neonate's learning in utero and may be influencing prenatal brain development (Dobbing, 1990; deCasper, Lecaunet, Busnel, Granier-Deferre, & Maugeais, 1991, 1994; Fifer & Moon, 1994). This has led to the recognition that the infant has well-established behavioral endowments at birth and the infant's development is influenced by both biological and environmental influences from the beginning.

These studies have also yielded an extensive taxonomy of newborn and infant behavior, showing that, for example, the newborn can visually track (Dannemiller & Freedland, 1991; Laplante, Orr, Neville, Vorkapich, & Sasso, 1996; Slater, Morison, Town, & Rose, 1985), hear and locate sounds (Muir & Field, 1979), and remember speech sounds (Swain, Zelazo, & Clifton, 1993). This body of research also demonstrates that the newborn infant is a social organism, predisposed to interact with his or her caregiver from the beginning and able to elicit the kind of caregiving necessary for his or her successful adaptation. The newborn seems to prefer the mother's voice (deCasper & Spence, 1991; Spence & Freeman, 1996), can imitate facial expressions (Field, Woodson, Greenberg, & Cohen, 1982), and clearly discriminate her mother's face from that of a stranger (Pascalis, de Shonen, Morton, Deruelle, & Fabre-Grenet, 1995).

What the Brazelton Scale body of research has added to this is evidence for the baby's capacity for self-regulation and affective regulation. After two decades of intensive research on newborn behavior and development, the human newborn has emerged as competent, complexly organized, and playing an active role in shaping his or her own development. The Brazelton Scale, therefore, does not merely provide a catalog of newborn competencies but over the course of serial examinations over the first weeks of life, allows us to see how the baby's discrete behaviors are integrated into coherent patterns of behavior and identify what role the caregiver can play in facilitating the infant's adaptation and development.

The Developmental Agenda of the First Two Months: The Development of Self-Regulation

Development by definition, proceeds from a state of relative globality and lack of differentiation to a state of increasing differentiation, articulation, and hierarchic integration (Werner, 1948). The BNBAS was designed to describe this process of differentiation as the infant learns to control and organize his or her responses to the new environment over time. The scope of the Brazelton Scale extends from birth to the third month of life and is designed to describe the infant's adaptation and development, specifically the capacity for self-regulation over that period of time. The task of self-regulation must be successfully negotiated before the infant can maintain prolonged moments of mutual gaze with his or her caregiver and develop the capacity for shared mutual engagement that constitutes the major task of the next stage of development (Adamson, 1993; Stern, 1995). From this developmental perspective, the BNBAS enables us to systematically study behavioral changes over time by describing the process of hierarchic integration of the different domains or systems of behavior over the first two months. The newborn infant is seen to face a series of hierarchically organized developmental challenges as he or she attempts to adapt to his or her new extrauterine world, both the inanimate and animate world (Brazelton, 1981). This includes the infant's capacity to first regulate his or her physiological or autonomic system, then his or her state behavior, his or her motor behavior, and finally, his or her affective interactive behavior, that develops in a stagelike epigenetic progression over the first two months of life.

The first and basic task for the newborn is *to organize his or her autonomic or physiologic behavior.* This involves dealing with stress related to homeostatic adjustments of the central nervous system. It involves the task of stabilizing his or her breathing, reducing the number of startles and tremors, and being able to maintain temperature control. When this homeostatic adjustment has been achieved, the newborn can move on to the second task—that of *regulating or controlling his or her motor behavior.* This means gaining control over and inhibiting random motor movements, developing better muscle tone, and reducing excessive motor activity. Although these challenges may not develop in an absolute sequence and they may be contemporaneous, there is an assumption of a hierarchic progression, such that each precedes the next. The third challenge of this period is *state regulation.* This is the ability to modulate his or her states of consciousness. This includes the ability to develop robust and predictable sleep and wake states and what could be called sleep protection or the ability to screen out negative stimuli while asleep. State control means that the infant is able to deal with stress, either through self-regulation strategies such as hand-to-mouth maneuvers or is able to communicate with the caregiver through crying and be consoled with the caregiver's help. The final task for the newborn is the *regulation of his or her affective interactive or social behavior.* This involves the capacity to maintain prolonged alert periods, the ability to attend to visual and auditory stimuli within his or her range, and the ability to seek out and engage in social interaction with the caregiver.

The BNBAS can reveal where along this hierarchic continuum the individual baby falls and in which domain he or she needs support and what kind of support he or she may need. Nevertheless, this developmental agenda and the baby's capacity to protect his or her sleep and develop pre-

dictable sleep and wake states, cope with stress, and respond to his or her environment can only be achieved with the support of the caregiver. The Brazelton Scale is designed to help the clinician and caregiver together identify where the infant needs support and how they can provide this support. Management of crying and sleep are two of the most overwhelming concerns of parents in these early months (Anders, Halpern, & Hua, 1992; Barr, 1990; Wolke, Gray, & Meyer, 1994). The Brazelton Scale can be used as a tool in providing guidance to parents on the most appropriate ways to manage sleep and crying behavior in a way that is responsive to the individual baby's needs.

The First Two Months: The Task of Affective Mutual Regulation

There is a growing consensus that the period from birth to the beginning of the third month of life involves not only a major transformation in many neural functions (Hopkins, 1998) and is a major stage in the infant's behavioral adaptation to his or her new environment (Barr, 1998; Rochat, 1998), but also constitutes a major transition stage in the development of the parent-infant relationship (Brazelton, 1993; Emde & Robinson, 1979; Konner, 1998; Sander, Stechler, Burns, & Lee, 1979; Stern, 1995; Trevarthen, 1979). At this stage, the earliest patterns of interaction are taking shape, as infant and parent are in a heightened state of readiness to exchange their first communication signals in their efforts to achieve a mutually satisfying level of affective mutual regulation, what Stern (1985) refers to as "affective attunement." Over the first two months, the infant develops the capacity for shared attentiveness (Adamson, 1993), so that both parent and infant have already embarked on and are actively engaged in an interactive regulative system (Sander et al., 1979).

From the parent's perspective, these first months can be considered a normative crisis, a period characterized by rapid change, as parents search for "the goodness of fit" between themselves and their new baby (Thomas & Chess, 1977). In the case of mothers, Stern refers to this unique but normal psychological condition as the "motherhood constellation," a condition or stage that every mother experiences. With the birth of a baby, a mother passes into a new and unique psychic organization, that will determine "a new set of action tendencies, sensibilities, fantasies, fears and wishes" (Stern, 1995, p. 171). This new condition, in turn, demands that a clinician, using the BNBAS while he or she draws on the baby's behavior as the key informant in this intervention, must be aware of the challenges parents are facing at this time if they are to enter into an empathetic relationship with the mother and develop a therapeutic alliance with the parents. This normative stage in the transition to parenthood has its own protoclinical challenges, the resolution of which will have an impact on the ontogeny of the parent-child relationship, a stage that is potentially conducive of change in the mother's own life development. The core challenge for the new mother is to engage her baby in a way that "fosters the baby's development and in a way that is authentic to her" (Stern, 1995). This involves her ability to nurture and care for the baby, help the baby to grow and thrive physically, become at-

tached to the baby, and provide a secure environment for the baby. Although there is a wide range of cultural variation in the role fathers play in this early stage, it should be pointed out that in most societies, both partners have a unique role to play in the socialization process of the young infant (Nugent, Yogman, Lester, & Hoffmann, 1988).

In summary, the period from birth to three months can be considered a major transition stage in the newborn's adaptation and development. It is a period defined by specific developmental challenges as the newborn attempts to make a successful transition to his or her new extrauterine environment. What the BNBAS has revealed is that this process is highly individualized and there is a wide range of variability in how newborn infants adapt to their new environment over these first two months. This period can be considered a major transition stage in the development of the parent-infant relationship. From an interventionist point of view, it has become clear that this transition period provides the mental health clinician with a remarkable opportunity to play a supportive role in promoting the baby's self-regulation and facilitating the mutual affective regulation process between parent and infant.

The First Two Months: A Formative Period in the Development of the Family

The early months are also unique in that it constitutes a critical transition point in the evolution of the family as a system (Minuchin, 1985; Garbarino, 1992). Indeed, it can be added that these profound life changes are also ecological transitions, as Bronfenbrenner (1979) and Garbarino (1992) point out, in that the birth of a child will irrevocably influence the family system and the wider circle of systems, including the family and neighborhood, that will potentially influence the course of the new baby's future development.

The entry of a baby into an already functioning system irrevocably changes the dynamics of family functioning because the period following birth involves a vital redefinition of roles (Belsky, 1985; Minuchin, 1985). The task of the family system is to accommodate the new member while maintaining a viable relationship among its elements and with its environment. The task of the clinician, then, is to help the family maintain stability within its system and at the same time enable it to be flexible enough to adapt to and accommodate a new element into an already existing, integrated system. Following birth, all family members—mothers, fathers, siblings, and grandparents—have to adjust to the presence of the new family member and to renegotiate their family relationships and roles (Nugent, 1991). The BNBAS can facilitate this major developmental process by helping parents understand the differential effects of the infant on the family and how the infant's behavioral makeup may influence family roles and functioning (Beal, 1986; Fabre-Grenet, 1997; Garbarino, 1982; Murray, 1994; Murray & Cooper, 1997; Myers, 1982).

With the birth of a baby, the family becomes an open system. The mental health clinician has a unique opportunity to enter and become an integral part of the family support system. In high-risk settings, this entry point can provide the clinician with a unique opportunity to support the family and, thereby, counterbalance the risk present within the microsystem itself (Garbarino, 1982, 1992; Klaus, Kennell, & Klaus, 1995). With poor families, single-parent families, or families who feel isolated or have no support system, the mental health clinician can serve as a bridge between the family and the broader community and increase the availability of informal community support for the family and more formal family resource services in the community (Weissbourd & Kagan, 1989; Wolke et al., 1994). This can best be achieved by a long-term partnership between the clinician and family, as illustrated by the Touchpoints model (Stadtler, O'Brien, & Hornstein, 1995). The use of home visitors to provide this kind of support is especially common in Europe, while certain innovative programs in North America involve grandparents (Crockenberg, 1986), foster grandparents making home visits to isolated young mothers during these first months (Anisfield & Pincus, 1978), or peer support groups (Boger & Kornetz, 1985). In such settings, the BNBAS-based intervention sessions conducted in the home or clinic setting can not only serve to strengthen the relationship of the clinician and the family, but can also be used to strengthen the relationship between the family and community support systems.

Preventative Intervention in the Perinatal Period

Although acknowledging the complex web of biological and environmental transactions that influence human development over the life span, many researchers and clinicians believe that preventive intervention in infancy can positively affect later development (Als, 1984; Bottos, 1987; Brazelton & Nugent, 1987; Field, 1987; Konner, 1987; Sameroff, 1993). It is argued that especially under conditions of environmental stress, early intervention can prevent the compounding of problems which occur when the caregiving environment is unable to adjust adequately to meet the needs of the infant (Fabre-Grenet, 1997; Garbarino, 1982; Meisels, Dichtelmiller, & Fong-Ruey, 1993; Zigler & Frank, 1988).

We have presented evidence to suggest that the period from birth to the beginning of the third month of life constitutes a major transition stage in the infant's adaptation to his or her new environment and the development of the parent-infant relationship. That is the time when the earliest patterns of interaction are taking shape, as infant and parent exchange their first communication signals in their efforts to achieve a mutually satisfying level of affective mutual regulation. We argue that it also presents the infant mental health clinician with a unique opportunity to intervene through prevention and support the family, especially under conditions of environmental stress. Although the prenatal period can be seen as an opportune time for primary intervention (Brazelton, 1975; Barnard, Morisset, & Speiker, 1993; Field et al., 1985), it is the immediate postnatal period that presents the clinician with the first epiphany of the parent-infant relationship and thus, the first opportunity for an infant-centered and family-focused intervention. It has been called the intervention touchpoint par excellence (Brazelton, 1994), not only because it comes first in time in the infant's life, but also because it is a time when both infant and parents seem to be in a state of optimal availability for exploratory interaction and mutual exchange, as Stern (1995), De Chateau (1987), Klaus and colleagues (1995), Trevarthen (1979), and Gomes-Pedro and his colleagues (1984, 1995) have demonstrated.

While it can be argued, as Stern (1995) does, that basic clinically relevant issues such as self-regulation, trust, attachment, and individuation are life course issues, the assumption on which this approach to preventative intervention is based is that these issues are being actively negotiated by the infant from the very beginning. As the infant adapts to his new extrauterine environment, his capacity for relatedness is being refined and consolidated. From this perspective, the focus on intervention is to support the infant's efforts to regulate and integrate his or her autonomic, motor, state, and affective systems and thus, consolidate his or her affective interactive capacities so that he or she is ready for the next stage, when face-to-face interaction provides the primary clinical window (Tronick & Cohn, 1989; Weinberg & Tronick, 1997). The infant by then has consolidated his or her autonomic, motor, state, and affective systems so that he or she is ready to demonstrate the full richness of his or her social and affective system to enter face-to-face interaction.

While the scope of the Brazelton Scale per se is confined to descriptions of the baby's behavior, the goal of Brazelton-based intervention is to form a relationship with the mother (parent) in order to provide her with the support she needs to meet the needs of her baby and confirm her role as a mother, adequately meeting her baby's needs. Approaching the third month of life, we find that the infant is no longer challenged by tracking the red ball of the Brazelton Scale but is now more attracted by human stimulation since he or she can now maintain prolonged moments of mutual gaze with an adult caregiver. The infant has moved to a new level of communicative functioning, emerging with a new well-developed capacity for prolonged alertness, gaze modulation, and face-to-face interaction (Barr, 1998; Brazelton, Koslowski, & Main, 1974; Emde & Robinson, 1979; Konner, 1998; Papousek & Papousek, 1987; Stern 1985, 1995; Trevarthyn, 1979). Since the primary goal of the newborn during the first two months is to develop this capacity for shared attentiveness or the capacity to establish and maintain shared mutual engagement with the adult caregiver, the achievement of this level of interactive functioning marks the end of the scope of the Brazelton Scale as a form of assessment or intervention.

The Brazelton Scale

The BNBAS was first published 25 years ago. At the time when it was being developed (Brazelton, 1973), the neonate was still thought of as a passive recipient of environmental stimuli, while the validity of preventative intervention in infancy had yet to be proven and the field of infant mental health had yet to be established. The notion that the baby could indeed see, hear, and respond differentially to positive and negative stimuli was a new idea at time the BNBAS was being conceptualized. Moreover, there was little appreciation of the notion that the newborn infant had an active role to play in his own development from the very beginning and might have the capacity to influence the parent caregiving or the parent-child relationship.

The assessment of neonates was confined to Apgar scores, pediatric examinations of physical competence, and neurological evaluations. These scales were developed with the explicit goal of identifying problems or abnormalities as early as possible in the life cycle. Because they were not based on any particular model of development and lacked an appreciation of the remarkable self-regulation capacities which newborns exhibited, they contributed little to a clinical understanding of the infant or to the understanding that newborn behavior contributed to the development of the parent-child relationship. The Brazelton Scale begins where these scales left off.

Most of the earlier research studies of infancy (Gesell, 1946; Thomas & Chess, 1977; Mahler, 1968) began their observations and assessment of infant behavior at approximately three months. Yet, the explosion of newborn research beginning in the 1960s and 1970s demonstrated that infants were endowed with a wide range of capacities even at birth. In order to understand the baby's adjustment to his new world, clinicians needed a scale to help understand this organization as early as possible. The Graham Scale (Graham, Matarazzo, & Caldwell, 1956) and the Graham-Rosenblith Scale (Rosenblith, 1961) were the first to attempt to outline behavioral differences among neonates as they responded to stimuli. These scales revealed the infant's ability to shut out or handle stimuli by changing state to a habituated or sleep state and that an infant who had too low a threshold for the intake of stimuli (hypersensitivity) or was too disorganized to respond to stimuli was easily overwhelmed by environmental stimulation.

We had to develop a more comprehensive scale, which would document the newborn's marvelous capacity to control levels of stimulation through his or her capacity for state regulation. In working with high-risk infants, we learned that the task of handling psychophysiological stimulation could be a costly task for fragile babies. We surmised that such an infant would be difficult for his or her caretaker as well and might be at risk for neglect or even abuse from an unsupportive social environment. For that reason, from its inception, we recommended that the Brazelton Scale be used as a means of demonstrating the infant's competencies and his or her threshold for responding to environmental stimulation. We began to better understand the capacity of the neonate to reduce interfering and motor activity and control his states in order to respond with socially interactive behaviors. The ability of the neonate to monitor, utilize and control states of consciousness has become one of the most important insights into the marvelous capacities of the human neonate. A fragile newborn has severely diminished capacity in this area and without it

has less opportunity to respond appropriately to environmental cues. In addition, we wanted a clinical tool that would also be compelling to parents, helping parents better understand their baby as an individual and thus, promoting the mother's relationship with her new baby.

Perhaps the most important concept that contributed to a more complete understanding of the newborn and to the development of the Brazelton Scale was the notion of *"states of consciousness."* In 1959, Peter Wolff and later Prechtl (1977) described the following "states of consciousness": Deep (non-REM) and light (REM) sleep states, quiet alert and active alert states, and crying states. States of consciousness are made up of a constellation of behaviors that tend to occur together and can be reliably observed and identified. This discovery led to the important clinical principle that the newborn's states of consciousness inevitably influences the quality of the newborn infant's responses. This discovery presented evidence that the newborn was not at the mercy of his or her environment but that the behavior of the newborn had an inherent organizational structure. Moreover, the newborn infant had predictable—even unique—behavioral patterns. This led to the understanding that "state" was a critical matrix on which to assess all reactions—sensory as well as motor (Brazelton, 1973). In addition, the concept of "state" was to become a powerful concept for parents in helping them understand the appropriateness of their handling techniques or the quality of the stimulation they provided to meet the needs of their infants.

One of the most important conceptual breakthroughs from our clinical and empirical work in using the scale with frail or high-risk neonates has been the concept of a *"lowered threshold"* for taking in, utilizing, and responding to stimuli. A frail neonate or one whose physiological system is still frail has such a low threshold, coupled with an inability to habituate to negative unpredictable stimuli, that he or she is easily overwhelmed. Such a baby is likely to become disorganized, stop breathing, become active, or start crying in order to shut out these overwhelming stimuli. His or her efforts to manage his or her autonomic system mean that he or she will have little energy to modulate motor behavior or sleep and wake states. When he or she is disorganized, still struggling to organize his or her motor system, for example, he or she will be unable to focus on environmental cues. Hence, the opportunity to take in and learn from the environment is seriously endangered. We have learned that these infants can accept reduced stimuli, but with only one modality at a time—either touch, visual, auditory, or kinesthetic. They cannot deal with two modalities. Respecting this need for reduced input, the baby will learn over time to handle more complex stimuli and will organize his or her Central Nervous System (CNS) to interact with a more and more complex environment. Within the context of the BNBAS, parents can learn to respond to their infant in a way that is sensitive to his or her needs and provide the baby with an environment that is sensitive to his or her current level of functioning and will support future organization and development.

In developing the scale, we also recognized that the clinician's sensitivity to state meant designing a scale in which the examiner had to provide a containing and facilitating envelope that would assist the baby toward optimal performance. Could we devise an assessment which reproduced the neonate's response to their parent's best efforts? The concept of *"best performance,"* which is now an integral part of the Brazelton Scale administration, was introduced. Precisely for that reason, the examiner plays a critical role in the behavioral assessment of the newborn, and his or her ability to elicit "best performance" becomes the hallmark of the competent examiner.

Scope and Uses of the Brazelton Scale

The BNBAS can be described as a neurobehavioral assessment scale, designed to examine the newborn's responses to his or her new extrauterine environment (Brazelton & Nugent, 1995). It can be used with newborns from 37 weeks gestational age up to the end of the second month postterm. It attempts to describe the individual infant's behavior in a way that is highly individualized and comprehensive. Never conceptualized as an objective assessment in the classic psychometric or medical diagnostic tradition with an emphasis on pass/fail criteria, it is based on a broader appreciation of phenomenology of newborn behavior. The Brazelton Scale takes a more comprehensive approach to the human newborn and attempts to present a dynamic profile of newborn functioning by identifying individual differences in newborn behavior.

The Brazelton Scale is based on the assumption of the newborn infant as both competent and complexly organized. The BNBAS assumes that the newborn infant is a social organism, predisposed to interact with his or her caregiver. From the beginning, therefore, the Brazelton Scale was used to document the neonate's contribution to the parent-infant system. The scale can be described as an assessment of the infant in an interactional process, not as a simple assessment of the baby alone. It was never conceptualized as a series of discrete stimulus-response presentations but rather as an interactive assessment, in which the examiner plays a major role in facilitating the performance and organizational skills of the infant. In this way, the examiner-baby transactions simulate the parent-infant relationship and provide a window into the baby's contribution to the emerging parent-infant relationship. We consider the assessment in the neonatal period as providing only one glimpse into the continuum of the infant's adjustment to labor, delivery, and adaptation to his or her new environment. As such, it was expected to reflect his or her inborn characteristics and the behavioral responses that had already been shaped by the intrauterine environment. We believed that repeated examination would best demonstrate the infant's coping capacities and capacities for utilizing inner organization as he or she began to integrate and profit developmentally from the environmental stimulation. Serial examinations would better reflect the interaction between the infant's inborn charac-

teristics and the environmental influences over the first weeks of life.

The Brazelton Scale reveals that the newborn is capable of communicating his or her needs. The course of infant development depends to a great extent on the ability of the caregiver to read and respond to these communicative cues. The infant emerges as being both socialized and socializer at the same time. It is a bidirectional process, wherein the infant regulates, modulates, and refines the caregiver's behavior in the service of his or her own adaptation and the caregiver in turn provides the scaffolding to help promote the infant's successful adaptation (Sander et al., 1979; Vygotsky, 1987). Several studies have examined the contribution of newborn behavior to parent-infant interactions and future developmental outcome (Waters, Vaughn, & Egeland, 1980; Linn & Horowitz, 1983; Murray & Cooper, 1997; Crockenberg, 1981; Lester, 1984; Van den Boom, 1991). Horowitz and Linn (1984) point out that it is only if Brazelton Scale scores are combined with measures of the infant's environment that prediction to later developmental measures are enhanced.

From the beginning, the Brazelton Scale was used in studies of intrauterine growth-retarded infants and premature infants to assess the effects of a range of other pre- and perinatal factors on newborn behavior (Brazelton & Nugent, 1995 for a comprehensive review of these studies). The use of the BNBAS to investigate effects of maternal ingestion of toxins has become one of the most productive areas of research with the scale over the past 10 years, especially because it has contributed to a better understanding of the impact of behavior on the caregiving environment and thus, to a better understanding of the nature of the interventions necessary to support parents in their efforts to understand and meet the needs of their at-risk infants. While this body of research confirms the finding that exposure to toxic substances such as cocaine, alcohol, caffeine, and tobacco during pregnancy affect the newborn's performance, it also reveals that due to the number of social, medical, and psychological comorbidities associated with prenatal drug use exposed infants are very likely to have parents who are at high risk for parenting failure than are nonexposed infants (Beeghly & Tronick, 1995). The forces for failure in the parent-infant interaction may be present at birth, and that becomes the focus of Brazelton-based interventions. Because of his or her behavioral immaturity, the infant often has poor state regulation and is unable to maintain alert states and, therefore, requires a great deal of support from the caregiver to reach that level of organization. The long-term outcome for these infants depends on the degree to which interventions can be instituted to support the caregiver in her efforts to meet the needs of her recovering infant (Beckwith & Parmelee, 1989; Fabre-Grenet, 1997; Werner, 1989).

Behavioral Domains Covered by the Brazelton Scale

The Brazelton Scale assesses the newborn's behavioral repertoire on 28 behavioral items, each scored on a nine-point scale. The Brazelton also includes an assessment of the infant's neurological status on 20 items, each scored on a four-point scale. The reflex items will identify gross neurological abnormalities through deviant scores or patterns of scores, but they are not designed to provide a neurological diagnosis. In the two most recent editions (1984, 1995), a set of supplementary items was added in an attempt to better capture the range and quality of the behavior of fragile high-risk infants. These items attempt to summarize the quality of the baby's responsiveness, the cost of attending to the infant's organization, and the amount of input the infant needs from the examiner to organize his or her responses. The usefulness of these items has been confirmed by recent studies of high-risk infants (Dreher et al., 1994; Eyler et al. 1997).

One of the major problems for both the researcher and the clinician who wants to communicate the information to parents is how to summarize Brazelton Scale scores in a way that is conceptually meaningful and clinically relevant. Factor analysis has been used in many studies to group Brazelton Scale items based on their statistical relationships (Lester et al., 1976; Sostek, 1985; Jacobson et al., 1986; Horowitz et al., 1984; Azuma, Malee, Kavanagh, & Deddish, 1991). There is remarkable consistency in the kinds of behavioral dimensions that emerge across populations from such analyses. In an earlier study with the scale, we conducted repeated examinations over the first 10 days of life and were able to observe four dimensions of functioning in newborn behavior: Physiologic, motor, state, and attentional/interactional. These serial observations revealed how the systems were being integrated over time and how they were being affected by environmental factors. Furthermore, this integrative task seemed to proceed in a hierarchical fashion, with autonomic regulation preceding motor organization, followed by the task of state regulation, and finally, social interactive tasks.

The scoring summary is derived from the individual items on the BNBAS. *Autonomic stability*, for example, is exemplified by the presence or absence of tremulousness, startles, or the lability of skin color. *Motor organization* is determined by the status of the infant's tone, motor maturity, activity level, and the level of integrated motor movements such as hand-to-mouth activities or defensive movements. The reflexes were examined as a component of the infant's motor organization and CNS status. *State organization* is assessed by examining the lability of states, level of irritability, peak of excitement, capacity for shutting out negative stimuli while asleep, rapidity of build-up, and consolability and self-quieting capacities. *The quality of the infant's affective/interactive capacities* is observed in the infant's degree of alertness and his or her response to animate and inanimate visual and auditory stimuli.

A conceptually and empirically-based seven-cluster scoring method developed by Lester and Brazelton (1982) has become the most commonly used approach to data reduction with the Brazelton Scale. It reduces the behavioral and reflex items into seven clusters. The clusters were derived from previous factor-analytical stud-

ies and from the four a priori dimensions. Lester (1984) presents patterns of change across these seven clusters using "recovery curves," based on three BNBAS assessments (at 3, 14, and 30 days postpartum), which provide a profile of how neonates change over the first month of life. Longitudinal studies using the Brazelton Scale suggest that predictive validity depends on the use of repeated Brazelton tests as well as ongoing measures of the concurrent contributions of the infant's caregiving environment. The following are the seven BNBAS clusters:

- *Habituation:* Includes the ability to respond to and inhibit discrete stimuli while asleep.
- *Orientation:* Includes the ability to attend to visual and auditory stimuli and the quality of overall alertness.
- *Motor:* Measures motor performance and the quality of movement and tone.
- *Range of State:* Measures of infant arousal and state lability.
- *Regulation of State:* Measures the infant's ability to regulate his or her state in the face of increasing levels of stimulation.
- *Autonomic Stability:* Records signs of stress related to homeostatic adjustments of the central nervous system.
- *Reflexes:* Records the number of abnormal reflexes.

The process of neonatal adaptation can best be measured by studying the patterns of change across these domains over repeated Brazelton examinations (Steichen-Asch, Gleser, & Steichen, 1986). Although some consistency in scores can be expected from day to day, it may be more appropriate to think of fluctuations in scores as indicative of how the newborn is adapting to changing environmental demands. Change, not stability, characterizes healthy development in the newborn period (Emde & Robinson, 1979). What is especially adaptive from a biological perspective is variability and range of behavior.

Our understanding of the neonate suggests, then, that these patterns of change may be the clinician's best index of the infant's current status and that these patterns of change in turn become the best index for predicting future outcome. Again, it should not be surprising that the Brazelton Scale scores alone do not necessarily predict the developmental outcome as Linn and Horowitz (1984) point out. If one's model of development is based on the assumption that developmental outcome is a function of the interaction of organismic and environmental factors, it is unlikely that either one or the other alone will predict significant amounts of variance at later ages. There is growing evidence that when Brazelton scores are combined with measures of the caregiving environment prediction of later development is enhanced (Vaughn et al., 1980; Bakeman & Brown, 1980; Linn & Horowitz, 1983; Murray & Cooper, 1997; Nugent, 1991). This means that three or at least two assessments should be conducted before we can have any assurance that the scale is capturing the quality of the infant's current level of adaptation.

In summary, it can be said that the repeated use of the assessment over time (the first two months) to monitor the baby's progressive adaptation can provide a window into the reorganization of the CNS which has been influenced by, for example, intrauterine exposure. Genetic insults may be permanent and the baby's CNS will not recover, but the more temporary disorganizing effects of immaturity or of cocaine, nicotine, or alcohol will improve over time with appropriate intervention regimens. Planning for early intervention to assist the baby's recovery can be effected from understanding the plasticity and the potential for recovery of the nervous system in a nurturing environment (Dixon, 1994).

The BNBAS as a Form of Intervention: Empirical Evidence

Since the Brazelton Neonatal Behavioral Assessment Scale was first published, it has been used increasingly as a form of preventive intervention by practitioners in the field of infant mental health, pediatrics, nursing, psychiatry, physical and occupational therapy, and early intervention. Because one of the primary goals of preventative intervention is to foster parents sensitivity and responsibility to their infants in order to prevent interactive disturbances, many clinicians have come to believe that the behavioral examination of the newborn in the presence of his or her parents can serve as a mechanism for strengthening this powerful relationship. By attempting to identify the newborn's unique behavioral capacities through the administration and interpretation of the BNBAS, the clinician hopes to increase parents' awareness of their infant's competencies, form a relationship with the parents, and, thereby, positively influence parent-child interaction from the beginning.

While there have been many approaches to using the Brazelton Scale with families, all share the same assumption that behavior is the infant's primary mode of communication. Reading and interpreting these communication signals becomes the shared task of the clinician and parent in the BNBAS session (Nugent, 1985.) Crying, bright-eyed alertness, sleeping behavior, changes in skin color—all of these signals communicate information which must be interpreted in terms of the infant's social availability and overall organization. In offering interpretive information to parents, it is imperative that the clinician have a thorough understanding of the process of newborn organization and development. The clinician's developmental perspective enables him or her to assess and interpret the individual infant's current level of subsystem functioning and understand and describe the level of integration of the autonomic, motor, state, and social interactive systems.

A number of follow-up studies have consistently reported positive effects of exposure to the BNBAS on variables such as maternal confidence and self-esteem, paternal attitudes toward and involvement in caretaking, parent-infant interaction, and developmental outcome (Anderson & Sawin, 1983; Beal, 1986; Beeghley et al., 1995; Britt & Myers, 1994; Dolby, English, & Warren, 1982; Furr & Kirgis, 1982; Gomes-Pedro, de Almeida, & Costa Barbosa, 1984, 1989, 1995; Grimanis et al.,

1989; Liptak, Keller, Feldman, & Chamberlin, 1983; Myers, 1982; Nugent, Hoffman, Barrett, Censullo, & Brazelton, 1987; Nurcombe et al., 1990; Olsen, Olsen, Pernice, & Bloom, 1981; Parker, Zahr, Cole, & Braced, 1992; Szajnberg, Ward, Kraus, & Kessler, 1984; Warren, Dolby, Meade, & Heath, 1989; Widmayer & Field, 1980, 1991; Worobey & Belsky, 1982).

Several longitudinal studies have reported long-term effects of BNBAS-based intervention procedures on developmental outcome and the parent-child relationship. In the case of Rauh, Achenbach, Nurcombe, Howell, and Teti's (1988) work with low birth weight infants and their families, intervention effects were found on the child's cognitive functioning at 24 months and 36 months, as measured by the Bayley and McCarthy scales, respectively, while at four years, intervention mothers were significantly more confident in their parenting than mothers in the control group. The Brazelton-based "intervention" package consisted of a series of Brazelton sessions with the mother conducted in the Neonatal Intensive Care Unit (NICU). Over five days, serial examinations were conducted, emphasizing a different dimension of newborn functioning on each occasion, reflecting the challenges or the developmental agenda the high-risk newborn faces in his recovery. The baby's autonomic system was emphasized on the first day, since the stabilization of his or her physiological system is the first and basic challenge of the premature newborn. The clinician points out the signs of stress and the examination allows parent and clinician to identify the infant's threshold for taking in or responding to environmental stimuli. Then, in the following days, mother and clinician observed the baby's motor behavior, activity levels, quality of tone, and the kinds of facilitating techniques that could support motor organization, such as swaddling, holding during medical procedures, and so on. Then, the baby's range of states are identified, including the quality or robustness of these states. The scale reveals how easily the baby moves from sleep to wake states and what control he or she has over these states. What is the baby's level of self-organization? By the fourth day, clinician and mother are focusing on the baby's alerting capacities and how these social interactive capacities can be supported. As they move along, clinician and parent are constructing a profile of the baby's current level of functioning and are identifying the best kinds of facilitating strategies to help the baby recover and adapt to the new environment. On the last day, the profile is complete and mother and clinician construct an individualized plan to help support the baby in the areas still deemed to be vulnerable.

Widmayer and Field's (1981) intervention study with low socioeconomic status (SES) adolescent mothers also showed positive effects for intervention at 1, 4, and 12 months. Gomes-Pedro, Patricio, Carvalho, Goldschmidt, Torgal-Garcia, and Montiero (1995) were also able to demonstrate positive effects on mental development, as measured by the Bayley scales, up to the end of the second year of life in a sample of primiparous, lower middle class Portuguese mothers. In this case, Gomes-

Pedro and his colleagues conducted the Brazelton session in the context of a brief pediatric discharge visit. Acknowledging the concepts of Klaus, Kennell, and Klaus (1993), Gomes-Pedro maintains that it is the timing of the BNBAS intervention that enhances its effectiveness, taking place as it does at that sensitive postpartum period when an intervention designed to influence the parent-child relationship positively may have lasting effects.

Worobey and Belsky (1982), Myers (1982), Keefer (1995), and Cardone and Gilkerson (1990) point to the influence of parental involvement in the session as playing a key role in its effectiveness as an intervention tool. They argue that where parents are given the opportunity to play an active role in eliciting the newborn's behavior during the BNBAS, this active participation in the intervention session enhances parents' feelings of confidence in their ability to respond contingently to their newborn infants.

In our work with intrauterine growth-retarded infants and their families (n = 133), the BNBAS was used to help parents begin to read and decipher their infant's cues and guide them in modulating their responses to meet their infant's arousal needs, thus supporting them in the establishment of a mutually satisfying interaction pattern (Beeghly et al., 1995). Because the BNBAS is designed to help parents identify individual differences in affective responsiveness, we believe it can help lessen the risk for later affective disturbances. By identifying high and low thresholds to stimulation, signs of overarousal or underarousal, the autonomic or physiological cost of attention, the signs of social availability, and the subtle signs of stress, parents reported that the scale helped with the task of reading and responding appropriately to their infant's cues.

Grimanis' and colleagues (1989) work with the parents of low birth weight babies revealed that there were three domains of functioning in the BNBAS that were especially compelling to parents and were most helpful in their caregiving. These behaviors had to do with the development of good sleep and wake cycles, the management of crying, and the maintenance and promotion of social interaction. The state regulation items, especially the habituation items, were helpful to mothers in helping them support their baby's efforts to develop sleep and wake patterns. The crying and consolability items informed mothers about their infant's threshold for stimulation, how easily their baby was upset, and identified the best strategies to help the baby calm. Observing the baby's capacity for alertness helped parents to learn how to facilitate their baby's alertness and how to play and interact with their new baby.

Parker and colleagues (1992) in their work with a low SES sample of mothers, invited the mothers to actively participate in the behavioral assessment of the infant in a NICU setting. Mothers elicited some of the items, including orientation items such as response to the human voice and response to the face and voice. Compared to mothers of preterm infants who received standard postpartum care, mothers in the intervention group rated their infants as having less difficult temperaments at four and eight months. These infants had higher developmental quotients at four and eight months than the control group infants.

In their study in Australia, Warren and colleagues (1989) developed a comprehensive prevention program for low birth weight babies, based on the BNBAS scores and on information derived from structured interviews with the mothers. The results supported the premise that effective parent interaction may the strongest working factor to override the early negative consequences of preterm birth. The study also confirms the value of developing interventions that flow from the BNBAS and are designed to meet the individual needs of the high-risk infant.

However, it must be pointed out that for the clinician who works with infants and families, controlled intervention studies that compare group mean scores tend to mask within-group differences and thus, make it difficult to ascertain which individual children or families benefitted from the intervention. The effectiveness of the Brazelton Scale as a form of intervention depends on many factors, including the nature and goals of the session itself, the nature of the contract between clinician and family, number of sessions, risk status of the infant and family, quality of the clinician-parent relationship, the nature of their social support systems, and the nature of the follow-up treatment.

Nevertheless, although these intervention studies are often characterized by small sample sizes, the evidence for short-term positive effects of BNBAS-based interventions is consistent for both high-risk and low-risk samples. A recent meta-analysis of 13 parenting intervention studies based on the BNBAS by Das Eiden and Reifman (1996), containing a total of 668 families, concluded that the BNBAS interventions had beneficial effects on the quality of later parenting. Although the longitudinal data show positive effects, the results cannot be used to argue for *direct* long-term effects as an exclusive function of BNBAS-based interventions. In the case of the (1988) study by Rauh and colleagues, and the Widmayer and Field (1980; 1981) studies, for example, the initial BNBAS-based intervention was complemented by other interventions at later points. Rather, the evidence suggests to us that short-term changes in parental attitude and behavior in response to the BNBAS in the newborn period can serve to initiate or launch a positive cycle of interaction between parents and infants that may have long-term, albeit indirect, consequences. We can conclude that although there may not be persistent *direct* effects as a result of BNBAS-based interventions, long-term effects may derive from *indirect* transactional effects.

In summary, the Brazelton Scale presents the clinician with a significant clinical window into the parent-infant relationship, offering a unique opportunity to enter into a supportive partnership with parents at a time when they may feel vulnerable and in need of support. Since the period from birth to the beginning of the third month of life is not only a major stage in the infant's behavioral adaptation to his or her new environment but also marks a unique transition stage in the development in the parent-infant relationship, the aim of the Brazelton-based intervention is to facilitate the development of a positive par-

ent-infant relationship. In fact, the most recent edition of the BNBAS extends the scope of the scale from birth through the second month up to the third month of the infant's life. This presents clinicians with a wider window for using the BNBAS and the opportunity to combine hospital, clinical, and home sessions.

The Process of Intervention with the Brazelton Scale

While there are many different approaches to using the Brazelton Scale with families especially in terms of when, where, and why it is conducted, in addition to the baby's risk status and the parent's psychological availability (Brazelton & Nugent, 1995, p. 84), every Brazelton session begins with the baby's behavior. Administering the scale enables the clinician to elicit the baby's behavior, as he or she moves through sleep, wake, and crying states. It provides a telescopic view of the baby's overall extrauterine adaptation. For that reason, each session presents parents with the opportunity to observe the baby's level of physiological stability, motor development, state regulation, and capacity for affective interaction so that over the two months parents have the opportunity to observe the baby's progress over these dimensions. We have found that every Brazelton session can be broken into three sections: An introduction to the goals of the session, including the task of engaging the parents, followed by the observations of the baby's behavioral responses during the scale, and finally, the summary and interpretation and guidelines for caregiving.

A modal session begins by observing the baby's efforts to protect his or her sleep states in the face of unpredictable disturbing stimuli (a light, rattle, and bell are used). This provides the parents with a forum to begin a discussion of the development of the baby's sleep and wake states and above all, to discuss the kinds of handling techniques that can best promote the baby's development in this area. We have found that by the third week, management of sleep and decision-making about how to promote the baby's sleep is a central issue for parents. By examining the baby's reflexes and muscle tone and observing activity levels, clinician and parent can begin to formulate approaches to meet the baby's motor needs. Does the baby need to be swaddled more? Does the baby need more shoulder and neck support? How can I help the baby develop his or her hand-to-mouth facility? How does the baby like to be held? Particular attention is given to the baby's threshold levels to ascertain what may be overstimulating or what kind of handling he or she prefers. The baby's autonomic functioning is ascertained by observing the number of startles, tremors, or color changes.

Again, by the third week, we have found that management of crying is a matter of concern for many parents, since they may see the onset of colic and much of the attention in the scale is addressed to the state organization items. Throughout the session, as the baby is exposed to the different levels of stimulation or handling, clinician and parent observe the baby's threshold for stimulation and the amount of crying. Does the baby move easily from sleep to wake states, or does the baby remain in an insulated crying state? Can the baby wake up and look around? If the baby cries, can he or she be consoled easily? Finally, as the baby's capacity for alertness expands as the weeks go by, the clinician and parent can see how to promote the baby's attention, read his or her communication cues, and interact with the baby.

While there have been many clinical adaptations of the BNBAS from the time of its initial publication in 1973, there have been some recent adaptations.

The Combined Physical and Behavioral Neonatal Examination (Keefer, 1995), uses the physical examination of the newborn to educate parents about behavior and development by incorporating behavioral items from the BNBAS into the routine physical examination. This combined examination is designed for pediatric practitioners to enable them to assess the normality of the infant's behavior and generate an individual behavioral profile for parents. The examiner narrates the examination for the parents and actively draws them in to assure them about their child's physical state and enhance their understanding of the behavior, with a view to improving their self-confidence and strengthening the parent-infant relationship.

The Family Administered Neonatal Activities (FANA; Cardone & Gilkerson, 1990) is an adaptation of the Brazelton Scale, which integrates the practices of short-term psychodynamic interviewing with a "family empowerment approach." The BNBAS-based activities are contained within a guided process whereby a trained facilitator offers parents an opportunity to observe and interact with their baby. The primary goals of the FANA are to affirm and enhance parental capacities to observe and engage their infant and help them integrate their initial parent perceptions and expectations with the infant's present behavior. It serves as a supportive activity to promote competence and adaptation for families who are coping well with the transition to parenthood or where there are stresses around labor and delivery or issues about the family's ability to care for the infant at home.

The Clinical Neonatal Behavioral Assessment Scale (CLNBAS) (Nugent & Brazelton, in preparation) is an adaptation of the NBAS, developed especially for clinicians to be used in the care of families in hospital, clinic or home settings over the first two months of the infant's life. The goal of this flexible short-form version of the NBAS, the CLNBAS, is to promote a positive relationship between clinician and family and to strengthen the relationship between parents and their newborn baby. This shared observation session provides a forum for parents and clinician to observe and interpret the newborn's behavior and is designed to help parents make informed choices about caregiving. While the CLNBAS preserves the conceptual richness of the NBAS, and describes the baby's physiological, motor, state and social-interactive behavior, it retains only the items which are deemed to have an impact on parental caregiving, such as, sleep behavior, feeding cues, crying and consolability, activity level, the baby's threshold for stimulation and social interactive capacities.

Therapeutic Principles Governing the Use of the BNBAS in Clinical Settings

An Infant-Centered Approach: The Infant as Catalyst

What is unique about the BNBAS-based intervention is that the infant—the infant's behavior—is at the center of the treatment. It is through the infant that we hope to motivate and support parents in their efforts to understand and respond to their infants. The Brazelton Scale reveals the power of the infant to elicit from his or her caregiving environment the nurturing and caregiving he or she needs to to for successful adaptation. Selma Fraiberg wrote that "when a baby is at the center of the treatment something happens that has no other parallel in any other form of psychotherapy" (1980, p. 53). The baby, therefore, becomes the catalyst in intervention settings by providing a powerful motive for positive change in the parents. The baby represents parents' hopes and deepest longings. "He stands for the renewal of the self; his birth can be experienced as a psychological rebirth for his parents" (Fraiberg, 1980, p. 54). All parents want the best for their child, so that when the clinician shares this goal, the baby becomes the bond that unites the clinician and parents in bringing their hopes for the baby to fulfillment. In this way, the positive adaptive tendencies inherent in the infant-parent relationship can be mobilized in the service of the infant development.

Whereas all BNBAS-based interventions share the same treatment procedure, it is the capacity of the Newborn Behavioral Assessment Scale to bring out the individuality or temperament of each infant that may constitute its effectiveness as a form of intervention. For this reason it has been suggested that through the BNBAS session, while parents learn new information about their newborn's capacities, what is more important is the ability of the scale to reveal the baby's unique traits or style of adaptation or temperament. This new knowledge, in turn, better enables parents to understand and respond to their baby as a unique individual and learn the baby's communication cues, as Anderson and Sawin (1983), Beal (1984), Liptak and colleagues (1983), Olsen and colleagues (1981), and other investigators have suggested.

It is the individualized nature of the approach that places the BNBAS-based intervention outside the domain of main effects treatment modalities and renders it responsive to the particular needs of individual infants and families. By eliciting, describing, and interpreting the newborn's behavior, the clinician has the opportunity to participate with parents in identifying the kinds of demands the infant will make on his or her environment and the kinds of caregiving techniques that can best promote the infant's organization and development. The BNBAS, thus, offers the clinician and parent a forum to observe the infant's level of functioning over the first two months and together arrive at a behavioral profile that captures the infant's individuality. Although the immediate goal of the BNBAS is to help reveal to parents the baby's unique adaptive and coping capacities, the long-term clinical goal is to influ-

ence the infant-parent relationship positively by developing a supportive therapeutic alliance with the family at what could be called the formative moment in the development of the family system. The BNBAS is, thus, seen as the first stage in the development of a supportive relationship between clinician and parents, which should continue beyond the newborn period.

Behavior is the infant's primary mode of communication so that reading and interpreting these communication signals becomes the shared task of the clinician and parent in the BNBAS session (Nugent, 1985.) Crying, bright-eyed alertness, sleeping behavior, changes in skin color—all of these signals communicate information which must be interpreted in terms of the infant's social availability and overall organization. In offering interpretive information to parents, it is imperative that the clinician have a thorough understanding of the process of newborn organization and development. The clinician's developmental perspective enables him or her to assess and interpret the individual infant's current level of subsystem functioning and understand and describe the level of integration of the autonomic, motor, state, and social interactive systems.

The Brazelton Scale provides the baby with a "voice," with an opportunity to reveal his or her own profile of behavior, temperament, or behavioral style and thus, prevent the possibility of premature labeling based on a priori medical or social background data. However, an assumption of the BNBAS session is that the baby's temperament or behavioral profile is a coconstruction of both parent and clinician and baby. The baby's behavior is never objective data in the sense that it stands on its own and is self-explanatory. While it may be interpreted by the clinician, the clinician must be aware then of the mother's psychic processes and should recognize that her representations of herself and of her baby will shape her understanding of the baby's behavior during the Brazelton session, as Bruschwieler-Stern (1997) points out. (see Stern [1995] for a more detailed discussion of the transference/countertransference process in developing a therapeutic alliance.)

The Therapeutic Partnership: A Positive-Adaptive Approach to Infant and Parent

In order to enter into a therapeutic alliance with the family, we propose using a model of intervention that is a positive-adaptive model rather than a pathological one (Brazelton, 1982). This positive approach may be particularly difficult for some mental health clinicians, as Cramer (1987) points out, due to the nonadaptive bias of our psychoanalytically inspired models. This is reflected in the persistence of the notion of the young infant as helpless and autistic (Mahler, Pine, & Bergman, 1975) and in the emphasis on the parent as the solitary contributor to the infant's development.

While the BNBAS-based intervention approach is built on the recognition and appreciation of the integrative capacities of newborn infants, this positive-adaptive approach is extended to our understanding of the caregiver's repertoire in meeting the needs of the young infant. The recognition of parents' capacities for nurturance is reinforced by our own microanalytic analyses of early parent-infant interactions (Brazelton et al., 1974; Lester, Hoffman, & Brazelton, 1985; Tronick, Als, & Brazelton, 1980; Weinberg & Tronick, 1997). These data demonstrate that the social stimulation provided by caregivers is rich, multimodal, and reciprocal. Papousek and Papousek (1987) assign these behaviors the position of intuitive behaviors because they seem to assume an intermediate position between categories of innate reflexes and responses that require rational decisions. The idea that human parental behaviors may be selected during evolution and that parents have endogenous parenting capacities demands that clinicians working with parents have a respectful, nondidactic, and nonjudgmental attitude toward parents. Belsky's (1986) reanalysis of his previous data and our own work with small-for-gestational-age (SGA) infants and their families (Nugent et al., 1987) suggest that the efficacy of BNBAS-based intervention is mediated by parental involvement and interest and lies as much in the quality of the clinician-parent relationship as it does in the demonstration of newborn behavioral capacities.

The quality of our relationship with parents is crucial because it is intended to have a transforming effect on the parent's relationship with her own child. The parameters of respect, concern, accommodation, and basic positive regard become crucial as the envelope of the entire "treatment" process. The more concerned or anxious the parent is, the more crucial does this reliable emotional context become. While the nature of the relationship will change over time, the quality of respect and mutuality must remain in order to withstand the unanticipated problems that inevitably occur. This aspect of the parent-clinician relationship can provide parents with what Lieberman (1991) refers to as a "corrective attachment figure" which contrasts with the criticisms they may be experiencing from other sources in their lives. By valuing the parent's attempts to reach out and understand her child, we provide the parent with a more nurturing and supportive relationship. Our hope is that this positive, nurturant, nonjudgmental experience becomes gradually internalized and incorporated in to the parent's own internal representation of herself as a parent and of her child. For parents who are feeling alone and vulnerable, "meeting with" a clinician who is supportive and caring can be the first step in enhancing a parent's sense of worth. This in turn is an important condition in helping the parents become more positively invested in their child.

Shaping the Development of Maternal Representations

It is in the immediate postnatal period that parents' perceptions of the infant begin to consolidate (Brazelton, 1982; Bruschweiler-Stern, 1997; Cramer, 1987; Stern, 1995; Zeanah et al., 1995). Although parents begin to develop perceptions of their infants during pregnancy by translating fetal movement patterns in behavioral terms such as, "She's very active," "He is so

good," or "She is very angry with me," it is only in the newborn period that they can test these attributions in light of the child's observable patterns of behavior. The BN-BAS can help parents develop realistic perceptions of their infants and help them modify their prenatal perceptions in response to their infant's objectively observed behavior patterns. Cramer (1987) maintains that parents' perceptions of infant behavior play a crucial role in determining the unfolding of the parent-infant relationship.

Many parents may tend to have unrealistic perceptions of their newborns, although Freedman (1980), Hinde (1976), and Kaye (1982) argue that a certain amount of "adultomorphism" or overestimation of the baby's capacities (e.g., "She has a mind of her own," "He understands everything I say") can be adaptive in that it motivates parents in their attempts to communicate with their infants, with the expectation of engaging in reciprocal interaction (Brazelton et al., 1974; Cohn & Tronick, 1983). On the other hand, negative attributions such as, "He doesn't seem to like me," or "Every time I look at her, she looks away," present important clinical information to the clinician and may suggest that the parent-infant dyad could be at risk for future interactive disturbances.

Stern (1995, 1997), Cramer (1987), and Bruschweiler-Stern's (1997) work clearly indicate that the task of influencing parents' perceptions of their infant is a complex one because the meanings parents attribute to their infant's behavior may have their origin in the parents' personal history and unconscious. Whereas the resolution of such distorted perceptions may be prolonged and painstaking, the BNBAS intervention can begin to contribute to the resolution of such perceptions by enabling parents to observe their infants' own unique behavioral makeup and the infants' own interaction capacities, thus helping to prevent the development of noncontingent interaction patterns. (see Bruschweiler-Stern, 1997, Stern, 1985, 1995, and Cramer, 1987, for a more comprehensive treatment of the meaning attribution process in parent-infant relations.) Fraiberg (1980) illustrates this in her work on "ghosts in the nursery," in which she demonstrates how conflicts from earlier relationships may intrude on and interfere with the parents' current relationship with their infant. For example, a child may become a replacement for a deceased or lost object so that the parent is reacting to an imaginary child and not to the real infant before him or her. We recognize Fraiberg's view that parents often repeat with their infants their own childhood traumas "in terrible and exacting detail" (Fraiberg, 1980, p. 165). The result of such distorted perceptions may lead to what Stern (1985) refers to as "parental misattunements," and it is proposed here that the scale can be used to prevent this from happening.

Building a Therapeutic Alliance with Parents

The establishment of a relationship of trust between clinician and family is the cornerstone for the development of this *therapeutic alliance,* as Greenspan (1981) and Stern (1995) point out. As argued earlier,

we believe that the infant-centered nature of the BNBAS-based intervention is better suited to facilitating parents' involvement at a pace consistent with their own degree of readiness. We have found that parents' involvement and participation increases over the course of the serial sessions. By the third month, the parents and clinician have come to know the infant more as an individual, as they have observed the baby's recovery and development over that period on the scale. By that time, the clinician hopes to have laid the foundation for an enduring, supportive relationship with the family as a system that will continue to grow as the neonate moves into infancy.

We would argue that in contrast to an exclusively parent-centered, verbally-mediated approach to intervention, this infant-centered, behaviorally-based form of intervention may be particularly effective in working with families under stress. In the context of the BNBAS, the baby becomes the key informant, and the clinician accepts whatever level of information or participation parents offer, at the pace at which they offer it. Our approach underscores the importance of respecting parents' defenses by neither directly eliciting clinical material nor predetermining the nature and extent of their involvement at this time of transition in their lives. We have found that by following this approach, parents' degree of involvement and participation in the intervention tended to increase during the course of the interventions over the first month (Nugent et al., 1987).

The clinician's predominant attitude toward parents is, therefore, both respectful and supportive. The clinician must be able to listen empathically for parent's questions and observations (Boukydis, 1986; Hirschberg, 1993; McDonough, 1993). In Cramer's (1987) view, paying attention to a mother's verbal reports and what she thinks about her baby is crucial because these attributes play a significant role in determining the unfolding of the mother-infant relationship. The Brazelton Scale should always provide parents with the opportunity to share their perceptions of their infant and relate their experience of becoming a parent, in what Zeanah and McDonagh (1989) refer to as the "family story."

In high-risk settings where families are under stress, however, parents may be unable to respond contingently to their newborn's eliciting behaviors. Where there is maternal depression or when parents are affectively unresponsive or unavailable, then interactive disturbances may occur (Field, 1987; Murray, 1994; Murray & Cooper, 1997). If, in turn, the infant's communication cues are difficult to decipher or if the infant is affectively unresponsive, then these factors compound the already existing risk status of the parents and together are likely to result in interactive disturbances. Helping parents read their baby's cues or merely confirming the validity of their own observations and providing parents with feedback on how their babies respond to them can help mobilize confidence in their efforts to communicate with their young infants. During the BNBAS session, we try to give parents an opportunity both to observe and interact with their infants. Parents have a chance to elicit

these behaviors from their own infants and in this way, they have an opportunity, with the facilitation and support of the clinician, to experience the sense of efficacy in eliciting these responses (Munck, 1985; Munck, Mirdal, & Marner, 1991).

A Systems Perspective: The BNBAS in a Family/Community Context

The transactional view of development with its emphasis on the bidirectional nature of parent-infant relations must be complemented by an understanding of the newborn as an active participant in a larger social network. The application of systems theory to parent-infant relations demands that we extend our focus from the mother-infant dyad to the family system in order to understand better the transforming effects of the infant on the family system and the effects of the various elements of the family system on the infant's adaptation and development. The infant is necessarily at the center of the BNBAS-based intervention.

The Brazelton Scale is, therefore, best done in a family context, which provides an opportunity to focus on the potential role of the infant in influencing mother, father, grandparents, neighbors, or whoever makes up the informal network of relatives or friends that has an investment in the growth and well-being of this new baby. The family and the entire network of family interactions becomes the focus of the Brazelton Scale approach in clinical settings. While the baby and his or her behavior is the focus of the Brazelton Scale session, it is the family that becomes, what Stern refers to as, the "port of entry" for the clinician using the Brazelton Scale (Stern, 1995). From this *systems perspective,* the Brazelton Scale attempts to assess the contribution of the new infant to family interactions and at the same time work with the family to learn what the family has to do to incorporate this new element into its system.

Using the BNBAS in such settings requires what Robert Emde (1987, p. 1314) refers to as *"systems sensitivity,"* which he defines as "the empathic registration by the therapist of the quality of functioning of complex personality subsystems and their interactions." Within the context of the BNBAS, this means that the clinician must be able to understand and assess ongoing interactions with the family system, between parent and infant as well as between the parents themselves. The BNBAS intervention is taking place at different levels so that for the clinician it requires an appreciation of the simultaneous operation of multiple systems within the intervention setting. At one level, the clinician is interacting with the infant as he or she attempts to assess the infant's interaction capacities and potential influence on the parents' caregiving. At another level, the clinician is interacting with the parents in an effort to develop a supportive and trusting relationship with them around their infant. The systems-sensitive clinician is equally aware that the quality of the parents' own relationship, their attitudes toward the infant, and their relationship with the clinician all affect the emotional climate of the session and will play a role in influencing the outcome.

We must also recognize that the new-born infant enters into a social network that may be made up of parents, grandparents, siblings, and friends, all of whom can exercise a significant influence on the infant. Although the newborn period often provides the clinician with a unique opportunity to develop a relationship with the infant's father (Beal, 1984; Myers, 1982), the effectiveness of the BNBAS session can benefit from the inclusion of the siblings, grandparents, or other important elements of the infant's social network because they all need to adjust to the presence of the new family member (Minuchin, 1985). Expanding the scope of the intervention to include a broader range of potentially supportive allies is particularly important when working with families under stress, such as economically disadvantaged families, single-parent families, adolescent parents, families with premature or SGA infants, or families with infants who are behaviorally irritable and difficult to handle (Barr 1990; Boukydis, 1986; Crockenberg, 1981; Field, 1987; Lester, Hoffman, & Brazelton, 1985; Wolke et al., 1994; Zigler & Frank, 1988). In this way, we use the BNBAS intervention to try to bridge the gap between the family and support networks within the community.

Using the BNBAS with Diverse Populations: Cultural Sensitivity

From the time it was first published, one of the most common uses of the Brazelton has been the examination of neonatal differences and their natural variations in different cultural settings (Brazelton, Robey, & Collier, 1969; Freedman & Freedman,

1969; Brazelton, Koslowski, & Tronick, 1977). Many of these studies have been reviewed by Lester and Brazelton (1982) and Super and Harkness (1982), and we have described studies using the Brazelton Scale from 38 different cultural settings (Nugent, Lester, & Brazelton, 1989, 1991, in press). Our cross-cultural research on early parent-infant transactions (Brazelton et al., 1977; Brazelton et al., 1969; Brazelton, Tronick, Lechtig, Lasky, & Klein, 1977; Dixon, Tronick, Keefer, & Brazelton, 1982; Nugent et al., 1989, 1991) constitutes a fraction of the growing canon of cross-cultural studies which together demonstrate the wide range of variability in parent-infant interaction patterns and child-rearing philosophies (Levine, 1980; Whiting & Edwards, 1988). These data suggest that whereas, the basic organizational processes in infancy may be universal, the range and form of these adaptations are shaped by the demands of each individual culture.

There have been a number of studies which have examined the cultural context of newborn behavior with a view to documenting cultural neonatal behavioral differences. The BNBAS was not normed or standardized, nor was the scoring based on any specific regional or national sample, but was designed in a way that made it possible for individual differences and cultural differences to be presented in descriptive rather than normative terms. These include studies of newborn behavior from European countries such as Italy (Paludetto, Mansi, Rinaldi, Margara-Paludetto, & Faggiano-Perfetto, 1991; Bottos, Dalla Barba, & Tronick, in press),

Denmark (Munck et al., (1991), Germany (Grossmann & Grossmann, 1991), Sweden, (Wells-Nystrom, 1991), Netherlands (Van den Boom, 1991; Van Baar, in press), France (Stoleru & Morales-Huet, 1991), Switzerland (Fricker, Hindermann, & Bruppacher, 1991), Portugal (Gomes-Pedro, 1989), Great Britain (Hawthorne-Amick, 1989; Hopkins, 1989; Murray, in press), Ireland (Nugent, Greene, & Wieczorek-Deering, & O'Mahony, in press), Spain, (Cantavella, Leonhardt, & Tolosa, in press).

In Asia, the Brazelton Scale has been used in India (Gathwala & Narayan, 1990), while Landers (1989) examined the cultural context of development and the role of the environment on behavior in her follow-up study of a sample on infants in South India. While Kato (1991) has studied a sample of Japanese infants in Tokyo, Akiyama and his colleagues (Akiyama et al., in press; Ogi, 1993; Kawasaki, Nugent, Miyashita, Miyahara, & Brazelton, 1994) have been conducting a longitudinal study on the social and behavioral factors that influence development in a sample of infants born on the Goto Islands. Studies of the cultural context of newborn behavior have also been conducted in Malaysia (Woodson & da Costa, 1989), Nepal (Walsh-Escarce, 1989), and Indonesia (Piessens, 1989). Byoung Hi Park Synn (in press) described the behavior of a sample of Korean infants and the influence of social support patterns on newborn behavior and the parent-child relationship. The behavior of third-generation Israeli infants belonging to two ethnic groups, Ashkenazi and Sephardic, and the behavior of a group of Panamian infants were compared in a study by Tirosh, Abadi, Harel, Berger, and Cohen (1992). Using item by item comparisons, they found significant differences between Ashkenazi and Sephardic infants in auditory habituation, whereas the Panamanian infants differed on motor, range of state, and autonomic cluster items.

In Central and South America, there have been studies by Saco-Pollitt (1989) describing newborn behavior in the Peruvian Andes, in Mexico (Atkin, del Carmen Olvera, Givaudan, & Landeros, 1989), and in Puerto Rico (Garcia-Coll, 1989). Dreher and colleagues (1994) and Hayes, Lampart, Dreher, and Morgan (1991), in their reports on the effects of maternal marijuana use on newborn behavior in Jamaica, describe their results in terms of the unique cultural and economic characteristics that mediate the use of marijuana in pregnancy in Jamaica. Studies in Africa include Kenya (Keefer, Dixon, Tronick, & Brazelton, 1991), Zaire (Winn, Tronick, & Morelli, 1989), and South Africa (Niestroj, 1989). In Israel, Auerbach, Greenbaum, Nowick, Guttman, Margolin, and Horowitz (1991) reported on the effects of different cultural and social class settings and examined their impact on newborn behavior. Nester and colleagues (in press) have examined newborn behavior in Saudi Arabia.

In addition, this series of studies describes studies of behavioral differences in different cultural groups in North America. Chisholm (1989) examines the relation between biology, culture, and the development of temperament in his study of

Navajo infants. Rosser and Randolph (1989), in the Howard University normative study, describe the behavior of a sample of healthy, full-term black infants and the influence of child-rearing practices on outcome. Muret-Wagstaff and Moore (1989) describe newborn behavior and child-rearing practices in the Hmong in a Minneapolis setting. Choi (1986) compared a sample of Korean and United States infants on the Brazelton Scale and reported that the Korean infants had higher scores on habituation and state regulation, although no differences were found on mother-child interaction assessments.

In summary, the studies of newborn behavior in different cultural contexts confirm the bidirectional nature of development while they expand our understanding of the range of variability in newborn behavioral patterns and the diversity of child-rearing practices and belief systems. These studies reveal the universals and the specifics of human behavior, what may be biologically based and unchangeable and what is environmentally induced and, therefore, by nature, variable. They may tell us what is phylogenetically programmed, what is culturally programmed, what is "bred in the bone," and what is shaped by parents and society (Nugent, 1994).

However, the heuristic value of the Brazelton Scale when used in different cultural settings goes beyond the simple description or documentation of different patterns of behavior in strange or exotic cultures. For clinicians who use the scale with infants and families from different cultures, it serves to challenge assumptions about the very nature of infant development and sensitizes clinicians to the different trajectories of infant development, from birth on. It forces practitioners to revise and broaden their definitions of what is considered "normal or typical" behavior and what is considered "abnormal or atypical." Studies with the Brazelton Scale demonstrate that the notion of risk is a cultural construction. This reminds us as clinicians, that we always have to examine the validity of the databases on which many of our at-risk categories and diagnoses are based. Risk categories have to be contextualized, and the only valid risk inventories are those that emerge from and are constructed from the communities which we serve. The BNBAS can serve to challenge our core assumption about the nature of development, about what we think of as "good," what is "optimal," what is "normal," or what is "abnormal." The concepts of normality and risk are, therefore, revealed as cultural constructions which may not have validity in cultures other than in the one in which the concept was constructed.

In addition, using the BNBAS with families from different cultures allows us to better understand the nature of infant development and the needs of infants and families from a wide range of cultural backgrounds. It enables us to broaden our understanding of the role of the baby in mediating the whole process of socialization. It also helps us identify the particular kinds of culturally-defined experiences that affect development, the role of mothers and fathers in the socialization process in soci-

eties where a larger family network is responsible for child care, and the role of different kinds of discipline or child-rearing practices, and in general, describe the range of cultural settings in which development takes place.

For those reasons, using the BNBAS in such clinical settings can serve to challenge the validity of our current assumptions about human behavior and to free us from our own unconscious ethnocentrism. This form of ethnocentrism can be called unconscious or latent because it is not readily accessible to our conscious reasoning and it plays a subtle and often unconscious role in our interactions with families from cultures other than our own (Nugent, 1994). This means that infant mental programs cannot be based on a priori goals that bear little relation to the cultural background of the families in which the programs are set. By emphasizing the primacy of context, this approach leads us the question the appropriateness of program goals and to reexamine the kinds of assessment tools we use to evaluate children, in light of the cultural background of the children and families in the program. From this perspective, each program must challenge itself to develop a set of strategies to meet the unique culturally-mediated goals of the population being served and ultimately to develop program goals that are inclusive and culturally comprehensive.

In summary, cross-cultural examples challenge our assumptions about the nature of development. They urge introspection as they force us to examine our own belief systems and unmask our own cultural biases by reviewing our attitudes toward children and toward families. Without an awareness and appreciation of our own culture or without a firm sense of identity with our own culture, it will be extremely difficult to be sensitive to or open to the nuances of another culture. It will be equally difficult to have access to our own biases and prejudices. Paradoxically, it is only in our engagement with other cultures that our understanding of our own culture is refined and our appreciation of other cultures is simultaneously enriched. Crosscultural experiences can serve to challenge the very essence of our beliefs about what we are doing and the efficacy of our intervention programs. Our cross-cultural studies demonstrate that the notion of risk is a cultural construction. We always have to examine the validity of the databases on which many of our at-risk categories and diagnoses are based. Risk categories have to be contextualized, and the only valid risk inventories are those that emerge from and are constructed from the communities which we serve. Listening to and searching for the authentic voices of infants and their families through the BNBAS is an invaluable opportunity in becoming a culturally-sensitive clinician (Finn, 1994).

Conclusion

We have proposed a model of development that emphasizes the transactional nature of early newborn environment relations and the significance of the first months of life as a major transitional stage in the infant-parent relationship, as a conceptual basis for using the BNBAS in clinical settings (Brazelton, 1982; Nugent & Brazelton, 1987). The newborn is conceptualized as competent and complex but also as a social organism, innately predisposed to interact with the environment in order to elicit from it the caregiving necessary for its survival and successful adaptation. In contrast to the classic psychoanalytic approach to working with infants and parents, where the infant is seen as asocial and the parent-infant relationship is viewed as asymmetrical, this approach stresses the bidirectional nature of the relationship and the powerful effects of the infant on the caregiver, as well as the effects of the caregiver on the infant.

The focus of the BNBAS as a form of intervention is on the parent-infant relationship and promoting the relationship between infant and caregiver. Our model emphasizes the role of both internal and external feedback systems in providing energy for the infant's healthy developmental progress (Brazelton, 1982). The infant's own unique behavioral predispositions toward successful adaptation conspire with the powerful influences of the caregiving environment in providing the internal and external feedback which produces new levels of organization and which cannot be predicted in any linear model. Both infant *and* parent *and* the family become, therefore, the focus of preventive intervention with the BNBAS. The goal becomes one of promoting infant adaptation by facilitating parent-infant interaction through the shared exploration and observation of the baby's behavioral organization.

The BNBAS is, thus, seen as the first

stage in the development of a supportive relationship between clinician and parents, which should continue beyond the newborn period. The unique characteristic of BNBAS-based interventions is that the infant is at the center of the treatment, and it is through the infant we hope to motivate and support parents in their efforts to understand and respond to their infants. We have argued that the infant-centered but family-focused form of intervention holds promise for early screening and intervention in preventing affective disturbances in the parent-infant relationship and can thus, serve as the first stage for a comprehensive follow-up program of support for infants and families.

Although not invoking the critical period hypothesis, we have argued that the first two months could be called a unique transition stage in the infant's behavioral development and in the development of the parent-child relationship. We have presented evidence to show that it is a major transition stage in the evolution of the parent-child relationship, a time when parents and infants are in a state of heightened readiness for social exchange and a time when the earliest parent-infant interaction patterns are being laid down. It is also a time when the family system is in a formative stage of its evolution as it prepares to accommodate the new infant into its system, a time when the family system provides a unique entree to the supportive clinician, and a time when the newborn, as he or she selectively engages his or her environment, is actively forming a sense of an emergent self, a sense of self that will remain active for the rest of the child's life

(Stern, 1985). The newborn period is undoubtedly a formative moment in the life of the infant, parents, and family and as such presents an invaluable opportunity to the clinician to intervene in a way that has potentially lasting effects on the parent-child relationship.

We have presented a model of intervention based on the development of a supportive therapeutic relationship between clinician and parents, beginning in the newborn period. Recognizing the integrity of parents' own parenting capacities, the clinician can invite them to explore the individual adaptive capacities of their infant and the kinds of caregiving techniques that can promote the infant's development. It is the infant, however, revealed in all his or her complexity and individuality through the BNBAS, who becomes the bond uniting clinicians and parents in this supportive alliance in such a way that the positive adaptive tendencies inherent in the parent-infant relationship can be mobilized in the service of the infant and his or her family.

The main goal of this chapter has been to present a model for preventive intervention for the first months of life based on the Brazelton Neonatal Behavioral Assessment Scale. The model is, by nature, both adaptive and flexible. Our hope, then, is that the systematic testing of the model leads to a refinement of our understanding of this model and thus enable mental health clinicians to give infants and their families the best possible start in life by maintaining both a constructive and a humane role in their lives from the very beginning.

References

Adamson, L. B. (1993). *Communication development during infancy.* Madison, WI: Brown and Benchmark.

Akiyama, T., Kawasaki, C., Goto, Y., Turusaki, T., Ohgi, S., Nakamura, M., Kawaguchi, Y., Nugent, J. K., & Brazelton, T. B. (In press) The relationship between neonatal behavior and development outcome at seven years of age in a sample of Japanese infants. In J. K. Nugent, B. M. Lester, & T. B. Brazelton (Eds.), *The cultural context of infancy: Vol. 3.* Norwood, NJ: Ablex.

Als, H. (1984). Newborn behavioral assessment. In W. J. Burns & J. Lavigne (Eds.), *Progress in pediatric psychology* (pp. 1–46) New York: Grune & Stratton.

Als, H., Lester, B. M., Tronick, E., & Brazelton, T. B. (1982). Manual for the assessment of preterm infants' behavior (APIB). In H. E. Fitzgerald, B. M. Lester, & M. Yogman (Eds.), *Theory and research in behavioral pediatrics:* Vol. 1 (pp. 65–132). New York: Plenum.

Anders, T., Halpern, L., & Hua, J. (1992). Sleeping through the night: a developmental perspective. *Pediatrics, 90,* 554–590.

Anderson, C. J., & Sawin D. (1983). Enhancing responsiveness in mother-infant interaction. *Infant Behavior and Development,* 6(3), 361–368.

Anisfield, E., & Pincus, M. (1978). The postpartum support project: Serving young mothers and older women through home visiting. *Zero to Three, 8,* 13–15.

Atkins, C., Olvera, M. C., Givaudan, M., & Landeros, G. (1991). Neonatal behavior and maternal perceptions of urban Mexican infants. In J. K. Nugent, B. M. Lester, & T. B. Brazelton (Eds.), *The cultural context of infancy: Vol. 2. Multicultural and interdisciplinary approaches to parent-infant relations* (pp. 201–236). Norwood, NJ: Ablex.

Auerbach, J. G., Hans, S. L., Marcus, J., & Maeir, S. (1992). Maternal psychotropic medication and neonatal behavior. *Neurotoxicology and Teratology, 14,* 399–406.

Azuma, S. D., Malee, K. M., Kavanagh, J. A., & Deddish, R. B. (1991). Confirmatory factor analysis with preterm NBAS data: A comparison of four data reduction models. *Infant Behavior and Development, 14,* 209–225.

Barnard, K. E., Morisset, C. E., & Speiker, S. (1993). Preventive interventions: Enhancing parent-infant relationships. In C. H. Zeanah (Ed.), *Handbook of infant mental health,* New York/London: Guilford.

Barr, R. (1998). Reflections on N-shaped curves in early infancy: Regulated or reorganized development? [Special Issue]. *Infant Behavior and Development, 21,* 184.

Barr, R. G. (1990). The normal crying curve: What do we really know? *Developmental Medicine and Child Neurology, 32,* 356–362.

Beal, J. A. (1986). The Brazelton Neonatal Behavioral Assessment: A tool to enhance parental attachment. *Journal of Pediatric Nursing, 1,* 170–177.

Beckwith, L., & Parmelee, A. (1989). EEG patterns in preterm infants: Home environment and later IQ. *Child Development, 57,* 777–789.

Beeghly, M., Nugent, J. K., Burroughs, E., & Brazelton, T. B. (1988). Effects of intrauterine growth retardation on infant behavior and development in the family [Special ICIS issue]. *Infant Behavior and Development, 11,* 21.

Beeghly, M., Brazelton, T. B., Flannery, K., Nugent, J. K., Barrett, D., & Tronick, E. Z. (1995). Specificity of preventative pediatric intervention effects in early infancy. *Journal of Developmental and Behavioral Pediatrics, 16*(3), 158–166.

Beeghly, M., & Tronick, E. Z. (1994). Effects of prenatal exposure to cocaine in early infancy: Toxic effects on the process of mutual regulation. *Infant Mental Health, 15*(2), 158–175.

Belsky, J. (1985). Experimenting with the family in the newborn period. *Child Development, 56,* 407–414.

Belsky, J. (1986). Tale of two variances: Between and within. *Child Development, 57,* 1301–1305.

Boger, K., & Kurnetz, R. (1985). Perinatal positive parenting: Hospital-based support for first-time parents. *Pediatric Basics, 41,* 4–15.

Bottos, M. (1987). *Paralisi cerebrale infantile.* Milano: Ghedini Editore.

Bottos, M., Dalla Barba, B., & Tronick, E. Z. (in press). The culture of handicap. In J. K. Nugent, B. M. Lester, & T. B. Brazelton (Eds.), *The cultural context of infancy: Vol. 3.* Norwood, NJ: Ablex.

Boukydis, C. F. Z. (Ed.). (1986). *Supports for parents and infants.* New York: Routledge & Kegan Paul.

Brazelton, T. B. (1973). *Neonatal behavioral assessment scale:* Clinics in developmental medicine, No. 50. London: Wm. Heinemann Medical Books.

Brazelton, T. B. (1984). *Neonatal behavioral assessment scale:* Spastics International Medical Publications. London: Blackwell Scientific. Philadelphia: Lippincott.

Brazelton, T. B. (1982). Early intervention: What does it mean? In H. E. Fitzgerald, B. M. Lester, & M. W. Yogman (Eds.), *The-*

ory and research in behavioral pediatrics: Vol. 1 (pp. 1–34). New York: Plenum.

Brazelton, T. B. (1992). *Touchpoints.* Reading, MA: Addison-Wesley.

Brazelton, T. B., Koslowski, B., & Main, M. (1974). The origins of reciprocity: The early mother-infant interaction. In M. Lewis & L. Rosenblum (Eds.), *The effect of the infant on its caregivers* (pp. 49–77). New York: Wiley Interscience.

Brazelton, T. B., Koslowski, B., & Tronick, E. (1977). Neonatal behavior among urban Zambians and Americans. *Annual Progress in Child Psychiatry, 15,* 97–107.

Brazelton, T. B., & Nugent, J. K. (1987). Neonatal assessment as intervention. In H. Rauh & H. C. Steinhausen (Eds.), *Psychobiology and early development* (pp. 215–229). Amsterdam: North Holland.

Brazelton, T. B., & Nugent, J. K. (1995). *The newborn behavioral assessment scale.* London: McKeith Press.

Brazelton, T. B., Nugent, J. K., & Lester, B. M. (1987). The neonatal behavioral assessment scale. In J. Osofsky (Ed.), *The handbook of infant development* (2nd ed., pp. 780–817). New York: Wiley.

Brazelton, T. B., Robey, J. S., & Collier, G. A. (1969). Infant behavior in the Zinancanteco Indians in southern Mexico. *Pediatrics, 44,* 274–281.

Brazelton, T. B., Tronick, E., Lechtig, A., Lasky, R., & Klein, R. (1977). The behavior of nutritionally deprived Guatemalan infants. *Developmental Medicine and Child Neurology, 19,* 364–372.

Bronfenbrenner, U. (1979). *The ecology of human development: Experiments by nature and design.* Cambridge, MA: Harvard University Press.

Bruschweiler-Stern, N. (1997). Mere a terme et mere premature. In M. Dugnat (Ed.),

Le monde relationnel du bebe (pp. 19–24). Ramonville Saint-Agne: ERES.

Candilis-Huisman, D. (1997). La NBAS, un paradigme pour l'etude des premieres relations du nouveau-ne. In M. Dugnat (Ed.), *Le monde relationnel du bebe* (pp. 93–100). Ramonville Saint-Agne: ERES.

Cardone, I. A., & Gilkerson, L. (1990). Family administered neonatal activities: A first step in the integration of parental perceptions and newborn behavior. *Infant Mental Health Journal, 11,* 127–131.

Chasnoff, I., Griffith, D. R., MacGregor, S., Dirkes, K., & Burns, K. A. (1989). Temporal patterns of cocaine use in pregnancy: Perinatal outcome. *Journal of the American Medical Association, 261,* 1741–1744.

Chisholm, J. (1989). Biology, culture, and the development of temperament: A Navajo example. In J. K. Nugent, B. M. Lester, & T. B. Brazelton (Eds.), *The cultural context of infancy: Vol. 1* (pp. 341–345). Norwood, NJ: Ablex.

Choi, E. S., & Hamilton, R. K. (1986). The effects of culture on mother-infant interaction. *Journal of obstetric, gynecologic, and neonatal nursing, 15,* 256–61.

Cohn, J. F., & Tronick, E. (1983). Three-month-old infants' reaction to simulated maternal depression. *Child Development, 54,* 185–193.

Coles, C. D., Platzman, K. A., Smith, I., James, M. E., & Falek, A. (1992). Effects of cocaine and alcohol use in pregnancy on neonatal growth and neurobehavioral status. *Neurotoxicology and Teratology, 14,* 23–33.

Cramer, B. (1987). Objective and subjective aspects of parent-infant relations. In J. Osofsky (Ed.), *The handbook of infant development* (2nd ed., pp. 1037–1059). New York: Wiley.

Crockenberg, S. (1981). Infant irritability, mother responsiveness, and social support influences on the security of infant-mother attachment. *Child Development, 52,* 857–865.

Crockenberg, S. (1986). Professional support for adolescent mothers: Who gives it, how adolescent mothers evaluate it, what they would prefer. *Infant Mental Health Journal, 7*(1), 49–58.

Dannemiller, J. L., & Freedland, R. L. (1991). Detection of relative motion by human infants. *Developmental Psychology, 27,* 67–78.

Das Eiden, R., & Reifman, A. (1996). Effects of Brazelton demonstrations on later parenting. *Journal of Pediatric Psychology, 21*(6), 857–868.

DeCasper, A. J., Lecaunet, J. P., Busnel, M. C., Granier-Deferre, C., & Maugeais, (1994). Fetal reactions to recurrent maternal speech. *Infant Behavior and Development, 17,* 159–164.

DeCasper, A. J., Spence, M. J. (1991). Auditorially mediated behavior during the perinatal period: A cognitive view. In M. J. S. Weiss & P. R. Zelazo (Eds.), *Newborn attention: Biological constraints and the influence of experience.* Norwood, NJ: Ablex.

De Chateau, P. (1987). Parent-infant socialization in several Western European countries. In J. Osofsky (Ed.), *Handbook of infant development* (2nd ed., pp. 642–668). New York: Wiley.

Dixon, S., Tronick, E. Z., Keefer, C., & Brazelton, T. B. (1982). Perinatal circumstances and newborn outcome among the Gusii of Kenya: Assessment of risk. *Infant Behavior and Development, 5,* 11–37.

Dobbing, J. (1990). Vulnerable periods in the developing brain. In J. Dobbing (Ed.),

Brain, behavior, and iron in the infant diet (pp. 1–25). London: Springer-Verlag.

Dolby, R., English, B., & Warren, B. (1982, March). *Brazelton demonstrations for mothers and fathers: Impact on the developing parent-child relationship.* Paper presented at the International Conference on Infant Studies, Austin, TX.

Dreher, M., Nugent, J. K., & Hudgins, R. (1994). Prenatal marijuana exposure and neonatal outcomes in Jamaica: An ethnographic study. *Pediatrics, 93,* 254–260.

Emde, R. N., & Robinson, J. (1979). The first two months: Recent research in developmental psychobiology and the changing view of the newborn. In J. Noshpitz (Ed.), *Basic handbook of child psychiatry* (pp. 72–105). New York: Basic Books.

Emde, R. (1987). Infant mental health: Clinical dilemmas, the expansion of meaning and opportunities. In J. Osofsky (Ed.), *The handbook of infant development* (2nd ed., pp. 1297–1320). New York: Wiley.

Eyler, F. D., Behnke, M., Conlon, M., Woods, N. S., & Wobie, K. (1997). Birth outcome from a prospective, matched study of prenatal crack/cocaine use: II. Interactive and dose effects on neurobehavioral assessment. *Pediatrics, 101,* 237–241.

Fabre-Grenet, M. (1997). L'echelle de Brazelton au quotidien dans un service de neonatologie. Le point de vue du pediatre. In M. Dugnat (Ed.), *Le monde relationnel du bebe* (pp. 101–8). Ramonville, Saint-Agne: ERES.

Field, T. (1987). Affective and interactive disturbances in infants. In J. Osofsky (Ed.), *The handbook of infant development* (2nd ed., pp. 972–1005). New York: Wiley.

Field, T., Woodson, R., Greenberg, R., & Cohen, C. (1992). Discrimination and imitation of facial expressions in newborns. *Science, 218,* 179–181.

Fifer, W. P., & Moon, C. M. (1994). The role of mother's voice in the organization of brain function in the newborn. *Acta Paediatrica* (Suppl. 397), 86–93.

Finn, C. (1994, September). *Irish mothers' perception of parenting a handicapped infant.* Paper presented at the 14th Annual Conference of the Society for Reproductive and Infant Psychology, Dublin, Ireland.

Fraiberg, S. (1980). *Clinical studies in infant mental health: The first year of life.* New York: Basic Books.

Freedman, D. (1980). Maturational and developmental issues in the first year. In S. I. Greenspan & G. H. Pollock (Eds.), *The course of life: Vol. 1. Infancy and early childhood* (pp. 78–786). Washington, DC: Government Printing Office.

Fricker, H. S., Hindermann, R., & Bruuppacher, R. (1989). The Aarau study on pregnancy and the newborn: An epidemiologic investigation of the course of pregnancy in 996 Swiss women, and its influence on newborn behavior using the Brazelton scale. In J. K. Nugent, B. M. Lester, & T. B. Brazelton (Eds.), *The cultural context of infancy: Vol. 1. Biology, culture, and infant development* (pp. 27–63). Norwood, NJ: Ablex.

Fried, P., & Makin, J. E. (1986). Neonatal behavioral correlates of prenatal exposure to marijuana, cigarettes and alcohol in a low-risk population. *Neurotoxicology and Teratology, 9,* 1–7.

Furr, P. M., & Kirgis, C. A. (1982, September–October). A nurse midwifery approach to early mother infant acquaintance. *Journal of Nurse Midwifery, 27*(5), 10–15.

Garbarino, J. (1982). Sociocultural risk: Dangers to competence. In C. B. Kopp & J. B. Crakow (Eds.), *The child: Development in a social context* (pp. 630–687). Reading, MA: Addison-Wesley.

Garbarino, J. (1992). *Children and families in the social environment.* New York: Aldine de Gruyter.

Garcia-Coll, C. (1989). The consequences of teenage childbearing in traditional Puerto Rican culture. In J. K. Nugent, B. M. Lester, & T. B. Brazelton (Eds.), *The cultural context of infancy: Vol. 1. Biology, culture, and infant development* (pp. 111–132). Norwood, NJ: Ablex.

Gathwala, G., & Narayan, I. (1990). Cesarean section and delayed contact: Effect on baby's behaviour. *Indian Pediatrics, 27,* 1295–1299.

Gessell, A. L. (1946). The ontogenesis of infant behavior. In L. Carmichael (Ed.), *Manual of Child Psychology* (pp. 295–331). New York: Wiley.

Gomes-Pedro, J., de Almeida, J. B., & Costa Barbosa, A. (1984). Influence of early mother-infant contact on synaptic behavior during the first month of life. *Developmental Medicine and Child Neurology, 26,* 657–664.

Gomes-Pedro, J., Monteiro, M., Patricio, M., Carvalho, A., & Torgal-Garcia, F. (1988). Early intervention and mother-infant behavior: A longitudinal perspective. In J. K. Nugent (Chair), *Cultural contexts of parent-infant relations.* Symposium presented at the Third Biennial Meeting of the International Association for Infant Mental Health, Providence, RI.

Gomes-Pedro, J., Patricio, M., Carvalho, A., Goldschmidt, T., Torgal-Garcia, F., & Monteiro, M. B. (1995). Early intervention with Portuguese mothers: A two year follow-up. *Developmental and Behavioral Pediatrics, 16,* 21–28.

Graham, F. K., Matarazzo, R. G., & Caldwell, B. M. (1956). Behavioral differences between normal and traumatized newborns: 1. The test procedures. *Psychological Monographs, 70,* (21, Whole No. 428).

Greene, S. (in press). Child development: Old themes and new directions. In J. Gomes-Pedro, J. K. Nugent, J. G. Young, & T. B. Brazelton (Eds.), *The infant and family in the 21st century.* New York: Brunner-Mazel.

Greenspan, S. I. (1981). *The clinical interview of the child.* New York: McGraw-Hill.

Grossmann, K., & Grossmann, K. E. (1991). Newborn behavior, the quality of early parenting and later toddler-parent relationships in a group of German infants. In J. K. Nugent, B. M. Lester, & T. B. Brazelton (Eds.), *The cultural context of infancy: Vol. 2. Multicultural and interdisciplinary approaches to parent-infant relations.* (pp. 3–38). Norwood, NJ: Ablex.

Hawthorne-Amick, J. A. (1989). The effects of different routines in a special care baby unit on the mother-infant relationship. In J. K. Nugent, B. M. Lester, & T. B. Brazelton (Eds.), *The cultural context of infancy: Vol. 1. Biology, culture and infant development* (pp. 237–267). Norwood, NJ: Ablex.

Hayes, J. S., Lampart, R., Dreher, M. C., & Morgan, L. (1991). Five-year follow-up of rural Jamaican children whose mothers used marijuana during pregnancy. *West Indian Medical Journal, 40,* 120–123.

Hinde, R. (1976). On describing relationships. *Journal of Child Psychology and Psychiatry, 17,* 1–19.

Hirshberg, L. M. (1993). Clinical interviews with infants and their families. In C. H. Zeanah (Ed.), *Handbook of infant mental health* (pp. 173–90). London/New York: Guilford Press.

Hopkins, B. (1991). Facilitating early motor

development: An intracultural study of West Indian mothers living in Britain. In J. K. Nugent, B. M. Lester, & T. B. Brazelton (Eds.), *The cultural context of infancy: Vol. 2. Multicultural and interdisciplinary approaches to parent-infant relations* (pp. 93–143). Norwood, NJ: Ablex.

Hopkins, B. (1998). Moving into the two-month revolution: An action-based account [Special Issue]. *Infant Behavior and Development, 21,* p. 183.

Jacobson, J. J., Fein, G. G., Jacobson, S. W., & Schwartz, P. M. (1984). Factors and clusters for the Brazelton Scale: An investigation of the dimensions of neonatal behavior. *Developmental Psychology, 20,* 339–353.

Kato, T. (1991). Follow-up study on the behavioral development of Japanese neonates. *Biology of the Neonate, 60* (Suppl. 1), 75–85.

Kawasaki, K., Nugent, J. K., Miyashita, H., Miyahara, H., & Brazelton, T. B. (1994). The cultural organization of infant's sleep. *Children's Environments, 11,* 134–141.

Kaye, K. (1982). *The mental and social life of babies.* Chicago: University of Chicago Press.

Keefer, C., Tronick, E., Dixon, S., & Brazelton, T. B. (1982). Specific differences in motor performance between Gusii and American newborns and a modification of the neonatal behavioral assessment scale. *Child Development, 53,* 554–559.

Keefer, C. H. (1995). The combined physical and behavioral neonatal examination: A parent-centered approach to pediatric care. In T. B. Brazelton & J. K. Nugent (Eds.), *The Neonatal behavioral assessment scale.* London: McKeith Press.

Keefer, C. H., Dixon, S., Tronick, E. Z., & Brazelton, T. B. (1991). Cultural mediation between newborn behavior and later development: Implications for methodology in cross-cultural research. In J. K. Nugent, B. M. Lester, & T. B. Brazelton (Eds.), *The cultural context of infancy: Vol. 2. Multicultural and interdisciplinary approaches to parent-infant relations* (pp. 39–61). Norwood, NJ: Ablex.

Klaus, M. H., Kennell, J. H., & Klaus, P. H. (1995). *Bonding.* Reading, MA: Addison-Wesley.

Konner, M. (1998). Behavioral changes around two months of age in a population of African Hunter-Gatherers [Special issue]. *Infant Behavior and Development, 21,* p. 185.

Korner, A. (1987). Preventive intervention with high-risk newborns. In J. Osofsky (Ed.), *The handbook of infant development* (2nd ed., pp. 1006–1036). New York: Wiley.

Landers, C. (1989). A psychological study of infant development in South India. In J. K. Nugent, B. M. Lester, & T. B. Brazelton (Eds.), *The cultural context of infancy: Vol. 1. Biology, culture, and infant development* (pp. 169–207). Norwood, NJ: Ablex.

Laplante, D., Orr, R., Neville, K., Vorkapich, L., & Sasso, D. (1996). Discrimination of stimulus rotations by newborns. *Infant Behavior and Development, 19*(3), 271–279.

Lester, B. M. (1984). Data analysis and prediction. In T. B. Brazelton, *Neonatal behavioral assessment scale* (2nd ed.). London: MacKeith Press.

Lester, B. M., & Brazelton, T. B. (1982). Cross-cultural assessment of newborn behavior. In D. Wagner & H. Stevenson (Eds.), *Cultural perspectives on child development* (pp. 20–53). San Francisco: W. H. Freeman.

Lester, B. M., Hoffman, J., & Brazelton,

T. B. (1985). The rhythmic structure of mother-infant interaction in term and preterm infants. *Child Development, 51,* 15–27.

LeVine, R. A. (1980). Cross-cultural perspectives on parenting. In M. Fantini & R. Cardinas (Eds.), *Parenting in a multicultural society* (pp. 17–26). New York: Longman.

Lieberman, A. F. (1991). Attachment theory and infant-parent psychotherapy: Some conceptual, clinical and research considerations. In D. Cicchetti & S. Toth (Eds.), *Models and integrations Rochester symposium on developmental psychopathology: Vol. 3* (pp. 261–288). Hillsdale NJ: Erlbaum.

Linn, P. L., & Horowitz, F. D. (1984). The relationship between infant individual differences and mother-infant interaction in the neonatal period. *Infant Behavior and Development, 6,* 415–427.

Liptak, G. S., Keller, B. B., Feldman, A. W., & Chamberlin, R. W. (1983, July). Enhancing infant development and parent-practitioner interaction with the Brazelton neonatal assessment scale. *Pediatrics,* 72(1), 71–77.

MacDonough, S. C. (1993). Interaction guidance: Understanding and treating early infant-caregiver disturbances. In C. Zeanah (Ed.), *Handbook of infant mental health.* New York/London: Guilford Press.

Mahler, M., Pine, F., & Bergman, A. (1975). *The psychological birth of the human infant.* New York: Basic Books.

Meisels, S., Dichtelmiller, M., & Fong-Ruey L. (1993). A multidimensional analysis of early childhood intervention programs. In C. Zeanah (Ed.), *Handbook of infant mental health.* New York/London: Guilford Press.

Minuchin, B. (1985). Families and individual development: Provocations from the field of family therapy. *Child Development, 59,* 289–302.

Muir, D., & Field, J. (1979). Newborn infants orient to sounds. *Child Development, 50,* 431–436.

Munck, H. (1985, January). *Reflections on qualitative aspects in a study of preterm infants and their parents.* Paper presented at the International Symposium on Psychobiology and Early Development, West Berlin, Germany.

Munck, H., Mirdal, G., & Marner, G. (1991). Mother-infant interaction in Denmark. In J. K. Nugent, B. M. Lester, & T. B. Brazelton (Eds.), *The cultural context of infancy: Vol. 2. Multicultural and interdisciplinary approaches to parent-infant relations* (pp. 169–199). Norwood, NJ: Ablex.

Muret-Wagstaff, S., & Moore, S. (1989). The Hmong in America. In J. K. Nugent, B. M. Lester, & T. B. Brazelton (Eds.), *The cultural context of infancy: Vol. 1. Biology, culture, and infant development* (pp. 319–339). Norwood, NJ: Ablex.

Murray, L. (1994, June). *The infant's contribution to the mother-infant relationship in the context of postnatal depression.* Paper presented at the 9th International Conference on Infant Studies, Paris, France.

Murray, L., & Cooper, P. J. (1997). The role of infant and maternal factors in postpartum depression, mother-infant interactions, and infant outcomes. In L. Murray & P. J. Cooper (Eds.), *Postpartum depression and child development* (pp. 111–35). New York/London: Guilford Press.

Myers, B. J. (1982). Early intervention using Brazelton training with middle class mothers and fathers of newborns. *Child Development, 53,* 462–471.

Niestroj, B. H. E. (1991). Fetal nutrition: A study of its effect on behavior in Zulu newborns. In J. K. Nugent, B. M. Lester, & T. B. Brazelton (Eds.), *The cultural context of infancy: Vol. 2. Multicultural and interdisciplinary approaches to parent-infant relations* (pp. 321–352). Norwood, NJ: Ablex.

Nugent, J. K. (1985). *Using the NBAS with infants and their families: Guidelines for intervention.* White Plains, NY: March of Dimes Birth Defects Foundation.

Nugent, J. K. (1991). Cultural and psychological influences on the father's role in infant development. *Journal of Marriage and the Family, 53*(2), 475–485.

Nugent, J. K. (1994). Cross-cultural studies of child development: Implications for clinicians. *Zero to Three, 15*(2), 1–8.

Nugent, J. K., & Brazelton, T. B. (1989). Preventive intervention with infants and families: The NBAS model. *Infant Mental Health Journal, 10,* 84–99.

Nugent, J. K., Greene, S., Wieczorek-Deering, D., & O'Mahony, P. (In press). Parent-infant relations: The transition to parenthood in a sample of Irish families. In J. K. Nugent, B. M. Lester, & T. B. Brazelton (Eds.), *The cultural context of infancy* (Vol. 3). Norwood, NJ: Ablex.

Nugent, J. K., Hoffman, J., Barrett, D., Censullo, M., & Brazelton, T. B. (1987, April). *The effects of early intervention on IUGR infants.* Presented at the Biennial Meeting of the Society for Research in Child Development, Baltimore, MD.

Nugent, J. K., Lester, B. M., & Brazelton, T. B. (Eds.). (1989). *The cultural context of infancy* (Vol. 1). Norwood, NJ: Ablex.

Nugent, J. K., Lester, B. M., & Brazelton, T. B. (Eds.). (1991). *The cultural context of infancy: Vol. 2. Multicultural and interdisciplinary approaches to parent-infant relations.* Norwood, NJ: Ablex.

Nugent, J. K., Lester, B. M., & Brazelton, T. B. (In press). *The cultural context of infancy* (Vol. 3). Norwood, NJ: Ablex.

Nugent, J. K., & Brazelton, T. B. (In preparation). *The Clinical Neonatal Behavioral Assessment Scale.* The Brazelton Institute, Children's Hospital, Boston.

Nurcombe, B., Howell, D. C., Rauh, V. A., Teti, D. M., Ruoff, P., & Brennan, J. (1984). An intervention program for mothers of low birthweight infants: Preliminary results. *Journal of the American Academy of Child Psychiatry, 23*(3), 319–325.

Ohgi, S., Tsurasaki, T., Kawasaki, C., & Akiyama, T. (1993, October). *Using the NBAS as a therapeutic intervention in the neonatal intensive care unit.* Paper presented at the Conference on the Brazelton Scale, University of Nagasaki, Japan.

Olsen, R. D., Olsen, G., Pernice, J., & Bloom, K. (1981, April). *The use of the Brazelton newborn assessment as an intervention with high-risk mothers in the newborn period.* Paper presented at the joint session of Ambulatory Pediatric Association and Society for Pediatric Research, San Francisco, CA.

Osofsky, J. (Ed.). (1987). *The handbook of infant development.* New York: 1987.

Oyemade, U. J., Cole, O. J., Johnson, A. A., Knight, E. M., Westney, O. E., Lareya, H., Hill, G., Cannon, E., & Fumufod, A. (1994). Prenatal substance abuse and pregnancy outcomes among African American women. *Journal of Nutrition, 124* (Suppl. 6), 1000S–1005S.

Paludetto, R., Mansi, G., Rinaldi, P., Margara-Paludetto, P., & Faggiano-Perfetto, M. (1991). Working toward a humanized neonatal care system in Naples: Interactions between parents, infants and health care personnel. In J. K. Nugent, B. M. Lester, & T. B. Brazelton (Eds.),

The cultural context of infancy: Vol. 2. Multicultural and interdisciplinary approaches to parent-infant relations (pp. 239–270). Norwood, NJ: Ablex.

Papousek, H., & Papousek, M. (1987). Intuitive parenting: A dialectic counterpart to the infant's integrative competence. In J. Osofsky (Ed.), *The handbook of infant development* (2nd ed., pp. 669–720). New York: Wiley.

Park-Synn, B. (In press). A comparison of the transition to parenthood in nuclear and traditional families in Korea. In J. K. Nugent, B. M. Lester, & T. B. Brazelton (Eds.), *The cultural context of infancy: Vol. 3.* Norwood, NJ: Ablex.

Parker, S., Zahr, L. K., Cole, J. C. D., & Braced, M. L. (1992). Outcomes after developmental intervention in the neonatal intensive care unit for mothers of preterm infants with low socioeconomic status. *Journal of Pediatrics, 120,* 780–785.

Pascalis, O., de Schonen, S., Morton, J., Deruelle, C., & Fabre-Grenet, M. (1995). Mother's face recognition by neonates: A replication and an extension. *Infant Behavior and Development, 18,* 79–85.

Piessens, P. W. (1991). Newborn behavior and development in Indonesia. In J. K. Nugent, B. M. Lester, & T. B. Brazelton (Eds.), *The cultural context of infancy: Vol. 2. Multicultural and interdisciplinary approaches to parent-infant relations* (pp. 271–298). Norwood, NJ: Ablex.

Prechtl, H. F. R. (1977). *The neurological examination of the full-term newborn infant* (2nd ed.). London: William Heinemann; Philadelphia: Lippincott.

Rauh, V., Achenbach, T., Nurcombe, B., Howell, C., & Teti, D. (1988). Minimizing adverse effects of low birthweight: Four-year results of an early intervention program. *Child Development, 59,* S44–553.

Rochat, P. (1998). The newly objectified world of 2-month olds. [Special Issue] *Infant Behavior and Development, 21,* 182.

Rosenblith, J. F. (1961). The modified Graham behavior test for neonates: Test retest reliability, normative data, and hypotheses for future work. *Biologica Neonatorum, 3,* 174–193.

Rosser, P., & Randolph, S. (1989). Black American infants. In J. K. Nugent, B. M. Lester, & T. B. Brazelton (1989). *The cultural context of infancy* (Vol. 1). Norwood, NJ: Ablex.

Sacco-Pollitt, C. (1989). Ecological context of development risk. In J. K. Nugent, B. M. Lester, & T. B. Brazelton (Eds.), *The cultural context of infancy: Vol. 1. Biology, culture, and infant development* (pp. 3–25). Norwood, NJ: Ablex.

Sameroff, A. J. (1993). Models of development and developmental risk. In C. H. Zeanah (Ed.), *Handbook of infant mental health* (pp. 1–13). New York/London: Guilford Press.

Sameroff, A. J., & Emde, R. N. (Eds.). (1989). *Relationship disturbances in early childhood.* New York: Basic Books.

Sander, L. W., Stechler, G., Burns, P., & Lee, A. (1979). Change in infant caregiver variables over the first two months of life: Integration of action in early development. In E. B. Thoman (Ed.), *Origins of the infant's social responsiveness* (pp. 349–407). Hillsdale, NJ: Erlbaum.

Sepkoski, C. M., Lester, B. M., Ostheimer, G. W., & Brazelton, T. B. (1992). The effects of maternal epidural anesthesia on neonatal behavior during the first month. *Developmental Medicine and Child Neurology, 34,* 1072–1080.

Slater, A., Morison, V., Town, C., & Rose, D. (1985). Movement perception and identity constancy in the new-born baby.

British Journal of Developmental Psychology, 3, 211–220.

Sostek, A. M. (1985). On the use of a priori cluster scales for the Brazelton neonatal behavioral assessment scale: A response to Maier et al. (1983). *Infant Behavior and Development, 8,* 245–246.

Spence, M. J., & Freeman, M. S. (1996). Newborn infants prefer the maternal low-pass filtered voice, but not the maternal whispered voice. *Infant Behavior and Development, 19,* 199–212.

Stadtler, A., O'Brien, M. A., & Hornstein, J. (1995). The Touchpoints Model: Building supportive alliances between parents and professionals. *Zero to Three, 15*(1), 24–28.

Stern, D. N. (1985). *The interpersonal world of the infant.* New York: Basic Books.

Stern, D. N. (1995). *The motherhood constellation.* New York: Basic Books.

Stoleru, S., & Morales-Huet, M. (1991). Parental attitudes and mother-infant interaction in mothers from Maghreb living in France. In J. K. Nugent, B. M. Lester, & T. B. Brazelton (Eds.), *The cultural context of infancy: Vol. 2. Multicultural and interdisciplinary approaches to parent-infant relations* (pp. 299–320). Norwood, NJ: Ablex.

Super, C., & Harkness, S. (1982). The infant's niche in rural Kenya and metropolitan America. In L. Adler (Ed.), *Cross-cultural research at issue.* New York: Academic.

Swain, I., Zelazo, P., & Clifton, R. (1993). Newborn infants' memory for speech sounds retained over 24 hours. *Developmental Psychology, 29,* 312–323.

Szajnberg, N., Ward, M. J., Kraus, A., & Kessler, D. (1984, April). *Low birthweight prematures: Preventive intervention and maternal attitude.* Paper presented at the International Conference on Infant Studies, New York, NY.

Thomas, A., & Chess, S. (1977). *Temperament and Development.* New York: Brunner/Mazel.

Tirosh, E., Abadi, J., Harel, J., Berger, A., & Cohen, A. (1992). Neonatal behavior of Panamanian and Israeli infants: A cross-cultural study. *Israel Journal of Medical Sciences, 28,* 87–90.

Trevarthen, C. (1979). Communication and cooperation in early infancy: A description of early subjectivity. In M. Bullowa (Ed.), *Before speech: The beginning of interpersonal communication.* Cambridge, England: Cambridge University Press.

Tronick, E., Als, H., & Brazelton, T. B. (1980). Monadic phases: A structural descriptive analysis of infant-mother face-to-face interaction. *Merrill-Palmer Quarterly, 26,* 3–13.

Tronick, E. Z., & Cohn, J. F. (1989). Infant-mother face-to-face interaction: Age and gender differences in coordination and occurrence of miscordination. *Child Development, 60,* 85–92.

Van Baar, A. (In press). Development of infants of drug-dependent mothers in the Netherlands. In J. K. Nugent, B. M. Lester, & T. B. Brazelton (Eds.), *The cultural context of infancy* (Vol. 3). Norwood, NJ: Ablex.

Van den Boom, D. (1991). The influence of infant irritability on the development of the mother-infant relationship in the first 6 months of life. In J. K. Nugent, B. M. Lester, & T. B. Brazelton (Eds.), *The cultural context of infancy* (Vol. 2). (pp. 63–89) Norwood, NJ: Ablex.

Vygotsky, L. S. (1987). *The collected works of L. S. Vygotsky: Vol. 1. Problems of general psychology.* New York: Plenum.

Walsh-Escarce, E. (1989). Across-cultural

study of Nepalese neonatal behavior. In J. K. Nugent, B. M. Lester, & T. B. Brazelton (Eds.), *The cultural context of infancy: Vol. 1. Biology, culture, and infant development* (pp. 65–86). Norwood, NJ: Ablex.

Warren, B., Dolby, R., Meade, V., & Heath, J. (1989). A preventive care program for low birthweight infants which incorporates parents needs. In M. Bottos, T. B. Brazelton, A. Ferrari, B. Dalla Barba, & F. Zachello (Eds.), *Neurological lesions in infancy: Early diagnosis and intervention* (pp. 265–68). Padova: Liviana Edrice.

Waters, E., Vaughn, B. E., & Egeland, B. (1980). Individual differences in infant-mother attachment relationships at age one: Antecedents in neonatal behavior in an urban, economically disadvantaged sample. *Child Development, 51,* 208–216.

Weinberg, M. K., & Tronick, E. Z. (1996). Infant affective reactions to the resumption of maternal interaction after the still-face. *Child Development, 67,* 905–914.

Weissbourd, B., & Kagan, S. (1989). Family support programs: Catalysts for change. *American Journal of Orthopsychiatry, 59,* 20–31.

Welles-Nystrom, B. L. (1991). The mature primipara and her infant in Sweden: A life course study. In J. K. Nugent, B. M. Lester, & T. B. Brazelton (Eds.), *The cultural context of infancy: Vol. 2. Multicultural and interdisciplinary approaches to parent-infant relations* (pp. 145–168). Norwood, NJ: Ablex.

Whiting, B., & Edwards, C. P. (1988). *Children of different worlds: The formation of social behavior.* Cambridge, MA: Harvard University Press.

Widmayer, S., & Field, T. (1980). Effects of Brazelton demonstrations on early interaction of preterm infants and their

teenage mothers. *Infant Behavior and Development, 3,* 79–89.

Widmayer, S., & Field, T. (1981). Effects of Brazelton demonstrations for mothers on the development of preterm infants. *Pediatrics, 67,* 711–714.

Winn, S., Tronick, E. Z., & Morelli, G. (1989). The infant and the group: A look at Efe caretaking practices in Zaire. In J. K. Nugent, B. M. Lester, & T. B. Brazelton (Eds.), *The cultural context of infancy: Vol. 1. Biology, culture, and infant development* (pp. 87–109). Norwood, NJ: Ablex.

Wolff, P. (1959). Observations on human infants. *Psychosomatic Medicine, 221,* 110–118.

Wolke, D., Gray, P., & Meyer, R. (1994). Excessive infant crying: A controlled study of mothers helping mothers. *Pediatrics, 94,* 322.

Woodson, R. H., & da Costa, E. (1989). The behavior of Chinese, Malay, and Tamil newborns from Malaysia. In J. K. Nugent, B. M. Lester, & T. B. Brazelton (Eds.), *The cultural context of infancy: Vol. 1. Biology, culture, and infant development* (pp. 295–317). Norwood, NJ: Ablex.

Worobey, J. (1985). A review of Brazelton-based interventions to enhance parent-infant interactions. *Journal of Reproductive and Infant Psychology, 3,* 64–73.

Worobey, J., & Belsky, J. (1982). Employing the Brazelton scale to influence mothering: An experimental comparison of three strategies. *Developmental Psychology, 18*(5), 736–743.

Worobey, J., & Brazelton, T. B. (1986). Experimenting with the family in the newborn period: A commentary. *Child Development, 57,* 1298–1300.

Zeanah, C. H. (Ed.). (1993). *Handbook of infant mental health.* New York/London: Guilford.

Zeanah, C. H., Boris, N. W., & Larrieu, J. A. (1997). Infant development and developmental risk: A review of the past ten years. *Journal of the American Academy of Child and Adolescent Psychiatry, 36*(2), 165–178.

Zeanah, C. H., & McDonough, S. C. (1989). Clinical approaches to families in early intervention. *Seminars in Perinatology, 13,* 513–522.

Zigler, E., & Frank, M. (1988). Conclusion. In E. Zigler & M. Frank (Eds.), *The parental leave crisis.* New Haven: Yale University Press.

6

The Assessment and Diagnosis of
Infant Disorders: Developmental
Level, Individual Differences, and
Relationship-Based Interactions

Stanley I. Greenspan and Serena Wieder

6

Introduction

The evaluation of infants, young children, and their families is both simple and complex. Infants and young children are very direct; what you see is what there is. An 8-month-old doesn't disguise his true feelings; he is either engaged and related or aloof and withdrawn. But there are many factors influencing behavior and many aspects of development that all relate to one another. For example, an aloof and withdrawn 8-month-old will be influenced by the relationship with the child's caregiver and by family functioning, as well as the child's own physical tendencies (e.g., over- or undersensitivity to sound or touch). This child will also be influenced by the relationships between the different aspects of his or her development, including his sensory, motor, language, cognitive, affective, and interpersonal capacities.

The evaluation of emotional and developmental disorders in infants and young children requires the clinician to take into account all facets of the child's experience. It is therefore necessary to have a model with which to examine the ways constitutional-maturational (i.e., regulatory), family, and interactive factors work together as the child progresses through each development phase.

The Basic Model

The developmental model can be visualized with the infant's constitutional-maturational patterns on one side and the infant's environment (including caregivers, family, community, and culture) on the other side. Both of these sets of factors operate through the infant-caregiver relationship, which can be pictured in the middle. These two sets of factors and the infant-caregiver relationship. In turn contribute to the organization of experience at each of six different developmental levels, which may be pictured just beneath the infant-caregiver relationship.

Each developmental level involves different tasks or goals. The relative effect of the constitutional-maturational, environmental, or interactive variables will therefore depend on and can only be understood in the context of the developmental level to which they relate. The influencing variables are best understood not as they might be traditionally, as general influences on development or behavior, but as distinct and different influences on the six different developmental and experiential levels. For example, as a child is engaging, or negotiating the formation of a relationship, the child's mother's tendency to be very intellectual and prefer talking over holding may make it relatively harder for the child to become deeply engaged in emotional terms. If the child has slightly lower than average muscle tone and is hyposensitive with regard to touch and sound, the mother's intellectual and slightly aloof style may be doubly difficult for both, as neither she nor the child is able to take the initiative in engaging the other.

Developmental Levels

In this model, there are six developmental levels. They include the infant or child's ability to accomplish the following:

1. Attend to multisensory affective experience and at the same time organize a calm, regulated state and experience pleasure.
2. Engage with and evidence affective preference and pleasure for a caregiver.
3. Initiate and respond to two-way presymbolic gestural communication.
4. Organize chains of two-way communication (opening and closing many circles of communication in a row), maintain communication across space, integrate affective polarities, and synthesize an emerging prerepresentational organization of self and other.
5. Represent (symbolize) affective experience (e.g., pretend play, functional use of language). It should be noted that this ability calls for higher level auditory and verbal sequencing ability.
6. Create representational (symbolic) categories and gradually build conceptual bridges between these categories. This ability creates the foundation for such basic personality functions as reality testing, impulse control, self-other representational differentiation, affect labeling and discrimination, stable mood, and a sense of time and space that allows for logical planning. It should be noted that this ability rests not only on complex auditory and verbal processing abilities, but visual-spatial abstracting capacities as well.

The theoretical, clinical, and empirical rationale for these developmental levels is discussed in *The Development of the Ego* (Greenspan, 1989).

At each of these levels, one looks at the range of emotional themes organized (e.g., can the child play out only dependency themes and not aggressive ones; is aggression "behaved" out?). One also looks at the stability of each level. Does minor stress lead a child to lose his ability to represent, interact, engage, or attend?

Constitutional-Maturational Patterns

Constitutional-maturational characteristics are the result of genetic, prenatal, perinatal, and maturational variations and/or deficits. They can be observed as part of the following patterns:

1. Sensory reactivity, including hypo- and hyperreactivity in each sensory modality (tactile, auditory, visual, vestibular, olfactory).
2. Sensory processing in each sensory modality (e.g., the capacity to decode sequences, configurations, or abstract patterns).
3. Sensory affective reactivity and processing in each modality (e.g., the ability to process and react to degrees of affective intensity in a stable manner).
4. Motor tone.
5. Motor planning and sequencing.

An instrument to clinically assess aspects of sensory functions in a reliable manner has been developed and is available (DeGangi & Greenspan, 1988, 1989a, b). The following section will further consider the constitutional and maturational patterns.

Sensory reactivity (hypo- or hyper-) and sensory processing can be observed clinically. Is the child hyper- or hyposensitive to touch or sound? The same question must be asked in terms of vision and movement in space. In each sensory modality, does the 4-month-old child "process" a complicated pattern of information input or only a simple one? Does the 4½-year-old have a receptive language problem and is the child unable to sequence words together or follow complex directions? Is the 3-year-old an early comprehender and talker, but slow at visual-spatial processing? If spatial patterns are poorly comprehended, a child may be facile with words and sensitive to every emotional nuance, but the child may have no context and never see the big picture (the "forest"); such children get lost in the "trees." In the clinician's office, such a child may forget where the door is or have a hard time picturing that his or her mother is only a few feet away in the waiting room.

In addition to straightforward "pictures" of spatial relationship (i.e., how to get to the playground), they may also have difficulty with seeing the emotional big "picture." If the mother is angry, the child may desperately feel as if the earth is opening up and he is falling in because he cannot comprehend that she was nice before and that she will probably be nice again. Such a child may be strong on the auditory processing side, but weak on the visual-spatial processing side.

Our impression is that children with a lag in the visual-spatial area can become overwhelmed by the affect of the moment. This is often intensified by precocious auditory-verbal skills. The child, in a sense, overloads him or herself, and does not have the ability to see how a situation all fits to-

gether. Thus, at a minimum, it is necessary to have a sense of how the child reacts in each sensory modality, how he or she processes information in each modality, and (particularly as the child gets older) a sense of the auditory-verbal processing skills in comparison to visual-spatial processing skills.

It is also necessary to look at the child's motor system, including motor tone, motor planning (fine and gross), and postural control. Observing how a child sits, crawls, or runs; maintains posture; holds a crayon; hops, scribbles, or draws; and makes rapid alternating movements will provide a picture of the child's motor system. His security in regulating and controlling his body plays an important role in how he uses gestures to communicate his ability to regulate dependency (being close or far away); his confidence in regulating aggression ("Can I control my hand that wants to hit?"); and his overall physical sense of self.

Other constitutional and maturational variables have to do with movement in space, attention, and dealing with transitions.

Parent and Family Contributions

In addition to constitutional and maturational factors, it is important to describe the family contribution with regard to each developmental level. If a family system is aloof, it may not negotiate engagement well; if a family system is intrusive, it may overwhelm or overstimulate a baby. Obviously, if a baby is already overly sensitive to touch or sound, a caregiver's intrusiveness will be more difficult for the child to handle. We see, therefore, the interaction between the maturational pattern and the family pattern.

A family system may throw so many meanings at a child that he or she is unable to organize a sense of reality. Categories of me/not-me may become confused, because one day a feeling is the child's, and the next day it is the mother's, and the next day it is the father's, and the day after it is the little brother's; anger may turn into dependency, and vice versa. If meanings shift too quickly, a child may be unable to reach the fourth level—emotional thinking. A child with difficulties in auditory-verbal sequencing will have an especially difficult time (Greenspan, 1989).

The couple is a unit in itself. How do husband and wife operate—not only with each other, but how do they negotiate on behalf of the children, in terms of developmental processes? A couple with marital problems could still successfully negotiate shared attention, engagement, two-way communication, shared meanings, and emotional thinking with their children. But marital difficulties could disrupt any one or more of these developmental processes.

Each parent is also an individual. How does each personality operate vis-à-vis these processes? While it may be desirable to have a general mental health diagnosis for each caregiver, one also needs to functionally observe which of these levels each caregiver can naturally and easily support. Is the parent engaged, warm, and interactive (a good reader of cues)? Is he or she oriented toward symbolic meanings (verbalizing meanings) and engaging in pre-

tend play? Can the caregiver organize feelings and thoughts, or does one or the other get lost between reality and fantasy? Are there limitations within these levels, and if so, what are they?

Each parent also has specific fantasies that may be projected onto the children and may interfere with any of the levels. Does a mother see her motorically active, distractible, labile baby as a menace and therefore overcontrol, overintrude, or withdraw? Her fantasy may govern her behavior. Does a father, whose son has low motor tone, see his boy as passive and inept, and therefore pull away from him or impatiently rev him up?

In working only with the parent-child interaction, and not the parent's fantasy, one may be dealing with only the tip of the iceberg. The father may be worried that he has a homosexual son, or the mother may be worried that she has a monster for a daughter (who reminds her of her retarded sister). All these feelings may be simmering beneath the surface of a parent, and they can drive parent-child interactions.

Infant-Caregiver Relationship Patterns

It is the caregiver-infant relationship that mediates these other variables and, in addition, determines whether each of the developmental processes is successfully or unsuccessfully negotiated. Often, parents will bring a baby in, and we will watch the parent-infant interaction in the first session, while we are hearing about their concerns. With an older child, a four-year-old, for example, we will have the parents wait to bring the child in, because we want them to talk freely from the beginning.

Usually, we let each parent play with the child for at least fifteen or twenty minutes, and then we will play with the child for about the same amount of time. We look for a pattern of interaction in the context of the developmental processes. We observe which levels are present and not present, and also look for the range of emotional themes in each of the core processes and the stability of these processes. For example, a four-year-old may be playing out wonderful fantasies of fairy princesses going off to a castle and being tied up by an evil witch and then being saved by the hero. While we are interested in the content, we first observe how the child is relating with his or her caregiver (and later on with us), the breadth of emotion, and the stability of the relationship.

Therefore, for each of the developmental levels or core processes, it is necessary to look at the child's constitutional and maturational status, the family, parent, and couple patterns, and the actual caregiver/parent-infant interaction. For each level one must look at what is influencing the successful or compromised negotiation at that level. Therefore, a therapist wants to be able to reach a conclusion about a child three years and older on all levels, and for the child less than three years, on the levels they should have attained (e.g., for a 2½-year-old, through the first three levels; for a 14-month-old, the first two levels—attention and engagement, and two-way communication).

The Process of Clinical Assessment

Each clinician may develop his own way of doing an evaluation. However, any assessment should (1) encompass certain baseline data; (2) organize data by indicating how each factor contributes to the baby's ability to develop; and (3) suggest methods of treatment. A comprehensive assessment usually involves the following elements: presenting "complaints," developmental history, family patterns, child and parent sessions, additional consultations, and formulation.

Presenting Complaints (Overall Picture)

We frequently spend a whole session on the presenting complaints or picture, which includes the development of the problems, the infant's and family's current functioning, and preliminary observation of the infant or child both with the caregiver(s) or, in the case of a child over three, without them as well.

We will usually suggest that the parents bring the baby with them to the first session. Even though we spend most of the time talking to the parents, we have our eyes on the baby and we watch what is going on spontaneously between parents and baby. If an older child (three or four years of age) is involved, we will have the parents leave the child at home the first time, if possible, so the parents can talk more freely.

We begin by asking the parents how we can help and we listen to their responses.

We encourage the parents to elaborate about the child's problem: whether it has to do with sleeping, eating, or being too aggressive or withdrawn. If we ask a question, it is usually to clarify something they have said, such as, "Can you give me some examples of that?" or "How is this different now from what it was six months ago, and when wasn't it a problem?" We try to find out when the problem started, how it evolved, and the problem's nature and scope. For example, if a 2½-year-old is aggressive with peers, we want to know whether the aggression occurs with all peers or only certain children. We are interested in what precipitated the problem and what may be contributing to it. Was there a change within the family, such as a parent getting a new job? Was there marital tension? Were new developmental abilities emerging which paradoxically were stressful to the child?

When the parents say, "Well, I think we have told you everything about the problem," we will then ask, "Is there more to tell about Johnny or Susie that would help clarify the picture?" It is much more helpful to ask open-ended questions than to ask specific questions about cognitive, language, or motor development at this point. One gathers together more relevant information when the parents elaborate spontaneously. Parents also reveal their own feelings and private family matters if the therapist is empathetic as he or she helps them describe their child. Therefore, a clinician should strive to be unstructured; ask facilitating, elaborative questions rather than "yes or no" or defining questions; and never be in a hurry to fill out a checklist.

The initial session also should establish rapport with the family and child in order to begin a collaborative process. The developmental process discussed earlier in relation to the child—mutual attention, engagement, gestural communication, shared meanings, and the categorizing and connecting of meanings—may occur between an empathetic clinician and the child's parents. How the clinician relates to the parents should reflect how the parents will be encouraged to relate to their baby. If the therapist asks hurried questions with yes or no answers, he or she sets up an untherapeutic model. It usually takes parents a long time to decide to come for help. They should be able to tell their stories without being hurried or criticized.

As part of this presenting picture, it is important to learn about all the areas of the child's current functioning. If the primary focus is initially on aggression and distractibility, the therapist should still try to learn the child's other age-expected capacities. One determines if the child is at the age-appropriate developmental level and, if so, whether the child displays the full range of emotional inclinations. Is the 8-month-old capable of reciprocal cause-and-effect interchanges? Is a 4-month-old wooing and engaging? Is a 2½-year-old exhibiting symbolic or representational capacities? Does he pretend play? Does he use language functionally? How does he negotiate his needs? At each of these levels, how is he dealing with dependency, pleasure, assertiveness, anger, and so forth?

Toward the end of the first session, we may fill in more gaps by asking questions about sensory, language, cognitive, and fine and gross motor functioning. Usually, we have a sense of these capacities and patterns from anecdotes and more general descriptions of behavior. We listen for indications of the child's ability to retain information; how he or she follows or does not follow commands; word retrieval skills; word association skills; fine and gross motor skills; and motor planning skills.

Some clinicians write down what parents say right after the session; others write during the session. Taking notes need not be an interference if one stops throughout to make good contact. We take detailed notes during the first fifteen or twenty minutes because we want as much information as we can get in the parents' words.

By the end of the first session, one has a sense of "where the child is" developmentally. One has a sense of the range of emotional themes the child can deal with at his developmental level. One has an awareness of the support, or lack of support, the child gets from his fine and gross motor, speech and language, and cognitive abilities. One also forms an impression of the support the child gets from his parents. One observes how the parents communicate and organize their thinking, the quality of their engagement, their emotional availability, and their interest in the child. One has a good sense of their relative comfort or discomfort with each emotional theme. In general, the therapist observes how the parents attend, engage, intentionally communicate, construct and organize ideas, and are able or not able to incorporate a range of emotional themes into their ideas as they relate to the therapist.

Developmental History

In the second session, we construct a developmental history for the child. (However, sometimes marital or other family problems show themselves during the first session. The parents may be at each other's throats; the mother and/or the father may be extremely depressed. In such cases, we will focus on individual parent problems as well as family functioning in the second session.)

We will usually start the session in an unstructured manner. We want to hear how development unfolded and what the parents thought was important. We encourage them to alternate between what the baby was like at different stages and what they felt was going on (both as a family and as individuals) in each of those stages. We try to start with the planning for the baby and to progress through the pregnancy and delivery. Next, we cover the six developmental levels, outlined earlier, in order to organize the developmental history.

Family Patterns

The next session focuses in greater depth on the functioning of the caregiver and family at each developmental phase. For example, a parent may admit that he or she was a little depressed or angry, or that there were marital problems, at different stages in the child's development.

Sometimes clinicians who are only beginning to work with infants and family may feel reluctant to talk to the parents about issues within the marriage. However, an open and supportive approach can elicit relevant information. One might ask,

"What can you tell me about yourselves as people, as a married couple, as a family?" We are also interested in concrete details of a history of mental illness, learning disabilities, or special developmental patterns in either of the parents' families.

Some families will not hesitate to discuss marital difficulties or other problems. Sometimes there will be discussion of how the child relates to the parents in terms of power struggles. If they describe a pattern, for example, between mother and child or father and child, we are likely to ask, "Does that same pattern operate in other family relationships—between mother and father, for example?" Is the pattern a carry-over from one of the parents' own families? By following the couple's lead, we try to develop a picture of the marriage, the careers of one or both parents, the relationships with other children and between all the children, the parents' relationship with their own families of origin, as well as friendships and community ties.

Sometimes the family as a whole functions in a very fragmented, presymbolic way. They gesture, "behave at" each other, overwhelm each other, and withdraw from one another, but they don't share any meanings with one another. Nothing is negotiated at a symbolic level. Even though each individual may be capable of functioning on a symbolic level, something about the family dynamics cancels out that ability. In this context, we want to know how the family handles dependency, excitement, sexuality, anger, assertiveness, empathy, and love.

For each unit of the family—the parents, each parent-child relationship, and the family as a whole—we want to find out how the different emotional themes were originally dealt with at different developmental levels and how they continue to be dealt with.

Child (or Infant) and Parent Sessions

We spend the next two sessions with a focus on the child or infant. We conduct the session differently with an older child (a three- or four-year-old, for example) than with an infant. With an infant, we may ask the parent to play with the baby to "show me how you like to be with or play with your baby or child." The parents may ask, "What do you want me to do?" "Anything you like" is our response. We offer the use of the toys in the office and tell them they may bring a special toy from home if they choose.

We watch each parent with the child, playing in an unstructured way, for about fifteen or twenty minutes. We are looking for the developmental level; the range of emotional themes at each level; the use of motor, language, sensory, and cognitive skills; and the support that the child is able to derive from such skills. We are also watching for the parents' abilities to support or undermine the developmental level; their range in that level; and use of sensory, language, and motor systems. After we watch the mother and father separately, we watch the three of them together to see how they interact as a group, because sometimes the group situation is more challenging. Later, we will join them and start to play with the child (briefly in the first session, and for a longer period in the second session).

During this time, we want to see how the child relates to a new person whom he or she knows only slightly. In addition, we want to determine how to bring out the highest developmental level at which the child can function. For example, if the parents do not support symbolic functioning in their three-year-old, we will try to get pretend play going. If an 8-month-old is being overstimulated, we will try to get cause-and-effect interactions going. If a 4-month-old looks withdrawn, we will try to flirt to pull him or her in. We will try to calm down a fussy 5-month-old with visual or vocal support, gentle tactile pressure, and a change of positions. We will work hands-on with an infant to explore his or her tactile sensitivity, motor tone, motor planning, and preference for patterns of movement in space.

One can learn a great deal through observation. For example, one could say to a child who is moving a train, "Oh boy, I can see that you know how to make this train go." The child may put a doll on the train, make the doll a conductor, and add a passenger. The passenger may have a baby while the train is going through a tunnel, and at the same time a doctor makes sure the baby is all right. A 3-year-old who generates such a "drama" is cognitively sophisticated and evidences a rich fantasy life.

With children 2½ to 3 years and older, depending on the child's comfort in being separated from his or her caregiver, we may reverse the sequence. We may have the first session with the child alone to explore how he or she engages, attends, initiates intentional two-way communication, and shares and categorizes meanings.

During this time alone, a 3½-year-old may stand in the middle of the room and look the clinicians over, while we look at the child. If we don't try to control the situation too quickly and can tolerate ten or fifteen seconds of ambiguity, the child may start to play, ask us a question about the toys, or talk about his or her family. What the child has to say without us saying, "Tell me what your mother told you about why you are here" or "Do you want to play with the toys?" can be very valuable. A child may look around and say, "I heard there were toys here. Where are they?" Such a statement indicates an organized, intentional child who has figured out why he or she is there and acts on this understanding. Another child may look puzzled and, after a silence, ask in a formal manner, "Can I sit down?"

Some 4-year-olds will talk to us through the session. We can have an almost adult-to-adult kind of dialogue about school or home, nightmares or worries, or just a chat about anything, as one might have with a neighbor. Other children will behave aggressively and want to jump on us or wrestle. They become too familiar too quickly.

During interaction with a child, we note the child's appearance, speech and language, gross and fine motor skills, and general state of health and mood. We observe the way the child relates to us, that is, the quality of engagement—overly familiar, overly cautious, or warm. We look for how intentional he or she is in the use of gestures and how well he or she sizes up the situation and us (without words). We try to determine his emotional range and his way of dealing with anxiety (e.g., does he become aggressive or withdrawn?).

The next step is to learn what is on the child's mind. One looks at the content of the play and dialogue, as well as the sequence of themes that emerge from them. The therapist's job is to be reasonably warm, supportive, and skillful in engaging the child and helping him or her to elaborate. If the therapist makes the interaction too easy by being overly seductive, he or she will not learn about the child's problems in relating. On the other hand, because the experience is new and scary to the child, the therapist should not make the interaction too hard.

With older children, we will have the parent come in, either toward the end of the first session or in the second session, in order to watch the therapist play with the child. If the parents come in first, the child may not want to play with the therapist alone because he or she is used to his parents being in the room. If the child comes in alone, because he or she is curious about the room and toys, he or she often establishes a primary relationship with the therapist. If the child is at all cautious, however, one may say, "Would you rather have mommy or daddy come in, too?" If the child elects to have the parents come in, have the parents and child play and talk first, then join them later.

Additional Consultations

As part of a complete evaluation, a child should have a pediatric evaluation to rule out physical illness. Suspected metabolic or genetic disorders should be investigated as well. If there is a question about a neurologic disorder, one should consider having a pediatric neurologist look at the child. If there are problems with receptive language, including word retrieval, word association, sequencing, or expressive language, a speech pathologist should be consulted. For questions about motor or sensory functioning (reactivity and processing), an occupational therapist should be consulted. If motor and language testing and clinical observation leave questions about cognitive or psychological capacities, a cognitive and/or psychological assessment may be considered.

Formulation

After learning about the child's current functioning and history and after observing the child and family firsthand, there should be a convergence of impressions. If a picture is not emerging, one may need to spend another session or two developing the history or observing further.

One then asks oneself a number of questions. How high up in the developmental progression has the child advanced, in terms of (1) attending, regulating, and engaging; (2) establishing two-way intentional communication; (3) preverbal problem-solving chains; (4) sharing meanings; and (5) emotional thinking? How well are the earlier phases mastered and, if not fully mastered, what are the unresolved issues? For example, does a child still have challenges in terms of his or her attention capacities, quality of engagement, and/or intentional abilities?

Determining the developmental level

tells you how the child organizes experience. To use a metaphor, it provides a picture of the "stage" upon which a child plays out his or her "drama." The presenting symptoms—nightmares, waking up at night, refusal to eat, and other concerns and inclinations—make up the drama; the stage may be age-appropriate. For example, a 4-year-old, who can categorize representational experience, has a drama of being aggressive to other children, but this drama is being played out on a stage that is age-appropriate. This child has the capacity to comprehend the nature of his aggression and use ideas to figure out his behavior. On the other hand, there may be major deficits in the stage (i.e., attending, being intentional, representing experience, or differentiating experience). If there are flaws in the stage, one wants to pinpoint the nature of those flaws.

For example, if a child is not engaged with other people, he or she may be aggressive because the child basically has no regard for other people's feelings. He or she may not even see people as human. Alternatively, another child may be aggressive because he or she cannot represent feelings and therefore acts them out. Still another child may represent and differentiate his or her feelings, but have conflicts about dependency needs.

One also looks at the range of experience organized at a particular developmental level. If a child is at an age-appropriate developmental level, does he or she accommodate such things as dependency, assertiveness, curiosity, sexuality, and aggression at that level? On the other hand,

even if a child is at the right developmental level, the stage may be narrow. In other words, the child might be only at that developmental stage when it comes to assertiveness, but when it comes to dependency, he or she is not quite there; and when it comes to excitement, he or she may function at a much lower level. In other words, if the child dances the wrong step, he or she could fall off the stage. One also looks at the stability of the developmental organization. Does even a little stress lead to a loss of function or are the functions stable?

Therefore, if the stage has cracks or holes in it because there are major problems from earlier developmental issues, we will say there are defects in the stage. If the stage is solid (no defects), it is either very flexible and wide or very narrow and constricted (e.g., it will tolerate a drama of assertiveness but not one of intimacy or excitement). In addition, the stage is either stable or unstable.

Next, the clinician wants to know about the contributing factors. One set of factors relates to observations about family functioning; the other set of factors relates to the assessment of the child's individual differences. The parent-child interactions are the mediating factors.

Developmental Diagnoses

The framework for the developmental diagnoses was discussed earlier. The goal is to profile each child as a unique individual in terms of his or her developmental level, interactive patterns, constitutional-maturational contributions, and family-environmental contributions. The clinician may wish to follow the following format.

The clinician should make a determination regarding each of the six developmental levels in terms of whether they have been successfully negotiated or not, and whether there is a deficit at any level that has not been successfully negotiated. Sometimes these levels have been successfully negotiated, but are not applied to the full range of emotional themes. For example, a toddler may use two-way gestural communication to negotiate assertiveness and exploration, for example, by pointing at a certain toy and vocalizing for his parent to play. The same child may either withdraw or cry in a disorganized way when he or she wishes for increased closeness and dependency instead of, for example, reaching out to be picked up or coming over and initiating a cuddle. This would indicate a constriction at that level.

Sometimes children are able to negotiate a level with one parent and not the other, with one sibling and not another, or with one substitute caregiver and not another. If it should reasonably be expected that a particular relationship is secure and stable enough to support a certain developmental level, but that level is not evident in that relationship, then there is a constriction at that level as well.

It is useful to indicate which areas or relationships are not incorporated into the developmental level. Consider the following areas of expected emotional range: dependency (closeness, pleasure, assertiveness [exploration], curiosity, anger, empathy [for children over 3½ years]); stable forms of love; self-limit-setting (for children over 18 months); interest and collaboration with peers (for children over 2 years); participation in a peer group (for children over 2½ years); and the ability to deal with competition and rivalry (for children over 3½ years).

If the child has reached a developmental level, but the slightest stress (such as being tired, having a mild illness (e.g., a cold), or playing with a new peer) leads to a loss of that level, then there is an *instability* at that level.

A child may have a defect, constriction, or instability at more than one level. Also, a child may have a defect at one level and a constriction or instability at another. Therefore, the clinician should make a "developmental" judgment based on the following developmental levels (See Table 6.1).

TABLE 6.1

Developmental Level	Defect	Constriction	Instability
1. Regulation and interest in the world			
2. Attachment			
3. Intentional communication			
4. Behavioral organization (complex sense of self)			
5. Representational elaboration			
6. Representational differentiation			

Symptom-Oriented and Phenomenologically-Based Diagnoses

In addition to the developmental profile, it is also useful to have an approach to symptom-oriented diagnoses. Three broad categories are suggested, under which most symptoms and patterns can be listed. While for each symptom-oriented diagnosis one must understand the developmental processes that are involved and the contribution of the constitutional-maturational and interactive and family dynamics, the descriptive diagnoses are helpful for administrative and some clinical purposes.

Descriptive symptom-oriented diagnoses may be divided into three general categories, each of which has its specific developmental roots and preventively oriented psychotherapeutic approaches. These three categories are interactive disorders, regulatory disorders, and multisystem disorders. These three categories were integrated into *Diagnostic Classification 0–3* (DC 0–3, 1994), developed by the Diagnostic Classification Task Force and established by Zero to Three/National Center for Infants, Toddlers and Families. This multidisciplinary Task Force sought to address the need for a systematic, developmentally based approach to the classification of mental health and developmental difficulties in the first four years of life. It met for almost eight years in order to develop a more appropriate and multifaceted approach to diagnosis, because in infancy and early childhood, prognosis may be

more optimistic if effective diagnosis and early intervention can occur.

Diagnostic Classification 0–3

The development of *Diagnostic Classification 0–3* (DC 0–3, 1994) is innovative in several important ways. First, its categories take into account constitutional and maturational variations, including individual differences in motor, sensory, language, cognitive, and affective patterns and their influence on infant/caregiver interaction patterns (Axis I). Second, it describes the earliest manifestations of the relationship between interaction patterns and maladaptive emotional and developmental patterns which have been identified among older children and adults but have not been fully described in infants and young children, such as trauma and affect disorders (Axis I). Third, it offers a relationship axis which helps differentiate when an infant's problem is part of a specific relationship which may not be able to support the infant's development, such as with a depressed or abusive parent (Axis II). Fourth, it examines symptoms with respect to how an infant might express distress and highlights the importance of considering the infant's reactions to trauma, grief, or deprivation (Axis I, Axis IV). Fifth, it considers sources of stress in terms of the infant's experience and takes into account protective and resilience factors (Axis IV). Sixth, it examines the infant's developmental level as described above with guidelines as to what interactive, relationship, and cognitive capacities to expect at each developmental level. Last, it identifies other related diagnoses in DSM-IV and ICD-9 under Axis III.

DC 0–3 also developed guidelines to help the clinician sort through the possible contributions to the presenting symptom picture. This was necessary because infants and young children present a limited number of behavioral patterns or symptoms, such as sleep or feeding disorders, and these same symptoms may be part of several diagnostic categories. It is recommended the clinician consider the various disorders in the following order: trauma, constitutionally based regulatory difficulties, adjustment reactions, mood and affect disorders, multiple delays (including communication and social relatedness difficulties), and relationship disorders.

Axis

The three categories include: problems that are part of the infant-caregiver patterns (interactive disorders), problems that are part of regulatory difficulties or disorders, and problems that are part of multiproblem or multisystem pervasive developmental difficulties which result in disorders of relating and communicating. Within these groups, one can classify all the DC 0–3 disorders as well as most of the DSM-IV infant and early childhood mental health disorders. These three broad categories have implications for therapy and prevention discussed below.

Interactive Disorders

Interactive disorders are characterized by a particular caregiver-child interaction or by the way the child perceives and experiences his emotional world. In the first category, difficulties that are a part of the infant-caregiver interaction pattern, there are only minimal contributions, if any, from constitutional-maturational differences and there are no significant irregularities, delays, or dysfunctions in such core areas of functioning as motor, sensory, language, and cognition. In other words, in this category the primary difficulty is in the interactions between the child and the caregiver.

The caregiver's own personality, fantasies, and intentions; the child's own emerging organization of experience; and the way these come together through the interactions will be the primary focus for understanding the nature of the difficulty and for intervention. Symptoms in this category include anxiety, fears, behavioral control problems, and sleeping and eating difficulties. This category, because it involves symptoms stemming from interactive patterns, also includes situational reactions of a transient nature, such as a mother returning to work or certain responses to trauma where the response does not involve multiple aspects of development.

The interactive disorders in Axis I, the primary diagnosis, include:

- Traumatic stress disorder
- Disorders of affect
- Anxiety disorders
- Mood disorders: prolonged bereavement/grief reaction and depression
- Mixed disorder of emotional expressiveness
- Childhood gender identity disorder

- Reactive attachment deprivation/maltreatment disorder
- Adjustment disorders

Regulatory Disorders

The second category, regulatory disorders, focuses on a group of infants and young children where there are significant and clearly demonstrable constitutional and maturational factors (Greenspan, 1989). They also have an interactive component. In this type of disorder sensory over- or underreactivity, sensory processing, or motor tone and motor planning difficulties, along with the child-caregiver interaction, the caregiver's personality and fantasies, and the family dynamics are part of the problem. These disorders include attentional and behavioral problems, such as irritability, aggression, distractibility, poor frustration tolerance, tantrums, and sleeping and eating difficulties.

The regulatory disorders include four types:

I. Hypersensitive—a. fearful and cautious, b. negative and defiant
II. Underreactive—a. withdrawn and difficult to engage, b. self-absorbed
III. Motorically disorganized, impulsive (overreactive defiant, underreactive stimulus craving)
IV. Other behavioral pattern (e.g., inattentive type)

In addition, sleep behavior and eating behavior disorders, so common in the early years, are included as separate classifications when there are no known sensory reactivity or sensory processing difficulties.

One may argue that all infants and children have unique constitutional and maturational variations, including the first group where the focus is the caregiver-infant interaction. This statement, in a relative sense, is true. The distinction is that, for the regulatory disorders, the constitutional and maturational factors are not just present as individual differences, but are a significant part of the child's problem. Therefore, in the second group, one wants not just to understand individual differences as part of the nature of the caregiver-infant interaction patterns, one wants to make the constitutional and maturational factors a major focus in their own right (alongside the interaction patterns and the family dynamics). Here, where possible, one will utilize intervention strategies that help the infant strengthen or organize constitutional and maturational variations in a more adaptive way. One will also seek to understand how the infant's constitutional and maturational variations are a stimulus for the parents' particular fantasies and how the infant's constitutional and maturational variations bring out certain maladaptive personality dynamics in the caregivers, parents, or family as a unit.

Disorders of Relating and Communicating—Multisystem Developmental Disorders

The third category of disorders involves multiple aspects of development and multisystem developmental disorders (MSDD), including social relationships and language, cognitive, motor, and sensory functioning. The extreme end of the continuum of these disorders is autism. Some of these types of disorders fall into the DSM-IV category of pervasive developmental disorders (PDD). The main distinction between MSDD and PDD is that children with MSDD reveal capacities or potential for engagement and closeness in relating but may be showing difficulties in relating and communicating *secondary* to sensory processing, regulatory, and motor planning difficulties. These children are quite responsive to comprehensive intervention, and they become relatively quickly engaged and interactive.

Before describing this third group of disorders, it is important to note that another type of disorder which involves multiple aspects of development is one in which an environmental stress or trauma leads to a global disruption in multiple areas of functioning. For example, when an infant evidences a failure-to-thrive syndrome, motor, cognitive, language, affective, and physical growth may slow down or cease altogether. Persistent types of neglect or abuse may produce a similar global disruption in functioning.

This third group of multisystem and pervasive developmental problems includes those groups of infants and young children that, in addition to variations in constitutional and maturational patterns, have significant delays or dysfunctions in multiple core areas of functioning, such as language, motor, sensory, and cognition. Here difficulties exist at a number of levels. The child evidences problems in infant-caregiver interaction patterns, parent perceptions, and family dynamics.

It is important to distinguish how regu-latory disorders differ from developmental disorders. Developmental disorders derail communication and relating, while regulatory disorders affect processing capacities but do not derail overall relating and communicating. Within developmental disorders there are also regulatory difficulties in terms of significant contributions from constitutional and maturational variations. Furthermore, either these regulatory patterns are so extreme that they are consistent with significant delays in sensory, motor, cognitive, or language patterns, or they are associated with significant delays in these core areas of functioning. In this third category, therefore, there are three broad areas of concern and focus for intervention: interactive, including family and caregiver variables; regulatory factors; and delays and dysfunctions in core areas of functioning.

One may question if, in this group, the main difficulty isn't only delays and dysfunctions in multiple core areas of functioning in the child. We suggest that there are almost always difficulties in the interactive patterns and caregiver and family dynamics. It is rare, even with the most flexible and adaptive parents, that the infant or young child's developmental challenges do not result in difficulties in the caregiver-infant interaction or in the family dynamics. The nature of the challenge the infant or young child presents, and the lack of expectable feedback due to language and visual-spatial-motor processing difficulties, almost always creates a significant stress on the interaction patterns and the family dynamics. Most families and caregivers seem prepared for certain types of communication patterns with infants and young children. When these biologically expectable interaction patterns are not forthcoming, special approaches are often needed. The degree of family contribution will vary considerably depending on the infant or child and the family's and caregiver's preexisting patterns. With this last group, therefore, interventions must focus simultaneously on the family dynamics, infant-caregiver interaction patterns, regulatory patterns, and developmental delays and dysfunctions in core areas, such as motor, language, cognition, and sensory functions.

In summary then, the three types of disorders are (1) interactive; (2) regulatory; and (3) multisystem developmental disorders (for which we propose an expanded classification below). Within these groups, one can classify the DC 0–3 disorders as well as most of the DSM-IV infant and early childhood mental health disorders. These three categories include problems that are part of the infant-caregiver patterns, problems that are part of regulatory difficulties or disorders, and problems that are part of multiproblem or multisystem pervasive developmental difficulties.

Axis II–Axis V

Axis II of DC 0–3 is the first classification system to consider disorders specific to a relationship when the parent-infant relationship goes awry and becomes fraught with difficulties. It examines the quality of the relationship with respect to behavior (of the parent and child), affective tone, and psychological involvement (attitudes and perceptions of the parent to the child).

Relationships may be characterized in the following ways: overinvolved, underinvolved, anxious/tense, angry/hostile, mixed, abusive, verbally abusive, physically abusive, and sexually abusive.

Axis III of DC 0–3 reports other medical and developmental disorders and conditions.

Axis IV reports psychosocial stressors of acute and enduring nature and take into account the severity of the stressor, the developmental level of the child, and the availability and capacity of adults in the caregiving environment to serve as a protective buffer and help the child deal with the stressor. In addition to expectable stressors, the stress index includes those specific to infants and young children, such as separation, a parent starting work, a child starting school, adoption, birth of a sibling, parent illness, frequent moves, and so on.

Axis V of DC 0–3 addresses the way in which the infant organizes affective, interactive, communicative, cognitive, motor, and sensory experiences as reflected in his or her functioning or developmental level. This has been described at length above and will only be summarized here under the headings used in Axis V: mutual attention, mutual engagement, interactive intentionality and reciprocity, representational/affective communication, representational elaboration, and representational differentiation I and II.

At this time, the DC 0–3 Classification Task Force is conducting reliability and validity studies of the classification system. For a further discussion of evaluation/diagnostic challenges and related intervention strategies, see DC 0–3, Infancy and Early

Childhood, The Child With Special Needs, The Challenging Child. The next section will propose an expanded conceptualization of MSDD.

Neurodevelopmental Disorders of Relating and Communicating

In the five years since the publication of DC 0–3 and the proposal of multisystem developmental disorders, we have collected diagnostic, treatment, and outcome data on several hundred more children diagnosed with severe disorders of relating and communicating. We may be able to improve our interventions and our research strategies even further to the degree that we can be specific on the subtypes and capture both the clinical features (such as the degree to which a child can relate, communicate with gestures, and interact with peers) as well as the underlying processing differences (such as the relative strengths in visual-spatial or auditory processing or motor planning). Based on this extensive clinical information, we have been able to broaden and add subtypes to both the classification of multisystem developmental disorder and the classification of autistic spectrum disorders.

The following dimensions are considered for each group, and together they provide a multidimensional profile of each child:

- The child's ability to connect affect (intent) and sequences of behavior and/or symbols. The affect serves as a signaling system telling the motor what to do and allows the child to initiate, be spontaneous, and engage in meaningful gestures and symbolic acts.
- The child's functional level—the child's ability to engage in complex problem solving through gestures and early ideas.
- The child's engagement, as evidenced by mutual or shared attention and mutual pleasure.
- Motor planning—the child's ability to both imitate or have an idea, plan how to execute it, and then sequence the steps necessary to do or express what he or she wants or is thinking.
- Auditory-verbal processing—this includes memory, comprehension (receptive understanding, e.g., semantics, reasoning, and logic), and expression (e.g., retrieval, pragmatics, etc.).
- Visual-spatial processing—memory and comprehension, including part-whole discrimination, organization, tracking, directional stability, time sense, visual-motor, construction-sequencing, and so on.
- Sensory reactivity and regulation—this includes sensory registration, orientation, interpretation, and responding or reacting (under- and overreactive or well modulated) to different sensory modalities.
- Symbolic thinking and rate of progress— the more rapidly the child climbs the symbolic ladder becoming an imaginative, representational, and abstract thinker, the better the rate of progress.

We propose the following classification involving subtypes under the broad heading of neurodevelopmental disorders in relating and communicating. The revised subtypes are based on the child's presenting profile and his or her early response to a comprehensive, developmentally based intervention program. We have identified five broad groups, some of which can be divided into a number of smaller groupings. Each will be described with respect to the dimensions described above.

Group I

This group tends to make very rapid progress over the course of two or three years, often moving from patterns of perseveration, self-stimulation, and self-absorption to warm, emotionally pleasurable engagement, spontaneous use of language, and abstract levels of symbolic play, with healthy peer relationships and solid academic skills. This group includes four subtypes to be described below, with the overall group characterized by the following patterns. These are also the criteria for identifying Group I.

1. Evidences difficulty connecting affect (or intent) to motor planning, sequencing, and symbol formation; therefore, behavior tends to be repetitive, self-stimulatory, fragmented, or to lack clear meaning or purpose.
2. Either partially has, or within the first few months of intervention acquires, the ability to engage in preverbal, gestural problem-solving interactions with caregivers (e.g., taking a caregiver by the hand, leading them to the toy room, and showing the caregiver the desired toy).

3. Either partially has, or in the first few months of intervention acquires, the capacity for warm engagement with positive affect, as evidenced by affectionate behavior with smiles and looks of delight with primary caregivers.
4. Relatively strong motor planning, though not age-appropriate (e.g., the child can sequence three or more motor actions, including sounds or words, such as taking a car and putting it in the garage, taking it out and having it go around the house).
5. Either has, or within the first few months of intervention acquires, solid imitative skills for motor actions, sounds, and/or words (e.g., can imitate "touch your nose" or "touch your head" as well as simple sounds and words, for example, "up" or "go"). Uses this to get into early stages of imaginative play over time.

The time intervals may vary, depending on when intensive intervention begins and the subtypes described below.

Group I also tends to be characterized by the following criteria, which are not necessarily early identifying criteria.

1. Hypersensitivity to sensation, such as touch and sound—although there is often some underreactivity to movement and occasionally to pain; the overall tendency of the child is to be overreactive rather than underreactive.
2. Visual/spatial processing tends to be a relative strength for some of the children and a relative weakness for others, as will be discussed below.

3. Auditory processing impairment tends to be relatively mild to moderate with good progress once intervention begins.
4. All the children in this group progress into imaginative play quickly, climbing the symbolic ladder from pretending real-life experiences to representational play, and are able to build logical bridges between ideas and become abstract thinkers.

SEQUENCE OF PROGRESS

Often there is rapid improvement in engagement, purposeful gesturing, range of affect expressed, and shared attention with caregivers and over time with peers. There is also rapid improvement in imitative skills because of better motor planning abilities, which lead to language and imaginative play sequences. Over time, during the first year or two of intervention, many of the children become excited with their emerging language skills and enter a stage of hyper-ideation where they talk about everything, but do so in a very fragmented (free-associative) manner. Over time, they learn to be more logical as the environment challenges them to build bridges between their ideas. During the early stage of becoming more logical, they tend to continue some preoccupations and perseverative tendencies with special interests, topics of conversation, or playthings (e.g., roads, cars, certain types of visual displays, etc.). During this phase, some may fit the description similar to that of Asperger's syndrome. With an emphasis on creative interactions and dialogues (e.g., using their interests as

a take-off for creative interactions), however, they gradually become more spontaneous, flexible, creative, and empathetic, and, over time, progress to higher and higher levels of abstract reasoning and social skills.

There are four different patterns under Group I.

Group I-A: Relatively strong auditory, visual-spatial, and motor planning, and reactive to sensation.

1. Meets the basic criteria described above and tends to make the most rapid progress. By the time they go to school, they may even show evidence of precocious academic skills (e.g., abstract thinking, reading, or arithmetic).
2. Tends to have relatively strong short-term auditory memory and expressive abilities (e.g., recites the alphabet and numbers, fills in the blanks to songs and stories, later memorizes scripts from TV shows or books, and so on).
3. Has relatively strong visual-spatial memory skills (e.g., knows where things are, good sense of direction, good at puzzles, recognizes letters and shapes).
4. Tends to be more reactive to sensation and emotional states, showing more intense joy and frustration, but develops better modulation over time.

Group I-B: Relative strong auditory processing but weaker visual spatial and motor planning with a tendency to be under-reactive.

1. Meets the basic criteria above. While also making rapid progress, children in

this group tend to remain more fragmented in their thinking and may have a harder time learning math (especially word problems), interpreting the meaning of what they read, and "seeing the forest for the trees" intellectually and socially.

2. Relatively strong short-term auditory memory.
3. Relatively weaker visual-spatial memory and processing capacities than I-A.
4. Relatively weaker motor planning abilities than I-A.
5. Tends to be more underreactive, with some sensory hypersensitivity. Has a longer fuse but also tends to process information more slowly.

Group I-C: Relatively stronger visual-spatial and motor planning, but weaker auditory processing and tendency to sensory underreactivity.

1. Meets the criteria above. Tends to make solid, consistent progress, but not quite as rapid as types A and B above. Tends to take a longer time, especially to learn to use words, but can use symbolic toys as a language to express many ideas. Also tends not to show evidence of a dramatic hyperideation learning phase since language develops more slowly, but is able to elaborate and sequence ideas through the use of toys and gestures aided by better motor planning abilities.
2. Visual-spatial memory and processing tends to be relatively stronger.
3. Auditory processing and memory retrieval tends to be relatively weaker.
4. Tends toward sensory underreactivity

but may get more emotional, especially when more frustrated or frightened because of weaker auditory processing and poor verbal communication.

Group I-D: Relatively strong auditory verbal and visual-spatial memory, but relatively weaker verbal and visual-spatial comprehension and motor planning. Tends to be overreactive and become overloaded.

1. Meets the criteria above. Tends to make consistent progress with good rote verbal skills, but has a narrower range of ideas, does not usually go through the hyperideation phase, and is weaker on his or her ability for higher-level processing of auditory and visual information. Also has a narrower range of acceptable emotions. Unless the environment can be more soothing and interactive, this child tends to be more rigid and anxious. Because they are more oversensitive, children in this group can become more easily overloaded without the resources to comprehend and integrate, thus resorting to constrictions and rigidity, and are more anxious and fearful, with more challenges with reality testing. This is the subtype that has many similarities to what others have described as Asperger's.
2. Both auditory and visual spatial memory are relative strengths.
3. Auditory and visual-spatial comprehension tends to be relatively weaker.
4. Motor planning tends to be relatively weaker.
5. Tends to be more overreactive, especially to unexpected sensations or events,

but also underreactive in some modalities, and may have reduced muscle tone.

CASE ILLUSTRATION

A 2½-year-old boy presented with self-absorption, perseveration, and self-stimulation, no peer play, and lack of eye contact and pleasure in relating to parents. During his evaluation, David spent most of his time reciting numbers in a rote sequence, spinning and jumping around aimlessly and randomly, and lining up toys and cars, all the while making self-stimulatory sounds. There were occasional shows of affection with some hugs.

David, however, showed strengths in his ability to show others what he wanted, when extremely motivated; his intimate shows of affection; the capacity to imitate actions, sounds, and words; and the ability to recognize pictures and shapes. With a comprehensive program, he quickly became more engaged and began imitating some pretend-oriented sequences, and he gradually began using his language purposefully and creatively. He then went through the pattern described above and, at present, is in a regular school excelling in reading and English as well as math. He has a number of close friends, a sense of humor, and insights into other people's feelings. His remaining challenges are with fine motor sequencing (penmanship) and with becoming somewhat anxious and argumentative when in a competitive situation.

Group II

Children in this group have greater challenges than Group I children do. They make slower but consistent progress. Each hurdle requires a great deal of work and is time consuming. Typically, these children can initially engage a little bit and be partially purposeful, and intermittently can do some problem solving. However, they take much longer to be able to become consistent, preverbal problem-solvers and to learn to use imitation as a basis for language and imaginative play. When they achieve these milestones, they do not generally go through a stage of hyperideation and rapid learning, but rather move through each new capacity very gradually. While many children in this group are still making progress, most are not able to participate in all the activities of a regular classroom with a large class size, as are the children in Group I above, but can benefit from appropriately staffed inclusion or integrated programs, or special needs language-based classrooms where the other children are interactive and verbal.

The characteristics and criteria for Group II include:

1. Evidences difficulty connecting affect (or intent) to motor planning, sequencing, and symbol formation; therefore, behavior tends to be repetitive, self-stimulatory, fragmented, or to lack clear meaning or purpose.

2. Can be partially purposeful, often oriented to basic needs, but not yet with solid mastery of preverbal, gestural problem-solving capacities (i.e., cannot do twenty-plus circles of problem-solving interaction and communication in a row).

3. Intermittent, but not full, capacity to

engage with caregivers. Initially, these children rely on more sensory motor stimulation. When self-absorbed or avoidant, these children need to be wooed and pursued.

4. Motor planning tends to be limited to two or less sequential actions (e.g., putting the car in the garage and taking it out, rolling the car toward a single destination).

5. Spontaneous imitative skills are not yet in evidence, other than perhaps some occasional ability to copy a familiar motor pattern, like knocking or building.

6. Relatively limited auditory processing capacities; can verbally express what they want better than they understand what others say, and rely on greater use of scripts.

Group II also tends to be characterized by the following criteria, which are not necessarily early identifying criteria.

1. Mixed reactivity to sensation with a tendency toward being underreactive and self-absorbed and/or underreactive and craving, as well as mixtures of the two, with some children tending to be more reactive.

2. Relative degrees of compromise in visual-spatial processing but may have good visual memory, and sooner or later learn to read but with weak comprehension.

SEQUENCE OF PROGRESS
Children in this group have the capacity to become joyfully engaged, but they may require wooing and persistent pursuit. They also have the capacity to move from simple, purposeful gestures to complex, problem-solving preverbal interactions and, eventually, to the use of imitation as the basis for learning words and becoming involved in pretend play. They learn primarily through what they see and may get very immersed in videos and books (before being encouraged to do more interactive work). They also may borrow scripts and scenes to embark on symbolic play as well. Each of these steps, from engagement to simple and then complex gestures to words and ideas, however, tend to be mastered very gradually and take a long period of time. Children in this group may evidence a large range of patterns of progress in the transition from preverbal gesturing to use of ideas. Some children in this group take a long time going beyond intermittent need-based short verbal phrases. Some of the children who are not able to develop imitative skills readily benefit from more semistructured challenges around the capacity to imitate actions, sounds, and words. This work, however, must be a part of a comprehensive program. As the children in this group develop language, the steps from creative elaboration to logical discussion also are a gradual and time-consuming process. The children in this group can easily become mired in the use of more fragmented, concrete, and early types of logic, and may have great difficulty in comparison to the children in Group I in progressing to more abstract and creative thinking. Some learn to read before they are fluent and conversant. Peer relationships are both possible and desired, but develop very gradually in parallel with their functional thinking ca-

pacities, benefiting from semistructured sensorimotor games before moving onto symbolic levels. Their capacities for experiencing warmth and pleasure with another child often precede their abilities to creatively interact and communicate. Nonetheless, with continued work, progress appears to continue.

There are two different patterns under Group II.

Group II-A: Relatively strong visual-spatial memory; other visual processing, auditory processing, and motor planning are relative weaknesses. Tends to be more reactive.

Meets the general criteria for Group II above and is more easily engaged and spontaneous. Tends to have moderate compromises in auditory processing (very difficult to respond to the words of others) but develops language, retrieves often-used phrases, and borrows fragments of scripts from books and videos which he or she uses for symbolic play. While language develops slowly and tends to be descriptive of what is seen or associative, this subtype slowly becomes more logical and able to reason over time. This subtype also speaks more spontaneously, which is related to their more reactive and often demanding nature.

1. Moderate compromises in visual-spatial processing (easily lost, poor sense of direction, can't find things) but relatively strong visual memory.
2. Moderate compromises in auditory processing.
3. Moderate compromises in motor planning.

4. Tend to be more reactive and intermittently sensation-seeking.

Group II-B: Relatively strong visual-spatial memory (like Group II-A), while other visual-spatial processing moderately impaired. Moderate to severe auditory processing and motor planning problems. Differs from Group II-A in that the child is underreactive with overreactivity to certain sounds.

Meets the general criteria of Group II above but tends to be more self-absorbed and avoidant, requiring more encouragement to speak. Tends to have moderate compromises in auditory processing but does learn to speak, with greater difficulty in understanding the unpredictable speech of others and retrieval difficulties; and relies on often-repeated phrases and scripts. Early conversations tend to be short and repetitive. Unlike Group II-A, this subtype is more underreactive and more self-absorbed, and has to be wooed to respond. This subtype also benefits from visual communication strategies and often learns to read sooner than speaking more fluently or spontaneously.

1. Moderate compromises in visual-spatial processing (easily lost, poor sense of direction, can't find things) but relatively strong visual memory.
2. Moderate to severe compromises in auditory processing.
3. Moderate to severe difficulties with motor planning and low muscle tone.
4. Hypersensitive and overreactive to sensation, with some sensation-seeking behavior.

CASE ILLUSTRATION

Three-year-old Joey presented with a great deal of avoidant behavior, always moving away from his caregivers, only fleeting eye contact, and a great deal of very simple perseverative and self-stimulatory behavior, such as rapidly turning the pages of his books or pushing his Thomas train around and around the track. He could purposefully reach for his juice or take a block from his parents, but he was not able to negotiate complex preverbal interactions or, for that matter, imitate sounds or words. Joey's progress at 6½, almost four years after his program began, showed abilities to relate with real pleasure and joy, use complex gestures to lead his parents to places, and describe what he wanted in sentences, such as, "Give me juice now!" Joey also showed ability to respond to simple questions, such as, "What do you want to do?": "Play with my trains!" and have short sequences of back-and-forth communication with four or five exchanges of short phrases. He is also able to engage in early imaginative play, making his action figures fly around the room with great joy and delight. He is not yet, however, able to consistently answer "why" questions and is only able to play with peers with some adult involvement where there is action or a structured game. However, he continues to make progress at a consistent but slow pace. Interestingly, Joey's perseverative, self-stimulatory patterns are only in evidence occasionally.

Group III

Moderate to severe auditory processing and visual-spatial processing, but more severe motor planning impedes purposeful communication and problem solving.

Children in this group are capable of intermittent problem solving interactions but cannot sustain their interactions. They are intermittently purposeful with self-absorbtion and/or aimless behavior. It is this "in and out" quality, with presymbolic islands of problem solving, that characterizes this group. These islands may involve the use of words, pictures, signs, and other 2- to 3-step gestures and/or actions to communicate basic needs. Receptive language of often-used phrases in routines and/or when coupled with visual cues or gestures is a relative strength. Some children will also use toys as if they are real as long as they are the actors but do not usually represent themselves or others through figures (e.g., they will eat pretend foods or feed a life-size baby doll, or put their feet into a pretend swimming pool as if they could go swimming). Some children with severe oral motor dyspraxia will not speak more than a few ritualized words, if they speak at all, but may show evidence of preverbal communication through a few signs, or picture communication, or the use of a favorite toy. Some children learn to recognize logos and may read words.

The characteristics and criteria for Group III include:

1. Very intermittently purposeful at the presymbolic level seen in islands of problem solving, but cannot sustain interactions (i.e., cannot do more than 4 to 5 circles of problem-solving interaction).

2. Very intermittent capacity to engage with caregivers; usually engagement involves sensory motor stimulation but tends to break off into aimless, self-absorbed, or avoidant behavior.

3. Auditory processing is a relative strength; may say a few words or phrases when in need or desiring of something. Receptive language is relatively stronger when accompanied by visual support and context. More severe motor planning, oral motor and/or visual-spatial challenges make it difficult for the child to convey/express just what they understand (receptively).

4. Motor planning tends to be limited to two or three sequential actions which are often repeated again and again, and the child often seeks hand-over-hand assistance for actions.

5. Do not imitate spontaneously and learn only through tremendous repetition.

6. Visual-spatial processing is relatively weak (e.g., disorganized, poor discrimination, poor searching, easily lost), but visual memory relatively stronger.

7. Mixed reactivity to sensation with a tendency toward being underreactive and self-absorbed and/or underreactive and craving, as well as mixtures of the two, with some children tending to be more passive and to have low muscle tone.

SEQUENCE OF PROGRESS

These children tend to progress slowly given the severity of their processing difficulties and only intermittent engagement and problem solving. The key is to "bring them in" to more sustained pleasurable interactions through persistent pursuit, playing simple games such as peek-a-boo, hide and seek, chase, tickling, horsie rides, and other sensory motor fun activities. More consistent engagement will create more motivation and lead to more interactive problem solving. The heightened affect inherent in having a "problem," such as getting a parent to do more roughhousing, finding a treasured Thomas train, getting more cookies, or going outside to play, motivate the child to process more information or input, be it visual or auditory. For example, a child will learn the sequence needed to get shoes, coat, keys, and Mom's purse in order to go outside. Once engaged, the caregiver's affect cueing will help the child expand his or her perceptions as well as sustain attention to the input, and the child's desire or objections will motivate them to go beyond her motor planning constraints and respond in some form. With more sustained engagement and interactions, children in this group also become more responsive to complex imitation, visual communication strategies, and practiced learning, and can go onto early levels of symbolic play.

CASE ILLUSTRATION

Sarah ran in looking for Winnie the Pooh and climbed up on the stool in front of the shelves, but could not move the little figures in the basket around to search for her beloved character. The next moment the basket was pulled off the shelf and all the figures fell out. She then looked in the next basket without bothering to look further on the floor. Her mom ran over before the second basket was dropped and offered to help. Sarah echoed, "Help!" and grabbed her mother's hands and put it in the basket. Her mother had to point to Winnie before Sarah actually saw the figure. She grabbed it and ran off to lie on the couch. Mom then came over with Tigger to say hello, and Sarah grabbed Tigger and ran to the other side of the room. She held her figures tightly and turned away when Mom came over again. Mom then took another related figure, Eeyore, and started to sing "Ring around the rosie," moving her figure up and down. This time Sarah looked and filled in the lyric "down" to "all fall down." But then Sarah moved rapidly away and went over to the mirror. This pattern of flight and avoidance after getting what she wanted, followed by not knowing what to do next, was typical. Sarah slowly learned the labels for things she wanted and how to protest. She recognized and could express familiar phrases: to come and eat, to go out, to bathe, etc. She became quite engaged with sensory motor play and loved to be swung and tickled. She even began to play with toys, first dipping her toes into the water of the play pool and then letting Winnie "jump" in. She began to imitate more words and actions, and tried to solve problems to get her figures, but only when very motivated or very mad, and usually only after energetic sensory motor play had pulled her in. Her expressive language expanded to more and more phrases indicating what she wanted, but it was difficult for her to answer any questions (weak receptive processing) and relied on visual and affect cues to understand what was said to her. This progressed to puppet play and even simple roleplay as a cook or doctor. Problem solving also advanced very slowly

because of her poor motor planning, but she became more easily engaged and more responsive to semistructured and structured learning approaches. Between ages four and five Sarah learned to count and identify colors, and loved to paint and cut with scissors. Sarah, who also began intervention at age three, demonstrated some pre-academic abilities able to read some sight words at 6½. She enjoys being with other children and joins the crowd in running around, hiding, and chasing, but does not yet play interactively even though she has learned the various social rituals of greetings, sharing, protesting, and so on. Sarah can also spontaneously communicate with a big smile, "Feel happy," or with a frown, "Feel mad."

Group IV

Very severe motor planning problems, as well as significant auditory and visual-spatial processing difficulties

Children in Group IV fall into two subgroups. Both subgroups are distinguished from Group III by having more severe challenges in all processing areas and especially motor planning, which includes oral motor dyspraxia. As a consequence, their progress is very uneven, with the most difficulty in developing expressive language and motor planning, and the most success in becoming warmly engaged and interactive through gestures and action games.

Children in Group IV-A evidence intermittent capacities for engaging with caregivers. Initially they tend to be very avoidant from having difficulty understanding what others want of them and difficulty being purposeful. They may wander around aimlessly or lie down passively, with intermittent bursts of sensory-seeking behavior. Severe motor planning impedes more than one- or two-step sequences, usually initiated to have basic needs met. With very persistent pursuit, Group IV-A children will eventually respond to and even initiate playful sensory motor activities. Because motor planning is so weak, they need a great deal of affect and motivation to propel them into purposeful gestures and problem solving when they want something. Complex imitation, however, is harder for them to master because it involves longer motor planning sequences. Some do eventually learn to say or sign some words through much practice and repetition. They also participate in presymbolic play when toys relating to real-life experiences (e.g., baby doll, slide, pool, school bus) are readily in sight and modeled, but they do not usually find or organize the toys themselves. Structural and visual communication strategies are very helpful in learning pre-academic and adaptive skills. They sometimes show evidence of symbolic understanding (seen in attachments to video and TV figures and desires for specific books and videos) but very poor motor planning impedes purposeful play.

Children in Group IV-B tend to evidence patterns of regression or greater neurological involvement (e.g., persistent seizures). This subgroup usually begins with enormous amount of challenges and make very limited progress, no progress at all, or have vacillations where there is a little progress followed by regression. These children tend to have severe processing challenges in all areas and yet, at the same time, they can show improvement in the areas of becoming happier and more engaged and, in learning to be partially purposeful, to solve problems when they want something. It is hard for this group to progress consistently into complex preverbal problem solving strategies or into the use of ideas, words, or complex spatial problem solving. During better times they may move into Group IV-A or Group III.

The characteristics and criteria for Group IV-A include:

1. Very intermittent ability to be purposeful (usually need-based) but still very dependent on adult actions to obtain what they want, even though very persistent in communicating their desires through simple and eventually more complex gestures.

2. Imitation and motor planning tends to be very limited; usually only single-step actions with objects such as throwing, pushing, or pulling with intent. May learn to enjoy simple puzzles and cause-and-effect toys, as well as presymbolic play.

3. Visual-spatial processing is a relative strength with moderate compromises. These children have better visual memory but weaker organization and visual-motor abilities (easily lost, poor sense of direction, can't find things, poor discrimination).

4. Severe auditory processing difficulties. May learn some need-based words but rely on visual cues to understand what others say. Some children with more se-

vere oral motor dyspraxia do not speak but have a narrow range of meaningful visual symbolic schema (such as cars or trains) they may enjoy and use repeatedly.

5. Show a wide range of reactivity and tend to be primarily overreactive or underreactive to sensation, with a greater tendency to be avoidant rather than self-absorbed.

Group IV-B is characterized by:

1. Only fleeting to intermittent engagement.
2. Fleeting to intermittent purposeful behavior related to very strong needs.
3. Severe motor planning difficulties. May intermittently use cause-and-effect toy brought to them (e.g., simple pop-up toy), but often only repetitive touching, banging, or self-stimulation are evidenced. Also shows severe oral motor dyspraxia. Little or no imitative ability is in evidence.
4. Auditory processing capacity is extremely limited.
5. Visual-spatial processing is extremely limited.
6. Tends to be underreactive to sensation. Often evidences low muscle tone and passivity.
7. May also evidence more overt neurological symptoms.

SEQUENCE OF PROGRESS—GROUP IV-A
With intensive pursuit these children can become more engaged, enjoy being around their families, and can become better problem solvers to get what they want. Because

of severe motor planning difficulties, they do not often initiate purposeful steps but can readily undo what they do not want, and then have difficulty knowing what to do next, often resorting to the repetition of the ideas (e.g., simple sequences with favorite toys, such as pushing a train on tracks through the tunnel). These children may learn words, usually through ritualized phrases, songs, and filling in blanks, but eventually retrieve the words for highly desired objects or objections in high affect states. Some children show visual-spatial learning on semistructured tasks such as matching, pointing to pictures, and easy puzzles, but cannot sequence actions to express ideas independently and function at a presymbolic level. Other children do not appear able to retain even repetitive learning, but do best when work focuses on their natural interests (e.g., to go outside, get food, play horsie, and so on). Relative visual-spatial strengths occasionally allow some of the children to read logos and words, but receptive understanding remains highly dependent on visual cues and context. With work on pleasure and consistent engagement, frustration, self-destruction, and aggression can be diminished and adaptation to surroundings and expectations can increase. Over time some children show evidence of unexpected strengths, moving on to presymbolic problem solving and an increased rate of learning.

CASE ILLUSTRATION FOR GROUP IV-A
Harold was able to progress only very slowly to imitating sounds and words, even with an intensive program organized to facilitate imitation. He could say one or two

words spontaneously when mad or insistent on getting something, but otherwise had to be prompted and pushed to speak. Every utterance was extremely difficult and he would sometimes stare at a caregiver's mouth to try to form the same movements. His severe dyspraxia also interfered with his evidencing pretend play, although from the different facial expressions and the gleam in his eye when he engaged in playful interactions with his parents, it appeared he was playing little "tricks." He sometimes held onto toy objects such as a Nerf sword or magic wand and used them in ritualized ways, but could not use toys to sequence new ideas. He showed an ability to get engaged, and even initiated sensory motor interactions in which pleasure and affection got expressed. While games with his brother had to be orchestrated, he did enjoy running around the school yard and the pool with other children. In the second year of intervention, he was able to interact and communicate with three or four back-and-forth exchanges about what he wanted, pulling his dad over to the fridge and finding the hot dogs. He could even retrieve a few words at such moments: "Hot dog." "What else?" "French fries." Harold became more consistently engaged over time, with islands of presymbolic ability, and became tuned in to more of what was going on around him. He no longer wandered aimlessly and could be observed picking up trucks to push or other cause-and-effect toys and simple puzzles. He let others join him, but invariably turned the interaction into sensory-motor play which brought him great pleasure. Pre-academic progress was also very slow even with lots of

structure, repetition, and practice, but he did make progress learning to complete "work" and self-care.

SEQUENCE OF PROGRESS—GROUP IV-B
These children, with a comprehensive program, can become happier and more purposeful, but often find it hard to move into complex preverbal problem solving. Over time, they are able to learn to be intermittently purposeful, engaged, and involved in preverbal, gestural problem solving, but they are not able to develop symbolic capacities. With structure, visual communication strategies, repetition, and practice, they can develop basic adaptive skills for home and school.

CASE ILLUSTRATION FOR GROUP IV-B
Margaret had severe perinatal complications and evidenced low muscle tone from shortly after birth. Her motor milestones were very slow: sitting up at nine months, crawling at twelve months, and walking at seventeen months with some asymmetry noted. Other than showing some pleasure in cuddling during the first year and some purposeful mouthing towards the end of the first year, she did not progress into consistent, purposeful interaction or complex preverbal problem solving. She tended to perseveratively rub a favorite spot on the carpet and stare toward the light, but could smile and show some fleeting pleasure with sensory-based play. With a comprehensive program, she has been able to make a little progress and become more robustly engaged, with deeper smiles, pleasure, more purposeful reaching, and some exchange of facial expressions, as well as indicating

preferences with facial expressions. At present, however, she has not progressed into complex behavioral problem solving interactions and recently began evidencing a seizure disorder for which she has been placed on medication.

Conclusion

This chapter presented an integrated developmental model for the clinical assessment and diagnosis of disorders of infancy and early childhood. In order to understand the full nature of an infant's difficulties, it is necessary to take three critical dimensions into account simultaneously: the developmental level, individual differences (constitutional and maturational factors), and relationships within the family and environment. The process of clinical assessment leading to a developmental as well as symptom-based diagnosis helps to identify the potential for adaptive functioning and appropriate interventions. As our clinical experience expands, we are able to conceptualize multidimensional models which can

be further evaluated for validity and reliability through research. We have also proposed an expanded classification of neurodevelopmental disorders based on the functional developmental level and various processing capacities described in this paper. This classification will provide the specificity needed to look at the full range of developmental disorders, guide the interventions needed, and examine outcomes.

References

DeGangi, G., & Greenspan, S. I. (1988). The development of sensory functioning in infants. *Journal of Physical and Occupational Therapy in Pediatrics, 8*(3).

DeGangi, G., & Greenspan, S. I. (1989a). The assessment of sensory functioning in infants. *Journal of Physical and Occupational Therapy in Pediatrics, 9,* 21–33.

DeGangi, G., & Greenspan, S. I. (1989b). *Test of sensory functions in infants.* Los Angeles: Western Psychology Services.

Diagnostic Classification Task Force, Stanley Greenspan, M.D., Chair., Serena Wieder, Ph.D.

7

Clinical Assessment of Infant Psychopathology Challenges and Methods

Maria Cordeiro

7

Introduction

In this chapter, the challenges and methods of clinical assessment, taking for granted that it is an indispensable, difficult, and time-consuming task, are discussed. It requires clinical experience and a wide range of skills and competencies from professionals, namely in normal child development, infant, and interaction observation. Clinical interview in a parent-child context and a basic knowledge and practice of adult psychopathology are also required. A theoretical framework, based on a psychodynamically oriented comprehensive understanding, and the capacity for self-observation and self-analysis are other indispensable requirements in this practice. Moreover, in spite of the tremendous growth of knowledge in the field of infant development and in the ontogenesis of psychic life during the last two decades, the lack of specificity of the risk factors in mental health, variability of the manifestations of clinical disorders during childhood, and inherent subjectivity of the process increase the difficulties. In general terms, assessment involves two different processes: Research and clinical practice.

Research in developmental psychopathology pertains to the study of the origins and course of patterns of behavioral maladaptation (Sroufe & Rutter, 1984) by comparing controlled variables in groups of normal and clinical populations. It is based on structured or laboratory/experimental situations which can be replicated and require instruments allowing data quantification and statistical inferences.

Clinical assessment refers to the infant in his or her individuality and specific environment and is based on as natural a situation as possible. A special relationship of mutual observation between the consultees and the observer is established, introducing elements of the observer's own subjectivity that make the situation unique and unable to be repeated. It starts with the concerns of the parents or other adults, professionals or not, who are responsible for the infant's well-being and whose primary objective is therapeutic orientation.

Consider the following issues specific to the clinical assessment in infancy:

- Growth and developmental changes are particularly rapid during the first years of life and the need to understand the perturbation in its developmental context is more compelling in infancy than later on, when developmental shifts are not so dramatic.
- The infant's physical and psychological

dependency on the caregiver makes the infant's manifestations meaningful and understandable only in the interactional context with the caregiver.

- Infant psychopathology is seen, in the great majority of cases, "as a manifestation of disturbance between individuals," rather than "within the individual" (Sameroff & Emde, 1989; Zeanah, Boris, & Scheeringa, 1997), considering the influence of relationship disturbances on infant development.
- The importance of past relationships of the parents in the organization of the caregiving system and the way the parents' relational patterns mold the infant's psychic life, in the first three years of life.
- The importance of familial context and support for competent parenting.
- The need to involve the parents in a therapeutic process from the beginning of the assessment (Bradley-Johnson, 1982).

All these issues make clinical assessment a multifactorial process, whereby the vulnerabilities and the strengths of both the parents and the child need to be considered for a therapeutic decision to be made.

Challenges

The Object of the Assessment

The first challenge is the diversity of the factors influencing clinical manifestations and its evolution. We have considered the infant, relationships, and social and familial context as the object of the assessment.

THE INFANT IN THE EVOLUTIONARY PROCESS

The changes occurring during the evolutionary process interfere, modify, or even resolve the psychopathological process and need to be taken into account in clinical assessment. In fact, the same risk factors can determine different clinical manifestations, depending on the developmental phase as well as on the infant's temperamental characteristics and competencies. Also, identical symptoms or maladaptive behaviors can be linked to different pathological processes and have different meanings according to the developmental phase and tasks.

Since birth, infants show individual differences that influence their capacity to adapt to the environment. These individual characteristics reveal themselves in physical features, activity levels, and reactivity to stimulation, as well as in the organization of sleeping, eating, or behavioral patterns. They are, to a large extent, influenced by maturational age and genetic differences, but the role played by the environment cannot be ignored. Individual differences in responsiveness and reactivity form the basis for identifying temperamental characteristics (Berger, 1985). However, Dunn and Kendrick's research, quoted by Berger (1985), underlined the idea that temperament cannot be seen as an independent factor from the child-family relationship.

Greenspan and Wieder (1993) also stressed the importance of individual differences in self-regulation. The authors described significant constitutional and maturational variations in infants' sensorial processing and/or motor planning that influence the way babies perceive and organize their experience and ability to negotiate and adjust to caregiving patterns. Moreover, individual characteristics and competencies of the infant play an important role by influencing the caregiver's behavior and responses to his or her manifestations. Numerous studies over the last 30 years have demonstrated not only infant competencies, but overall, the highly complex behavioral organization of the infant. This is evident in several domains, such as achieving biological rhythms, regulating interactive sequences by displaying approach-withdrawal cycles, and showing affective states. The latter are manifested by facial expressions, vocalizations, motor agitation, or changing behavior patterns in response to interactive pleasure or displeasure that do or do not elicit responses from the caregiver (Stern, 1980; Brazelton, 1981, 1983; Papousek & Papousek, 1983; Emde & Sorce, 1983; Sander, 1983, 1989; Fraiberg, 1987; Emde, 1989). For instance, Brazelton (1981) showed that it is possible from three weeks of age to distinguish different kinds of attention and behavior in an infant when placed in different situations or with different persons (mother, father, or stranger). It means that the infant is able to learn and to adapt readily, generating feedback from adults and new possibilities of learning during interactions. The caregiver's behavior, adapted to the infant cycles of attention, promotes reciprocity, negotiation, and development.

The way an infant's individual characteristics interact with the developmental stage and impinge on the infant's subjective experience has been a source of different theoretical assumptions. Sroufe and Rutter (1984) selected some "salient developmental issues" based on the formulations of several researchers, showing that maturational steps and achievements in social, cognitive, or behavioral domains are strongly influenced and blended by relationships and the child's subjective experience. These issues are biological regulation (harmonious dyadic interaction/formation of an effective attachment relationship during the first year of life), exploration (experimentation and mastery of the object world), individuation and autonomy (responding to external control of impulses between 12 and 30 months), and initiative (self-reliance, identification, and gender concept after 36 months).

Moreover, the achievement of each developmental level constitutes the ground for the next ones, in the subsequent phases. In a structuralistic approach, each phase of development is characterized by an expected level of organization, integrating both an individual maturational program and the child's age-appropriate experience, which progresses to higher levels of complexity as the individual achieves maturity (Greenspan & Porges, 1984; Greenspan, 1989).

Therefore, clinical assessment of the infant needs to take into consideration the infant's capacities in the sensorial, motor, and cognitive spheres and capacity to organize experience to the age-appropriate developmental level in several domains, such as: (1) biological cycle regularity and self-regulation, (2) affective regulation and signaling, (3) attachment relationships and socialization, (4) interest and exploration of the external of world, and (5) symbolic activity and play.

PARENT-CHILD RELATIONSHIP

Most of the infancy syndromes are related to the infant-relational context. As normal infant development is enhanced by healthy relationships, disturbed relationships compromise individual functioning. There is empirical evidence that even when developmental changes occur in the child's behavior, the quality of the interactions are relatively stable and can be predictive of future relationships, meaning that in early development, "the assessment of the relationships can be more predictive than individual assessment" (Sroufe, 1989). Zeanah and colleagues (1997) argued that the risk factors that most influence the outcome and the psychopathology in infancy are those "which most directly compromise the quality of parenting." The assessment of parent-child relationships in infant psychopathology is a major issue facing researchers and clinicians because of its vital influence on early development and on the adaptation of an infant's experiences. Several theoretical approaches have been developed in order to understand and evaluate interactions and relationships.

One possible way to assess relationships is based on the concepts of regulation and adaptation. The regulatory model of development postulated by Sameroff (1989) considers that development "is conditioned by a number of regulatory systems acting on different levels of organization," namely the biological and social system in order to achieve adaptation and self-regulation. During infancy, the social system is represented by transactions with the caregivers.

In a classical assessment approach, the disturbance of the infant with difficulties lies in the child, whereas in a regulatory and transactional assessment approach, the disturbance, if there is any, lies in the regulatory system (Sameroff, 1993). If parents do not adapt to the infant's needs and do not adequately regulate necessary stimulation, disturbances to the infant's adaptation can occur. Anders (1989) considered that regulation during interaction implies a dynamic equilibrium of inhibitory and excitatory mechanisms crucial for the physical and psychological well-being of both mother and infant. "Disruptions in the regulatory function are associated with pathology in relationships" (Anders, 1989). Reciprocity and mutuality in exchanges between parent and child are an essential feature for achieving regulation in relationships. Anders (1989) considered five patterns of regulatory disorders (overregulation, underregulation, inappropriate, irregular, and chaotic).

Several authors have discussed different ways to characterize the relationship between parent and infant. To enhance the infant's learning and communication, Papousek and Papousek (1983) described a set of behaviors to enable parents to respond adequately to the needs of the infant and provide the infant with the necessary stimulation by adapting their behavior to the conditions of maturational capacities of the newborn. The authors stressed the biological prevailing basis of these behaviors and called them "primary parenting," because they are intuitive and outside of rational thinking.

Stern (1980) beautifully demonstrated affect attunement by showing how the infant's and caregiver's repertoire matched or did not match in order to attain affective regulation and communication and how by means of internalization and sequences of interactions relationships are formed. The transmission and role of the affect signals during mother-infant interactive sequences has been described and emphasized by Stern (1985) and Emde and Sorce (1983) among others.

Emde (1989) defined the parent-infant relationship in terms of its functions. According to this author, each functional domain of the relationship, biologically determined, has complementary aspects in the parent and in the child (attachment/ bonding, vigilance/protection, physiological regulation/provision of organized structures, responsiveness to needs, affect regulation and sharing/empathic responsiveness, learning/teaching, play/play, and self-control/discipline). He also stressed the importance of the maternal affective availability and affect signalization for the organization of the infant's relational experience.

Kreisler (1987) considered affective richness ("plenitude"), flexibility ("souplesse"), and stability to be the essential interactive qualities for preventing infants from psychosomatic failure. Mazet and Stoleru (1983) pointed to the importance of the postural and tonic exchanges, the "tonic dialogue," between mother and child. These exchanges, influenced either by the mother's state of mind or by the infant's global or local tonic reactions can affect communication during interaction.

Greenspan and Lieberman (1989) considered contingency during interaction as an important feature in understanding the meaning of the interactive behavior and in promoting the infant differentiation process (differentiation of persons, somatic discomfort from mental states, and different kinds of communication coming from the caregiver). Contingency implies the attribution of meaning to the behavior of others and responding adequately to it. In turn, the attribution of meaning implies the concept of mental representation.

It is important to bear in mind that quality, content, and regulation of interactions are guided by mental representations. In the beginning of infant life, they are oriented mostly by maternal representations. Progressively, as the infant's psychic life becomes more organized, the infant's representations of the mother, her intentions and affects, and the representations of the infant's relationship with her also guide interactive behavior. Because empirical evidence exists that mental representations of the mother are one of the major features influencing the mother's sensitivity and availability to her child and, consequently, the mother-child relationship, their influence on infant development and psychopathology has been one of the most important areas of concern for clinicians and researchers. The assessment of maternal representations is a crucial feature in infant mental health.

Stern (1991) described a set of maternal representations whose influence on mother-infant interaction is clinically important. This author considers that after birth the maternal representations and, consequently, mother-infant relationships are greatly determined by a new psychic constellation "the motherhood constellation," the core of which is the mother's relationship with her own mother (Stern, 1995). In fact, the use of a structured interview in assessing parent's internal representations of the child (Working Model of the Child Interview–WMCI) showed a significant concordance between some characteristics of mothers' representations of their infants and the infants' attachment (Zeanah, Benoit, Hirscherg, Barton, & Regan, 1994).

Bowlby's attachment theory and Ainsworth's strange situation allowing the operationalization of the attachment concept as well as the concept of internal working model (Bowlby, 1988) gave rise to numerous studies, greatly increasing our knowledge about the influence of relationships on human development. The initial findings of Ainsworth and her colleagues (Ainsworth, Bell, & Stayton, 1971) concerning the correlation between child's attachment patterns at the age of 12 months and the sensitivity of mother' responses during the first year of life found strong confirmations in other studies (Grossman, Spangler, Suess, & Unzuer, 1985). Moreover, longitudinal studies (Main, Kaplan, & Cassidy, 1985; Erickson, Stroufe, & Egeland, 1985) showed not only the relative stability of the characteristics of attachment patterns across toddlerhood, but also the internalization and generalization of relationship patterns at six years of age.

Since the study of Main and colleagues (1985) moving from the behavioral level to a representational level of attachment relationships, many other studies, based on the internal working model concept, were undertaken on a transgenerational perspective, showing how the transmission of patterns of attachment relationships operates and opening new perspectives for preventive interventions. The use by several groups of researchers of the Main's Adult Attachment Interview showed significant correlation between the characteristics of childhood attachment relationships, as recalled by parents, and attachment patterns displayed by the child. Bretherton (1990) stated the importance of the ill effects of rejecting or neglecting experiences from parents' childhood onto their attachment patterns, provoking low sensitivity in their interactive behavior and consequently, interfering with the construction of the child's internal working model. Also, Fonagy, Steele, Steele, Moran, and Higgitt (1991) found significant correlations between mothers' attachment patterns before birth and the childs' attachment patterns at 12 and 18 months of age.

In spite of the evidence of the influence of attachment patterns on infant development, we need to examine perspectives concerning other domains of mental functioning, namely the unconscious level of representations and conflicts. We would, therefore, like to stress a point of view first developed by Selma Fraiberg and followed by French-speaking authors based on clinical evidence and case studies. These authors point to the transmission of unconscious conflicts of the infantile past of the parents into the relationship with their baby. The latter may represent one of the parents, a brother, or even part of the infantile self of the parent, and these images invade the place of the actual baby in the relationship (Fraiberg, Adelson, & Shapiro, 1980). These conflicts are activated by the presence of the baby and "acted" in the interactions with the baby, influencing their affective quality, contingency, and content, provoking interactive discomfort and leading to pathological defenses in the infant (Fraiberg, 1987) and subsequent psychopathology. The parental interactive behaviors based more on projective identification mechanisms than on identification mechanisms and empathy were called "symptomatic interactive sequences (SIS)" (Cramer & Espasa, 1993). This transfer of unconscious conflicts and fantasies from parents to infants corresponds to the so-called, "intergenerational mandate" (Lebovici, 1988). For Lebovici, the child is "mandated" by his or her parents to convey the familial culture and beliefs and accomplish a destiny determined by parents' unconscious fantasies, centered on Oedipal conflict. The baby is, then, an object of parent's narcissistic, libidinal, and aggressive cathexis and consequently, parental representations have an intense affective charge, contributing to the attribution of the infant's role on the parent's mental life and in certain cases, disturbing the perception of the actual baby. The fantasmatic baby and the fantasmatic interaction impose their reality over the infant actually born and his manifestations.

Because of the importance of this fantasmatic interaction (Kreisler & Cramer, 1981; Lebovici, 1988) in the background of an observable interactive scenario, the past relationships of the parents and the fantasmatic role attributed to the baby needs to be included in the assessment process, in order to better understand the dynamic meaning of the relational maladaptation.

PARENTS/CHILD—
OBSERVER RELATIONSHIP

Subjectivity in the clinical assessment process can be considered an important tool for diagnostic purposes, contrary to the usual scientific methodology pointing to the need for measurement, quantification, and objectivity. The observer's subjectivity is not only inevitable, but also necessary, and it needs to be taken into account very seriously for the accuracy of the assessment process.

Subjectivity is *inevitable* because nobody can escape the emotional climate aroused by the presence of the parents and their babies. Moreover, in clinical practice, the urge to understand is inherent to the process and leads the observer to identify both with the parents and the child, very often provoking contradictory identificatory movements. Countertransferential positions, in which the observer's ego is totally involved in the emotional experience and identified only to one element of the dyad/triad, distort the listening of the parent-child communication, and the observer risks to "act" instead of to understand (Goncalves, 1994). On the other hand, when parents, distressed by their infant's manifestations, meet a mental health professional, strong and frequently mixed feelings toward that person emerge immediately, depending on the representation of the help they possibly get from him or her.

The child, as young as he or she may be, is also prone to establish relationships with the observer, not only due to the fact that the child feels the observer is an important person for his or her parents, but also because the observer tends to establish a special relationship with the baby by identifying himself or herself with the "ideal mother." In fact, because of their primary experience of caregiving, not only adults, but also babies bring inside themselves the idea of the "mothering" they need. We have observed toddlers looking for "mommy" when their mother is around. Also, very deprived infants who have not been mothered by any particular caregiver or autistic children do not build inside themselves the representation of mothering, leaving adults confused about their role as caregivers.

This transferential/contratransferential play provokes in the observer an activation of his or her own attachment representations, as well as an arousal of affects rooted in their infantile relationship. It is the special interest and awareness toward his or her subjectivity, as well as the predisposition to autoanalysis that prevent the observer from impinging his or her personal point of view on the patients and compromising the accuracy of the process by introducing a personal bias.

Complementary to this self-analysis attitude, the discussion of clinical material in regular staff meetings is another important filter, allowing the discrimination of subjective aspects of the assessment by con-

fronting the observer's impression with feelings and opinions aroused by the case among the group. Moreover, the group has a function of containing and holding anxieties aroused by the contact of the observer with babies in distress and their families. In some situations these anxieties, because their intensities impend over his or her capacity of thinking or seeing, undermine the judgment of the case (Trowell & Rustin, 1991).

Subjectivity is *necessary* because the quality of the effects aroused by the parents and the child in the observer are precious guidelines for the appreciation of the affective parent-child climate and understanding the meaning and the content of the interactions. As the parental affects and availability organize their experience with their child (Emde & Sorce, 1983; Emde, 1989), the observer's affects during observation organize his or her experience with this particular family and help in the assessment of the quality of the relationships and emotional availability for relationship of parents and child.

In clinical practice very often the observer's clinical impression obtained from the videotape observation of interactive sequences differs from the clinical impression of the same observer inside the room. Rather than contradictory, it means, in fact, that we cannot undervalue any of the approaches. We need to integrate these two different ways of catching reality to enrich and deepen our clinical knowledge.

FAMILIAL AND SOCIAL CONTEXT

The importance of familial context and social support for child development is underscored by many studies and authors. In a broader scope, the evaluation of the pathological phenomenon is not independent from the cultural background of the population. The characteristics of caregiving are deeply rooted in the familial culture and cultural values of the societies. Religion, traditions, beliefs, moral values, and family structure are important social references for characterizing upbringing in a specific society. In a more restrictive level, the parent's educational background, the support from the enlarged family, and the cultural and social integration of the family in the community influence the caregiving practices. Today, in Europe and particularly in Portugal, migrations are frequent from rural to urban communities or to other European countries with the consequent isolation, lack of familial support, and loss of cultural references, increasing the familial stress.

Sameroff and Seifer (1983) stated that the constellation of risk factors are more pervasive for development than one single risk factor. Poverty, for instance, is one situation which involves several ill circumstances for development (unemployment, bad housing, marital conflicts, poor academic skills, mental health problems, etc.). Child resiliency needs a competent and resilient environment to be effective and promote the child's capacities for coping with adversity (Demos, 1989), but the greater the risks, the less the child is able to cope, particularly in the early years.

It is quite obvious that adverse conditions, such as lack of marital or familial support, illness or death of close relatives, and overburdening from financial difficulties,

primarily influence the mother's state of mind and the quality of primary care and secondarily, the child's well-being. In addition, the father's presence and his capacity for sharing the caregiving tasks with the mother to support the mother-child relationship, as well as substitute for the mother when she is not available, is a protective factor in infant development. On the contrary, if the father acts as the mother's rival, preventing mother and baby's closeness or devaluing her maternal skills, his behavior constitutes a risk factor, increasing marital conflicts and familial distress.

The impact of parental mental illness on child development has been an important concern for clinicians and researchers. Seiffer and Dickstein (1993) remarked that children of mentally ill parents are at increased risk for mental health problems, not only because the mental illness is associated with other social risk factors, such as psychosocial stress, poverty, and marital conflicts, but also because of its impact on the mother-child relationship.

Maternal depression is one of the most pervasive conditions, quite often neither identified nor recognized as an illness condition. Kreisler (1987) stated that the insufficiency, excess, and incoherence of the caregiver's interactive behaviors are associated with maternal affect disorders, namely the mother's depression. Also, maternal postpartum depression studies show its negative influence upon the child's interactive behavior, cognitive skills, and mental functioning (Murray, 1991, 1996). Another group considered at risk are adolescent mothers. Osofsky, Hann, and Peebles

(1993) point to the importance of the developmental factors specific to adolescence, such as identity autonomy and self-esteem issues, which interact with parenting abilities.

From our clinical practice and from literature, it seems to us that environmental and psychosocial risk must be evaluated more in terms of the impact on parents and their caregiving skills, rather than in terms of the direct effects on infant functioning. In Portugal, for instance, the European country with the highest frequency of working woman and young children in day care, there is simultaneously a very traditional family system, centered in the woman's role as responsible for children's upbringing. These contradictory facts tremendously increase maternal stress, especially in families with lower socioeconomic status, decreasing maternal availability and sensitivity toward their children. It is not surprising that in similar conditions we found in our clinical population (n = 60) a high incidence (22 percent) of infant depression and reactive attachment disorders (Cordeiro, 1997).

The Nature of Mental Disorders in Infancy

The second challenge in the clinical assessment process is to define the pathology endangering infant development and later outcomes in terms of individual mental health. Two major issues concern clinicians. One is the assessment of risk factors which are likely to lead to infant developmental disorders. The other is the assessment of the actual disorder of the child, not only as a manifestation of psychic pain and distress, but also as psychopathological manifestations with specific outcomes or subsequent repercussions on child development. It is difficult to clearly define and conceptualize both issues.

The studies of developmental psychopathology based on the effect of the risk factors on later development have shown: (1) there is no direct association between the presence of specific risk factors in infancy and outcomes in later childhood in terms of behavioral adaptation, psychiatric disorder, or mental development, (2) there is more likelihood of later developmental disorders when there is an association of risk factors than when only one risk factor is present (Rutter, 1994a), and (3) the risk factors affecting parental competencies are more likely to affect infant development rather than risk factors directly affecting the infant (Zeanah et al., 1997).

The definition of what is a psychopathological manifestation in the infant is a somewhat controversial issue. On one hand, most infant disorders are primarily relationship disorders. In a sample of a clinical population (n = 60), 65 percent of the cases had a diagnosis in DC: 0–3 Axis II (DC: 0–3, 1994; Cordeiro, 1997). On the other hand, it is very difficult, at this early phase of life, to clearly distinguish between normal and abnormal mental functioning. The developmental changes and challenges that the child between zero and three years and the child's parents have to face are complex. The plasticity of the adaptive behaviors and manifestations of the infant, specificity of each infant's maturational schedule, lack of specificity of the clinical manifestations and psychopathological processes, and diversity of phenomenological behavioral or symptomatic manifestations along the course of development are examples of some of the difficulties that clinicians find in their work when they need to establish the border between normal and pathological conditions and foresee their evolution. We agree that the intensity, frequency, combination of symptoms (Gerber, 1984), and multiplicity of undermined areas of functioning, as well as the concern of the parents or the professionals are good indicators for establishing the difference.

Nevertheless, it is worthwhile looking at the underlying process of development and functioning of the child rather than at the external manifestations (behavior, symptoms, and developmental delays) to assess clinical disorders in infancy. In fact, Stroufe and Rutter (1984) emphasize that assessment needs to shift from symptoms and behavioral manifestations, both lacking in stability along development, to individual functioning and coping with developmental tasks or stressful events, that seem to be more stable and consistent than the former. Implicitly, it is assumed that the internal psychic processes are more elucidating than their external manifestations for the purpose of defining the clinical situation.

The difficulty in infant mental health of clearly limiting clinical syndromes, with its causal factors, homogeneous clinical manifestations, and foreseeable outcomes, makes the concepts of resiliency and vulnerability very helpful in this matter. In a broader sense, these issues examine the way the infant is able or not to overcome difficulties or changes in his or her external or internal reality, particularly those in which the child needs to strive for adaptation. Demos (1989) defined resiliency in terms of child's skills, (activity, persistence, flexibility, capacity to develop different strategies, and a range of interests and goals) which are, in most part, constitutional but which can be enhanced when interacting with certain family characteristics, such as empathy, family resiliency (flexibility and capacity to contain problems), and underaffective motivation. In fact, research has demonstrated that although temperament plays a role in some problem-solving situations, its effects are mediated through interpersonal relationships (Rutter, 1994b; Stroube, 1985) and influenced by the quality of the relational context. Bowlby (1989) linked resiliency and attachment patterns, part of the self, when he states that "the extent to which he or she (developing individual) becomes resilient to stressful life events is determined to a very significant degree by the relationship pattern developed during the early years." Bowlby refers to Grossman's experimental study, in Germany, that confirmed that securely attached children respond with "confidence to potential failures."

Current scientific knowledge proves that attachment is a very powerful factor in influencing social adaptation, affect regulation, and cognitive competencies. The studies of Erickson et al., (1985) mentioned previously show some correlation between attachment patterns at 12 and 18 months of age and the later development of the child. Infants with a secure attachment have a greater "ego-resiliency" manifested by greater autonomy, persistence, enthusiasm in solving problems at the age of 42 months, and more capacity to interact with peers and teachers in school than those with an insecure attachment. The group of children with this same pattern of attachment studied by Main and colleagues (1985) at the age of six displayed more capacity to express feelings, namely about the separation situation, and better social and cognitive competencies than the other group.

Stern (1985) considered the sense of self a central issue for understanding coronal and impaired interpersonal development. He described both the sense of self as a primary organizational principle and the emergence of different senses of the self along evolutive progression as the reorganization of the subjective experience under the influence of the development of new skills and capacities.

Fonagy and colleagues (1991) distinguished two different kinds of functioning of the self, according to the developmental age of the child or in adults, according to their level of functioning or even psychopathological conditions: The prereflexive self and the reflexive self. They found some evidence that infant security, seen by these authors as an internal quality of the self, relied on the parents' capacity to understand infant mental states. This ability to observe and understand mental states in oneself and in others is a function of the reflexive self. It constitutes a protective factor either for adult mental disability or for the development of a secure attachment pattern between the child and the mother in the first year of life.

If we agree that infant mental health relates to the concepts of resiliency and vulnerability, we can assume that the level of self-development underlies psychopathology in infancy. It is the quality of the early emotional experiences of the infant and the degree of the achievement of the inner organization of the self (a separate, coherent, and constant sense of the individual's subjective experience) that provides the necessary mechanisms to deal with new facts and new persons, as well as to cope with stressful events or in others words, regulates the balance between resiliency and vulnerability (Cordeiro, 1997). In terms of psychopathology and in order to be useful to therapeutic purposes, clinical assessment needs to focus on assessing the level of functioning of the psychic structures, namely self-organization and ego development, underlying the clinical disorder more than on the external manifestation of the disorder.

The Classification of Mental Disorders in Infancy

Because of the difficulties in characterizing psychopathology in infancy, a third challenge is the diagnostic classification of infant mental health disorders. It involves clinical, theoretical, and cultural issues. This is indeed a very controversial question. Many clinicians, especially those psychoanalytically oriented, as many are in Europe, are very critical about using diagnostic classifications in infancy. There are several problems in establishing clear definitions of clinical syndromes. Because such syndromes are developmentally determined, they change rapidly, and causal factors lack specificity. Increasing the complexity of diagnosis are the contribution of relationship disorders to infant psychopathology, the paramount importance of psychic functioning over the overt clinical manifestations (see preceding) as expressed by the diversity of evolution and outcomes, the importance of the preventive issues in the infant mental health field, and the danger of "labeling" infants (Emde, Bingham, & Harmon, 1993). Also, diagnostic classification efforts undertaken by clinicians are considered, and often they are influenced by the observer's affects and involvement during the clinical process, undermining the evolution of the assessment process and so, the understanding of the psychopathology (Cordeiro & Caldeira da Silva, 1998).

Diagnostic classification is an important part of the clinical process following the assessment process. They are both part of the diagnostic process, but they have different objectives and "the distinction between assessment of individuals and classification of disorders help to avoid a pitfall" (Emde, 1998). If we have a theoretical framework for understanding psychopathology, we can help infants and their families without referring to a diagnostic classification system, but we can hardly generalize our experience and communicate it appropriately to others. Let us briefly examine the advantages of diagnostic classification. Basically, it fulfills the urge to communicate knowledge among professionals and to advance research in determining the etiology and the course of the disorders (Emde et al., 1993), as well as to organize data collection (Thomas & Harmon, 1998). It provides us with the structure to develop follow-up studies and assess therapeutic efficacy. Moreover, our communication with other agencies dealing with infant well-being (courts, adoption services, and welfare services) is also very much facilitated and more accurate (Cordeiro & Caldeira da Silva, 1998).

Another important consequence is political in establishing priorities in infant health programs and in giving arguments to health authorities to create infant and family mental health facilities. Generally, infants' rights to get mental health care are not more easily recognized by politicians and health insurance companies. Moreover, the diagnostic process also involves cultural issues. As a matter of fact, diagnostic classifications are not supposed to consider specific cultural contexts (Guedeney & Lebovici, 1997). Classifications need to be designed in order to be applied commonly by all professionals involved, achieving the criteria that make them acceptable (coverage, usefulness, reliability, and validity) (Emde, 1998). Nevertheless, the accuracy of assessment, in which diagnostic classification and assessment modalities are based, relies much more on cultural specificities and similarities between the assessor and families (Guedeney & Lebovici, 1997). The values, beliefs, expectations, and language shared by the observer and the family in a specific cultural and political context paramountly influence not only risk evaluation and the understanding of illnesses (Emde, 1998), but also the process itself, its procedures and instruments. This is one more reason why diagnostic classification and assessment must remain different approaches.

If we obtain valid and correctly interpreted information from assessment, even in different settings, we can always share the diagnostic classification commonly chosen with other professionals. In our case, this is the Diagnostic Classification of Mental Health and Disorders of Development of Infancy and Early Childhood, DC: 0–3 (DC: 0–3, 1994) because it fulfills the general acceptable criteria for classification and respects infancy specificities.

Methods

We now present the assessment procedures conducted in our infant mental health unit by a multidisciplinary team in an outpatient-based clinic setting and involving a Portuguese urban population.

The Assessment Process

The assessment process in infant mental health includes the evaluation of infants' mental functioning and development, parents' aspects and familial constellation, and the interactive and relational context of the child with his key caregivers. In order to collect all this information we created an observation setting in the Infancy Unit (Unidade da Primeira Infancia) that includes an interview with parents, direct and videotaped interaction observation, direct observation of the child, and eventually, developmental observation with standard tests and/or home visit (Cordeiro, 1997).

From our first contact with families, the assessment goal is doubled by a therapeutic concern meaning that there is no clear separation between assessment and intervention (Rabouan & Renard, 1986). All our interventions, even in the diagnostic phase, are based on our endeavor to establish an empathic communication with the parents and the baby by listening, trying to understand them, and containing their distress. It is only in the context of a dynamic exchange with the parents that we can obtain significant information about the child and the family (Hirschberg, 1993).

The family is introduced to the assessment procedure by our nurse. She welcomes the family to the unit, explains to the parents the way in which the observation will take place, and establishes the continuity between the different steps of the assessment process.

THE INTERVIEW

In infancy, the presence of the infant during the interview with the parents lends a "special climate" to the session. Although the objective of the interview is to obtain information about the child's developmental history and symptoms, familial context, and the history of parent relationships, the dialogue between the parents and the observer is blended by the shared comments on the observation of the child's behavior in the room. This observation provokes free associations, arouses affects either in parents or in the observer, and guides the course of the interview. This means that the observer has in mind a certain number of issues that need to be dealt with, but the way and the timing for doing so is very much determined by what is going on with the baby, the parents' state of mind, and the quality of parental discourse. For instance, if a baby needs to be calmed down or fed and his mother is angry or anxious about it, the observer must be available to adapt to this new situation. "Watch, wait and wonder" (Muir, 1992) is central to developing empathy with the parents and to helping to establish a therapeutic alliance.

The interview is based on a mutual agreement between the parents and the observer: Parents need to feel accepted and validated in their difficulties. In turn, the observer needs to accept that he or her will be observed and evaluated by parents without imposing his or her own beliefs, principles, or technical rules. This does not mean, of course, to get involved with parents or to forget the ethical recommendations. Neutrality and avoidance of acting are good principles to bear in mind if we want to be helpful toward our patients. During the initial part, the interview is nondirective, focusing on mutual engagement and allowing parents to present the problem in the way chosen by them. Our interventions are more supportive and follow the affect displayed by parents and the latent meaning of their speech. The questions are formulated in order to clarify some aspects, such as some inconsistencies in the parents' report, their interpretation of the symptoms or a particular behavior of the child, differences between the way parents describe the baby and our observation during the session, or even the relationship between the current and past events. Moreover, we try to be attentive to their deeper attitude toward the consultation and the consultant (submission versus rivalry, depression and guilt ver-

sus omnipotence and persecution) their self-representation and the self with others representation, and their availability to be involved with their child and to adapt to changes.

In a second phase, we try to ask direct questions about development, daily life, illnesses, and significant familial events, always bearing in mind the need to follow the parents' discourse and affect. As Hirschberg (1993) puts it, the issue is to achieve the "history making rather than history taking." We are aware of the fact that the parents' attitude during the interview and toward the baby depend very much on the quality of their relationship with the interviewer. The data collection, besides providing relevant and relatively objective information about the child, allows us to obtain a better idea about the parents' involvement and their subjective attitude toward the child through the richness and accuracy of their recollections, the changing affective tone of their speech, and their degree of pleasure and pride about the child's capacities and performances. With certain very inhibited or depressed parents, it is helpful not to dwell too long on the initial phase because asking direct and precise questions about the child helps them to organize their speech and to feel more comfortable during the interview. Contrarily, in other cases with parents who are more detached from their child and forgetful about important aspects of child development and life or yet, with more persecutory feelings, the direct questions can be understood as an inquiry. It can provoke aggression towards the observer and/or premature interruption in the clinical process because unbearable feelings of guilt or intrusion arise. Therefore, the management of the interview needs flexibility on the part of the observer based on his or her skills acquired during professional training about adult mental health and the self-analysis of contratransferential feelings.

Our clinical file includes the following sections:

- A. Child's identification, motive for referral, pathways followed by the parents since the beginning of the problems, and identification of the family's background and socioeconomic status.
- B. Parents' free speech during the nonoriented part of the interview focusing on their complaints, perceptions of the child's manifestations and problems, and the quality and intensity of their involvement.
- C. Systematic collection of the data, referring to the following items:

1. Previous pregnancies and deliveries: Number, birth control, medical assistance, evolution and abortions or hospitalizations during pregnancy, pre- or perinatal complications, and duration of the hospitalization.
2. Present pregnancy: Birth control, evolution and existence or not of medical complications, the moment of the fetus' first movements, evolution of parents' expectations and representations of the baby, gender preference and time of knowledge of gender and reactions, life events during pregnancy, and psychic conditions of both parents.

3. Delivery: Characteristics (site, term, type, fetus presentation), newborn's vital signs and characteristics, and resuscitation procedures, if any.
4. Newborn period: Perinatal complications, duration of the stay at hospital and reasons (newborn/mother or both), newborn's isolation, if any, and motives, first contact with the baby (when, how, rooming-in), and first reactions to the "actual" baby and to his manifestations.

Throughout items 1 through 4, the objective is the identification of previous stressful events or medical conditions influencing the quality and the intensity of the involvement with the baby, as well as the screening of relevant medical conditions through obstetrical history. Previous abortions and perinatal troubles were significantly more frequent in our clinical population than in a nonclinical population and 51 percent of our cases had a separation of mother and newborn during the 48 hours (Cordeiro, 1990).

Also, the evaluation of the evolution of the mental representation of the baby ("imaginary baby") during pregnancy and the affective reaction to the actual baby's reality and appearance are assessed through the following data.

5. Mother/infant early relationship: Mother's description of the baby's manifestations, needs, and reactions, infant caregiving and caregivers, at home, and role of the father and maternal grandmother or other members of the family.
6. History of caregiving: Caregiving characteristics and caregivers, chronologi-

cal evolution, infant's reactions to changes and adaptation to transitions, and separations (age, motives, and duration) and infant's and parents' reactions.

Items 5 and 6 attempt to evaluate the mother's state of mind and capacity for caregiving, identify symptoms of depression and the degree of mother/infant pleasure and empathy, and evaluate the parents' adaptation to their parental function and to the new baby with his specific characteristics and reactivity. Also, familial support to the mother and familial context are important issues to be taken into account. We usually interpret the successive changes in caregiving as a sign of lack of consistency in parent involvement beyond the circumstances of life.

7. Medical history: Infant's health bulletin (mental deficiency screening, vaccination schedule), acute or chronic diseases, hospitalizations or operations and motives, accidents (frequency, severity, home accidents, and so on), and sensorial impairment, if any.

Item 7, simultaneously with the identification of relevant medical conditions, tries to identify the somatic vulnerability and the accident-proneness of the child, which is eventually linked to parental negligence and infant's depression as well as parental incapacity to protect the child's health.

8. Feeding and eating evolution: Breast feeding, bottle feeding, spoon feeding, and self-feeding (age, characteristics,

and adaptation), problems (refusal, vomiting, selectivity, rituals, and colic), and parental attitude and procedures and interpretation.

9. Sleeping evolution: Early sleep pattern and rhythm, environmental conditions, sleeping problems (insomnia, nocturnal agitation, hypersomnia, and fears), and parental attitude and procedures and interpretation.

10. Motor development: Developmental markers, global motor activity and muscle tone, abnormal movements and habits, and parental attitude and interpretation.

11. Toilet training: Age of the beginning of training by parents or others and full acquisition, delays and/or problems, and parental attitudes and procedures.

12. Language and speech development: Interest and capacity for verbal communication, onset of vocalizing, first words, phrases, and self-designation, capacity for expressing desires, affects, and symbolic thoughts, delays and/or specific troubles, and parental attitudes.

13. Socialization: Social markers (social smile, strange anxiety, and separation anxiety), capacity for social relating with adults, peers, in groups, inside or outside, and known and familial environments, and withdrawal or isolation behavior.

14. Affect expression: Readiness for expressing emotions, variety and adaptation to situations, and affect inversion or inadequate variation.

15. Sexuality development: Curiosity, interest in, and reactions to gender dif-

ferences, self-erotic activities, and parental beliefs and attitudes.

16. Child's particular attitudes, interests, and behavior: Temper tantrums, aggressive manifestations, impulse control, fears, stubbornness, repetitive/stereotyped activity or interest, autostimulation activities, and so on.

Items 8 through 16 identify the possible troubles in corresponding areas that can indicate difficulties in ego and self-development, as well as possible environmental and parental attitudes, being not only inappropriate but leading to reinforcement of the difficulty.

17. Description of one day in the child's life: This can indicate the degree of coherence and the variety of child's experience, according to his age and maturity.

18. Family history: Health condition, psychiatric care, if any, parents' biography and evolution of relationship with their own parents, relevant life events in parents' life for their position as parents of this particular child, and sibling's history and role in the family.

Items 17 and 18 attempt to identify the incapacitating conditions of parents to caregiving that put the child at risk, the anomalous familial situations leading eventually to child maltreatment and abuse, or contrarily, the integration of the nuclear family in a broader familial context. We also try to understand parental attitudes in terms of an unconscious tendency to repeat the parents' childhood experiences and relationship in the relationship with their child and the prevalence of projective identification over identification mechanisms. The balance of parent involvement with the other children in the family is also evaluated, even in the case of a dead child. In short, we try to understand the link between the baby's problem and the personal history of his parents, the caregiving, and the parents' mental functioning (narcissistic equilibrium, object relationship quality, and dominant defense mechanisms).

OBSERVATION OF THE INTERACTION

During the interview with the both parents or with only the mother/caregiver, we usually register the interaction with the infant. It is a twofold observation, with a direct observation made by an observer in the room and a videotaped sequence. An independent observer not involved in the consultation process stays in the room and tries to catch the movements, affective nuances, and dialogue between the mother/father and the infant, without intervening actively. A written report of an initial period of 15 to 20 minutes is given. This kind of observation is closer to the affective climate displayed by parents and the child and its impact on the evaluators and allows a deeper discussion in terms of the quality of affects of the interaction, also associated with the speech of the parents about the child. Moreover, we try to assess the mother's capacity to monitor the child's activity and respond to the child's needs, as well as the quality of her attention while engaging in a particular situation such as the interview. This procedure attempts to reproduce home situations in which mothers need to share their attention between caring for the child and other tasks with which they are involved. Whenever fathers come to the consultations, which is more and more frequent, the observation of the interaction includes both parents and the baby. Although not so systematic as the Lausane Triadic Play Method (Signal, 1995), we evaluate the father-child interaction, the father's attitudes toward the dyad, and communication between both parents.

The timing of the videotaped sequence depends on the evaluation of the infant's state of mind and the parents' availability for playing with the child. In general, it happens in the last part of the consultation after the interview. Parents are asked to be available for the child during free activity, without being very active or demanding and after that, leave the room for a short period (no more than three to four minutes). Then they come back and play with the child, as they are "used to doing at home." This kind of observation allows an analysis of the interactive behavior and transactions in different situations and the evaluation of the characteristics of the child's behavior, namely his or her reaction to separation/reunion and modes of adaptation.

During these sequences, some important clinical aspects of mother/father-child interaction can be observed that allow the quality of the relationships to be assessed. They are as follows:

- The use by the child of the mother/father as a reference figure and mother's response to that behavior.

- The diversity of the child's developmentally appropriate modalities of approach and initiative.
- The diversity of mother/father modalities of approach and initiative in engaging the child.
- Mother/child postures and movements and their adaptability.
- Mother's/father's and child's capacity to focus attention together in the external world, as well as capacity to develop circles of increasingly complex interaction and degree of mutual pleasure.
- Mother's and child's predominant affective modes and changes, according to specific situations or behaviors.
- Mother's/father's capacity to calm the child down or to introduce age-appropriate frustration without provoking distress in the child.
- Child's capacity to recognize and deal with frustration, seek help from the mother/father/other available, or to calm himself down.
- Content, affective quality, and adaptation of mother's/father's speech to child's manifestations and their free association.
- Impact of the observation on the observer(s) during the consultation and after the videotape observation.

The data of both written reports and videotaped sequences are analyzed in group discussions especially designed for the assessment of the interaction. We systematically address issues: Reciprocity and contingency of mother/father/child behavior (Greenspan & Lieberman, 1989), appropriate mirroring and affective attunement (Stern, 1985), mutual pleasure, regulation of the interactive behaviors (Anders, 1989), tonal dialogue (Mazes & Stoleru, 1993), existence of symptomatic interactive sequences (SIS) (Cramer & Espasa, 1993), and the coherence of maternal communication. In fact, we observed that mother-child communication is enhanced whenever the different components of the interactive sequence (sensorial, psychomotor, postural, and verbal) carry on the same affective tonality. On the contrary, if the components of the observable interaction transmit multiple and contradictory messages to the baby, the mother's communication cannot be understood by the child, and the child reacts with avoidant or even disorganized behaviors. In a group of anorexic toddlers, these particular kind of interactions were related to maternal ambivalent feelings toward the child (Cordeiro, Rodrigues, & Caldeira da Silva, 1993).

Although we abandoned standardized and scored evaluations of interaction, most of them usually used in research contexts because of their relative reductionism and usefulness for strictly clinical purposes (Crowell & Fleishman, 1993), our final evaluation includes the use of the PIR GAS scale (Zero to Three, 1994) for classifying the relationship during the diagnostic classification phase of the clinical process.

OBSERVATION OF THE CHILD
During this time-consuming consultation, there is plenty of time for the observation of the child's behavior with parents, during the parents' absence and with the observer. According to the age-expected capacities, we assess:

- The modalities of integrating and processing sensorial stimulation, the stimuli-reactivity threshold, and under which conditions of stimulation (social or sensorial) the child displays disorganized or withdrawn behaviors.
- Capacity for motor planning, degree of maturity, and integration of psychomotor activity.
- Balance between pleasure/displeasure during activities and predominant mode of expression of the effects—their appropriateness and variety.
- Modes of dealing with frustration (when disappointed, shows distress, ignores it, or changes behavior without apparent emotional variation).
- Responses and attitudes in accordance with the mother's/father's state of mind or parent's speech content during the consultation (e.g., when the mother suddenly begins to cry, a two-year-old interrupts his or her own play to give the mother his or her toy).
- Modes of dealing with a new situation, new person, new space, and new objects (inhibition, negativism, or excessive easiness in adaptation) and the evolution of behavior during the session.
- Capacity to establish different relationships with different persons, according to the person or the situation (e.g., a toddler asks the assessor when he or she wants an object from the room, but asks mother for help or an infant shows more curiosity with the person interacting with the mother than with the observer who is writing the observation).
- Capacity and interest in the exploration

of the room by the child when the mother is engaged with the assessor.

- Type of play and function (imitative, functional, repetitive, or symbolic) and capacity to play alone in the presence of an adult.
- Level of language and interest in verbal communication.
- Child's behavior during separation and reunion and capacity to use others during mother's absence (e.g., a walking toddler is distressed when his or her mother leaves the room and is unable to get up and approach the door or another toddler shows perplexity and sadness, but slowly begins to handle a toy, usually the one the mother played with and finally, looks at the observer and grins).

In summary, bearing in mind not only the understanding of psychopathology, but also the role of the baby in it, we evaluate the maturational/constitutional characteristics of a child's competencies (reactivity, motor, and sensorial processing, capacity to organize the experience), as well as several parameters of age-appropriate mental functioning. The interest in the environment and in others, level of language, play, modes of adaptation, modes of dealing with anxiety or distress, and affect expression are good indicators for the degree of self-autonomy (differentiation of the mental representations of the self and the self with others), symbolic activity, and cognitive development. Reactions to mother's separation and reunion allow us to obtain some addi-

tional information about the quality of the child's attachment.

Concluding Formulations Guiding Therapeutic Orientations

The conclusions of our assessment are discussed with the parents in a session planned for that purpose and scheduled for one or two weeks later. We think there are some advantages in this procedure, not only by giving time to the professionals to elaborate, organize, and discuss all the information collected, but also for parents to work through their difficulties.

The professionals involved need time to internally organize the information they received before making a more schematic presentation and discussion. Also, the parent's elaboration of what went on during the assessment needs time and provokes some changes. It can be premature to invade them with solutions, the scope and aim of which they cannot readily totally understand.

The positive effects of assessment on the family are frequent and show their availability for therapeutic changes. These therapeutic benefits are based, in our opinion, on some features occurring during the assessment session(s). One of them is the *surprise* effect. Parents are often confronted with dramatic changes in the child's behavior during the consultation: The insomniac baby who falls asleep in his mother's lap or the excessive demanding 9-month-old that plays alone during a large part of the consultation without fussing. Also, the accent by our team on the positive aspects of the child's manifestations is a very surprising and rewarding situation for the parents.

A second feature is *curiosity* about the meaning of the child's manifestations (Cordeiro, 1997), aroused by our questions and curiosity about their baby, which makes them also question themselves after the consultation. Another one is the *interest* that the baby shows in the assessor and in playing. Very often, toddlers resist leaving the unit and show great pleasure in coming back, stimulating parents to continue with the consultations. Also, the fact that all the professionals involved in a specific assessment *share* the same empathic and understanding attitude toward the baby's problem gives the parents a feeling of mutual engagement and confidence in the team and in themselves. We must say that this effect is the result of an ongoing team effort involving all professionals.

In our group, the data collected during the assessment procedure are presented in a clinical meeting and discussed by the whole team. Therapeutic orientations arise from these discussions. The clinical discussion focuses on the dynamic meaning of the infant's psychopathology in his or her psychic organization and on the relationship with the caregivers, as well as on the level of the infant's self-organization separation/ individuation process, differentiation of the representations of the self and the self with others, and mechanisms of adaptation. Aware of the importance of the quality of the emotional experiences, we also evaluate the impact of the parents' past relationships and history on the representa-

tion they have of the actual child, as well as the severity of its distortions by projection mechanisms as they show up in the adequateness of interaction or in the frequency of SIS.

Because it is not always easy to differentiate what belongs constitutionally to the child from the consequences of the relational disorder, we also evaluate, as separately as possible, the part played by the infant from the part played by the parents. We do this through the infant's characteristics such as appearance, activity, expressiveness, proneness to engage socially, and capacity to deal with frustration.

The evaluation of the capacity for change of each partner is also imperative for the therapeutic orientation. In parents, personality disorders, narcissistic failures, balance between aggressive and libidinal impulses, rigidity of the defense mechanisms, capacity of the representation of their own mental states and of others', and the "reflective function of the self" (Fonagy et al., 1991) are important factors influencing their capacity to change. In the child, characteristics of resiliency and ability to adapt and change behavior in different situations help us to make our therapeutic decisions and assignments.

Very often, referrals for further assessment procedures are decided during these clinical discussions. For instance, home visits may be required in order to better understand the familial context and routines or a further evaluation of the child's development may be conducted by the use of standardized tests, usually the Griffiths test (Griffiths, 1970). The developmental profile analysis allowed by the use of this scale can be an important tool for differential diagnosis and therapeutic orientation. In fact, the application of the Griffiths developmental scales in our clinical population showed different developmental patterns through the comparison of the results in each subscale. Two main profile patterns were identified in children presenting multisystemic developmental disorders. One pattern, characterized by homogeneous results in the subscales, appeared in the group of children in which processing difficulties of cognitive information were dominant. A second pattern, characterized by heterogeneous results in the subscales determining a disharmonic profile, appeared in the group of children where the importance of affective and relationship disturbance was preponderant (Fornelos, Fornelos, Caldeira da Silva, & Cordeiro, 1996).

In specific groups, either because of clinical research objectives or reassessment objectives, some other standardized instruments are used. In the case of multisystemic developmental disorders, the CHAT (Check-list for Autism in Toddlers) (Baron-Cohen et al., 1996) is used. In the case of anorexic infants, the "Entretien-R" (Stern et al., 1989) is used (Cordeiro et al., 1993). However, in our unit the use of standardized instruments is not a very current practice. It is our experience that it overcharges the process. Parents feel themselves more as the object of investigation rather than concern, and it possibly overlaps therapeutic aims. In addition, a fragmented process of assessment can lead to multiple and separate therapies in the

same child, thereby, lacking a global understanding of psychopathology and consequently, a consistent and unified therapeutic orientation. In our opinion, standardized instruments must be used in very specific programs with well-defined objectives and the prior agreement and knowledge of the parents about the process in which they will be involved.

Nevertheless, even in clinical practice we need to organize our data in order to deepen our knowledge and understanding of psychopathology and therapeutic results. The use of DC: 0–3 (Zero to Three, 1994) helped us tremendously in this task, although we had to adapt our thinking namely about obtaining information on the child and separating it from information about parents. With this clarification, the use of DC: 0–3 Axes has been very helpful. In all our first cases, we discuss the diagnosis in DC: 0–3 Axis I and II. In reassessments (cases with six months therapy or more) Axes I, II, III, and IV are used, systematically. Axis V has been used specifically in MSDD cases. In other diagnosis and with our procedures, it has been hard to take advantage of this axis. Instead, we are creating our own Infant Global Functioning Scale, adapted from DSM–IV GAP (APA, 1995), which is now in an exploratory phase. It rates infant symptoms (quantity and quality), social relatedness, interest in external world, autonomy/independence, expression of affects (adequateness and range), cognitive and psychomotor development, communication (interest in verbal communication and level of verbal language), and play (age adequateness, flexibility, and function).

In conclusion, we consider that with both the dynamic evaluation of the infant psychopathology and the diagnostic process with DC 0–3 system, our procedure gives us an overview of the psychopathological process, and it is helpful for guiding therapeutic intervention. However, we are aware that this is a process in constant reformulation, such as the evolutionary process of the child, the relationships, and the environment as well as their evolving and mutual interactions.

The multidisciplinary ground of our clinical work and discussions constitutes a consistent training setting for professionals in infant mental health and promotes scientific knowledge and exchanges.

References

Ainsworth, M. D. S., Bell, S., & Stayton, D. J. (1971). Individual differences in strange situation behavior of one year olds. In H. R. Schaffer (Ed.), *The origins of human social relations* (pp. 17–57). London: Academic.

American Psychiatric Association. (1995). Diagnostic and statistical manual of mental disorders: International version (4th ed.). Washington, DC: Author.

Anders, F. A. (1989). Clinical syndromes, relationships disturbances and their assessment. In A. J. Sameroff & R. Emde (Eds.), *Relationship disturbances in early childhood* (pp. 125–144). New York: Basic Books.

Baron-Cohen, S., Cox, A., Baird, G., Swettenham, J., Nightingale, N., Morgan, K., Drew, A., & Charman, T. (1996). Psycho-logical marks in the detection of in infancy in a large population. *British Journal of Psychiatry, 168,* 158–163.

Berger, M. (1985). Temperament and individual differences. In M. Rutter & L. Hersov (Eds.), *Child and adolescent psychiatry: Modern approaches* (2nd ed., pp. 3–16). London: Blackwell Scientific Publications.

Bowlby, J. (1988). *A secure base: Clinical applications of attachment theory.* London: Routledge.

Bowlby, J. (1989). The role of attachment in personality development and psychopathology. In S. I. Greenspan & G. H. Pollock (Eds.), *The course of life: Vol. I. Infancy* (pp. 228–270). Madison, WI: International Universities Press.

Bradley-Johnson, S. (1982). Infant assessment as intervention and parent education. *Infant Mental Health Journal, 3,* 293–297.

Brazelton, T. B. (1981). Comportement et competence du nouveau-né. *Psychiatrie de l'Enfant, 24,* 375–396.

Brazelton, T. B. (1983). Assessment of techniques for enhancing development. In J. D. Call, E. Galenson, & R. L. Tyson (Eds.), *Frontiers of infant psychiatry* (pp. 347–361). New York: Basic Books.

Bretherton, I. (1990). Communication patterns, internal working models, and the intergenerational transmission of attachment relationships. *Infant Mental Health Journal, 11,* 237–252.

Cordeiro, M. (1997). Treating infants and mothers in psychic distress: A mental health program for *Infant Mental Health Journal, 18,* 145–157.

Cordeiro, M., & Caldeira da Silva, P. (1998) (In press). La classification diagnostique des troubles de la santé mentale du nourresson: une expérianee clinique. *Devenir.*

Cordeiro, M. J. (1990). Risk factors for the child development and mother-child interaction. Paper presented at the 5th Congress of the International Federation of Psychiatric Epidemiology, Montréal, Canada.

Cordeiro, M. J., Rodrigues, E., & Caldeira da Silva, P. (1993). L'anoréxie du nourrisson: Une étude clinique. *Devenir, 5,* 35–50.

Cramer, B., & Palacio-Espasa, F. (1993). *La practique des psychothérpies mère-bébé.* Paris: PUF.

Crowell, A., & Feischmann, A. (1993). Use of structured research procedures in clinical assessments of infants. In C. H. Zeanah (Ed.), *Handbook of infant mental health* (pp. 210–222). New York: Guilford.

Demos, E. V. (1989). Resiliency in infancy. In T. F. Dugan & R. Coles (Eds.), *The child in our times: Studies in development resiliency* (pp. 3–22). New York: Bruner/Mazel.

Emde, R. (1998) (In press). À propos des classifications diagnostiques de la petite infance: quelques principes. *Devenir.*

Emde, R., Bingham, D., & Harmon, J. (1993). Classification and the diagnostic process in infancy. In C. H. Zeanah (Ed.), *Handbook of infant mental health* (pp. 225–235). New York: Guilford.

Emde, R. N. (1989). The infant's relationship experience: Developmental and affective aspects. In A. J. Sameroff & R. N. Emde (Eds.), *Relationship disturbances in early childhood: A developmental approach* (pp. 33–52). New York: Basic Books.

Emde, R. N., & Sorce, J. F. (1983). The rewards of infancy: Emotional availability and maternal referencing. In J. D. Call, E. Galenson & R. L. Tyson, (Eds.), *Frontiers of infant psychiatry* (pp. 17–30). New York: Basic Books.

Erickson, M. F., Sroufe, A. L., & Egeland, B. (1985). The relationship between the quality of attachment and behavior problems in pre-school in a high-risk sample. In I. Bretherton & E. Waters (Eds.), Growing points of attachment theory and research (pp. 147–116). *Monographs of the Society for Research in Child Development, 50.*

Fonagy, P., Steele, M., Steele H., Moran, G. S., & Higgitt, A. C. (1991). The capacity for understanding mental states: The reflective self in parent and child and its significance for security of attachment. *Infant Mental Health Journal, 12,* 201–218.

Fornelos, M., Fornelos, J., Caldeira da Silva, P., & Cordeiro, M. (1996). *The use of Griffith's developmental scales in the differential diagnoses of pervasive developmental disorders.* Poster session presented at WAIMH, Sixth World Congress, Tampere.

Fraiberg, S. (1987). Pathological defences in infancy. In L. Fraiberg (Ed.), *Selected writings of Selma Fraiberg* (pp. 183–204). Columbus: Ohio State University Press.

Fraiberg, S., Adelson, E., & Shapiro, V. (1980). Treatment modalities. In S. Fraiberg (Ed.), *Clinical studies in infant mental health: The first year of life* (pp. 164–196). New York: Basic Books.

Garber, J. (1984). Classification of childhood psychopathology: A developmental perspective. *Child Development, 55,* 30–48.

Gonçalves, M. J. (1994). Identification et contre-transfert dans les psychothérapies mère-enfant. *Revue Française Psychanalise, 5,* 1669–1673.

Greenspan, S. I. (1989). The development of the ego: Insights from clinical work with infants and young children. In S. I. Greenspan & G. H. Pollock (Eds.), *The course of life: psychoanalytic contribu-*

tions toward understanding personality development: Vol. I. Infancy (pp. 85–163). Madison, WI: International Universities Press.

Greenspan, S. I., & Forges, S. W. (1984). Psychopathology in infancy and early childhood: Clinical perspective on the organization of sensory and affective thematic experience. *Child Development, 55,* 49–70.

Greenspan, S. I., & Lieberman, A. F. (1989). Infants, mothers and their interaction: A quantitative clinical approach to developmental assessment. In S. I. Greenspan & G. H. Pollock (Eds.), *The course of life: Vol. Infancy* (pp. 503–560). Madison, WI: International University Press.

Greenspan, S. I., & Weider, S. (1993). Regulatory Disorders. In C. H. Zeanah (Ed.), *Handbook of infant mental health* (pp. 280–290). New York/London: Guilford.

Griffiths, R. (1970). *The abilities of young children.* High Wyconse Test Agency.

Grossman, K., Grossman, K. E., Sprangler, G., & Unzner, L. (1985). Maternal sensitivity and newborn's orientation response, as related to quality of attachment in Northern Germany. In I. Bretherton & E. Waters (Eds.), Growing points of attachment theory and research (pp. 223–256). *Monographs of the Society for Research in Child Development, 50.*

Guédeney, A., & Lebovici, S. (1997). The importance of personal relationships in infant evaluation. *Infant Mental Health Journal, 18,* 171–178.

Hirschberg, M. (1993). Clinical interviews with infants and their families. In C. H. Zeanah (Ed.), *Handbook of infant mental health* (pp. 173–190). New York: Guilford.

Kreisler, L. (1987). *Le nouvel enfant du désordre psychossomatique.* Toulose: Privat.

Kreisler, L., & Cramer, B. (1981). Sur les bases cliniques de la psychiatrie du nourresson. *La Psychiatrie de l'enfant, 24,* 1–15.

Lebovici, S. (1988). Fantasmatic interaction and intergenerational transmission. *Infant Mental Health Journal, 9,* 10–19.

Main, M., Kaplan, N., & Cassidy, J. (1985). Security in infancy, childhood, and adulthood: A move to the level of representation. In I. Bretherton & E. Waters (Eds.), Growing points of attachment theory and research (pp. 66–72). *Monographs of the Society for Research in Child Development, 50.*

Mazet, P., & Stoleru, S. (1993). *Psychopathologie do nourrisson et du jeune enfant* (2nd ed.). Paris: Masson.

Muir, E. (1992). Watching, waiting and wondering: Applying psychoanalytic principles to mother-infant intervention. *Infant Mental Health Journal, 13,* 319–328.

Murray, L. (1991). Intersubjectivity, object relation theory and empirical evidence from mother-infant interactions. *Infant Mental Health Journal, 12,* 219–232.

Murray, L. (1996). *Post-partum depression and consequences on infant development.* Séance plénière. Colloque International de Psychiatrie Perinatale, Mónaco.

Osofsky, J. D., Hann, D. M., & Peebles, C. (1993). Adolescent parenthood: Risks and opportunities for mothers and infants. In C. H. Zeanah (Ed.), *Handbook of infant mental health* (pp. 280–290). New York/London: Guilford.

Papousek, H., & Papousek, M. (1983). Interactional failures: Their origin and significance in infant psychiatry. In J. D. Call, E. Galenson, & R. L. Tyson (Eds.), *Frontiers of infant psychiatry* (pp. 74–85). New York: Basic Books.

Rabouam, C., & Renard, L. (1986). Nécessité et Difficultés de L'evaluation dans l'intervention psycho-thérapeutique auprès de jeunes enfants. *Devenir, 8,* 7–19.

Rutter, M. (1994a). Stress research: Accomplishments and tasks ahead. In R. J. Haggerty, J. Robert, L. R. Sherrod, N. Garmezy, & M. Rutter (Eds.), *Stress, risk, and resilience in children and adolescents, processes mechanisms and interventions* (pp. 354–385). New York: Cambridge University Press.

Rutter, M. (1994b). Temperament: Changing concepts end implications. In W. B. Carey & McDevitt (Eds.), *Early intervention: Individual differences as risk factors for the mental health of children* (pp. 23–34). New York: Brunner/Mazel.

Sameroff, A. J. (1989). Principles of development and psychopathology. In A. J. Sameroff & R. N. Emde (Eds.), *Relationship disturbances in early childhood: A developmental approach* (pp. 17–32). New York: Basic Books.

Sameroff, A. J. (1993). Models of development and developmental risk. In C. H. Zeanah (Ed.), *Handbook of infant mental health* (pp. 3–13). New York/London: Guilford.

Sameroff, A. J., & Emde, R. N. (1989). *Relationship disturbance in early childhood.* New York: Basic Books.

Sameroff, A. J., & Seiffer (1983). *Familial risk and child competence, 54,* 1254–1268.

Sander, L. W. (1983). Polarity, paradox and the organizing process in development. In *Frontiers of infant psychiatry* (pp. 334–346). New York: Basic Books.

Sander, L. W. (1989). Investigation of the infant and its caregiving environment as a biological system. In S. I. Greenspan & G. H. Pollock (Eds.), *The course of life: Vol. I. Infancy* (pp. 359–391). Madison, WI: International University Press.

Seifer, R., & Orikstein, S. (1993). Parental mental illness and infant development. In C. H. Zeanah (Ed.), *Handbook of infant mental health* (pp. 120–142). New York/London: Guilford.

Sroufe, A. L. (1985). Attachment classification from the perspective on infant-caregiver relationships and infant temperament. *Child Development, 56,* 1–14.

Sroufe, A. L. (1989). Relationships and relationship disturbances. In A. J. Sameroff & R. N. Emde (Eds.), *Relationship disturbances in early childhood: A developmental approach* (pp. 97–124). New York: Basic Books.

Sroufe, A. L., & Rutter, M. (1984). The domain of developmental psychopathology. *Child Development, 55,* 17–29.

Stern, D. (1980). *The first relationship: Infant and mother* (3rd ed.). Cambridge, MA: Harvard University Press.

Stern, D. (1985). *The interpersonal world of the infancy: A view from psychoanalysis and developmental psychology.* New York: Basic Books.

Stern, D. (1991). Maternal representation: A clinical and subjective phenomological view. *Infant Mental Health Journal, 12,* 174–186.

Stern, D. (1995). *Motherhood constellation.* New York: Basic Books.

Stern, D. N., Robert-Tissot, Besson, G., Rusconi-Serps, S., Muralt, M., Cramer, B., & Palacio, F. (1989). L'Entretien—R: Une méthode d'évaluation des représentations maternelles. In S. Lebovici, P. Mazet, & J. P. Visier (Ed.), *L'évaluation des interactives précoces entre le bébé et ses partenaires* (pp. 151–178). Genève: Editions Eshel/Medecine et Hygiène.

Thomas, J., & Harmon, R. (1989). La classification diagnostique des troubles de la santé mentale du nourisson et du jeune enfant:

Un système dynamique pour la connaissance et letraitement nourrisions, des jeunes enfants et de leure families. *Devenir.*

Triangulations in relationships. (1995). *Signal, 3,*(2), 1–6.

Trowell, J., & Rustin, M. (1991). Developing the internal observer in professionals in training. *Infant Mental Health Journal, 12,* 233–245.

Zeanah, C., Benoft, D., Hirshberg, L., Barton, M. L., & Regan, C. (1994). Mother representations of their infants are concordant with infant attachment, classifications, developmental issues. *Developmental Issues in Psychiatry and Psychology, 1,* 9–18.

Zeanah, C. H., Boris, N. W., & Scheeringa, M. S. (1997). Psychopathology in infancy. *Journal of Child Psychology and Psychiatry, 38,* 81–99.

Zero to Three/National Center for Clinical Infant Programs. (1994). *Diagnostic classification of mental and developmental disorders of infancy and early childhood. DC: 0–3.* Arlington, VA: Author.

8

Evaluating Mother-
Infant Psychotherapies:
Bridging the Gap between
Clinicians and Researchers

Bertrand Cramer and Christiane Robert-Tissot

8

Introduction

This chapter illustrates ways in which demanding research can be realistically integrated into a child guidance clinic, how clinicians can learn to accept the intrusiveness of methodological constraints, and how researchers can manage to adapt their ways to the vagaries of therapeutic practice. Assessment is part of the daily routine of clinicians. They are used to evaluating diagnosis, treatment indications, and the many factors that contribute to pathology. While many assessment instruments have been created to help clinicians systematize their assessments and enhance reliability, a large contribution is left to what is called clinical experience. Clinical experience is very difficult to describe and analyze in a way allowing replication and systematic teaching. In clinical practice, the assessment of indications, active ingredients of technique, and outcome are left to the personal and, therefore, subjective evaluation of therapists.

The need for the systematic evaluation of these various aspects does not appear to be a main objective in training. Assessment of results and processes is generally considered to be part of the private relationship between therapists and patients. Clinical practice has, thus, somewhat eluded the requirements of systematic research and, indeed, most clinicians have not found that psychotherapy research brings valuable information to their practice. This failure to submit, in practice, various phases of psychotherapeutic endeavors to information and criticisms is partly due to the considerable difficulties in practicing methodologically sound research.

Difficulties in Assessing Psychotherapies

One should not underestimate the considerable difficulties in assessing outcome and process in psychotherapy. They have been well documented and aptly discussed (Parloff, 1982; Kazdin, 1994; Forrest Talley, Strupp, & Butler, 1994; Roth & Fonagy, 1996). A summarized review of these difficulties points to the following issues:

1. It is difficult to *enlist bona fide therapists* in collaborating with psychotherapy research. The therapeutic encounter is one of the most intimate forms of social intercourse. Its usual atmosphere is one of total confidentiality, needed to protect both patients and therapists. Therapists fear the intrusiveness of third party observation. Moreover, the constraints imposed by methodological requirements (standardization of technique, strict criteria for patient selection, systematic evaluation procedures, etc.) are experienced as altering the true nature of the therapeutic relationship.

2. It is difficult to *convince clinicians of the relevance of psychotherapy research.* Standards of methodological rigor are experienced as altering the therapeutic context of the research results. Some clinicians feel that studies conducted with flawless methods are unrelated to issues of deep clinical significance and that they merely reinforce existing theoretical beliefs, without changing practice (Widlocher, 1981; Spence, 1994; Greenberg, 1994). Indeed, surveys have shown that clinicians tend to ignore research reports (Rausch, 1974; Cohen, Sargent, & Set-Sechrest, 1986; Morrow-Bradley & Elliot, 1986).

3. Researchers and clinicians *have goals, epistemologies, and ethics that are different,* sometimes even opposite. Researchers systematize, standardize, and operationalize assessment procedures and psychotherapy techniques. They attempt to isolate and validate the essential ingredients of therapy-induced changes (Kiesler, 1994). To do so, they need to impose controls on the situation, isolate technical ingredients, and introduce objective, quantitative measures on data that is often mainly subjective in nature. They find it difficult to adapt strict methodological standards to suit the specificity of therapeutic formats and criticize therapists for their reluctance to submit their work to scientific inquiry. Therapists are essentially motivated by a wish to heal. They follow a "transformation project" aiming at modifying another human being through the effects of a relationship and the application of a highly prized theory. For them, understanding and searching for truth is in the service of an action: The cure of the patient. These and other discrepancies result in conflicts between researchers and therapists.

4. *Psychotherapy research accumulates many sources of nonvalidity.* It is very difficult to control the therapeutic situation, especially the active ingredients of technique. Isolating active ingredients may become artificial since they are all embedded in the therapeutic relationship that codetermines them. Causal links between ingredients of technique and outcome are difficult to demonstrate and consider truly valid. No two patients are exactly alike, making subject selection uneasy. Therapists are also very different

from each other. Therefore, strict technique adhesion is an illusion. Psychotherapy, like all human interaction, is responsive and hence nonlinear and chaotic. Therefore, prediction and control at the level of particular interventions seem exceedingly unlikely (Stiles, 1994; Kowalik, Schiepek, Kumpf, Roberts, & Elbert, 1997). Moreover, some of the most significant change occurring in therapy may not be observed at the time of posttherapy assessment but much later. Some changes might remain purely subjective or may not even be reported because they are unconscious. Information stemming from patients, therapists, and researchers may show little agreement. Many other sources of error could be added to this list and have prompted many clinicians to disqualify the research efforts in this field. Freud heralded this pessimistic view when he said to Rosenzweig that his efforts to do research in psychoanalysis "can do no harm" (letter to Dr. Saul Rosenzweig, 1934).

5. There are major *differences in existing psychotherapy research and practice* (Gérin, 1984; Kazdin, 1994; Robert-Tissot & Bachmann, 1995). In child therapy research, the majority of children (over 75 percent) are solicited as volunteers, while in practice they are spontaneously referred. This affects the levels of motivation and the types of problems referred. Methods of treatment differ. The majority of treatment studies focus on behavior modification and cognitive-behavioral techniques, while practice is based rather on psychodynamic, family therapy, relation-

ship therapy, and eclectic therapy. Duration of treatment is shorter in research studies, and therapists are often still in training. To seem valid for therapists "research must provide a therapeutic context to its interpretation" (Forrest Talley et al., 1994). This means that research must take place in a therapeutically "natural" context that is within a practice that does not depart from routine work. Moreover, therapists have to contribute to the research design by raising questions and testing hypotheses that correspond to their daily quandary.

In this chapter, we report on the experience we accumulated in the Geneva Child Guidance Clinic over a period of ten years, during which a research and clinical team attempted to produce sound research in the new field of mother-infant psychotherapy. These studies on outcome and processes in psychotherapy are rooted on a routine practice in its natural surroundings, with a population consulting for symptoms and difficulties in infants. We first describe our present views of infant pathologies, as they determine the processes of assessment. Then, we relate what forms of therapies are practiced in the clinic.

Therapies of Early Childhood Pathologies

Early appearing pathologies were first presented as new syndromes, such as autism (Kanner) and hospitalism (Spitz), and were described on a nosological basis. These manifestations were first noticed because of their great severity and because they foretold dire prognoses. While these entities still borrowed many terms from adult psychiatry, they heralded the concept of pathologies characteristic of infancy. Infant psychiatry in its own right was thus created. It became progressively apparent that the relationships between parents and infants played a crucial role in most infancy disorders. Spitz was the most powerful reference in this relational orientation. He proposed a classification of disorders according to the types of deviation in the mother-infant relations (Spitz, 1951). Mahler developed her tripartite model of treatment for childhood psychoses and focus on the symbiotic relationship that she elevated to the status of "normal phase," emphasizing the shaping influence of relationships on normal and pathological developments (Mahler, 1973; Mahler, Pine, & Bergman, 1975). Other authors also pioneered treatments via the parents (Furman, 1951) or with the mother-infant dyad (Fraiberg, Adelson, & Shapiro, 1980).

These developments contributed to a consecration of the relational conceptualization of most infant problems, eventually called "relationship disturbances" (Sameroff & Emde, 1989). What this means is that diagnostic assessments and treatments need to pay attention to the interaction between the infant's intrinsic characteristics and his milieu, mostly his immediate, familial environment (Osofsky, 1987). The focus on the relationship as the object of assessment is not without problems. It challenges the traditional medical model still largely based on a "within the organism diagnosis" (Emde, Birgham, & Harmon, 1993). The diagnosis becomes difficult to locate when several relationships are considered as cocreating the problems. Family studies have consistently proved that multigenerational dimension needs to be taken into account. What happened between the infant's parents and grandparents may weigh heavily on the present child. Cultural factors (as the immigrant status) may powerfully influence the relationships parents have with their baby. Even when multiaxial schemes of diagnosis are used, these "prehistoric" factors (as they played a determinant role even before the birth of the infant) are very difficult to include in diagnostic classification. Another difficulty appears because there is a lack of pathognomic signs of psychopathology in infancy. Most symptomatic behaviors in infancy are not specific of an underlying constitution or structure making difficult the use of discrete symptom-based disorders. This may be due to the rapid changes imposed on infant behaviors by developmental processes, but it also reflects the dependency of the infant who is highly sensitive to external influences. Many regulatory disorders seem to illustrate a problem of fit between the infant and his or her parents.

These difficulties explain why existing classifications (DSM–IV and ICD–10) have so few and imprecise diagnostic categories for infants and why more refined modes of classifying (Anders, 1989; Zero to Three, 1994) are still not easy to use for the clinician. New ways of conceptualizing diagnoses at this tender age have to be devised in order to take into account infant specificity such as the relational context, developmental changes, and importance of comorbidity. It has been suggested, for example, that childhood symptoms are better conceptualized as dimensional (i.e., as existing on a continuum with normality) than as categorical (i.e., viewing disorders as absent or present) (Emde et al., 1993). This would be one way of approaching disorders that remains totally elusive if one does not take into account the fluctuations of manifestations that are so powerfully influenced by maturational changes and interactional factors. Our work reflects the considerable difficulties in assessing infants. Taping interactive styles and configurations is still extremely uneasy, in spite of existing instruments (Clark, 1985; Zero to Three, 1994). Interactions, by their nature, fluctuate and attempts to define and classify them are as difficult as describing body movements. One has to resort to standardizing interactions in a set situation, such as is done in the Strange Situation procedure. However, much of the spontaneity of interrelations as they occur during sessions cannot be captured this way.

Our clinical experience indicates that while interactional factors remain very difficult to assess in a standardized measurable way, they still should always be taken into account in diagnostic and therapeutic endeavors. In most forms of mental retardation and in many cases of severe pervasive developmental disorders, interactional factors will not be considered the prime etiological factors and the main focus of intervention. We found that in cases where constitutional or temperamental factors seem to best explain symptoms,

such as early eczema, difficulties in consoling with constant crying, and early appearing withdrawal, a therapeutic approach focusing on parent-infant relational difficulties may cure the symptom. This does not necessarily mean that parent-infant conflicts were the cause of the symptoms, but that a resolution of the relational tension surrounding the symptom may actually cure it. This point of view, added to a generally accepted position that infant disorders need to be treated with the active participation of parents, confirms a basic therapeutic bias. It is the relationships between infants and parents that are the main target of therapeutic approaches.

Functional disorders (i.e., disorders involving somatic symptoms such as sleeping, eating, breathing, elimination, skin, etc.) have proved to be best understood and treated along interactional lines (Kreisler & Cramer, 1995). They are the most frequently presented problems in children between zero and three (Richman, Stevenson, & Graham, 1975), especially sleep disturbances. Moreover, in these functional disorders as well as in many behavioral problems (tantrums, aggression, separation difficulties), brief treatment of the mother-infant dyad brings considerable relief and symptom cessation. The rapid pace of curative change can also be seen as revealing the major influences of interactional factors in these disorders. When the major conflict between mother and child is treated, the symptoms are often lifted. To sum up our point of view on early childhood pathologies, we propose that while important contributing or etiological factors reside inside the infant's makeup or inside the parents psychic functioning (such as in the case of postpartum depression), most infant disorders are best understood and treated when it is the relationship that is taken as object of comprehension and intervention.

Psychotherapies in Infant Psychiatry

Treatment of young children via the parents has been long known and practiced (Furman, 1951). While systematic interventions with young children and parents have been practiced for 25 years (Cramer, 1974) and have been recommended as efficient and cost-effective approaches, these methods, in their different forms, have not yet become routine interventions in child guidance clinics (for a review on this subject, see Fonagy, 1996). In addition to their preventive and therapeutic effects, they are also powerful tools for teaching and represent a useful format for research. While the first formulations of these techniques were psychodynamically oriented, other approaches have also been developed such as behavior modification models or parent education approaches. Family interventions borrowing from systemic studies have been developed with applications in research (E. Fivaz, this series, vol. 3). Recently, the attachment paradigm has been used as a basis for "corrective attachment experience" for mothers (IJzendoorn, Lieberman, Weston, & Pawl, 1991; Van IJzendoorn, Juffer, Duyvesteyn, 1995).

Generally, it is now recognized that the psychiatric treatment of the infant needs to be carried out with the parents as active participants in the therapy. The growing experience in this area has opened a wide field of clinical research in what has come to be termed "the transgenerational dimension," or "transgenerational transmission" (Fonagy, 1994). The cross influences between parents and infants (and beyond, with the grandparents) has promoted original forms of technique (Cramer, 1998) and has forced researchers to find new concepts and tools for assessment, such as the Adult Attachment Interview (Main et al., 1985).

In the clinic, we started by developing techniques of mother-infant interventions on the basis of the psychodynamic therapy model (Cramer, 1974). When we embarked on outcome research of these therapies, we needed a comparative technique of therapy. We ruled out a control group (with no treatment) or a waiting list group, as they would not be tolerable in a regular child guidance clinic. Some of our colleagues were then trained in the United States by Susan McDonough and her group to learn the technique known as Interactional Guidance. Since then, we propose one of the two forms of treatments to our consulting population.

Parent-Infant Psychotherapies: A Brief Historical Review

The concepts underlying these approaches borrow from several sources. Theoretically, the basic focus is the infant's dependency on its mother for its physical survival, gratification of basic needs, protection against anxiety, development of attachment, and, last but not least, for the acquisition of communication and social skills (see the works of

Anna Freud on developmental lines, Melanie Klein on projective identifications, Margaret Mahler on the symbiotic phase, and Winnicott on the maternal preoccupation). Various clinicians developed therapeutic techniques tailored to the types of phenomenon (anxieties, projections, modes of relationships) found when a mother seeks help for symptoms in the infant (Fraiberg, 1980; Cramer, 1974; Lebovici, 1983; Lieberman & Pawl, 1993; Hopkins, 1992; Blos, 1985). Then came two developments, which brought new vistas in early relationships. The attachment paradigm (Ainsworth, Blehar, Waters, & Wall, 1978) allowed clinicians to use tools for the evaluation of attachment types and new modes of intervention (Liebermann, Weston, & Pawl, 1991). Simultaneously, what can be called the interactionist school provided new vistas in the development, regulation, and maintenance of communication in the dyad. The works of Brunner in the field of communication, Brazelton in the identification of reciprocity in social exchanges, Emde in the field of emotional exchanges and early conscience building, and Stern in the microanalytic study of interactions all provided profound insights into the working of parent-infant interactions. Sameroff and Emde's (1989) book on relational disturbances demonstrated that the best way to understand, classify, and treat infant's disturbances was to approach them from an interactive perspective. This brief review of the theoretical background of mother-infant psychotherapies demonstrates the variety of their conceptual underpinnings that influence their practice in their different forms. Psychodynamic theory focuses mainly on representations and subjective experience, while ethology-derived interactive studies define data at the level of overt behaviors. It must be stressed here that the reliance on objective data provided by microanalytic studies of interactions or by attachment studies have greatly enhanced the process of assessment, which was much more difficult within the sole domain of a psychodynamic framework.

Psychodynamic Brief Therapy with Mother and Infant

The approach we used was recently described exhaustively, at the levels of theory and practice by two members of our team (Cramer & Palacio, 1993) and in an abridged version in English (Cramer, 1995). Several concepts constitute the theoretical basis of this approach. First, while both the baby and the mother have, to very different extents, their own particular modes of functioning, there is an intermeshing of their psychic functioning, particularly during postpartum and what M. S. Mahler called the symbiotic phase. While we can only hypothesize how the baby represents the mother and their relationship, we know much more about the way that mothers construct their representation of the baby and the maternal role. A major principle is that of projective identifications, through which mothers imagine the fetus and then create a powerful maze of meaning attributions that lends intention, an identity theme, and even a fate to the baby. These attributions play a major role in maternal distress over a baby's symptom in addition to contributing to its development and maintenance. Hence, a basic technical device: Maternal interpretations of the baby will be thoroughly assessed and their source will be unraveled, leading secondarily to anxiety resolution and cessation of attenant pathogenic interactions.

The period of the postpartum which, according to some clinicians (Kumar & Brockington, 1988) can be extended to 12 or even 18 months, is characterized by at least two features. First, it can be characterized by maternal preoccupation that as a state of constant alertness and vigilance over the baby powerfully motivates mothers to find the best tactics to help the infant. Thus, they become highly motivated partners in a psychotherapeutic endeavor, creating mostly positive therapeutic alliances. Secondly, the period can be characterized by the "transparency" of maternal thoughts, fantasies, and feelings about the child and maternal role. This feature as recognized by many clinicians (Bibring, Dwyer, Huntington, & Valenstein, 1961; Bydlowsky, 1997; Cramer & Palacio, 1993) creates a unique freedom of associations provided by the mother, with a minimum of denial and other resistance. Technically, this is used as early as the first session, where therapist and mother work together toward an early definition of a focus that captures the essential problem at stake, its relationship to events, projective identifications, specific characteristics of the infant, and a basic form of anxiety in the mother, with its forerunners in the mother's childhood. A third factor, the presence of the infant, helps focus the mother and the therapist's hypothesis formation. The infant will start behaving in a way that illustrates and

sometimes validates inner scenarios that express the basic problem and the failing interactions. The infant thus materializes the problem allowing therapist and mother to better understand its development and maintenance. Technically, this requires dual attention from the therapist. The therapist hears the mother *and* watches the baby's behaviors and solicitations. At the level of assessment, this requires a special attention to what we called the "double agenda" of the clinicians.

Interventions aim mostly at deciphering maternal anxieties and projections and the style of relationships and attenant interactions. Particular attention is paid to the links between the actual behavior of the child and its distortions due to maternal infantile conflicts that were transferred onto the infant. The formulation of these various aspects evolves in the creation of a therapeutic focus, whose aim is to define the anxiety provoking "ghosts in the nursery" (Fraiberg, 1980) and decontaminate the representation of relationship from its conflictual underpinnings.

The term *focus* is a concept that was developed mostly in brief psychotherapies where it is necessary to rapidly obtain a basic hypothesis defining the main problem (Sifneos, 1972; Malan, 1976). It is a construct that has been labeled differently by various authors, for example, the "Core Conflictual Relationship Theme" (Luborsky, 1990; Luborsky, Barber, & Diguer, 1992). In brief mother-infant therapies, the focus is defined on the basis of the following constituting factors: The description of the infant's symptom (for example, temper tantrums), the main maternal projection onto the child and corresponding representations and anxieties (for example, "He is so willful that he turns me into a slave"), a main conflict and mode of relationship ("I can't tolerate to be exploited by him"), and a reference to the mother's past ("My father used to be tyrannical and frightening"). These factors considered together create a basic constellation typical for a dyad that orients the therapist's and the mother's inquiries, curiosity, and interpretations. The therapy aims at interpreting the focus and modifying the projections and conflicts in order to bring a new form of relationship with, when possible, cessation of the referral symptom. Transference to the therapist is not interpreted, but transference to the infant is a main focus of attention. Practical arrangements are: sessions occurring once a week, for one hour, over six weeks. Mother and child are encouraged to interact while mother reports her thoughts to the therapist. The infant may stay on the mother's lap or play on the ground. While in most cases, it is mothers who request the consultation and attend with the child, fathers may also attend. Our attention to the focus is worth stressing, because this construct became an important object of assessment.

Interactional Guidance

Interactional guidance was developed in the United States by Susan McDonough (1989, 1992, 1995) in a specific context. It was designed to help families nonamenable to classical, more verbally-oriented therapies. Those are often multiproblem families, with parents who are experiencing various forms of stress (economic, social, housing, etc.) and especially, deprivation. Their notions of child development and parental skills are lacking. This therapy was developed on the basis of various backgrounds: Family therapy, emotional-cognitive approaches, parent education, and so on. Its major aim is twofold: Demonstrating the profile of mother-infant interactions essentially from a developmental perspective and support of positive patterns. The main technical originality lies in the use of videotape recording of sessions of mother-infant play. Selected portions of these episodes are shown to mothers who are encouraged to refine their reading of the infant's cues. They are also asked to report on their own reactions and how they felt when they responded to the child. A main endeavor is the development of maternal sensitivity to the messages. The therapist seeks to empower families by identifying positive caregiving behavior and attends problems by suggesting alternative interpretations of the infant's behavior (for a thorough description, see McDonough, 1995; Rusconi Serpa, 1992). The therapist does not probe in the mother's past nor does he or she allude to her transference.

Interactional Guidance (IG) can be considered as a contrast therapy, mainly because its main ingredients are different from those used in psychodynamic (PD) approaches. The main difference lies in the lack of probing into the mother's unconscious fantasies, projections, or past history. The therapist remains in the "here and now" and capitalizes on a refined observation of interaction sequences that are problematic and reveal maternal misperceptions of the infant's signals. Moreover, the therapist will not seek to unearth unconscious maternal conflicts that distort perceptions. The therapist will rather reinforce, with encouragement, interactions that are favorable using mainly the impact of maternal behavior on the infant's functioning. Rather than interpreting the mother's conflicts, the therapist emphasizes the good outcomes to interactive difficulties. One may summarily describe these differences as interpreting negative representations in psychodynamic therapy, while supporting adaptive solutions in interactional guidance. In PD therapy, the main port of entry is representations, while it is interactions in IG (Stern-Bruchweiler & Stern, 1989).

Common Factors

While it was important to find a therapeutic technique that could serve as a real contrast to psychodynamic approaches, we found some *commonalties* between these differing approaches. Both therapies rely on constructing a focus for understanding the problematic material. The content of the focus is different according to each therapy, but the endeavors of finding a basic hypothesis is common. The creation of a working alliance is a basic goal common to both therapies. Both therapies share a theoretical model of interrelational factors causing and maintaining problems and choosing the relationship as main target of therapy (for commonalties between parent-infant interventions see Stern, 1995).

We have elaborated in some depth on the description of treatments themselves because we wanted to give the reader a

fairly good idea of the treatments that we have assessed. We do not dwell on diagnostic assessment per se or evaluation of severity of pathology. What we report on is the assessment of changes induced by therapy (Outcome Study[1]) and an attempt to assess what goes on during the sessions (Process Study[2]).

Outcome Study

First, we report on a standard outcome study where the main issue was to evaluate the results obtained at the end of the therapy compared with the status before treatment. Basically, this study attempted to answer questions such as: What can therapies modify in infant and mother-infant pathologies? Did the changes last? Did the results support the relational hypothesis concerning early functional problems? Is there any difference in results between the two types of treatment? Is the prognosis a good predictor of the therapeutic effects?

Introductory Phase

A single case study (Cramer & Stern, 1988) served as a pilot study wherein we tested a basic hypothesis: Therapy-induced changes can be observed at the level of overt behaviors and interactions in the dyad. A corollary hypothesis was that conflicting maternal representations about the mother and her infant contributed to symptom formation and maintenance. A coding system was developed to determine which conflicting themes in the mother were related to which pathogenic interactions and what changes in these two realms were produced during the six therapy sessions. Results showed important changes for the different behavioral indicators (frequency of aggressive acts and of acts of affection, for example) as treatment progressed. This single case study demonstrated which representational and interactive parameters needed to be studied and gave the impetus to embark on a large outcome study of brief mother-infant therapies involving more than 100 cases.

The Geneva Child Psychiatric Clinic specializes in infant psychiatry. More than half of the infants referred are sent by pediatricians from the city. They refer cases to the clinic when usual pediatric evaluation and counseling have failed to bring relief. We included in the study 109 mother-infant dyads (infants ages from 2 to 30 months, mean age 14.5 months, SD 7.54) consulting the Geneva Clinic of Child Psychiatry for sleeping (55 percent), eating (8 percent), relational problems (19 percent), or behavior problems (17 percent) such as constant crying, tantrums, and excessive aggression. Fifty-five percent of the infants were males. Cases were mostly (50 percent) referred by pediatricians.

Mother-infant dyads participated in a pretreatment and two post-treatment assessments (one week and six months after therapy termination) and met a list of inclusion/exclusion criteria for short-term mother-infant psychotherapy. The main counterindications were major psychopathology in mothers (severe depression,

psychotic functioning) or in infants (mental retardation, pervasive developmental disorders). The 109 dyads included in the study were assigned to Psychodynamic Therapy (63 dyads, 58 percent) or Interaction Guidance Therapy (46 dyads, 42 percent) and had an average of six therapy sessions.

Collaboration between Researchers and Clinicians: Procedure

Researchers and clinicians worked together at defining research design, procedures, and instruments. Regular conjoint meetings maintained cohesion in the unfolding of the project while researchers and clinicians had clearly defined specificity in their contributions. All *researchers* were psychologists. They established the first contact with the parents after the initial referral to the clinic. They informed them about the procedure, asked for written authorization, and conducted initial interviews and various evaluations (pretest and posttest treatment and six and twelve months later). They proposed the type of therapy to parents. Researchers needed to have a clinical training as they interviewed parents who were often acutely distressed. They needed to be tactful enough to carry out lengthy interviews and gather information without getting involved to the point of interfering with the therapeutic relationship that would unfold after the initial assessment, when therapists started the treatment per se. The *therapists* were in charge of formulating the indications (and counterindications) for treatment and prognosis. They applied the therapies.

The complete protocol of the study followed five basic phases: 1. The *pretreatment evaluation* (Evaluation 1) was done by the research team and was conducted with the infant and the mother (or both parents) during two 1½ hour interviews within one week of the mother's initial telephone call to the clinic. It consisted of a systematic procedure assessing various aspects of infant's and mother's functioning (described following); 2. The *indication of therapy and prognosis* for new cases was presented to the clinical team during regular weekly seminars. The clinical team discussed the indication for brief mother-infant therapy, completed the Indication Criteria Questionnaire, and provided a prognosis rating on a consensus base. If there was no counterindication, the case was randomly assigned to psychodynamic therapy or interaction guidance; 3. The *therapy* was conducted according to clinical criteria for each technique; 4. The *posttreatment assessment* was conducted by the same psychologists using the same instrument one week after the end of treatment (Evaluation 2); and 5. during the *follow-up* six months later (Evaluation 3).

Instruments of Assessment

INFANT'S DEVELOPMENT

The infant's development was evaluated with the help of the parents, using the Bayley Scale of Infant Development. Competencies were evaluated just as much as problems. While testing, members of the team evaluated not only the infant's performances, but also important aspects of parent-infant interactions (parental demands, support, and reinforcements).

SYMPTOMATIC MANIFESTATIONS OF THE INFANT

The Symptom Check-List (Robert-Tissot et al., 1989) was employed to measure the frequency, duration, and intensity of disturbances in the following areas: Problems affecting bodily functions (sleep, feeding, digestion, breathing, skin, allergies), behavior disorders (temper tantrums, negativism, crying spells, aggression), and fears and separation problems. Each problem area was addressed with open questions (description of problem, history of the problem, mode of parental intervention, etc.) and closed questions. This evaluation does not refer to norms. It reflects the mother's observations and her subjective experience of the impact caused by the infant's disturbances. The evaluation of severity involved 52 questions that could be quantified. Frequency, duration, and intensity of disturbance were evaluated over the previous four weeks by the mother on a five-point scale (ranging from 1 = never or not important to 5 = nearly always or very important). A summary score was computed for each area of symptoms.

Used by both parents together, this questionnaire allows the observation of interesting aspects of communication and role sharing in the couple (who the speaker is in the couple, the agreements or disagreements concerning the questions, the conflicting areas, etc.). The experience showed also that this interview prompts the parents to think the problem over and modify their point of view about their preoccupation. We clearly demonstrated our interest for "How are things going?" and "How do you understand the problem?" In fact, we tried to understand not only objective data, but also the representations, explanations, or theories the parents elaborated concerning the problem with their infant. These elements may constitute the "red threads" for the treatment.

MOTHER-INFANT INTERACTIONS

Mother and child were videotaped during a 20-minute structured series of episodes: (1) play without object, (2) play with toys, (3) teaching a task not yet mastered by the child, (4) ignoring the child, (5) separation, and (6) reunion. A split screen videotape technique was used. When both parents were present, mother-infant interactions were recorded first. The father was then asked to play with the infant. Sometimes we suggested that they play with the infant according to Fivaz' Lausanne Triadic Play (Corboz-Warnery, Fivaz-Depeursinge, Gertsch Bettens, & Favez, 1993). The videotapes were coded with two instruments developed for research purposes in the field of mother-infant interactions: (1) Maternal sensitivity (ability to read and respond appropriately to the infant signals) was rated on a five-point rating scale (from less to more sensitive) devised by Ainsworth et al. (1974) and (2) The quality of mother-infant interactions during play sequences with an object was rated with the Crittenden Experimental Index of Adult-Infant Relationships (Crittenden, 1981).

MATERNAL REPRESENTATIONS

The R-Interview was developed originally in collaboration with an international research group (Stern et al., 1989). The interview was done with the mother. It con-

tained 28 questions grouped into the following themes: The infant, the mother in her mothering role, the mother as a person, the mother's mother, the infant's father, affects, and self-esteem. Each theme was first investigated with an open-ended question, revealing spontaneous contents and descriptions. The mother was requested to illustrate the most significant descriptions with the report of a recently experienced event. The mother then evaluated, in each theme, a series of ad hoc descriptive adjectives presented on a bipolar scale (i.e., affectionate vs. affectionate, aggressive vs. nonaggressive, etc.). This data was quantified by calculating the distance (in millimeters) between the negative pole (i.e., unaffectionate) and the mother's mark. The scale of responses ranged between 0 (most negative) to 100 (most positive). A summary score was computed per theme. Important events in the infant's and the mother's own past were investigated but not submitted to a quantitative evaluation. Mothers were also asked to fill out the Beck Depression Inventory.

INDICATION CRITERIA AND PROGNOSIS

The Indication Criteria Questionnaire (presented in Appendix 2 and discussed in detail later in this chapter) was designed to assess the feasibility and prognosis of the therapy. Most questions concerned the mother's potential availability for therapeutic work (i.e., insight, resistance, transference, capacity to talk about inner world), while other questions concerned the existence of conflicting foci in the mother. Each criteria (C1 to C13) is presented as a statement, rated by the clinician on a four-point scale (definitely true, somewhat true, somewhat wrong, definitely wrong).

Results of the Outcome Study

Effects of Treatment

Brief mother-infant psychotherapy produced marked *symptom* relief (Cramer et al., 1990; Robert-Tissot et al., 1996a). All referral symptoms were improved by therapy, with a particularly high rate of cure for disorders of sleep that caused the reason for half of the consultations. We found that 80 percent of the subjects corresponded to the criteria of severe sleep disorder according to Richman's (1981) criteria. Three-quarters of treated infants returned to a level of functioning within the normal range on our measures of symptoms, and we did not find the emergence of replacement symptoms either at Evaluation 2 or in our six-month follow-up, as is often expected. While our intervention population does not match the severity of pathologies found in multirisk families often described in American or French intervention studies (Liebermann et al., 1991; Stoleru & Morales-Huet, 1989), this is a group showing symptoms and relationship disorders that are intense and protracted enough to warrant the label of pathology and the need for intervention. Behavior problems were correlated to infant's age both before and after treatment. However, repeated analysis of variance computed separately for the group consulting for a behavior problem showed a significant decrease in tantrums, negativism, and aggression.

Maternal sensitivity to infant's signals increased, while intrusive control decreased. The infants became more cooperative, less compulsive-compliant, and also showed an increase in happiness. A significant increase in the mother's self-esteem as well as several significant changes in *maternal representations* occurred between pretreatment and posttreatment assessments. The infant was perceived by the mother as less excited, more affectionate, more independent, and less aggressive. The mother rated herself as being happier, more active, more intelligent, and good-looking. Moreover, we found more correlation between mothers' maternal ratings of themselves and of their infants after treatment than before. This could indicate a better identification with the infant. Lastly, *affects* experienced by the mother in her relationship with the infant showed significantly less anxiety, guilt, sadness, and anger after treatment (see Figure 8.1).

Follow-Up

Improvement continued six months after the end of therapy, with some renewed improvements in interactions and no symptom replacement (Cramer et al., 1990; Robert-Tissot et al., 1996a). These findings demonstrate that therapy is effective and a major factor of change, confirming our clinical impression that mother-infant disturbances are particularly sensitive to therapeutic interventions. "Mother-infant dyads are an unstable system; they are highly sensitive to internal and external influences, and allow both a

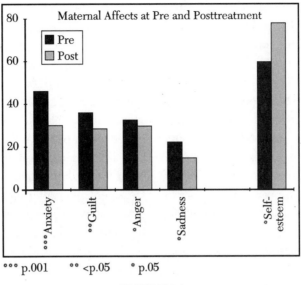

FIGURE 8.1

practice and a study of psychic modification" (Cramer & Palacio-Espasa, 1993, p. v).

Relational Hypothesis

The *relational hypothesis* about infants' functional disturbances received partial support from our data. Improvement of infants' disorders was associated with improvement of mother-infant interactions in more than 60 percent of the dyads. Moreover, we discovered a strong positive association between (1) sleeping problems, separation problems, and fear in infants and (2) a strong negative association between maternal sensitivity during interactions and infants' level of functional disorders.

Differences between Types of Therapy

The hypothesis that changes over time (between pretreatment and posttreatment as-

sessment) would differ for the outcome measures, according to the *type of therapy* examined. There were no significant differences in the area of symptoms, both therapies being equally effective. Concerning mother-infant interactions, IG cases made a greater improvement in maternal sensitivity than PD cases. Regarding maternal representations, PD cases showed a greater improvement in self-esteem than IG cases. Although these results are consistent with our expectations, the differences were very few. The impact of *maternal depression* before treatment was also considered (Cramer, 1993). Our results demonstrate greater improvements for more depressed mothers, rated as poor prognosis, than for mild or nondepressed mothers.

Prognosis of Therapeutic Effects

Clinicians' prognosis before treatment had started was rather good or definitely good for about 70 percent of cases and rather poor or definitely poor for 30 percent of cases. Predictability of prognosis regarding therapeutic effects was examined (Bachmann & Robert-Tissot, 1992). ANOVA testing for interaction between outcome measures and prognosis before therapy were insignificant. But ANOVA computation on change in scores (between pretreatment and posttreatment assessment) showed greater improvement for a poor indication than for a good indication. Using symptoms' and interactions' improvement for each case, we also observed that good prognosis did worse than expected while poor prognosis fared better than expected, as in the case of maternal depression.

Process Study

This study, still in progress, is aimed at exploring various aspects of therapeutic processes, such as the choice of treatment, development of therapist-patient alliance, types of verbal exchanges between therapist and patient, and impact of the infant on the session's unfolding. We hypothesized that the early determination and interpretation (during the first or second session) of a therapeutic focus was the essential agent of change (Cramer & Palacio-Espasa, 1993).

Choice of Treatment

Random allocation of patients to treatment conditions constitutes, with treatment integrity and statistical significance, the major *credo* of outcome research and intervention evaluation. However, the agreement between patient and therapist about the objectives of the treatment constitutes an important dimension of the therapeutic alliance (Frieswyk et al., 1986; Bachelor, Guérin, Théoret, Poitras, Tremblay, 1993; Hentschel & Bijleveld, 1995). We hypothesized that a patient's active collaboration with his or her treatment could be facilitated through participation in choosing treatment and exploring an alternative solution more appropriate to clinical standards than random assignment.

A subsample of 42 mother-infant dyads from the outcome study (described previously) was selected for this part of the study and participated in the choice of their treatment modality. Reason for consultation, inclusion criteria, and pretreatment and posttreatment assessments were the same for the whole sample.

Method

MOTHERS' CHOICE OF TREATMENT

At the end of the pretreatment assessment, a description of the treatments (Appendix 1) drawn up by the therapists was given to the mother. The mother was instructed to choose the treatment she preferred to use in case a brief therapy was indicated. One-half of the mothers received an A-B description, and one-half of the mothers received a B-A description to control for the effect of presentation order.

INDICATION OF TREATMENT

Therapists followed the indication process (described previously) and collectively provided a recommendation for the modality they considered best suited to the mother-infant dyad. They were blind to the mother's choice and had to reach a consensus.

Results

Results revealed (Robert-Tissot & Cramer, 1998) a very high agreement between the mother's choice and therapists' recommendation. Mothers' choice appeared to be significantly related with therapists' recommendation (Chi^2 = 17.30, p = .002). Taken altogether (PD choices, IG choices, and no choice), mothers' and therapists' opinion was congruent in 71 percent of the cases (N = 29). Within each treatment modality, mothers' choice and therapists' recommendation were congruent in 82 percent of the cases for PD therapy and in 67 percent of the cases for IG therapy. In the case of absence of choice (n = 5, 12 percent), mother and therapists shared the same opinion only once. Examination of patient and pretreatment variables showed no major differences between the two groups resulting from a choice of treatment procedure. The second treatment was more often chosen (68 percent) than the first (Chi^2 = 4.88, p = .02), and psychodynamic therapy was more often chosen by mothers and by therapists (52 percent) than interaction guidance (36 percent).

Mothers were not surprised to be offered a treatment choice. None of them asked for more information about the treatments, although the written presentation was not very detailed. Of particular interest was the finding that no mother asked for more information about therapist's sex, age, ethnicity, social background, experi-ence, values or cognitive style, and so on. None of the therapist variables generally submitted to investigation in psychotherapy research were referred to in our choice situation.

From a *research methodological* point of view there was, surprisingly, no major difference in the two treatment groups resulting from a choice of treatment procedure. Groups were balanced for the main patient variables (age, sex of infant, reason for consultation, referral source, socioeconomic status of families). Intensity of infant's symptoms and maternal depression, selected as pretreatment variables, proved also to be equivalent in the two groups. We can, therefore, conclude that the choice of treatment procedure allowed achieving internal validity, as did the random assignment procedure used in the first part of the study. In contrast to random assignment, the present procedure ensures external (and ecological) validity.

Therapists were clearly involved in a decision process. They had to decide the best way to help mother-infant dyads or "what to apply to whom" (Roth & Fonagy, 1996). Therapists' recommendations were significantly related to prognosis. Mothers considered as good candidates (i.e., with a good prognosis for both forms of treatment) were more likely to receive a recommendation for a psychodynamic therapy. Interaction guidance cases appeared as more difficult patients (and situations) in general. The worst prognosis found for IG cases is coherent with the objectives of this technique. This form of treatment was primarily designed for the treatment of multi-risk families, for whom prior classical therapy had failed (McDonough, 1995; Sameroff & Emde, 1989).

Mothers and therapists chose psychodynamic therapy more often than interaction guidance therapy. What does this mean? It may be that psychodynamic therapy, described explicitly to mothers as a "talking cure," still corresponds in our population to a prototypical representation of psychological treatments. This category appears to have a greater accessibility than interaction guidance therapy and functions as a prototypical exemplar of the natural category "psychotherapy." From the patients' point of view, one can imagine that innovation is not so attractive. That therapists' recommendation for psychodynamic therapy outnumbered interaction guidance reflects the main theoretical background of the clinic and also probably results from availability of therapists. Interestingly, the two treatment modalities, when offered as a result of a random assignment procedure (during the first phase), were found in equivalent proportion.

From a *clinical point of view*, the high level of agreement on treatment choice between patients and therapists was the most surprising and important finding of this study. Usually, clinicians tend to expect that patients will either object to psychotherapy or will resist any process uncovering either their hidden motivations or their interactional habits. Our findings do not only reveal a very high level of positive alliance with the therapeutic proposal but even more interesting, reveal that the mothers' intuitive choice matches the therapists' choice concerning the most appropriate form of therapy. This suggests that patients have intuitive knowledge about their own psychological functioning. Our results, although exploratory, support firstly, the validity of a choice of treatment procedure and secondly, provide information concerning human decisions in natural settings and tasks. They contribute to a better understanding of clinical activity, especially indication process and prognosis (Rock, Bransford, & Maisto, 1987). This study was conducted in a well-defined setting with specific patients and therapies. Thus, conclusions are restricted to this clinical context and cannot be generalized to psychotherapy research in general.

Therapeutic Alliance and Focus

We defined therapeutic alliance as a necessary condition to the elaboration and interpretation of a focus. The previous subsample (cf., choice of treatment) provided the opportunity to gather empirical data concerning this issue. We present some results concerning the relationships between the determination of a focus and therapeutic alliance at the onset of treatment.

Method

We used questionnaires filled out after each session separately by the therapist and by the mother (or parents). Questions concerning the focus, alliance, empathy, and overall impression of the session were rated on a four-point scale (from definitely true to definitely wrong). We consider here only the answers gathered after the first therapy sessions (n = 39).

Results: Focus and Alliance after the First Therapy Session

We found that in about one-half of first sessions there was a determination and interpretation of a focus. Concerning the overall rating of the session, most of the patients (75 percent) had a good session, while none had a bad session. Most of the therapists (52 percent) were half-satisfied, and 30 percent were unsatisfied. Therapists were less satisfied than patients, and agreement between them was not high, even if "it takes two to do therapy" (Hentschel & Bijleveld, 1995).

What leads up to the *therapist's impression* of a good or bad session? The therapist's rating of the session was mainly based on his or her success to elaborate and interpret a focus for a good session and the failure to do so for a bad session, as several analyses have demonstrated. We also found the therapist's evaluation of the alliance with the patient significantly associated with the determination of the focus (p = .004), as were other process variables such as resistance, transference, attractiveness (for the patient's variables) and empathy and confidence (for the therapist's variables). Inversely the *patient's* evaluation of the alliance with the therapist was not related to the presence or absence of a focus. Patients rely more on "feeling understood," "enough talking," and perceiving the treatment or the session as helpful. These factors, referred to as unrevealing, unconditional acceptance of the patient and as helping alliance (Luborsky, Crits-Christoph, Mintz, & Auerbach, 1988), were the first determinants of patient's overall rating of the first session, as revealed by regression analysis of the data.

These results show unequivocally that the therapist's and the patient's judgments are not based on the same criteria. They demonstrate once again that therapists are strongly influenced by the guidelines dictated by their theory. These results question the now classical notion that the therapeutic alliance is a necessary condition even prior to the development of therapeutic work. This latter proposition seems valid for patients but not for therapists. As we saw, therapists' evaluation of alliance is, in great part, determined by their possibilities and impossibilities to have been in a position allowing them to put to work the essential ingredients of their technique, which in our study is represented by the determination of a focus. When this determination was rated as present, patients received positive ratings. When it was absent, patients received negative ratings. The same was true when these questions were addressed to the therapists themselves.

In the literature, opposite ratings between therapists and patients appear as an irreducible contradiction, and classically, one does not know which of the two sources is trustworthy. In fact, the question should not be asked in terms of "who to trust." Our data show that both therapists and patients are right in their own way. They simply have different needs and goals. Patients seek first to be accepted and find a trusting relationship. Therapists are very intent on strictly applying their technique as the only way to provide truly professional help. From our point of view, it appears artificial to disentangle the alliance from the application of technical ingredients. In practice, these two aspects develop hand in hand. Therapists develop much more positive evaluation of their patients when they feel they have been allowed to successfully practice their technique. Patients are not interested in technical know-how but are sensitive to a relational climate. Ideally, the first sessions should help bring these two sets of goals closer, allowing for the development of truly shared purposes.

Therapist's and Patient's Verbal Interactions

This part of the study is a first attempt to describe and characterize therapeutic process, which brings about the determination of a focus. Our aim was to explore the verbal features that could possibly discriminate sessions, leading therapists and patients to share a working hypothesis (the focus) versus sessions where partners failed to achieve this goal. Particular attention was applied to the patterns of association between emotional and cognitive features during a session. Mergenthaler (1996) described several such patterns (relaxing, experiencing, connecting, and reflecting).

Method

We chose a bottom-up approach and used the Stuttgart Interactional Categories System (Czogalik & Mauthe, 1991) to code the complete verbatim transcriptions of first, second, and second to last sessions (from 700 to 1,800 sentences per session). The database generated by the multidimensional coding[3] allows for several analyses of therapeutic discourse (emotional involvement, speech acts and linguistic features, therapeutic interventions, content, temporal orientation). Until now, 40 sessions (including first, second, and second to last sessions) were completely coded. Analyses were computed according to therapeutic techniques and/or the determination of a focus or its absence during the session. First sessions of dropouts were extensively analyzed (Wasem, 1996).

Results: What Accounts for the Determination of a Focus during the First Session?

Therapeutic interventions, emotional involvement, and speech acts account for the determination of a focus during the session. We observed that interpretation does not appear in a vacuum. A working hypothesis, corresponding to the patient's material, is built upon the basis of intensive and joint exploring and comprehending activities. These activities of the therapist *and* the patient include affective displays and sharing of intimacy (Mergenthaler, 1996; Holzer, Pokorny, Kächele, & Luborsky, 1997). Content and temporal orientation appear to be linked to therapeutic techniques. When faced with unexpected difficulties or resistance, therapists use several strategies. Evolution of individual patterns during the first therapy session shed some light on the complex interaction between the different levels of analysis and particularly affect and emotion displays (Axis 1) and abstraction or "thinking" (Axis 3). Both aspects account for the determination of the therapeutic focus. Figure 8.2 shows the balance between both emotion and thinking occurring during the first, second, and second to last sessions for an easy or "good" case (401) and for a "difficult" one (410). The same therapist conducted both treatments.

Good sessions (a therapeutic focus was interpreted) are characterized by more emotional involvement and more self-disclosure of the patients and more therapeutic actions from the therapist and from

the patient (exploring, structuring, confronting, interpreting). The first session of case 401 (Figure 8.2) provides a good example of a connecting pattern where therapist and patient are in a state of connecting emotion, tone, and thinking. This leads to the interpretation of a focus.

Difficult sessions (no therapeutic focus could be identified) are characterized by a greater amount of speech from the therapist than from the patient, more questioning from the therapist and more refusing

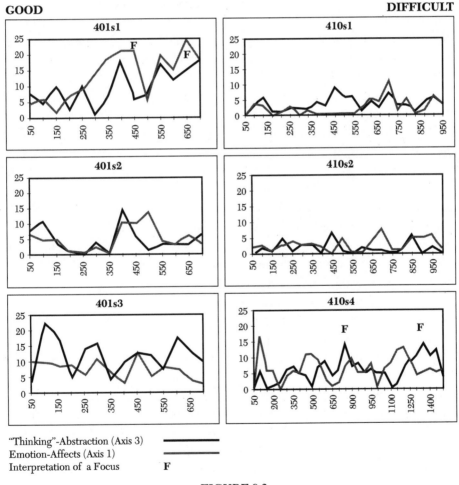

"Thinking"-Abstraction (Axis 3) _____
Emotion-Affects (Axis 1) _____
Interpretation of a Focus   F

FIGURE 8.2

from the patient, more conflictual connection between speakers, such as taking the floor with "no, but; yes, but . . . ," and less topic continuation between therapist and patient (Robert-Tissot et al., 1996b, 1996c; Cramer et al., 1997; Cramer, 1998). The first and second sessions of Case 410 (Figure 8.2) provides a good example of a relaxing pattern where patient and therapist do not show much emotion nor thinking. For these different aspects, we found a continuum rather than a clear-cut difference between good and difficult sessions and between techniques.

The *variability of techniques* we found between good and difficult cases is worthy of attention. It shows the distance between treatment manuals (guidelines) and real applications. The overall impression gathered by the verbal exchanges analyzed is that *treatments are closer to a strict adherence to techniques with good cases.* There is less difference between the two techniques in difficult cases, despite theoretical and technical disparities. For example, *psychodynamic technique* encourages the patient to deliver authentic and open information, information that reveal a certain degree of intimacy. It concerns especially the mother's report on past experiences with her own parental figures, and her memories of childhood and painful events. These are materials used to build a therapeutic focus. As expected, we found self-disclosure of the patient relatively high in PD good cases. In PD difficult cases, self-disclosure of the patient was equal or lower than in IG cases. On the other hand, *interaction guidance technique* aims at consolidating patient-child relationship and parental self-esteem. This should ap-

pear, at the verbal level, by more positive than negative qualifiers and more positive than negative emotion conveyed by the participants' statements. Again, this was found to be true, but only in IG good sessions. In difficult sessions, negative qualifiers were more important in both forms of treatment than positive qualifiers. In difficult sessions, the overall emotional involvement was weaker. Factual statements were more important than affective or cognitive statements, whatever the technique. We also found a *variability within the same therapist* according to good and difficult cases. With his good case (401), the therapist followed the mother's discourse with as much activity of reflecting (mirroring or repeating of partners' previous verbalizations), as of questioning. Mother's self-disclosure and emotional involvement was as important as were therapeutic interventions. Refusing was scarce. With his difficult case (410), the therapist's questioning reached about tenfold the proportion of reflecting, and refusing of patients increased conversely. Self-disclosure of parents and emotional involvement was scarce, as was reflecting on the part of the therapist.

Nonverbal Interactions: Participation of the Infant

Although infant's participation to therapeutic processes has been referred to in several clinical papers (Fraiberg et al., 1980; Cramer & Palacio-Espasa, 1993), no systematic studies have yet treated this issue. Therefore, an exploratory study is currently conducted in our clinic on the *infant's* contribution to the therapy. The main objective is to describe and analyze how the infant's interactive and symptomatic behavior during the session highlights the therapeutic process (Cramer, 1995; Cramer et al., 1997; Rusconi Serpa & Sancho, 1997). Selection and coding of behavioral sequences focus on visual attention between all the partners and on proxemics (body orientation and distance between participants). Until now, 33 sessions were completely coded for each partner, with a one-second unit of analysis.

Results show firstly that infants are interacting (behaviorally or verbally) with therapists and/or parents during about 50 percent of the duration of the sessions. Two categories of sequences deserve special mention: (1) "Joint attention" of therapist and parents focusing on the infant and (2) "Double-agenda" of therapist. "Joint attention" sequences occur in different situations or contexts and have several functions such as initiation/termination of the session, conversational pauses (particularly during high emotional involvement of partners), discontinuation of topics, and infant's symptomatic behavior. A close look regarding who initiates and who interrupts the joint attention sequences provided promising cues on changes in interactive patterns observed as the therapy proceeds. In some cases, for example, we found that mothers initiated most of joint attention at the onset of treatment, while it was the infant who took the lead in initiation toward the end of the treatment. This could be taken as an indicator of improvement. "Double-agenda" concerns the therapist's sharing of attention: He is simultaneously involved in a verbal exchange with the

mother or parents and in play with the infant. This technical particularity requires a special expertise in mother-infant therapy. The work on nonverbal interactions demonstrated that infants' contributions during sessions are essential to the determination of a therapeutic focus. Joint attention appeared as key moments in the process of therapy. They constitute observational markers, which should be taken into account in any attempt to understand parent-infant psychotherapies.

Clinicians and Researchers Working Together: How to Avoid Divorce

The aim of our research on outcome and process was to study the effects of mother-infant psychotherapies and explore the underlying change process. We learned much regarding the practice of psychotherapy, the psychopathology of young children, the interactional contribution to infant symptoms, and especially, the efficiency and limits of such therapeutic approaches. Thus, a primary goal was attained concerning many clinical issues in infant mental health. But as the process of our research unfolded over more than ten years, we simultaneously obtained precious experience and knowledge regarding the social, intellectual, and epistemological issues revealed when researchers and therapists cooperate in creating and developing a long-term common research. Each of these two professional families had their own logic, goals, and ethics, and these differences needed to be elaborated again and again, in order to work through conflicts that repeatedly threatened to tear the two teams apart.

We report on some of these issues, stressing the difficulties and their modes of resolution. We especially try to show how common work resulted, in some areas, in modifying each family's basic ideals and modes of functioning. This crossbreeding is particularly important in the field of psychotherapy research, because it has been repeatedly stressed that research brings little new insight or modification in the practice of psychotherapy.

Adhesion of Therapists to the Research Projects

While medical tradition considers research on therapeutic effectiveness (and safety) as a major form of clinical scientific endeavor, this is less the case when it comes to assessing the effectiveness of psychotherapy. While there is now a tradition of psychotherapy research, with meta-analytic reviews of hundreds of studies on psychotherapy (Smith, Glass, & Miller, 1980; Weisz, Weiss, Alicke, & Klotz, 1987), there are still important obstacles in this field. A main difficulty comes from the reluctance most therapists show toward exposing their practice to observations by a third party. External agents, such as health insurances and even members of the family of the patient, are usually experienced as interferences by therapists when information about the treatment is requested. Moreover, the paramount and visible influence of countertransference factors in the un-

folding of the therapy can provide external observers with "inside information" on the therapist's personal functioning, promoting suspicion toward research that needs precisely to tap the clinicians mental functioning.

Therapists generally believe that the main object of psychotherapy is in the realm of subjective factors, such as self-images, feelings, and very personal modes and themes of representations. To them, objective assessments of such elusive items appear like a reductionistic activity that mutilates subjective truth. It is thus, very reluctantly that they usually tolerate the objectification of the subjective. The fear of objectification is compounded because many therapists consider that the main target of psychotherapeutic change concerns unconscious factors, such as unconscious fantasies, affects, or defenses. This difficulty accounts for the scarcity of research on psychodynamic therapies, with some notable exceptions (Fonagy & Target, 1994; Target & Fonagy, 1994a, 1994b).

Adhesion of therapists to the project was, in spite of these difficulties, acquired and maintained (with the same original group for the duration of the whole project) for two principal reasons. First, the research project on evaluating the therapies practiced in the clinic was initiated by therapists and directed by the director of the clinic. This meant that the basic questions were raised by the therapists who supported an evaluation of their own practice, and the authority of the director maintained cohesion as he was convinced of the necessity of psychotherapy evaluation. Second, during innumerable meetings, conflictual views, such as those concerning indications and assessment of representations, were discussed and worked through until solutions acceptable to the two parties were devised.[4] Thus, we fairly frequently attained definitions of shared purposes which is the necessary precondition for a long, lasting "marriage between psychotherapists and psychotherapy researchers" (Elliott & Morrow-Bradley, 1994). Researchers learned to be particularly attentive to the therapists' fears that their therapy data might be altered beyond recognition by methodological constraints. Therapists, likewise, needed to accept that all their practices *and* their ideas (that are often preconceived in nature and highly idealized) had to be exposed to analysis and ultimately, operationalized in a way that allowed for valid and reliable assessment.

Modification of Usual Clinical Practice

Assessment of therapy effects requires a comparison between the state of the patient before and after treatment. This needs to be done in a systematic way with standardized instruments. In order to achieve this goal, therapists accepted that their usual practice be modified in the following way. The initial and the final assessments were done by the research team, while in standard clinical practice all phases of diagnosis and assessment were done by the therapist himself, patients needed to correspond to strict inclusion criteria, and patients had to be evaluated with standardized instruments.

Thus, in many ways, therapists had sacrificed total mastery of their usually well-protected relationship to patients. Patients were no longer exclusively *their* patients. They shared them with the research team, whose members often left a powerful impression on the mothers, especially since the first narration of the mother was trusted upon them. It is well known that the first contact, even if it is for evaluation purposes and not for therapy, creates an emotional bond and provides relief from anxiety. We found, indeed, that the first two interviews between mothers and assessment researchers were often followed by symptom removal. Thus, therapists could not consider themselves the sole providers of relief and of understanding the patients.

The main crises between teams occurred when researchers insisted on imposing onto therapists methods and procedures that insure optimal validity and reliability to a point that therapists found intrusive into their therapeutic relationship. A good example of this issue was the random assignment of patients to treatment modalities used during the first phase of the outcome study. This goes against the therapist's usual ways, since in usual practice it is the therapist who decides one-sidedly the form of therapy to recommend. The issue of selection of treatment became even more conflictual when we realized that outcomes were, on the whole, similar between the two forms of therapy, inducing a form of competition between therapists trained in psychodynamic therapy versus those trained in interactional guidance. When this conflict abated, therapists achieved a higher level of detachment.

They agreed to totally renounce ownership of the choice of treatment and even the choice of patients. This led us ultimately to leave patients (who were mothers most of the time) to select the type of therapy *they* considered best fit for them (as presented previously).

The Therapist as Source of Information

Optimal adhesion of therapists to the project was particularly important as they provide one of the three main sources of information, the other two being the patients and the external observers, that is, the research team. Therapy is not the result of the standard application of a technical product, as one can say of the administration of a pharmaceutical agent. Therapy is better defined as a truly interactive process, that is, a collaboration between partners contributing to the cocreation of a process that is oriented by the therapist's theory and technical skill and knowledge. This viewpoint promotes equal attention in research to the patient's and the therapist's thinking and productions. Therefore, the therapist's mode of functioning, including theory, ideas, intuitions, emotions, and verbal and behavioral productions, all become a crucial source of information.

Thus, we asked our therapists to answer a series of questions before therapy (indication criteria), during therapy (focus, main themes, and therapeutic alliance), and after therapy (evaluation of the success of the therapy). These questionnaires allowed us to analyze the therapist's expectations, their criteria, and the goals they set for themselves. They provided insights into the weight placed on the therapists by their own theory. This was particularly clear when we studied the assessment of therapist's satisfaction with the work done. We realized that the therapists rated their work according to a highly idealized concept of what a satisfactory therapy should be. This became all the more evident when we compared therapists' and mothers' posttreatment evaluation of satisfaction. Mothers were almost always more satisfied than therapists. This indicates that the goals of therapy are represented and experienced differently by patients and therapists.

Operationalization of Concepts

The principal requirement for research is not to rely on numbers but to rely on explicit statements which allow for public communication and replication (Reuchlin, 1981). Clinical practice, in general, and psychodynamic therapy, in particular, are based on highly complex concepts which are difficult to operationalize and therefore, often not based on or linked to empirical research evidence, especially in the psychodynamic realm. A main task in psychotherapy research is to find ways of operationalizing relevant aspects of clinical practice. This implies a long process of analyzing the components of clinical concepts, before research per se can begin. Operationalizing means first, to identify the basic concepts, second, to deconstruct concepts into their constitutive elements, and third, to find simple formulations in order to translate these elements into propositions or questions that can be understood and rated by different clinicians the same way for the same patient.

The process of *indication* for brief mother-infant psychotherapies is used here to illustrate the challenging process of operationalization and because the question of indication has not received the attention it deserves in psychotherapy research (von Benedek, 1989; Huber, 1996). Much more systematic research is needed to solve the ever-recurring question: "What treatment for which patient by which therapist?" (Luborsky et al., 1988; Roth & Fonagy, 1996). The process of indication includes indication criteria, prognosis, and prediction of therapy results. In our study, we went through the following steps:

a. Ask the clinicians to identify and list the elementary criteria that enter in their decision process concerning indication and prognosis for brief mother-infant psychotherapy.
b. Make sure that the elements that were determined were necessary and sufficient, meaning that nothing important was missed and no element was redundant with another.
c. Phrase each component into an explicit proposition or question.
d. Devise a rating system for each component.

When working on the identification of elementary criteria that constitute the basis for a clinical impression concerning positive or negative indication, clinicians had many disagreements. They found it difficult to agree among themselves about the nature and importance of criteria. For example,

was the mother's capacity for insight and ability to link the present and the past more decisive than her type of relationship to the infant and her theories about symptom formation? Reference to the literature concerning adult time-limited therapy provided some clues (Sifneos, 1972; Malan, 1976; Mann, 1983). After many hours of discussion between researchers and clinicians and several revisions of previous work, a list of 14 indication criteria was settled upon. The final list (Indication Criteria, Annex 2) covers the following topics: Feasibility of treatment (C1 and C2), mother's relationship to the child and understanding of symptomatology (C3 to C5), significant events in mother's and infant's history (C6 to C8), mother's potential for therapeutic work (C9 to C13), and prognosis (C14).

The list was applied during data collection of the Outcome Study, after pretreatment evaluation for each therapy indication (n = 103). At that stage, discrepancy arose between clinicians and researchers. Clinicians complained that researchers forced them to answer a questionnaire divided into too narrow items, while they were used to relying on holistic judgments about the various aspects of their patient's functioning. They found the items too rigid and not corresponding to the genuine, varied characteristics of mother-infant dyads. Much coaxing was needed to get clinicians to agree to submit to such an analytical approach and to write down precisely the ratings they attributed to each item. Clinicians were also reluctant to rate patients on the basis of information that they did not gather firsthand. According to the procedure (see preceding), the cases were described to them by the research team and then videotape excerpts were shown. They understood that an evaluation of the prediction of outcome needed to be done *before* treatment started, but they constantly claimed that it would be easier to determine prediction after several personal encounters with a patient. Researchers, on the other hand, were intent on questioning clinicians on their thinking and deciding processes in order to study the basis of clinical judgment.

What did we learn from the results? First, we discovered that clinicians are strongly faithful to what theory prescribes when posing an indication, at least before the treatment starts. When the indication is posed (after the pretreatment evaluation and before treatment has started), items such as positive transference, resistance, and insight appear as the main factors correlated to the prognosis of therapy (see Table 8.1), and this corresponds to what theory teaches about indications. Prognosis is essentially linked to the maternal potential for therapeutic work and her ability to go through a reflexive process (F1 and F2, see Table 8.2). Surprisingly, the specific components of the technique of mother-infant therapies which enable the therapist to elaborate a focus and an interpretation (significant events in the past history) and clinical feasibility appear as secondary factors (F3 and F4) in the indication process. Both aspects are not related to the prognosis. Clinicians' ratings seem to rely mainly on judging the potential mothers have for

TABLE 8.1

Indication Criteria and Prognosis before Treatment Has Started (N = 103)

			F1	F2	F3	F4
		Eigenvalue	3.29	2.65	1.64	1.71
		% of variance	23.5	18.9	11.7	12.2
F1	C13	Positive transference	.80	.05	.02	.27
	C12	Resistances	.78	.32	.07	.13
	C11	Insight	.74	.43	.09	.07
	C14	**Prognosis**	.73	.13	−.11	.29
	C8	Positive memories of the past	.51	−.23	−.41	−.05
F2	C9	Access to inner world	.50	.65	.02	−.11
	C4	Search for explanations of symptoms	.17	.83	.04	.16
	C5	Theories of symptoms available	−.05	.73	.15	.18
	C10	Links between present and past	.19	.72	.13	−.03
F3	C7	Traumatic events in infant's history	.04	.00	.81	−.15
	C8	Traumatic events in mother's history	−.05	.26	.77	.03
F4	C1	Nature of symptom suits mother-infant therapy	−.02	.17	−.29	.79
	C2	Time-limited treatment sufficent	.54	.07	−.12	.69
	C3	Positive investment of infant	.30	−.01	.23	.59

Factor Analysis (principal components, varimax rotation)

an ideal psychoanalytically-based treatment, rather than on the actual conditions for conducting a mother-infant therapy (Bachmann & Robert-Tissot, 1992). Clinicians' ratings reflect both reference to an ideal patient and neglect of the actual clinical evidence at hand.

Secondly, we discovered that as soon as the treatment had started the prognosis ratings (C14) were no longer explained by the ratings of the components of the indication, while the ratings of criteria themselves did not change drastically. After the first session, the prognosis was no longer linked to the availability and ability of the mother for therapeutic work (F1 and F2, see Table 8.2). Nor was it linked to any other factor or item on the list. One should also note that ratings specifically concerning the infant (traumatic elements and positive investment of the mother) surprisingly appeared to no longer be related to any other criteria. The first encounter between the therapist and the patient appeared, thus, to have a strong impact on clinical judgment about prognosis since the previously found association between prognosis and availability for a therapeutic work (F1) was no longer observed at that stage. It is noteworthy to outline that no rating of "poor prognosis" was given after the first therapy session, while it did appear before treatment started in 30.6 percent of the cases. Clinicians appear to have become more positive after the first session than before as if they made a bet on a positive evolution that detached them from theory-based indication criteria. We can

TABLE 8.2

Indication Criteria and Prognosis after First Therapy Session (N = 72)

				F1	F2	F3	F4
			% of variance	26.3	11.6	10.2	9.6
F1	C12	Resistances		**.87**	.18	.03	−.07
	C13	Positive transference		**.80**	.03	.13	.06
	C11	Insight		**.75**	.32	−.01	.00
F2	C9	Access to inner world		.24	**.75**	.09	−.09
	C5	Theories of symptoms available		−.05	**.75**	−.17	.27
	C4	Search for explanations of symptoms		.25	**.73**	−.04	−.02
	C10	Links between present and past		.11	**.65**	.48	−.01
F3	C8	Positive memories of the past		.00	.16	**−.88**	.03
	C6	Traumatic events in mother's history		.13	.25	**.61**	.16
F4	C1	Nature of symptom suits mother-infant therapy		−.15	.07	.09	**.85**
	C2	Time-limited treatment sufficent		.42	.23	−.04	**.67**
	C7	Traumatic events in infant's history		−.04	.10	.17	.13
	C3	Positive investment of infant		−.08	.29	.14	.05
	C14	**Prognosis**		.40	.04	−.01	.27

Factor Analysis (principal components, varimax rotation)

hypothesize that this modification in prognosis criteria after the first session actually reveals the powerful impact on the clinician's judgment of a relational factor, best described as the development of a therapeutic alliance. Once they engaged in the relational bond, therapists relied more on clinical impressions, based on the nature of the encounter, and no longer relied exclusively on theory-based criteria. The real patient has taken over the ideal patient.

Thirdly, as far as *prediction* is concerned, our procedure brought forth some interesting findings. Prediction of therapy results is well known for its weakness. Our data lead to the same results but only for the prognosis given before treatment has started. No significant association was found between prognosis before treatment and any measure of outcome at posttreatment evaluation. However, this was no longer true for prognosis given after the first session. Prognosis given by the therapist after the first session strongly predicted the symptomatic evolution of the infant. Furthermore, the prognoses given after the second session and third session was found to predict the improvement of maternal sensitivity during interactions with infant and modification of maternal affects (anxiety, anger).

We have given a fairly long account of the assessment of indications for treatment because it reveals the clinicians' implicit and explicit reasoning about indication and prediction, a major issue in the clinical field. This example also demonstrates how research methods and statistical analysis illuminates the clinical process of indication in addition to revealing the challenges involved in the collaboration of researchers and clinicians.

Conclusion

When we look back on the evolution of collaboration between clinicians and researchers, we can conclude that one of the main impacts of the research was a *modification of practice in our clinical and research teams*. Therapists had to give up total mastery over what they usually consider their exclusive province: The creation and maintenance of a therapeutic relationship with a (or with several) patient(s). This meant renouncing total ownership of decision-making, data gathering and analysis, and the exclusive intimate relationship with a patient. Simultaneously, researchers had to renounce total mastery over an assessment procedure that would follow pure rules of methodology. They came to realize that the application of a *pure* method could seriously alter the data that was researched and alienate the therapists when they felt too threatened by what they experienced as damaging intrusion. This working through process led to abandoning omnipotent control over each family's area of expertise, thus promoting a common goal of searching for truths that transcended individualistic ideologies. We were very gratified when we reached levels where partisan viewpoints were replaced by common endeavor to discover truths that had not been predicted by the usual ethos of each of the two teams. This has been an exercise of decentralization in thinking (in the Piagetian acception of the term). We recommend to colleagues who would want to enter this type of joint venture research to allow for ritual moments of common brainstorming. Thus, issues of what constitutes the basic differences in defining goals for researchers and clinicians and what could be the resolutions of conflicts in these two epistemologies could can be approached in common. As we found that therapists and patients work together on bringing their respective goals closer and achieve "shared purposes," clinicians and researchers need to follow the same path and develop common goals and working processes.

Notes

1. This part of the research program was funded by the Fonds National Suisse de la Recherche Scientifique, subsidies No 32-8949.86 ("Brief psychotherapies in children under 3 years of age: a quantitative study of therapeutic outcome"). The study was conducted at the Child Guidance Clinic (HUG, Geneva) in collaboration with B. Cramer, D. N. Stern, C. Robert-Tissot, F. Palacio-Espasa, J. P. Bachmann, D. Knauer, S. Serpa Rusconi, M. de Muralt, G. Besson, G. Mendiguren, and C. Berney.

2. This part of the research program was funded by the Fonds National Suisse de la Recherche Scientifique, subsidies No 32-031.323.91 and 32-40902.94. The study was conducted at the Child Guidance Clinic (HUG,

Geneva) in collaboration with B. Cramer, C. Robert-Tissot, F. Palacio-Espasa, J. P. Bachmann, D. Knauer, S. Serpa Rusconi, M. de Muralt, G. Mendiguren, C. Berney, O. Pous, F. Luethi, V. Wasem, K. Bachmann, and A. Sancho.

3. Each sentence (or verbal statement) is coded according to five dimensions: Axis 1. Emotional and cognitive involvement, Axis 2. Conversational regulation, Axis 3. Therapeutic techniques, Axis 4. Content, Axis 5. Temporal orientation.

4. One domain where therapists found it particularly difficult to accept the validity of objectification was the domain of representations. Mothers were asked (R-Interview) to graphically represent their evaluation of themselves in various domains such as self-esteem, affects such as sadness or joy, and maternal competence (as described previously). Mothers were asked to designate the point on a straight line that corresponded to their subjective assessment. While this proved to be a very valid instrument, therapists took a long time before they could accept this assessment as validly representing the very subjective nature of maternal self-evaluation.

Appendix 1: Description of the Two Treatment Modalities (AB form) (Robert-Tissot & Cramer, 1998)

A. Psychodynamic Therapy: The therapist will try to help you understand your problems and those of the child through discussions. He will ask you to speak as freely as possible about yourself, your family, and your child. On the basis of these discussions, the therapist will try to shed light on the relationships between your history and your child's problem.

B. Interaction Guidance Therapy: The therapist will invite you to play freely with your child. These interactions will then be observed by video during the session. These observations, with discussions, will allow you to have a new perception of your child's various behaviors and your modes of reacting to them. The therapist will then establish links with the problems which brought you to the therapist.

Appendix 2: Indication Criteria Questionnaire (Bachmann & Robert-Tissot, 1992)

Feasibility of brief mother-infant psychotherapy according to the clinical situation:

C1. The nature of the symptom suits brief psychotherapy.

C2. The clinical situation can be resolved in a time period of 10 sessions maximum.

Mother's relationship to the child and conception of symptomatology:

C3. The mother's investment in her child is sufficiently positive to enable its use in brief psychotherapy.

C4. The mother looks for explanations for her child's behavior and symptoms.

C5. The mother has some theories, even if rudimentary, concerning the possible cause of her child's problem.

Significant events in mother's and infant's history:

C6. Presence of traumatic events in the mother's personal history which can be brought into relation with the actual problem.

C7. Presence of traumatic events in the infant's personal history which can be brought into relation with the actual problem.

C8. The mother has sufficient positive memories of her own past; she is able to rely on it positively.

Mother's potential for therapeutic work:

C9. The mother can talk about her inner world (representations and affects) with relative ease.

C10. The mother makes spontaneous links between her past and her actual life.

C11. The mother has sufficient psychological insight to be able to benefit from a brief psychotherapy.

C12. The mother's resistances are weak and easily overcome, in order to allow brief psychotherapy.

C13. The mother appears to be able to establish the type and intensity of transference necessary for brief psychotherapy.

Prognosis:

C14. Overall impression for brief psychotherapy and expected effects.

Each proposition (C1 to C13) is rated on a four-point scale: 1. definitely true; 2. almost true; 3. almost wrong; 4. definitely wrong.

Prognosis (C14, overall impression) is rated as follows: 1. definitely good prognosis; 2. rather good; 3. rather poor; 4. definitely poor.

References

Ainsworth, M. S. D., Bell, S. M., & Stayton, D. J. (1974). Infant-mother attachment and social development: "Socialization" as a product of reciprocal responsiveness to signals. In M. P. M. Richards (Ed.), *The integration of a child into the social world* (pp. 99–135). London: Cambridge University Press.

Ainsworth, M. D. S., Blehar, M., Waters, E., & Wall, S. (1978). *Patterns of attachment: A psychological study of the strange situation.* Hillsdale, NJ: Erlbaum.

Anders, T. (1989). Clinical syndromes, relationship disturbances, and their assessment. In A. Sameroff & R. N. Emde (Eds.), *Relationship disturbances in early childhood: A developmental approach* (pp. 125–144). New York: Basic Books,

Bachelor, A., Guérin, M. C., Théoret, M., Poitras, J., & Tremblay, J. (1993). L'alliance thérapeutique: le point de vue des clients. *Psychothérapies, 3,* 171–178.

Bachmann, J. P., & Robert-Tissot, C. (1992). Le raisonnement du clinicien dans les indications aux psychothérapies brèves mère-bébé. *Psychothérapies, 2,* 99–109.

Bibring, G., Dwyer, T. F., Huntington, D. S., & Valenstein, A. F. (1961). A study of psychological processes in pregnancy of the earliest mother-child relationship. *The Psychoanalytic Study of the Child, 16,* 9–27.

Blos, P. J. (1985). Intergenerational separation—individuation: Treating the mother-infant pair. *The Psychoanalytic Study of the Child, 40,* 41–56.

Bydlowski, M. (1997). *La dette de vie.* Paris: PUF.

Clark, R. (1985). *The parent-child early relational assessment.* Madison, WI: Department of Psychiatry, University of Wisconsin Medical School.

Cohen, L. H., Sargent, M. M., & Set-Sechrest, L. B. (1986). Use of psychotherapy research by professional psychologists. *American Psychologist, 41,* 198–206.

Corboz-Warnery, A., Fivaz-Depeursinge, E., Gertsch Bettens, C., & Favez, N. (1993). The systemic analysis of father-mother-baby interactions: The Lausanne Triadic Play. *Infant Mental Health Journal, 14*(4), 298–313.

Cramer, B. (1974). Interventions thérapeutiques brèves parents et enfants. *Psychiatrie de l'Enfant, XVII*(1), 53–118.

Cramer, B. (1993). Are postpartum depressions a mother-infant relationship disorder? *Infant Mental Health Journal, 14*(4), 283–297.

Cramer, B. (1995). Short-term dynamic psychotherapy for infants and their parents. *Child and Adolescent Psychiatric Clinics of North America, 4*(3), 649–660.

Cramer, B. (1998). Mother-infant psychotherapies: a widening scope in technique. *Infant Mental Health Journal, 19*(2), 151–167.

Cramer, B., & Palacio-Espasa, F. (1993). *La pratique des psychothérapies mères-bébés.* Paris: PUF.

Cramer, B., Robert-Tissot, C., Rusconi Serpa, S., Luethi, F., Wasem, V., Sancho Rossignol, A., Bachmann, K., Champ, C., Genevay, S., Scippa, L. G., Palacio-Espasa, F., Knauer, D., & Berney, C. (1997). *Etude détaillée des processus dans huit thérapies parents-bébé.* Rapport scientifique N° 6, Subside FNRS N° 32–40902.94.

Cramer, B., Robert-Tissot, C., Stern, D. N., Serpa-Rusconi, S., De Muralt, M., Besson, G., Palacio-Espasa, F., Bachmann, J. P., Knauer, D., Berney, C., & d'Arcis, U. (1990). Outcome evaluation in brief mother-infant psychotherapy: A preliminary report. *Infant Mental Health Journal, 11*(3), 278–300.

Cramer, B., & Stern, D. N. (1988). Evaluation des changements relationnels au cours d'une psychothérapie brève mere-nourrisson. In B. Cramer (Dir.), *Psychiatrie du Bébé: Nouvelles Frontières* (pp. 31–70). Paris et Genève: Eshel et Editions Médecine et Hygiène.

Crittenden, P. M. (1981). Abusing, neglecting, problematic, and adequate dyads: Differentiating by patterns of interaction. *Merrill-Palmer Quarterly, 27,* 201–218.

Czogalik, D., & Mauthe, C. (1991). *Manual for the Stuttgart Interactional Categories System* (Research Report No. 10). Stuttgart: Center for Psychotherapy Research.

Elliott, R., & Morrow-Bradley, C. (1994). Developing a working marriage between psychotherapists and psychotherapy researchers: Identifying shared purposes. In P. Forrest Talley, H. H. Strupp, & S. F. Butler (Eds.), *Psychotherapy research and practice: Bridging the gap* (pp. 124–142). New York: Basic Books.

Emde, R. N., Birgham, R. D., & Harmon, R. J. (1993). Classification and the diagnostic process in infancy. In C. Zeanah (Ed.), *Handbook of infant mental health* (pp. 225–236). New York: Guilford.

Fonagy, P. (1994). Mental representations from an intergenerational cognitive science perspective. *Infant Mental Health Journal, 15*(1), 57–68.

Fonagy, P. (1996). *Prevention, the appropri-ate target of infant psychotherapy.* Plenary Address at the Sixth World Congress of the World Association for Infant Mental Health, Tampere, Finland.

Fonagy, P., & Target, M. (1994). The efficacy of psychoanalysis for children with disruptive disorders. *J. Am. Acad. Child Adolesc. Psychiatry, 33,* 45–55.

Forrest Talley, P., Strupp, H. H., & Butler, S. F. (Eds.). (1994). *Psychotherapy research and practice: Bridging the gap.* New York: Basic Books.

Fraiberg, S., Adelson, E., & Shapiro, V. (1980). Ghost in the nursery: a psychoanalytic approach to the problems of impaired infant-mother relationships. In S. Fraiberg (Ed.), *Clinical studies in infant mental health: The first year of life* (pp. 164–194). New York: Tavistock.

Frieswyk, S. H., Allen, J. G., Colson, D. B., Coyne, L., Gabbard, G. O., Horowitz, L., & Newsom, G. (1986). Therapeutic alliance: Its place as a process and outcome variable in dynamic psychotherapy research. *Journal of Consulting and Clinical Psychology, 54,* 32–38.

Furman, E. (1951). Treatment of under-five by way of their parents. *Psychoanalytic Study of the Child.* (Vol. XII, pp. 250–262). New York: International University Press.

Gérin, P. (1984). *L'evaluation des psychothérapies.* Paris: PUF (Nodules).

Greenberg, J. (1994). Psychotherapy research: A clinician's view. In P. Forrest-Talley, H. H. Strupp, & S. F. Butler (Eds.), *Psychotherapy research and practice: Bridging the gap* (pp. 1–18). New York: Basic Books.

Hentschel, U., & Bijleveld, C. (1995). It takes two to do therapy: On differential aspects in the formation of therapeutic alliance. *Psychotherapy Research, 5*(1), 22–32.

Holzer, M., Pokorny, D., Kächele, H., & Luborsky, L. (1997). The verbalization of emotions in the therapeutic dialogue: A correlate of therapeutic outcome. *Psychotherapy Research, 7*(2), 261–273.

Hopkins, J. (1992). Infant-parent psychotherapy. *Journal of Child Psychotherapy, 18,* 5–19.

Huber, W. (1996). Le problème de l'indication en psychothérapie. *Acta psychiat. belg.,* 135–153.

Kächele, H. (1992). Narration and observation in psychotherapy research: Reporting on a 20 year long journey from Qualitatif case reports to Quantitatif studies on the psychoanalytic process. *Psychotherapy Research, 2*(1), 1–15.

Kazdin, A. E. (1994). Psychotherapy for children and adolescents. In A. E. Bergin & S. L. Garfield (Eds.). *Handbook of psychotherapy and behavior change* (pp. 543–594). New York: Wiley.

Kiesler, D. J. (1994). Standardization of interventions: The tie that binds psychotherapy research and practice. In P. Forrest-Talley, H. H. Strupp, & S. F. Butler (Eds.), *Psychotherapy research and practice* (pp. 143–153). New York: Basic Books.

Kowalik, Z. J., Schiepek, G., Kumpf, K., Roberts, L. E., & Elbert, T. (1997). Psychotherapy as a chaotic process II: The application of nonlinear analysis methods on quasi time series of the client-therapist interaction: a nonstationary approach. *Psychotherapy Research 7*(3), 197–218.

Kreisler, L., & Cramer, B. (1995). Les bases cliniques de la psychiatrie du nourrisson. In S. Lebovici, R. Diatkine, & M. Soulé (Eds.). *Nouveau traité de psychiatrie de l'enfant et de l'adolescent* (pp. 1927–1952). Paris: PUF.

Kumar, R., & Brockington, I. F. (Eds.). (1998). *Motherhood and mental illness* (Vol. 2). London: Wright.

Lebovici, S. (1983). *Le nourrisson, la mère et le psychanalyste.* Paris: Le Centurion.

Lieberman, A. F., & Pawl, J. H. (1993). Infant-parent psychotherapy. In C. Zeanah (Ed.), *Handbook of infant mental health* (pp. 427–442). New York: Guilford.

Lieberman, A. F., Weston, D. R., & Pawl, J. H. (1991). Preventive intervention and outcome with anxiously attached dyads. *Child Development, 62,* 205–208.

Luborsky, L. (1990). A guide to CCRT method. In L. Luborsky & P. Crits-Christoph (Eds.), *Understanding transference: The CCRT method* (pp. 15–36). New York: Basic Books.

Luborsky, L., Barber, J. P., & Diguer, L. (1992). The meanings of narratives told during psychotherapy: The fruits of a new observational unit. *Psychotherapy Research, 2*(4), 277–290.

Luborsky, L., Crits-Christoph, P., Mintz, J., & Auerbach, A. (1988). Who will benefit from psychotherapy? *Predicting therapeutic outcomes.* New York: Basic Books.

Main, M., Kaplan, N., & Cassidy, J. (1985). Security in infancy, childhood and adulthood: A move to the level of representation. In I. Brettherton & E. Waters (Eds.), Growing points of attachment theory and research (pp. 66–104). *Monographs of the Society for Research in Child Development, 50*(1–2, Serial No. 209).

McDonough, S. C. (1989). *Interaction guidance: A technique for treating early relationships.* Paper presented at the Fourth World Congress of Infant Psychiatry and Allied Disciplines in Lugano, Switzerland.

McDonough, S. C. (1992). L'aiuto all'interazione: una tecnica per il trattamento dei disturbi relazionali precoci. In G. Fava

Viziello & D. N. Stern, (Eds.), *Dalle cure materne all'interpretazione: nuove terapie per i bambino et le sue relazioni: i clinici raccontano* (pp. 221–233). Milano: Raffaello Cortina.

McDonough, S. C. (1995). Promoting positive early parent-infant relationships through interaction guidance. *Child and Adolescent Psychiatry Clinics of North American, 4*(3), 661–672.

Mahler, M. S. (1973). *Psychose infantile: Symbiose humaine et individuation.* Paris: Payot.

Mahler, M. S., Pine, F., & Bergman, A. (1975). *The psychological birth of the human infant.* New York: Basic Books.

Malan, D. H. (1976). *The frontier of brief psychotherapy.* New York: Plenum.

Mann, J. (1983). *Time-limited psychotherapy.* Cambridge, MA: University Press.

Mergenthaler, E. (1996). Emotion-abstraction patterns in verbatim protocols: A new way of describing psychotherapeutic processes. *Journal of Consulting and Clinical Psychology, 64*(6), 1305–1315.

Morrow-Bradley, C., & Elliott, R. (1986). The utilization of psychotherapy research by practicing psychotherapists. *American Psychologists, 41,* 188–197.

Osofsky, J. D. (Ed.). (1987). *Handbook of infant development* (2nd ed.). New York: Wiley.

Parloff, M. B. (1982). Psychotherapy research evidence and reimbursement decisions: Bambi meets Godzilla. *American Journal of Psychiatry, 139*(6), 718–727.

Rausch, H. L. (1974). Research, practice, and accountability. *American Psychologist, 29,* 678–681.

Reuchlin, M. (1981). Options fondamentales et options superficielles. *Revue de Psychologie Appliquée, 31*(2), 96–115.

Richman, N. (1981). A community survey of the characteristics of the one- to two-year-old with sleep disruptions. *Journal of the American Academy of Child and Adolescent Psychiatry, 20,* 281–291.

Richman, N., Stevenson, J., & Graham, P. (1975). Prevalence of behavior problems in 3-year-old children: An epidemiological study in a London borough. *Journal of Child Psychology and Psychiatry 16,* 272–287.

Robert-Tissot, C., & Bachmann, J. P. (1995). L'evaluation des psychothérapies. In S. Lebovici, R. Diatkine, & M. Soulé (Eds.), *Nouveau Traité de Psychiatrie de l'Enfant et de l'Adolescent* (pp. 2103–2116). Paris: PUF.

Robert-Tissot, C., & Cramer, B. (1998). When patients contribute to the choice of their treatment. *Infant Mental Health Journal, 19*(2), 245–59.

Robert-Tissot, C., Cramer, B., Luethi, F., Wasem, V., Cramer, B., Bachmann, K., Bonzon, P. A., & Barraud, V. (1996b, July). Mother-infant psychotherapies: Good and difficult cases. Symposium on Early Therapeutic Interventions: Clinical and Research Issues. WAIMH VIth World Congress, Tampere, Finland.

Robert-Tissot, C., Cramer, B., Stern, D. N., Rusconi Serpa, S., Bachmann, J. P., Palacio-Espasa, F., Knaeur, D., de Muralt, M., Berney, C., & Mendiguren, G. (1996a). Outcome evaluation in brief mother-infant psychotherapies: Report on 75 Cases. *Infant Mental Health Journal, 17*(2), 97–114.

Robert-Tissot, C., Luethi, F., Wasem, V., Cramer, B., & Bachmann, K. (1996c, September). Verbal exchanges and early determination of a therapeutic focus. 5th European Society for Psychotherapy Research Meeting, Cernobbio (Côme), Italie.

Robert-Tissot, C., Serpa-Rusconi, S., Bachmann, J. P., Besson, G., Cramer, B., Knaeur, D., de Muralt, M., Palacio Espasa, F., & Stern, D. (1989). Le questionnaire "Symptom Check-List": Evaluation des troubles psycho-fonctionnels de la petite enfance. In S. Lebovici, P. Mazet, & J. P. Visier (Eds.), *L'evaluation des interactions précoces entre le bébé et ses partenaires* (pp. 179–186). Paris: Eshel. Genève: Médecine et Hygiène.

Rock, D. L., Bransford, J. D., & Maisto, S. A. (1987). The study of clinical judgement: an ecological approach. *Clinical Psychology Review, 7,* 645–661.

Roth, A., & Fonagy, P. (1996). *What works for whom? A critical review of psychotherapy research.* New York: Guilford.

Rusconi Serpa, S. (1992). La Guidance Interactive: les points essentiels du traitement. *Psychoscope, 13,* 7–10.

Rusconi Serpa, S., & Sancho-Rossignol, A. (1997, Septembre). Patterns interactifs et transmission intergénérationnelle. *Symposium les Filiations Psychiques.* Lausanne, Switzerland.

Sameroff, A. J., & Emde, R. (1989). *Relationship disturbances in early childhood: A developmental approach.* New York: Basic Books.

Sifneos, P. (1972). *Short-term psychotherapy and emotional crisis.* Cambridge, MA: Harvard University Press.

Smith, M. L., Glass, G. V., & Miller, T. I. (1980). *The benefits of psychotherapy.* Baltimore, MD: Johns Hopkins University Press.

Spence, D. P. (1994). The failure to ask the hard questions. In P. Forrest-Talley, H. H. Strupp & S. F. Butler (Eds.), *Psychotherapy research and practice: Bridging the gap* (pp. 19–38). New York: Basic Books.

Spitz, R. (1951). The psychogenic diseases in infancy: an attempt at their etiological classification. *The Psychoanalytic Study of the Child* (pp. 255–275). New York: International University Press.

Stern, D. N. (1995). *The motherhood constellation: A unified view of parent-infant psychotherapy.* New York: Basic Books.

Stern, D. N., Robert-Tissot, C., Besson, G., Serpa-Rusconi, S., de Muralt, M., Cramer, B., & Palacio-Espasa, F. (1989). L'Entretien "R": une méthode d'évaluation des représentations maternelles. In S. Lebovici, P. Mazet, & J. P. Visier (Eds.), *L'évaluation des interactions précoces entre le bébé et ses partenaires* (pp. 151–160). Paris: Eshel. Genève: Médecine et Hygiène.

Stern-Bruchweiler, N., & Stern, D. N. (1989). A model for conceptualizing the role of the mother's representational world in various mother-infant psychotherapies. *Infant Mental Health Journal, 10,* 142–156.

Stiles, W. B. (1994). Views of the chasm between psychotherapy research and practice. In P. Forrest-Talley, H. H. Strupp, & S. F. Butler (Eds.), *Psychotherapy research and practice: Bridging the gap* (pp. 154–166). New York: Basic Books.

Stoleru, S., & Morales-Huet, M. (1989). *Psychothérapies mère-nourrisson dans les familles à problèmes multiples.* Paris: PUF.

Target, M., & Fonagy, P. (1994a). The efficacy of psychoanalysis for children: Prediction of outcome in a developmental context. *Journal of the American Academy of Child and Adolescent Psychiatry, 33,* 1134–1144.

Target, M., & Fonagy, P. (1994b). The efficacy of psychoanalysis for children with emotional disorders. *Journal of the American Academy of Child and Adolescent Psychiatry, 33,* 361–371.

van Ijzendoorn, M. H., Juffer, F., & Duyvesteyn, M. G. C. (1995). Breaking the intergenerational cycle of insecure attachment: A review of the effects of attachment-based interventions on maternal sensitivity and infant security. *Journal of Child Psychology and Psychiatry, 36*(2), 225–248.

Von Benedek, L. (1989). *Le travail mental du psychanalyste.* Paris: Editions Universitaires, Bégédis.

Wasem, V. (1996). *Psychothérapie et rupture du traitement: Analyse des interactions verbales de deux premières séances de thérapie brève parents-bébé.* Mémoire, Diplôme d'Etudes Supérieures en psychologie clinique. FPSE: Université de Genève.

Weisz, J. R., Weiss, B., Alicke, M. D., & Klotz, M. L. (1987). Effectiveness of psychotherapy with children and adolescents: A meta-analysis for clinicians. *Journal of Consulting and Clinical Psychology, 55*(4), 542–549.

Wildlocher, D. (1981). Pratique clinique et recherche clinique. *Revue de Psychologie Appliquée, 31*(2), 117–129.

Zero to Three: Diagnostic classification of mental health and developmental disorders of infancy and early childhood. (1994). National Center for Clinical Infant Program.

9

Advanced Training in Infant Mental Health: A Multidisciplinary Perspective

Karen A. Frankel and Robert J. Harmon

9

Introduction

Evaluation and treatment of infants, toddlers, and their families can be provided from a number of different theoretical views and in a number of different clinical settings. Over the past 20 years at the University of Colorado School of Medicine (UCSM), Division of Child Psychiatry, we have developed an integrated clinical service and training program that interfaces with parents and infants in several different settings. In this chapter, we describe our programs, beginning with a history of how these programs naturally developed out of the interest and activities of the faculty. The history illustrates several key elements that have been crucial in the success of the infant psychiatry clinical and training programs. Next, a description follows of the current clinical and training services, philosophies, and models. The chapter concludes with recommendations regarding developing infant mental health programs within a medical school setting.

History

The First Site: Neonatal Intensive Care Unit

THE CONSULTATION PROGRAM

The first clinical program in infant mental health at UCSM was consultation to the Neonatal Intensive Care Unit, (NICU) which began in 1976. This consultation originated as part of a Child Psychiatry resident elective that provided assessment and treatment for parents who were having difficulties coping with the birth of a very low birth-weight infant. Previously, when a mother or family was having psychological difficulties or causing problems for the staff, a psychiatry fellow from the adult residency was contacted through the hospital consultation liaison service. Over time it became clear to the NICU staff and the psychiatry trainees/faculty that expertise in issues of infancy and parenting were necessary to appropriately intervene in this setting. This realization coincided with the admission of several fellows to the child psychiatry training program who had a particular interest in infancy.

There was a strong need for consultation to the NICU. Families were mostly of lower socioeconomic status whose infants were born at a state-supported, public university hospital. Families were easily overwhelmed by the environment and demands of the NICU. Many of the factors that were associated with the birth of a premature or developmentally disabled infant (substance abuse, poverty, domestic violence, and poor self- and prenatal care) continued to be problematic for families once the babies were born. Conflicts with staff and physicians were frequent. Initially, the focus of consultation was on supporting the families and assisting the staff and families in interacting. Fairly soon, however, the developmental needs of these premature high-risk infants also became apparent. Basic research ongoing in the infant development laboratories at UCSM (Emde, Gaensbauer, & Harmon, 1976; Emde & Harmon, 1972; Emde, Harmon, Metcalf, Koenig, & Wagonfeld, 1971; Emde, McCartney, & Harmon, 1971; Harmon, 1983; Harmon & Emde, 1972) was highlighting important aspects of neonatal development. It seemed crucial to bridge the gap between the laboratory and the clinical site. Understanding and assessment of infant state, sensitivity to diurnal cycles, and "entertainment" became integral parts of the psychosocial intervention with families and staff. Consultants introduced the use of neonatal behavioral assessment instruments to aid parents and staff in developing individualized behavioral intervention programs for the infants to optimize their development (Culp, Culp, & Harmon, 1989; Harmon, 1983).

In addition to directly serving the families and babies, the consultation program initiated a family-focused consultation to the staff of the NICU. As noted previously, the unit could often be a stressful place to work. Families were frequently low functioning and conflictual. Staff had to manage the intensely technical aspects of caring for a neonate in an intensive care unit and interfacing with the baby's family. Oftentimes, these two goals were at odds. To confront this stress and improve the quality of clinical care, the child psychiatry residents began conducting a weekly psychosocial conference where the coping strategies of the parents who had infants on the unit were discussed. These rounds were coordinated by the nursing staff and attended by a child psychiatrist, the social worker providing service to the unit, a public health nurse coordinator, a nutritionist, a physical therapist, and other appropriate allied health professionals offering assistance to the infants and families. An attempt was made each week to discuss all of the infants and their families. When the unit's census was high, the group would prioritize cases and focus on those infants and families with the greatest concerns. Case discussions focused on several factors thought to indicate the coping and/or risk patterns interaction of families (Prugh, 1983; Harmon, Glicken, & Good, 1982).

Staff were given guidelines and consultation on understanding types of interactions that would signal the development of a healthy and positive relationship, as well as how to recognize "red flags" for possible problems. For example, attention was paid to visiting patterns or, as is often the case if the family lives a great distance from the hospital, the number of times they called the unit to check on their infant. The conference focused on the developing "bond" of the parents with their infant. How parents interacted with and talked about their infants was seen as crucial. Since the NICU was usually staffed by experienced, well-trained nurses and social workers, they were often able to "sense" problems and use the psychosocial conference to help pinpoint and identify the exact concerns so an intervention plan could be developed. In general, the unit social worker attempted to evaluate all families in order to facilitate referrals and to offer support of therapeutic counseling. The psychiatry fellows followed families closely while their infants were on the unit and then often continued to provide outpatient follow-up after discharge.

THE FETAL DEMISE PROGRAM

As part of this consultation, child psychiatry fellows asked to become involved in working with parents whose infants had died. A number of clinical services and interventions were developed to help grieving families not only deal with the loss, but also to provide some preventive intervention related to healthy decision-making concerning subsequent pregnancies (Harmon, Glicken, & Siegel, 1984; Harmon & Graham-Cicchinelli, 1985; Porreco, Harmon, Murrow, Schultz, & Hendrix, 1995). (Harmon, Plummer, & Frankel, 2000). The approach providing systematic care for these families was similar to the service developed in the NICU. Protocols for clinical, medical, and nursing care outlined what staff should do before, during, and after an infant's death. Funding was made available for a "family room" in which families could spend their final time with their infant, aided by a nurse to talk with and about the baby, prepare mementos such as photos, and soothe and care for the infant as he or she died. These rituals and the support provided by staff helped the families with their sense of loss and enhanced their memories of their lost child (Davis, Stewart, & Harmon, 1988, 1989).

A weekly "fetal demise" conference was established in which all losses, spontaneous abortions, and fetal and neonatal losses that occurred on the inpatient services were discussed on a regular basis. Losses that occurred during the previous week were reviewed at the conference. Staff and family reactions, coping patterns, and experiences with the loss protocols were reviewed. The child psychiatry fellows provided in-service education to NICU and obstetrics staff on the effects of pregnancy loss, grief and bereavement, and how to help parents approach decision-making related to subsequent pregnancies.

As part of this work, in conjunction with the University Hospital chaplain, an annual memorial service was held for families who had suffered a pregnancy loss during the previous year. Interestingly, despite the fact that many of the fetal demise programs no longer exist due to funding and service changes, this service continues to the present time. Each spring, parents who named their lost children can have their child's name listed in a memorial bulletin for the nondenominational service. The list of names is read out loud as part of the service. Many families have found it to be useful to come to the service on a yearly basis, initially as a way to deal with their feelings of loss and grief and later as a way to remember the child and the life that was to be. The service is well attended by both parents and university faculty and staff.

The Second Site: Outpatient Infant Psychiatry Clinic

As noted earlier, these hospital-based services frequently resulted in referrals for follow-up mental health care. Families who developed a relationship with the child psychiatrist during the hospitalization wanted to have the continued support and guidance of the therapist after their infant was discharged to home and some of the true parenting challenges began. Many of the parents who were seen initially for bereavement counseling later returned for additional treatment for their anxiety during a subsequent pregnancy and their concerns about overprotection of their "replacement child."

In order to provide a structured setting in which to see these families and their infants, the Infant Psychiatry Clinic was officially established in 1981. This became the second clinical service of the infant psychiatry program. Faculty had actually been carrying outpatient "infant cases" from referrals for the consultation service and general outpatient referrals for several years prior to the development of the clinic. The clinic, therefore, began as a faculty clinical case conference in which selected members of the departmental faculty discussed their infant cases. The major goals of this case conference were to encourage peer supervision of clinical work with infants, toddlers, and their families and to develop a set of common principles for training child psychiatry residents and allied mental health professionals in clinical infant mental health. In July 1982, the Infant Psychiatry Clinic began as both a clinical service and a training site for child psychiatry residents. In 1984, training opportunities for psychology and social work were added. This clinic continues to the present as the mainstay of the infant psychiatry clinical and training program.

The Third Phase: Diversification

In the last several years, the clinical and training opportunities have been able to increase from a center-based only program to include community-based sites and statewide consultation. Through funding from a private foundation, the infant mental health program has been able to offer its own training positions to psychology, psychiatry, and social work postgraduate fellows. The following is a description of the sites that currently compose the infant mental health clinical and training program within the department of psychiatry.

Current Programs

The Outpatient Infant Psychiatry Clinic

CLINIC FORMAT

The outpatient clinic continues to be supported through the Division of Child Psychiatry at the medical school. Faculty in the clinic are both full-time university-based and adjunct clinical appointees in the disciplines of child psychiatry, psychology, and social work. Trainees from several mental health disciplines participate in the clinic, including predoctoral psychology externs, interns from the Clinical Psychology Internship, residents from the Child Psychiatry Training Program, and postdoctoral research fellows in developmental psychopathology. The "clinic" is, in fact, a weekly case conference and group supervision meeting (see following).

The clinic theoretical philosophy asserts that infant mental health is a relational construct that begins with the transition to parenthood (Harmon et al., 1982). Therefore, the clinic evaluates and treats expectant parents as well as infants and their families from birth to four years old. The framework is a developmental one from a psychodynamic orientation within a family systems perspective (Fraiberg, Adelson, & Shapiro, 1975; Harmon et al., 1990; Lieberman & Pawl, 1993; Sameroff & Emde, 1985). The model considers internal working models of relationships and sensitivity to attachment issues for all members of the family system.

The clinic takes an individualized case-based assessment and treatment approach. Individual infants and their families are assigned to a clinical trainee who serves as the primary clinician and case manager. This framework has been developed and refined over the years as both the field of infant mental health and our own practices have matured and become more sophisticated. The focus of the Infant Psychiatry Clinic

has been on behavioral problems of young children four years of age and younger. Four years was established the cutoff age based on our belief that children under four are qualitatively different from their older peers and that they present many unique problems with regard to assessment and treatment. The length of treatment varies from a single consultation up to several years of ongoing treatment. In some cases, the clinic has been involved with multiple members of the family, including several generations of parents. Presenting clinical problems vary widely and include regulatory disorders, psychic trauma disorders, attachment disorders, sleep problems, aggression, separation disorders, oppositional disorders, developmental deviations, autism, toileting difficulties, hyperactivity, psychophysiological disorders, parenting problems, and parental psychopathology to mention the most common (Harmon et al., 1990; Frankel et al., 1997).

When families call the child psychiatry outpatient clinic, a one-half hour screening appointment is given to the parents within one week after the call. This screening is done by a senior child and adolescent psychiatry resident and focuses on the chief complaint and the history of the present problem. A preliminary diagnosis is reached and appropriateness for Infant Psychiatry Clinic is established. In addition, necessary eligibility and financial issues are discussed. Each infant and family is then assigned to an infant psychiatry clinic trainee who serves as the primary clinician and case manager. The case is discussed in the Infant Psychiatry Clinic group supervision meeting after the intake screening interview and before being seen by the trainee. The faculty supervisors provide guidance as to how this particular case should be approached. In some cases, the parent(s) and infant are seen initially, whereas in others the parent(s) may need to be seen alone to clarify additional information about the presenting problem and/or to develop the alliance with the parents prior to seeing their young child.

The Infant Psychiatry Clinic is the center-based portion of our program. Families and their young children are seen by the trainees in their university clinic offices at any time during the week. A larger family therapy room and a video studio therapy room are also available on a sign-up basis. Home visitations and preschool/daycare observations or consultations are made by the clinician when clinically indicated. The clinician can also request specific evaluations from psychology, speech pathology, and occupational therapy/physical therapy as indicated. In general, trainees are encouraged to think of intervention as two phases that, while separate, are fluid and interrelated: The evaluation phase and the treatment phase.

Unlike some clinics that have a one-day interdisciplinary assessment approach, our model is a case-based approach, individually tailored and directed by the primary clinician. The clinician meets with the family and child, consults with other significant adults and settings (e.g., daycare, preschool, and grandparents), and determines whether assessments by other disciplines (e.g., speech language, developmental evaluation, or pharmacological evaluation) are necessary. If so, the primary clinician coordinates the additional assessments and joins with the family and consulting staff to provide feedback. Usually, the evaluation process takes four to eight sessions. The clinician works to formulate with the family a joint conceptualization of the difficulties that will help lead naturally to an agreed upon treatment approach. Treatment and/or intervention strategies may be tested during the evaluation phase to help both with diagnostic clarity and with illuminating treatment prognosis.

CLINICAL SUPERVISION

The Infant Psychiatry Clinic has a weekly case conference in which staffing and ongoing group supervision is provided for all trainees on the cases seen during the week. In addition, each trainee has at least one hour of individualized case supervision per week. Supervision is provided by faculty in the disciplines of child psychiatry and psychology. The clinical approach taught in the clinic focuses on psychodynamic (Zeanah, Anders, Seifer, & Stern, 1989) and family systems issues (Lyons-Ruth & Zeanah, 1993), as well as on the unique characteristics of the young child and his or her cultural context (Garcia-Coll & Meyer, 1993; Nugent, 1994). While trainees, especially new trainees, often wish for simple or formulaic approaches to diagnosis and treatment, we encourage them to "embrace complexity" which may temporarily raise anxiety levels in the clinicians. However, we believe it is crucial to have cultural, familial, developmental, and relationship contexts in which to see and treat the child for understanding and working with families of young children. They also receive individual and group relationship-based clinical supervision (Fenichel, 1992) in the process of individual child therapy, infant-parent psychotherapy, and family therapy.

Since the inception of the clinic, trainees have been encouraged to video-tape their sessions and bring the videotape to the group supervision. The university has a special video studio that is available on a sign-up basis. Tapes are shown un-edited, at whatever point in the session the faculty or trainee believes contains useful information. It has required some effort on the part of the faculty and time to build a tradition of videotape viewing in order to create a safe learning atmosphere where trainees and their supervisors can comfort-ably show videotapes of assessment and therapy sessions. Videotapes serve as pow-erful stimuli for discussion, as well as pro-vide both process and content supervision. Trainees with limited experience with in-fants (either personal or professional) find videotapes from faculty extremely helpful in decreasing their anxiety and exposing them to the "flow and feel" of a therapy ses-sion with very young children. Trainees bring videotapes from any point in the eval-uation and/or treatment and often give "regular updates" for discussion.

DIDACTIC COURSE WORK

Our training model attempts to give trainees the tools to evaluate and treat in-fants and their families from multiple per-spectives: Constitutional, developmental, family, cultural, interpersonal/psychody-namic, and pharmacological. This is a long and intensive process. Trainees participate in the program for a minimum of one year and more generally for two years on a weekly basis. The group supervision and clinical case discussions meetings are com-bined with readings and didactic lectures. Trainees are exposed to standardized methods of assessing cognitive develop-ment (Bayley, 1993), relationships and in-teractions (Hirshberg, 1993), sensory functioning (Anzalone, 1993), and child emotional functioning (Emde, 1989). Reading modules concentrate on the more common diagnostic problems seen in the clinic, including attachment (Bretherton, 1985), trauma (Drell, Siegel, & Gaens-bauer, 1993), adolescent parenting (Mu-sick, 1990), temperament (Bates, Wachs, & Emde, 1995), and child abuse (Cicchetti & Toth, 1995; Gaensbauer & Harmon, 1982). Specific training in developmental, cognitive, and socioemotional assessment of infants is available for the psychology trainees. For the child psychiatry resi-dents, didactic training and clinical super-vision in the appropriate and judicious use of psychotropic medications is provided (Harmon & Riggs, 1996).

Day Treatment Programs

Over the course of the first few years of the outpatient therapy work in the Infant Psy-chiatry Clinic, it became clear that there were a number of children with severe symptoms who could not be adequately treated through outpatient interventions alone. With that in mind, the program ex-panded to include two-day psychiatric hos-pital programs, one of which is for autistic children and the other is for children who have suffered severe physical and/or sexual abuse and neglect. Over time, the autism program has developed into a separate program with its own outpatient assessment and treatment service. The majority of children presenting at outpatient clinic initial screening interviews, who show problems consistent with pervasive developmental disorder, are now routinely referred to be evaluated and treated in that setting (Rogers & Lewis, 1989).

The community-based preschool/day hospital program (called the "therapeutic preschool") for physically and/or sexually abused and neglected young children has increasingly become an integrated component of the UCSM infant mental health program. Most of the children in the therapeutic preschool are of lower socioeconomic backgrounds, and the majority are living in foster adoptive homes. The preschool has treated approximately 160 children since 1974, with an equal number of boys and girls. The ethnic distribution is 50 percent African-American, 25 percent Hispanic, and 25 percent Caucasian. Most of the children have remained in the program for two years. Children generally enter the program at preschool age for their first year and then continue their attendance after entering kindergarten in their second year, spending half of each day in each setting (Harmon & Riggs, 1996; Oates, Gray, Schweitzer, Kempe, & Harmon, 1995). This allows the children to work on therapeutic issues in the preschool day treatment program in the morning and become part of mainstream kindergarten peer groups in the afternoon.

Children can be referred to the thera-peutic preschool either through the Infant Psychiatry Clinic following an evaluation or directly by a referring agency who has evaluated the child and determined the need for day treatment services. Children who begin treatment in the outpatient Infant Psychiatry Clinic are usually referred to the therapeutic preschool as the severity or nature of their symptoms becomes clear or if outpatient treatment is not sufficient to care for the needs of the child and family.

The preschool/day hospital is a therapeutic milieu involving a four hour, day treatment session with highly structured therapeutic and educational activities. The classroom is managed by a head teacher, with two staff teachers and several advanced-level trainee assistants or community volunteers. There is generally a 1:3 adult-to-child ratio. Classroom curricula cover both the standard preschool and prekindergarten academic activities, as well as a strong focus on programs to promote socioemotional development. Relationship building, safety promotion, and nonviolent conflict resolution are cornerstones of the classroom program (see Oates et al., 1995, for complete program description). Here, as in the Infant Psychiatry Clinic, there is a case-based approach. Each child is assigned an individual clinician who also serves as case manager. Cases are reviewed weekly by the entire treatment team (i.e., primary clinician, supervising child psychiatrist, supervising child psychologist, team social worker, pediatrician, and teachers). Therapeutic interventions include twice weekly individual psychotherapy, twice monthly family/parental therapy, pediatric medical assessment and management, and regular case manage-ment. Family work and liaison to social service agencies is regularly provided by the program social worker.

As the therapeutic preschool serves as a training site for both infant mental health programs, there are concomitant training and service activities. Children are fol-lowed in therapy by psychology externs, psychology postdoctoral fellows, and child/adolescent psychiatry residents who serve as primary clinicians. Both individual and group supervision is provided to the clinicians. Supervision is both clinical, case-based and didactic. There is training in psychological and developmental test-ing available to psychology trainees. Child psychiatry residents receive training in psychopharmacological management of young traumatized children (Harmon & Riggs, 1996).

Community-Based Sites

The training programs are beginning to co-ordinate training and clinical service provi-sion to infants and toddlers within the com-munity. Early Head Start is now providing an opportunity for infant mental health consultation to a wide range of settings and families. Two Denver sites have initiated pilot programs with our trainees to provide mental health consultation at their sites. This collaboration will hopefully serve the needs of these newly developing programs for infants and their families. While cogni-tive and socioemotional needs have always been a focus of Head Start, mental health needs are now being reevaluated with a new critical eye. We hope to cooperate in

developing consultation to staff, families, and children that will increase both profes-sional and public awareness about infant mental health.

Community mental health centers statewide and the developmental disability and early childhood education providers are also seeking collaboration with the ex-panding infant mental health services. Re-cently, there has been a mandate in the state to begin providing mental health services to infants and toddlers through the public sector programs. Unfortunately, these programs are not yet equipped to handle the needs of young children and their families, either from a programmatic or a technical perspective. The effort to link these providers to experts in infant mental health and offer training and ongo-ing supervision is underway. Finally, as in many states, Colorado is becoming aware of the importance of linking infant mental health and infant day care services.

Training Issues

There are two major training tracks within the Division of Child and Adolescent Psy-chiatry related to infancy: (1) the child and adolescent psychiatry residency and (2) the infant mental health postgraduate training program. Both of these training experi-ences are designed for advanced practi-tioners in mental health fields. The inten-tion of the training programs at the Univer-sity of Colorado School of Medicine is to train professionals who will teach and con-sult to infant programs and their staff, as well as provide direct intervention. Infant mental health fellows are expected to go on to work in academic and training settings, teaching, supervising, consulting, and pursuing clinical research. It is the value of the program that there is an important role for highly trained infant mental health specialists to consult, teach, educate, and provide supervision and direct clinical service to programs that serve infants, toddlers, and their families.

In the residency program, trainees are all exposed to extensive work with infants through the Outpatient Infant Psychiatry Clinic as described previously. Several residents can also elect to receive additional experience through a minor rotation placement at either of the therapeutic day treatment programs Fellows in the infant mental health program receive a more intensive training experience solely in the area of infancy. They are placed at a major rotation site (any of the previously mentioned programs) and can, if time and interest permit, be placed in a minor rotation as well. As part of the training program, these fellows receive extensive didactic course work in core issues of infant mental health. Intensive clinical supervision in groups and individually constitutes the third component of the fellows' training experience.

In each of the training programs there are several key components that are the cornerstones of training in infant mental health: Assessment, differential diagnosis, intervention, and academic scholarship. There are also several basic tenets of training that are core to this program. It is the philosophy of the training program to assert that all infant mental health professionals need to know how to understand the emotional, developmental, biological, temperamental, and interactional capabilities of an infant and their partner. Infant mental health professional trainees are required to become proficient in observation of an infant and their caregiver, in order to understand the nature of each partner and unravel the meanings of their interactions. It is essential that infant mental health professionals are skilled in assessing adults and adolescents from a psychosocial and psychobiological perspective, since these individuals are fully one-half of the caregiver-infant system. It is a requirement of the trainees in each program that they have good prior training in general adult and child mental health before entering the training programs. Trainees are expected to understand general child and adult development and psychopathology. They need to be solid clinicians familiar with several different ways of intervening with adults, children, and families before entering the infancy training program. With these requirements satisfied, the training in the residency and fellowship can focus on training in infant development and mental health and parent-infant interaction. Therefore, the training in assessment, differential diagnosis, intervention, and scholarship focuses on infant mental health issues.

Assessment

Assessment is taught through didactic course work, group supervision of cases, and observing the faculty conducting assessments. All fellows are taught the general principals of assessment from a psychometric and psychiatric perspective (Sattler, 1992; Hirshberg, 1993; Greenspan & Meisels, 1994). Fellows are taught how to use standardized infant and parent-infant assessment tools (Bayley, 1993). Time is spent observing infants and their families and discussing the observations. As described previously, in the infant clinic and in other settings where video facilities are available, trainees are strongly encouraged to videotape sessions with infants and bring them to their appropriate supervision groups for viewing. In viewing the videotapes, the framework suggested by Hirschberg (1993, adapted from Emde, 1989) has been a helpful guide to focus discussions and remind trainees of the multiple domains of observation necessary to begin to know and clearly understand a particular infant. Fellows are also familiarized with several research paradigms that aid in teaching keen observation skills. For example, they are shown videotapes and scoring samples of infants engaging in the Strange Situation Paradigm of Ainsworth (Ainsworth & Wittig, 1969) in order to learn about assessing attachment relationships. They have the opportunity to view infants participating in Mastery Motivation tasks (Morgan & Harmon, 1984) to learn about another important developmental drive. Experience viewing clinical material with a normative developmental "eye" is invaluable to the infant clinician.

For psychiatry residents, training in assessment of infants for psychotropic medications is crucial. It is the philosophy of the programs that there are a circumscribed number of cases in children under the age of four where medications are appropriate when used judiciously. Since there are limited opportunities for most child psychia-trists to obtain expertise in this area (and this has not necessarily limited practice), we have a strong belief in responsible education, supervision, and clinical research in the assessment for and administration of medication with young children. Therefore, training in psychopharmacology is also in the form of didactic course work and individual and group clinical supervision. Finally, for all assessment procedures the impact of culture is explored through articles and supervision, as well as first-hand experience with infants and families of color.

Differential Diagnosis

Differential diagnosis is another important training tool in both the fellowship and residency program. Approaching families from a family-centered and family-strengths perspective is crucial. However, it is also important for the advancement of infant mental health to endeavor to understand the difficulties, challenges, and disorders that afflict infants and their families from a diagnostic point of view. Conceptualizing an infant's case from a diagnostic perspective allows clinicians to build a common language to talk about children with both parents and other professionals. A common language is sorely needed in the quickly growing field of infant/preschool mental health. Common reference points can lead the way toward developing more effective, disorder-specific forms of treatment intervention (Harmon, 1995).

Since the introduction of the *Diagnostic Classification of Mental Health and Developmental Disorders of Infancy and Early*

Childhood (DC: 0–3) (Zero to Three/National Center for Clinical Infant Programs, 1994), trainees have received extensive training in using the diagnostic system and its accompanying data record. This is done for several reasons (Harmon, 1995). In order to use the diagnostic system's five axes, the clinician is almost required to do a thorough evaluation of the child and family from all of the perspectives. The system helps to guide clinicians in asking about all areas of functioning (e.g., emotional, developmental, biological, temperamental, and interactional capabilities), not only those they are most comfortable with or about which they have the most expertise. The exercise of discussing a differential diagnosis and then determining and carrying out the evaluation process necessary to arrive at a final diagnostic formulation is considered one of the most enriching training experiences for both fellows and residents. Diagnostic discussions challenge trainees and supervisors alike to think about different etiologic scenarios and consider what treatment options would be indicated for different conceptualizations.

Intervention

Through their experiences in learning assessment and differential diagnosis, trainees begin to become familiar with the various disorders and difficulties faced by infants and their families. The training program then continues with in-depth training about the entire range of problems seen in infancy (e.g., all DC: 0–3 diagnostic categories, all applicable DSM–IV diagnoses, and problems such as child abuse, being the infant of a teen or addicted parent, being an infant in a violent family, or the difficult challenges of foster care, etc.). For this portion of training, fellows and residents learn through peer-reviewed articles, book chapters, visiting "experts," and clinical group supervision of cases. Training highlights what is known about the etiology and phenomenology of disorders, what assessment tools and pathognomonic signs can help identify the disorder, and what is known about the natural history and treatment experiences of infants with the various problems. Fellows and faculty are encouraged to provide case examples of each problem that is being discussed to give the trainees the "feel" of working with infants and families who exemplify the challenges about which they are reading. The key, often, for these well-trained fellows and residents is to integrate their understanding of pathology of older children and adults with knowledge of infancy and infant development to become well-versed in how disorders manifest themselves at the earliest ages. A developmental psychopathology framework (Cicchetti & Cohen, 1995) is crucial in learning to think in this way. It takes almost one full year of weekly classes to cover the spectrum of difficulties applicable to infancy in appropriate depth, though trainees often wish there was more time and more readings.

As mentioned previously a key process in learning intervention skills is group supervision of clinical cases. The training model within the psychiatry department adheres to a "learning by doing" model. The program generally uses a reflective supervision model in teaching and in consultation (Fenichel, 1992). While this approach is not unusual in mental health settings and in fact, is what trainees have come to expect, it is very helpful to elucidate the principles of reflective supervision so that the fellows can learn to use them in their clinical rotations. All trainees carry a caseload commensurate with their experience and skill level that increases as training progresses. Group supervision is an invaluable tool in infant mental health training and is especially useful in the multidisciplinary training program. Trainees learn as much from each other—with their extensive and varied training histories—as they do from program faculty.

Additionally, the faculty's experience of many years in training students of varying levels of expertise to work in infant mental health has repeatedly highlighted the anxiety and trepidation that the great majority of trainees encounter when embarking on this kind of clinical work. Trainees, especially those who have not yet had their own infants, show a high level of anxiety that the program faculty have recognized over the years as an expectable reaction to beginning training in a form of therapy that most often does not rely on words—*words* which to date had been the trainees main psychotherapeutic tool. It initially appears to trainees to be a daunting task to communicate with and understand a being who does not use the trainee's primary mode of communication. Group supervision, again, is a powerful tool in helping trainees to share and learn to overcome their initial feelings of trepidation and incompetence. It is an arena where they can share with one another their subjective experiences and stumbling blocks, as well as the good coping strategies they have found to confront the challenges.

In the portion of training that concentrates on intervention, there is a certain amount of "technique" that is taught. Fellows are exposed to the classic articles in infant mental health (Fraiberg, Adelson, & Shapiro, 1975) as well as to the different schools of therapy most commonly used with infants and families. The training highlights parent-infant psychotherapy (Lieberman & Pawl, 1993), parent-guidance (McDonough, 1995), early intervention (Barnard, Morisset, & Spieker, 1993), and family supportive therapy (Weissbourd, 1993). Specific treatment protocols that have been shown successful with particular disorders are reviewed as the disorder is taught (e.g., attachment and behavior, by Speltz, 1990). As with the training in assessment, the influence of context and culture is emphasized through the use of articles and case examples. Each fellow is encouraged to synthesize the learning materials and develop an intervention style that "fits" with their own therapeutic style and personality. It is important for fellows to identify their strengths and weaknesses and the types of infant mental health work that are most compelling for them (e.g., consultation, dyadic therapy, early intervention, etc.) to enable them to set future professional goals.

Scholarship

Because the training programs are designed for advanced degree professionals who plan to continue in an academically-oriented career, the program also encompasses a certain amount of scholarly activities. All fellows take an active role in planning and evaluating course curricula. Each module is jointly designed by faculty and fellows to address the training interests and highlight the current state of knowledge. Fellows learn library and computer literature searching skills in order to seek out the most timely and comprehensive articles, books, and chapters for each topic. When studying research articles, faculty focus on helping trainees with limited prior training in research to become competent consumers of clinical and developmental empirical works. It is the expectation of the program that the fellows will become astute critical consumers of clinical and developmental research. It is expected that they will integrate and apply research information into their interventions and philosophical thinking about infants and infant mental health.

For fellows who are particularly interested in research and expecting to embark on an academic or academic medical career, training and experience in clinical research is offered. Fellows may design and implement their own circumscribed research project or join any of the several ongoing projects in infant development and mental health available within the psychiatry department. For example, previous fellows have chosen to study post traumatic stress and attachment in maltreated children (Rudnick, Schwietzer, Hathaway, & Harmon, 1995), to conduct a clinical medication trial with children with trauma-induced symptoms (Harmon & Riggs, 1996), or to identify a possible measure of

hypervigilance in maltreated children (Frankel, Boetsch, & Harmon, in press). Some fellows have concurrent research postdoctoral training and work in both basic and clinical research (Kelsay, 1998a, 1998b). Alternately, several fellows have joined in an ongoing project looking retrospectively at the data from over 15 years of clinical cases seen in the Infant Psychiatry Clinic (Frankel et al., 1997).

Conclusion

The infant mental health training programs at the University of Colorado School of Medicine encompasses a continuum of care and training which has focused on outpatient evaluation and treatment, hospital-based consultation, and therapeutic day programs. With the development of more family and community-centered interventions, the program has now expanded to include nonuniversity affiliated sites, building a sorely needed consultation service to community daycare, Head Start, and mental health agencies. In summary, the infant mental health program at UCSM has grown from a hospital-based consultation program to an integrated program of service and training. The program trains child psychiatry residents, psychology pre- and postdoctoral trainees, and social work trainees.

The child and adolescent psychiatry residents and the infant mental health fellows learn through a combination of clinical experience, didactic seminars, and ongoing supervision. Assessment, developmentally appropriate differential diagnosis, intervention techniques, and the development of scholarship are the key elements of the training program. Supervision, both group and individual, has been an essential teaching component.

Although there may be many models of training in infant mental health, the UCSM program has focused on training advanced mental health practitioners. Experience has demonstrated an important role for highly trained infant mental health specialists to consult, teach, educate, and provide supervision and direct clinical service to programs for infants and toddlers and their families.

References

Ainsworth, M. D. S., & Witting, B. (1969). Attachment and exploratory behavior of one-year-olds in a strange situation. In B. M. Foss (Ed.), *Determinants of infant behavior: Vol. 4* (pp. 113–136). New York: Wiley.

Anzalone, M. E. (1993). Sensory contributions to action: A sensory integrative approach. *Zero to Three, 14*(2), 17–20.

Barnard, K. E., Morisset, C. E., & Spieker, S. (1993). Preventive interventions: Enhancing parent-infant relationships. In C. H. Zeanah (Ed.), *Handbook of infant mental health* (pp. 386–401). New York: Guilford.

Bates, J. E., Wachs, T. D., & Emde, R. (1995). Toward practical uses for biological concepts of temperament. In J. E. Bates & T. D. Wachs (Eds.), *Temperament: Individual differences at the interface of biology and behavior* (pp.

275–306). Washington, DC: American Psychological Association.

Bayley, N. (1993). *Bayley Scales of Infant Development* (2nd ed.). San Antonio: The Psychological Corporation.

Bretherton, I. (1985). Attachment theory: Retrospect and prospect. In I. Bretherton & E. Waters (Eds.), Growing points in attachment theory and research. *Monographs of the Society for Research in Child Development, 50*(1), 3–35.

Cicchetti, D., & Cohen, D. (Eds.). (1995). *Developmental psychopathology: Vol. 2. Risk, disorder, and adaption.* New York: Wiley.

Cicchetti, D. & Toth, S. L. (1995). A developmental psychopathology perspective on child abuse and neglect. *Journal of the American Academy of Child and Adolescent Psychiatry, 34,* 541–565.

Culp, R. E., Culp, A. M., & Harmon, R. J. (1989). A tool for educating parents about their premature infants. *Birth, 16,* 23–26.

Davis, D. L., Stewart, M., & Harmon, R. J. (1988). Perinatal loss: Providing emotional support for bereaved parents. *Birth, 15,* 242–246.

Davis, D. L., Stewart, M., & Harmon, R. J. (1989). Pregnancy after perinatal death: Perspectives on doctor's advice. *Journal of the American Academy of Child and Adolescent Psychiatry, 28*(3), 481–487.

Drell, M. J., Siegel, C. H., & Gaensbauer, T. J. (1993). Post-traumatic stress disorder. In C. H. Zeanah (Ed.), *Handbook of infant mental health* (pp. 291–304). New York: Guilford.

Emde, R. N. (1989). The infant's relationship experience: Developmental and affective aspects. In A. J. Sameroff & R. N. Emde (Eds.), *Relationship disturbances in early childhood: A developmental approach* (pp. 33–51). New York: Basic Books.

Emde, R. N., Gaensbauer, T. J., & Harmon, R. J. (1976). Emotional expression in infancy: A biobehavioral study. *Psychological Issues, 10,* 1–200.

Emde, R. N., & Harmon R. J. (1972). Endogenous and exogenous smiling systems in early infancy. *Journal of the American Academy of Child Psychiatry, 11,* 177–200.

Emde, R. N., Harmon, R. J., Metcalf, D. R., Koenig, K. L., & Wagonfeld, S. (1971). Stress and neonatal sleep. *Psychosomatic Medicine, 33,* 491–497.

Emde, R. N., McCartney, R. D., & Harmon, R. J. (1971). Neonatal smiling in REM states, IV: Premature study. *Child Development, 42,* 1657–1661.

Fenichel, E. (Ed.). (1992). *Learning through supervision and mentorship to support the development of infants, toddlers and their families. A source book.* Arlington. VA: Zero to Three/National Center for Clinical Infant Programs.

Fraiberg, S., Adelson, E., & Shapiro, V. (1975). Ghosts in the nursery: A psychoanalytic approach to the problems of impaired infant-mother relationships. *Journal of the American Academy of Child Psychiatry, 14*(3), 387–422.

Frankel, K. A., Boetsch, E. A., Bennett, E., Harmon, R. J., Gavin, L. A., & Boyum, L. A. (1997, December). *Fifteen years in an infant psychiatry clinic.* Paper presented at the 12th National Training Institute of Zero to Three/National Center for Infants, Toddlers and Families, Nashville, TN.

Frankel, K. A., Boetsch, E. A., & Harmon, R. J. (in press). Elevated picture completion scores: A possible indicator of hypervigilance in maltreated preschoolers. [Special Issue]. *Child Abuse & Neglect.*

Gaensbauer, T. J., & Harmon, R. J. (1982). Attachment behavior in abused/neglected and premature infants. In R. N. Emde & R. J. Harmon, *The development of attachment and affiliative systems* (pp. 263–279). New York: Plenum.

Garcia-Coll, C., & Meyer, E. (1993). The sociocultural context of infant development. In C. H. Zeanah (Ed.), *Handbook of infant mental health* (pp. 56–59). New York: Guilford.

Greenspan, S. I., & Meisels, S. J. (1996). Toward a new vision for the developmental assessment of infants and young children. In S. J. Meisels & E. Fenichel (Eds.), *New Visions for the Developmental Assessment of Infants and Young Children.* (pp. 11–26). Washington, DC: Zero to Three/National Center for Infants, Toddlers, and Families.

Harmon, R. J. (1983). Infant behavior and family development. In L. Sonstegaard, G. Jennings, & K. Kowalski (Eds.), *Primary health care of women* (pp. 327–343). New York: Grune and Stratton.

Harmon, R. J. (1995). Diagnostic thinking about mental health and developmental disorders in infancy and early childhood: A core skill for infant/family professionals. [Special Issue]. *Zero to Three 15*(3), 11–15.

Harmon, R. J., & Emde, R. N. (1972). Spontaneous REM behavior in a microcephalic infant: A clinical anatomical study. *Child Development, 34,* 827–833.

Harmon, R. J., Glicken, A. D., & Good, W. V. (1982). A new look at maternal infant bonding: implications for prenatal practice. *Perinatology-Neonatology, Sept.–Oct.,* 27–31.

Harmon, R. J., Glicken, A. D., & Siegel, R. E. (1984). Neonatal loss in the intensive care nursery: Effects on maternal grieving and a program for intervention.

Journal of the American Academy of Child Psychiatry, 23, 68–71.

Harmon, R. J., & Graham-Cicchinelli, D. (1985). Fetal and neonatal loss. In R. C. Simons (Ed.), *Understanding human behavior in health and illness* (3rd ed., pp. 151–157). Baltimore: Williams and Wilkins.

Harmon, R. J., & Riggs, P. D. (1996). Clonidine for posttraumatic stress disorder in preschool children. *Journal of the American Academy of Child and Adolescent Psychiatry, 35*(9), 1247–1249.

Harmon, R. J., Plummer, N. S., & Frankel, K. A. (2000). Perinatal loss: Parental grieving, family impact, and intervention services. In J. D. Osofsky & H. E. Fitzgerald (Eds.), *WAIMH handbook of infant mental health, Vol. 4: Infant mental health in groups at high risk.* New York: Wiley.

Harmon, R. J., Stall, P. J., Emde, R. N., Siegel, C., Kempe, R. S., Margolin, M. H., McGehee, R., & Frederick, S. R. (1990). Unresolved grief: A two-year-old brings her mother for treatment. *Infant Mental Health Journal, 11*(2), 97–112.

Hirshberg, L. (1993). Clinical interviews with infants and their families. In C. H. Zeanah (Ed.), *Handbook of infant mental health* (pp. 173–190). New York: Guilford.

Kelsay, K. (1998a, February). *Postdoctoral grant preview: The relationship between the inner world of preschoolers and their engagement in play therapy.* Presented at the Developmental Psychobiology Research Group Seminar, University Colorado School of Medicine, Denver, CO.

Kelsay, K. (1998b, February). *Early childhood narratives: Collaborative research and prospects for clinical assessment.* Presented at the Department of Psychiatry Grand Rounds, University of Colorado School of Medicine, Denver, CO.

Lieberman, A. F., & Pawl, J. H. (1993). Infant-parent psychotherapy. In C. H. Zeanah (Ed.), *Handbook of infant mental health* (pp. 427–442). New York: Guilford.

Lyons-Ruth, K., & Zeanah, C. H. (1993). The family context of infant mental health: Affective development in the primary caregiving relationship. In C. H. Zeanah (Ed.), *Handbook of infant mental health* (pp. 14–37). New York: Guilford.

McDonough, S. C. (1995). Promoting positive early parent-infant relationships through interaction guidance. *Child and Adolescent Psychiatric Clinics of North America, 4,* 661–672.

Morgan, G. A., & Harmon, R. J. (1984). Developmental transformations in mastery motivation: measurement and validation. In R. N. Emde & R. J. Harmon (Eds.), *Continuities and discontinuities in development* (pp. 263–291). New York: Plenum.

Musick, J. (1990). Adolescents as mothers: The being and the doing. *Zero to Three, 11*(2), 21–28.

Nugent, J. K. (1994). Cross-cultural studies of child development: Implications for clinicians. *Zero to Three, 15*(2), 1–8.

Oates, R. K., Gray, J., Schweitzer, L., Kempe, R. S., & Harmon, R. J. (1995). A therapeutic preschool for abused children: The KEEPSAFE project. *Child Abuse & Neglect, 19*(11), 1379–1386.

Porreco, R. P., Harmon, R. J., Murrow, N. S., Schultz, L. A., & Hendrix, M. L. (1995). Parental choices in grand multiple gestation: Psychological considerations. *The Journal of Maternal-Fetal Medicine, 4,* 111–114.

Prugh, D. G. (1983). Appendix B: Identifying high-risk parent infant relationships: The "five questions" approach. In *The psychosocial aspects of pediatrics* (pp. 669–673). Philadelphia: Lea & Febiger.

Rogers, S. J., & Lewis, H. (1989). An effective day treatment model for young children with pervasive developmental disorders. *Journal of the American Academy of Child and Adolescent Psychiatry, 28*(2), 207–214.

Rudnick, L., Schweitzer, L., Hathaway, P., & Harmon, R. J. (1995, May). Aggression and post traumatic stress disorder in abused preschoolers: Diagnosis, management and treatment. In R. J. Harmon (Chair), *Aggression and violence: Developmental pathways.* Seminar presented at the 23rd Annual Child Abuse and Neglect Symposium, Keystone, CO.

Sameroff, A., & Emde, R. (1985). *Relationship disturbances in early childhood: A developmental approach.* New York: Basic Books.

Sattler, J. M. (1992). *Assessment of children* (4th ed.). San Diego: Author.

Speltz, M. (1990). The treatment of preschool conduct problems. In M. Greenberg & D. Cicchetti (Eds.), *Attachment in the pre-school years* (pp. 399–426). Chicago: University of Chicago Press.

Weissbourd, B. (1993). Family support programs. In C. H. Zeanah (Ed.), *Handbook of infant mental health* (pp. 402–413). New York: Guilford.

Zeanah, C. H., Anders, T. F., Seifer, R., & Stern, D. N. (1989). Implications of research on infant development for psychodynamic theory and practice. *Journal of the American Academy of Child and Adolescent Psychiatry, 28,*(5), 657–668.

Zero to Three/National Center for Clinical Infant Programs. (1994). *Diagnostic classification of mental health and developmental disorders of infancy and early childhood.* Washington, DC: Author.

10

Assessing the Risks and Strengths of Infants and Families in Community-Based Programs

Sarah Landy

10

Introduction

In North America, a growing number of infants and young children contend with a variety of risk factors that can compromise their development. Although the statistics may differ in Canada and the United States, the trends are similar. Due to multiple changes in the societal context, fewer families have extended family supports available, largely due to high mobility, and increasing numbers of families are experiencing feelings of being unsupported and isolated. Due to government cutbacks in funding, many communities have less services available for families and as a result this can increase their sense of isolation (Garbarino, 1992; Steinhauer, 1996).

In both Canada and the United States, an increasing number of infants and young children live in families with incomes below the poverty line. In Canada, in 1994, 21.3 percent of children under seven were living in poverty (Doherty, 1997). This compares to 25 percent of children under three with families with incomes below the poverty line in the United States (Carnegie Task Force on Meeting the Needs of Young Children, 1994). Income rates are linked to the unemployment rate, another risk factor that can create stress and can cause marital dissatisfaction and negatively impact on parents' interactions with their children (Doherty, 1997; Shaw, Vondra, Hammerding, Keenan, & Dunn, 1994).

A growing number of babies in the United States are born to single mothers, many of them teenagers. Divorce rates are increasing, and in the United States almost 50 percent of children live for some years in a single-parent household (Glick, 1988). In Canada, young children in single-parent homes are significantly more likely to live in poverty (Hanvey, Avard, & Graham, 1994). The number of families in which both parents work due to economic necessity has increased dramatically in recent years. More than 50 percent of children in Canada live in two-parent families where both parents are employed or are students. This leaves many parents exhausted from the demands of work and home, with little opportunity or energy to spend needed time with their children (Hewlett, 1991; Steinhauer, 1996).

This trend toward two-parent working families means that millions of children in North America spend most of their waking hours in the care of people other than their parents (Lero, Goelman, Pence, Brockman, & Nuttall, 1992). Unfortunately, much of this care is substandard, whether it is in day care centers, family care homes, or by relatives (Pence & Goelman, 1991). In Canada, only 33 percent of children are in regulated day care facilities (Pepper & Stuart, 1992).

In many communities across North America, a large proportion of the residents are new immigrants or refugees. Much of the clinical literature on the development of immigrant children concludes that the stresses experienced by these groups are extensive. They include insufficient preparation for school, loss of familiar persons, customs, clothing, and family, little or no ability to comprehend the language, and reduced involvement with parents who are often stressed and preoccupied with getting settled (Sluzki, 1979). Moreover, some may experience post-traumatic stress from the victimization they received in their country of origin. Some ethnic groups may have somewhat less informal and formal social networks than the more established groups, and this can adversely affect their adjustment (Rabkin, 1979). Finally, nonwhite ethnic groups are more likely to be victims

of discrimination (Lalonde, Majumder, & Parris, 1995).

With increased stress experienced by families, the numbers of children who are abused and neglected and experience removal into foster care continues to increase. In the United States, there were an estimated 46 reports of suspected child maltreatment per thousand children in 1995 (Lung & Daro, 1996). Many incidences of abuse and neglect go unreported because they remain undetected or are not reported, so it is likely that official statistics underestimate the incidence (Ards & Harrell, 1993; Trocme, McPhee, Tam, & Hay, 1994; Wolfner & Gelles, 1993). Surveys of adults about abuse during childhood indicate that as many as 21 to 31 percent report experiencing physical abuse (e.g., MacMillan, Fleming, & Trocme, 1997). Children who experience abuse and neglect suffer from consequences that impair later functioning and have been associated with psychiatric disorders, antisocial behaviour, problems with relationships, and impaired functioning (Cicchetti & Rizley, 1981; Aber, Allen, & Carlson, 1989; Egeland & Sroufe, 1981; Lewis, 1992; Malinosky-Rummell & Hansen, 1993). Family violence has reached epidemic proportions. Almost one million Canadian women are victims of abuse by their husbands, boyfriends, or former spouses (Canadian Centre for Justice, 1992). In the United States, where broader definitions of violence are used (such as pushing, slapping, grabbing, or throwing an object), the incidence of family violence has been estimated in various surveys to be as high as 25 to 45 percent (Jouriles, Murphy, &

O'Leary, 1980; O'Leary, 1987; Strauss, Gelles, & Steinmetz, 1980). Not only are the effects devastating for adults, witnessing abuse can negatively impact on the development of children (Finkelhor & Dziuba-Leatherman, 1994; Jouriles et al., 1989).

In some neighborhoods with a high incidence of unemployment and low income families, there are concentrations of extreme risk factors and limited resources to combat them. Particularly in urban areas, families are often exposed to high rates of crime, drug abuse, and violent juvenile gangs, making parents reluctant to leave their homes for fear of exposing their children to injury or even death (Garbarino, Kostelny, & Dubrow, 1991). Statistics for premature births, accidents and injuries to infants and young children, child abuse, and domestic violence are excessively high in such neighborhoods.

Because of the multiple needs of families in many communities, a growing number of prevention and early intervention programs in these areas provide multidimensional programming intended to meet the extreme needs of many families. Sometimes called multicomponent or multigenerational programs, they attempt to provide services directly to infants and young children, as well as to their parents. Because of the economic hardships faced by many parents in high-risk neighborhoods, these programs provide services both to improve parenting capacity and reduce isolation, as well as increase parents' sense of competence and their involvement in the community (St. Pierre, Layzer, & Barnes, 1995).

Because these programs are provided in the community, frequently in the home,

and to multiethnic populations, they present multiple challenges for assessment of children and families. In this chapter, the goals and objectives and clinical approaches of community-based programs are described. This is followed by a description of approaches to the assessment of risk and protective factors, and program examples are provided. The chapter closes with conclusions and recommendations for the development of optimal methods of assessment in these community-based, multidimensional programs.

Community-Based Programs

Types of Community-Based Programs

One of the main characteristics of community-based programs is that they are offered in the community, typically with services offered in the home. This is to reach families who would not usually attend clinics and for the convenience of parents by removing barriers of transportation and child care (Gomby, Larson, Lewit, & Behrman, 1993). Program organizers often emphasize how important home visiting can be in order to evaluate and really understand the family's interactions in the home and the neighborhood environment with which the family is contending. Home visiting may also be crucial when a family is in crisis, to bring needed support and concrete help in order to alleviate a particular situation (Weiss, 1993). As well, community-based programs typically encourage the participation of parents in the initiation, planning, and presentation of various program components (Halpern, 1990). Most community-based programs, in addition to an outreach component, provide a strong in-center component with a variety of groups offered, some developed by staff and others at the request of participating parents. These usually emphasize, for example, the reduction of stress and isolation (drop-in centers), enhancement of parenting capacities (parenting groups of various kinds), improving parents' sense of competence by providing skills (e.g., job training), and encouraging parents' involvement in their community (various community groups and organizations) (Ramey, Ramey, Gaines, & Blair, 1994). Programs may provide all of these in-center components themselves or may refer parents to other community agencies to avoid duplication of services (St. Pierre et al., 1995; Wasik, Ramey, Bryant, & Sparling, 1990).

Apart from these core principles of operation, community-based programs often differ significantly in terms of the populations they work with, the services that are offered, and their philosophies and staffing. Often operating in high-risk areas, programs may target the whole population within the geographic boundaries or a particular group within it, such as teenage mothers, a particular ethnic group, or infants and young children identified with developmental delays or physical problems.

Perhaps the greatest variation in community-based programs comes from their philosophies and beliefs about the mechanisms of change. As discussed by Dunst, Trivette and Deal (1988), different models can be distinguished by their "attributions about causes for both problems and solutions." Many programs are family-focused and concentrate on the provision of social support for families involved (Crnic & Stormshak, 1997). Social support is a complex concept and can include the provision of understanding and empathy, concrete assistance and information needed by the family (Crnic, Greenberg, & Slough, 1986; Dumas, 1986). The philosophy of the need for such services has arisen partly out of the lack of natural support networks that many families in high-risk communities currently experience. Many recent programs use an enabling and empowerment model with the service provider, adopting an approach which emphasizes the strengths of parents and promotes their efforts to meet the family's own identified needs, aspirations, and directions for growth (Dunst & Trivette, 1987; Dunst et al., 1988). The basic philosophy and belief about change is that seeing the family as competent, rather than needing treatment or efforts to prevent problems, results in parents being able to deal with future problems and plans more effectively, and the "interventions" will be likely to be associated with positive effects (Brickman et al., 1983). More clinically oriented, psychodynamic or infant mental health programs may also adopt some of these approaches but will focus on efforts to build the relationships between parent and child, as well as service provider and parents. Workers will also try to bring insight and resolve internal conflicts of the parents caused by previous history that may be getting in the way of an infant or child and parent having a mutually satisfying relationship. These

341

may or may not be identified as areas for change by the parent. A fourth approach which has been adopted, particularly by public health nurses, is that of health promotion that aims to provide information and developmental guidance around such issues as childbirth, breast-feeding, safety, birth control, nutrition, parenting, and other health-related issues (Landy, 1996).

The focus of the program will often determine the composition of the staff, with those with a health promotion emphasis relying primarily on public health nurses, more clinical or mental health approaches utilizing clinicians of various kinds such as social workers, psychologists, and psychiatrists, and with many social support and empowerment-focused programs having a growing tendency to use community mothers with some training and supervision. These community mothers often come from the same neighborhood, cultural background, speak the same language, and have similar histories to the families they visit.

In summary, community-based programs may differ in a number of aspects of their service provision but, in reality, workers may shift naturally between these approaches according to the predominant needs identified by the family and the service provider at a particular time.

Goals and Objectives of Community-Based Programs

In spite of their complexity, community-based early intervention and prevention projects provide programs with the goal of enhancing the development of infants and young children in the population they serve.

Although in the past child outcomes were usually assessed using Development Quotients (DQ) or Intelligence Quotients (IQ), there is a growing understanding that consideration should be given to a far broader range of aspects of development, particularly those that contribute to a child's competence and especially to their ability both to initially adjust to and later continue successfully in school. These capacities include such abilities as frustration tolerance, concentration, social skills, and affect regulation, (Landy, in press). Considering these skills and abilities has been particularly important in order to demonstrate the effectiveness of programs, especially when children are followed-up through high school and beyond (White, 1984; Zigler & Weiss, 1985). See Table 10.1 for a list of some capacities that may be considered and their effect on the child's early adjustment in school.

Besides the overall goal of enhancing child health and development, early intervention programs offered in the community usually have objectives that emphasize the areas of parenting capacity (such as sensitivity to the child, parenting knowledge, and the home environment), parents' sense of competence (e.g., increasing a sense of social support and obtaining employment), and involvement in their community.

Whatever the main objectives of community-based programs, many of their activities can be seen as efforts to reduce risk factors and enhance protective factors and strengths of families, so that a positive balance is achieved and as a consequence, the development of infants and young children enhanced. In order to be able to provide optimal interventions, the risks and strengths

TABLE 10.1
The Competent Child

Capacity	Effect in School/Home
Emotion regulation	• Communicates feelings and wants in a socially appropriate way • Controls aggression and anxiety • Controls aggression and anxiety • Does not become easily frustrated and is not impulsive
Social skills	• Cooperates with the group • Successful peer interactions • Can access sources of social support
Attention and concentration	• Can follow directions • Can stay at task long enough to complete it • Is not distracted by what is going on around him or her
Secure attachment	• Has a sense of trust of people • Can manage and function away from attachment figures for appropriate length of time • Able to explore environment without excessive anxiety
Positive self-esteem and self-confidence	• Affective balance with a generally positive mood • Confidence in achieving
Adequate verbal skills	• Can listen to and communicate effectively with adults and peers
Achievement motivation	• Has a desire to learn • Keeps trying even when a task or situation is difficult
Coping skills	• Can problem-solve • Can overcome obstacles • Hs strategies to seek help when necessary

of individual families need to be assessed, understood, and integrated into the types of services offered.

Assessment in Community-Based Programs

Risk and Protective Factors

Risk factors are variables that have been found to be associated with the develop-ment of intellectual delays and/or mental or physical health problems in children. They are usually organized under four general headings: Child characteristics, interactional or parenting variables, parental history and current functioning, and sociodemographic and societal factors. See Table 10.2 for a list of some of the aspects of these broad categories which are usually considered in assessing families.

One of the most significant risks for infants is extreme prematurity or low birth weight. The lower the weight, the greater the risk for the child having ongoing health and developmental problems (Allen, Donohue, & Dusman, 1993; Hack, Taylor, & Klein, 1994). Other biological and/or genetic conditions are also significant risks in terms of cognitive and other developmental areas. Chronic medical conditions and repeated illnesses have also been found to be related to later psychosocial difficulties (Offord, Boyle, Fleming, & Blum, 1989; Schultz-Jøgensen, Kyng, Maar, Rasmussen, & Højlund, 1987). Medical conditions and illnesses are often difficult for families to handle, and the children may have academic and social difficulties when they enter school. Very difficult temperament can challenge parents' caretaking of their child and can include a very high or low level of response to various stimuli, which can in turn lead to persistent arousal of the sympathetic nervous system, anxiety, irritability, intensity of response, and other reactions (Thomas, Chess, & Birch, 1968; Coll, Kagan, & Resnick, 1984).

Many researchers suggest that interactional and parental variables are the most important to consider in predicting child outcomes (Rutter, 1989; Werner, 1989, 1993). In a variety of longitudinal prospective studies with large cohorts (Sameroff & Fiese, 1990; Egeland & Erickson, 1990) and in a smaller study of high-risk families (Greenspan et al., 1987), the later impact of early parent-child interactions on development has been found to be highly significant. For example, lack of sensitivity, responsiveness, and attunement to the infant's cues and negative affect toward the child can lead to the development of an in-

secure attachment, a known risk factor for the development of later emotional and social difficulties (Ainsworth, Blehar, Waters, & Wall, 1978; Main & Goldwyn, 1984). For some parents lack of knowledge about expected developmental milestones and parenting techniques can lead to difficulties with discipline and failure to encourage language and other areas of development (Crockenberg & Litman, 1990).

Parent characteristics that can place the infant or child at risk include families in which one or both parents have a psychiatric condition. Whether the parental mental illness undermines the child's development depends on such factors as the nature and severity of the illness and whether there is another caregiver in the home to buffer the child from the effects of the parent's illness (Anthony, 1982; Bell & Pearl, 1982; Phares & Compas, 1983; Wieder, Jasnow, Greenspan, & Strauss, 1983). Significant levels of depression in a parent, particularly the mother, can increase the child's vulnerability to both anxiety and behavioral disorders (Beardslee, Bemporad, Keller, & Klerman, 1983; Carro, Grant, Gotlib, & Compas, 1993; Pape, Byrne, & Ivask, 1996). Other significant risk factors include having less than average intelligence (Luthar & Zigler, 1992), drug or alcohol abuse (Reich, Earls, Frankel, & Shayka, 1993), and criminality of either parent (Fisher, 1995; Gobel & Shindledecker, 1993). It is also clear that some less obvious or latent variables, such as the parents' experience of their relationships and upbringing, especially if it was traumatic and included abuse, neglect, or significant loss, can impact dramatically on

TABLE 10.2
Risk Factors

The Child	Interactional or Parenting Variables	Parental History and Current Functioning	Sociodemographic and Societal Factors
Low birth weight/pre-maturity	Lack of sensitivity or at-tunement to infant's cries or signals	Mental illness or depression	Chronic unemployment
Failure-to-thrive/feed-ing difficulties	Negative affect toward child	Serious medical condition	Inadequate income/housing
Developmental delays	Lack of vocalization to child	Parents seem incoherent or confused	Frequent moves/no telephone
Congenital abnormali-ties/illnesses	Lack of eye-to-eye con-tact	Developmental delay	Less than Grade 10 education
Very difficult tempera-ment/extreme crying	Negative attributions to-ward child	Criminal or young of-fender's record	Single teenage mother
Very lethargic/nonre-sponsive	Lack of preparation dur-ing pregnancy	Previous child has been in foster care	Violence reported in the family
Low or high muscle tone	Lacks parenting knowl-edge	Mother experienced loss of previous child	Severe family dysfunc-tion
Resists holding/hyper-sensitive to touch	Infant not brought for regular medical care	Previous child has be-havior problems	Lack of support/isolation
	Infant dirty and un-kempt	Alcohol and drug abuse	Recent life stresses (death, job loss, immi-gration)
	Very punitive toward child	Background with severe abuse, neglect, or loss in childhood	
	Does not encourage child's development		

their ability to parent and the attachment security of their children (Benoit & Parker, 1994; Main & Goldwyn, 1984).

Variables that are more sociodemo-graphic or relate to the family environment can also significantly increase the risk for later child problems. Low socioeconomic status, particularly if the family is living be-low the poverty line or in "deep poverty," has been shown frequently to be a signifi-cant risk factor (Offord & Lipman, 1996;

Zyblock, 1996). Living at this level of poverty means that the family is constantly struggling to provide children with their basic needs for food, shelter, and clothing. Poverty may also mean living in subsidized, substandard housing, in violent neigh-borhoods, found in some studies to be an important predictor of later child psychopathology (Dubrow & Garbarino, 1989; Offord et al., 1989). Children from homeless families have a particularly high incidence of dysfunction (Dail, 1990; Schfeingart, Molnar, Klein, & Lowe, 1997). Not only do parents living in poverty find it difficult to meet their children's basic needs, they often find it difficult to talk to, spend time with, and read to their children. Nurturing interactions may be difficult to provide as parents may be depleted and have feelings of hopelessness and depression (McLoyd & Wilson, 1991). Adolescent parenting increases children's risk for having both physical and emotional complications (Weinman, Robinson, Simmons, Schreiber, & Stafford, 1989). When other risk factors such as poverty, depression, and drug and alcohol abuse are also present, the risk rises substantially (Hechtman, 1989). Other significant risks include severe family dysfunction, especially if it results in spousal abuse (Fergusson, Horwood, & Lynskey, 1992; Pedersen, 1994). Isolation and lack of social supports can also result from such situations and can also contribute to their ongoing maintenance (Allen, Bruin, & Finlay, 1992; Moroney, 1992). As well, chronic family adversity, stresses, or "hassles" have been found to correlate with infant attachment security, although the researchers found variables related to personality risk to be the most powerful predictors of insecure attachment (Shaw & Vondra, 1993). To summarize, a variety of variables have been found to be associated with poor outcomes for children, but there are multiple pathways and processes which determine the ultimate patterns of adaptation or maladaption (Cicchetti & Rogosch, 1996; Zeanah, Boris, & Larrieu, 1997). One of the reasons for the divergency in outcomes is the in-

fluence of a variety of protective factors which interact complexly with the risk factors discussed previously.

Protective factors refer to conditions which can improve resistance to risk factors and contribute to successful outcomes, adaptation, and child resiliency. They are typically seen as falling into three main categories: (1) personal characteristics within the child such as high intelligence, good social skills, and positive temperament qualities, (2) relationship variables which provide the children with a secure relationship with a warm empathetic adult either within the family or community, and (3) a social environment or community that reinforces and supports positive efforts made by the child. For young children, this is most likely to occur in a day care setting.

The relationship between risk and protective factors and the development of child resiliency is complex and does not involve straightforward linear relationships. However, some writers have described protective factors as the opposite of risk variables, whereby isolation, for example, would be a risk factor and the opposite, having a strong family network or support system within the community could act as a protective factor. Rutter (1990) and Werner (1995), rather than describing protective factors, have elaborated upon possible protective mechanisms that may occur to create resilience in children. Rutter (1990) describes a variety of ways that involvement in risk conditions or negative effects of exposure to risk can be reduced and which serve to avoid the perpetuation of the risk effects. Situations that enhance the child's feelings of self-esteem and self-confidence and opportunities that are provided for the child are also seen as possible pathways to resilience.

UNDERSTANDING OUTCOME PATTERNS
Since there are many factors which contribute to outcomes in any individual and myriad pathways to any particular outcome, adaptive or maladaptive, predicting a child's developmental trajectory or assessing potential for difficulties at a time in the future, such as school entry, is extremely challenging. However, there is a growing understanding about the contribution of risk and protective factors and their influence on development that can and should be used when considering the assessment of children and their families in community-based settings.

Perhaps the most important and consistent finding from longitudinal studies of development has been the understanding that one or two risk factors, unless they are extreme, rarely negatively impact on development. As the number of risk factors increases, the negative effect has been found to enlarge disproportionately. For example, having four or more risk factors can lead to a tenfold increase in difficulties, a result that has been replicated in a number of studies (Sanson, Oberklaid, Pedlow, & Prior, 1991; Rutter, 1979; Sameroff, Seifer, Barocas, Zax, & Greenspan, 1987). More recently, researchers have also been considering the number of protective factors in the same way and have identified what has been called a "cumulative protection index" consisting of three or more protective factors as contributing to early re-

siliency (Bradley, Whiteside, Mundfrom, & Casey, 1994).

Other researchers have gone beyond looking at the number of risk and protective factors and have emphasized the importance of considering the types of factors that are impacting on a child (Sanson et al., 1991; Zeanah et al., 1997). It is also crucial to consider not only the predictive factors but the outcomes being considered. For example, in considering children with severe developmental delays and a limited number of mental disorders, biological and genetic factors are strongly implicated (Werner, 1993). On the other hand for children with mild delays and behavioral and emotional difficulties, factors in the environment may be far more critical (Offord et al., 1989; Sameroff et al., 1987).

In determining the environmental factors that are most important, a number of issues with current research have made it difficult to draw relevant conclusions. Many epidemiological studies have been limited to variables that can be collected by survey instruments, sometimes using a telephone. This has meant that data has often been missing such as parent-infant or child interactions, parental attributions of their child, parents' subjective experience of their childhood, and maternal stress and depression. This has clearly limited the implications of the findings. Certain studies of children in low socioeconomic families have failed both to distinguish those families in the lowest quartile of poverty or in chronic situations of poverty from those families in less adverse situations. As well, few researchers have considered the other variables that contribute significantly in these homes, such as the teaching style of the parents, their own experience of being parented, discipline style, and maternal personality. In fact, in studies that have considered these variables, they have often been found to be more crucial and important predictors of later outcome than socioeconomic level alone (Davies & Cummings, 1994; Hart & Risley, 1995; Mantini-Atkinson, 1993; Werner, 1993).

Another finding that has major implications for assessment in community-based settings is that different factors within the environment and family are important at different ages and certain developmental events in the child can constitute turning points that can be negative or positive for a child's development. Becoming a toddler, for example, can be either viewed by parents as a positive gain or a period of rejection which can influence its effect on later outcomes.

In conclusion, in infancy and early childhood, variables that have the most effect on development are likely to be those that are most proximal or closest to the child, such as the parent-child interactions. The nature of the influence of other more distal variables, such as stressful life events, poverty, single-parent status, and marital distress is poorly understood as it may be direct in that it sensitizes the child to negative affect expressions or may be more indirect because of their impact on parenting behavior and interactions. The implications of these findings for conducting assessments in community-based settings would appear to be that face-to-face assessments that consider the more latent and interactional variables are crucial, assessments need to take place at more than one point during the child's early

years, and assessments need to consider the type and balance of risk and protective factors in making recommendations about relevant interventions. Figure 10.1 suggests a model for consideration of risk and protective factors and for suggested interventions.

Measures of Risk and Protective Factors

Introduction

For use in community settings an assessment tool is needed that can be administered in a home setting. It must also be acceptable and able to be administered by a number of staff, not require extensive videotaping and analysis, and able to be adapted for use with families who may be resistant, suspicious, or use a language or have cultural practices that are unfamiliar to staff members. The measure needs to consider both risk and protective factors and should have some way to weight the variables into an index that balances them to estimate the potential for compromised development. Although the primary use will be clinical, it is also useful if the tool can be used for short-term program evaluation and estimate long-term program outcomes. Interestingly, there appear to be very few measures available that meet these criteria, and there is very little consensus as to which can be used to identify families in order to specify relevant intervention strategies. Even more difficult is that those measures that are available and have sound psychometric properties with good reliability and validity have primarily

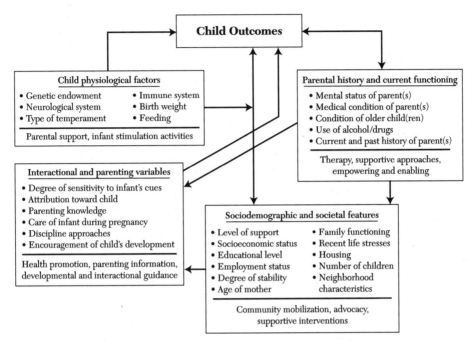

FIGURE 10.1

Risk and Protective Factors: Improving Outcomes

been used to predict abuse and neglect (Sims-Jones, Stewart, Hanvey, & McDonald, 1997). Some of these measures are described following.

Measures Used Primarily to Identify Abuse and Neglect

The Family Stress Checklist (FSC) (Murphy, Orkow, & Nicola, 1985) consists of ten items which can be used to rate families based on their responses to an interview during the prenatal period. When responses to the items are added together, they place a child at "no risk," "moderate," or "high" risk of abuse or neglect. The measure has good predictive validity and successfully predicted cases of failure-to-thrive, abuse, or neglect. The sensitivity of

the test or percent of correct negatives was rated at .89 using a group of 587 women assessed during pregnancy, with 100 of those considered "at risk" followed up two to 25 years later and compared to 100 mothers who had been considered to be at "no risk."

The Child Abuse Potential Inventory (Milner, Gold, Ayoub, & Jacewitz, 1984) takes about 15 to 20 minutes to administer by interview to an adult family member and consists of about 160 self-report items. The measure has been tested over several years and has high test-retest reliability over a day of .91 and over three months of .75. In one study, it was found to correctly identify families 95 percent of the time.

The Michigan Screening Profile of Parenting (MSPP) (Helfer, Hoffmeister, & Schneider, 1978) is an interesting measure which explores some areas of parenting not considered in other scales. These include whether the emotional needs of parents are met, relationships with their parents, coping strategies, and expectations of the child. There are 74 items which are completed by parents. The test developers suggest that the screen only be used in order to identify individuals for further assessment. Substantial support for the discriminant and concurrent validity of the dimension of whether emotional needs are met is presented, with sensitivity rates between 78 to 90 percent and specificity rates between 80 to 85 percent.

The Washington Assessment of Risk Model (WARM) (Miller, Williams, English, & Olmstead 1987) is an assessment tool which has 37 items clustered in seven domains, namely child characteristics, parent characteristics, environmental factors, characteristics of maltreatment, if present, family characteristics, and parent-child interactions.

The New York Risk Assessment Model (New York State Department of Social Services, 1991) is an instrument that has 12 factors in the preliminary assessment of safety and 25 other risk factors that are considered. The items and their weightings were chosen by a working group from Protection Services, Cornell University, and a National Risk Assessment Advisory Committee. The assessment model considers the following scales: Caretaker influence, child influence, family influence, intervention influence, and abuse/maltreatment influence. Summary scores of level of risk and safety are obtained. The assessment model has been field tested and has been quite widely used.

The Dysfunctional Parenting Scale (Larson, Collet, & Hanley, 1987) is The Postpartum Inventory and is a screening test developed to assist in the identification of "high-risk" families. It uses a small number of questions which address mother's age and education, whether she attended prenatal classes, neonatal illness, source of milk, and neonatal sleep problems. Criterion validity was calculated for 584 subjects within a heterogeneous, urban community who were assessed prenatally and postpartum or within 17 days by telephone and then followed up with observation in the home at six weeks and six months postpartum. The Home Observation for Measurement of the Environment (HOME) inventory and a maternal behavior scale were completed at that time. The test's sensitivity was estimated as .81 and specificity as .67.

The Family Risk Scales (Magura, Moses, & Jones, 1987) were developed to assess the risk of a child entering foster care. The scales consist of 26 individual rating scales with four to six levels that range from adequacy to increasing degrees of inadequacy. They emphasize parental coping skills such as knowledge of child care and development, supervision of children, and preparation for parenthood. The scales include six of the scales from the Child Well-Being Scales. An internal consistency coefficient of reliability was computed for each of the scales and were all around .8. The scales were normed on a representative sample of 1,158 families, and the scores obtained can be used for comparisons with other populations.

As will be noted, the majority of these measures concentrate on the identification of risk factors, while few look for protective factors or any index of the strengths of the family. However, they are all relatively simple to administer and score and do provide a risk index which has been shown to have current or predictive validity. In the next section, information on a number of tests that can provide additional information in a number of areas is listed.

Tests of the Child

It is clear that no in-home assessment conducted without adequate medical tests can be used to identify or diagnose complex medical or genetic conditions. However, developmental tests used as a screen can often identify infants or young children who need further assessment by specialists or early intervention for delays. The tests listed can be administered by professionals or paraprofessionals in the home if necessary and have at least some sound psychometric qualities.

The Diagnostic Inventory for Screening Children (DISC) (Amdur, Mainland, & Parker, 1990) was standardized on a Canadian population and assesses children ages three months to five years in the following areas of development: Gross and fine motor, receptive and expressive language, auditory and visual perception and memory, and social and self-help skills. Split-half reliabilities range from .98 to .99 across the eight scales. Concurrent validity shows the scale can distinguish those children requiring further attention for developmental delay and has adequate correlations with the Stanford Binet (.64) and the Denver Developmental Scales (.68).

The Ages and Stages Questionnaires (ASQ) (Bricker, Potter, & Bricker, 1995) are parent-completed questionnaires that can be completed at home or in the office at four- or six-month intervals. Each questionnaire has about 30 questions about the child's abilities in the areas of gross motor, fine motor, communication, personal-social, and problem-solving. Each only takes about 10 minutes to complete. The system can be used for tracking children's development and as a basis for further assessment or referral. Test-retest reliability completed by 175 parents at two-week intervals was 94 percent agreement and interobserver reliability by 112 parents and examiners was 94 percent. Concurrent validity as measured by comparing results to other standardized infant tests ranged according to age from 75 to 91 percent agreement. Specificity of the questionnaires was 96 percent and sensitivity averaged 75 percent.

The Child Development Inventory (CDI) (Ireton, 1992) was designed to obtain child development information from parents. However, another caregiver or teacher who has observed the child extensively can complete the inventory. The CDI provides a profile of the child's development in the areas of gross motor, fine motor, expressive language, language comprehension, self-help, social, and letters and numbers. There is also a measure of overall development or the general development scale. Items are organized under these general areas. The inventory has been used to identify and assess children with developmental problems, as well as measure developmental progress with normal children. It has been the subject of research over the last 20 years and was revised and renamed from the Minnesota Child Development Inventory recently. It is best used for children from 15 months to six years. The age norms are based on an "average sample" of 568 children, one to six years, three months old. The relationship between the CDI and the child's subsequent school performance was studied for 132 kindergarten students. Correlations with CDI scores and reading and math scores were significant for all areas except social and gross motor scales. General development scores were most significant (.69 and .59). For 26 children who had completed the CDI and who later required early intervention programs, all were identified on the CDI in one area or another. The expressive language, language comprehension, and general development scales showed the highest reliabilities or internal consistency, but all are considered adequate. They range from .42 to .95.

Interactional or Parenting Variables

Home Observation Measurement of the Environment (HOME) (Caldwell & Bradley, 1984) is a measure that evaluates constructs, such as maternal responsiveness, involvement and acceptance of her child, organization of the infant's physical environment, and opportunities for variety of stimulation. There are two versions, one for infants from birth to three years and one for preschoolers from three to six years. It has been used with a number of cultural groups and information is collected in the home by observation and interview. Interrater reliabilities range from .75 to .95, and HOME scores correlate substantially with children's scores on cognitive tests. For example, the HOME correlated at age three years with the Stanford Binet (r = .59) and at three years with the Illinois Test of Psycholinguistic Abilities scores, .57 for black children and .74 for white children.

The Pediatric Review and Observation of Children's Environmental Support and Stimulation (PROCESS) (Casey, Bradley, Nelson, & Whaley, 1988) can be used with infants from two to 18 months of age and the results used to provide developmental guidance. It can be used during pediatric or nursing examinations in the clinic or the home. After an extensive content validation, the final inventory has 24 items completed by the parents and 20 items which are rated by the clinician. There is also a list of toys available in the home completed by the parent. Items are scored from 1 to 4, and a total score is obtained. Concurrent validity has been established with the HOME and observed parent-child interactions. Correlations obtained were .84 and .86, respectively. No significant correlations were found between the measure and infant development over a four month follow-up.

The Massey-Campbell Scale of Mother-Infant Attachment Indicators During Stress (ADS) (Massie & Campbell, 1984) is a one-page guide to observation of mother-infant interactions during a stressful situation such as a medical examination. It has been used from birth to 18 months. There are six basic measures: Gazing, vocalizing, touching, holding, affect, and proximity for mother and baby, as well as a total score. It is described by the authors as easily taught to nurses and has yielded scale agreements between examiners of .83 to .99. In a small pilot study of cases which were followed from birth to 3½ years, it was found that infants assessed at birth as below average were assessed as less happy, had more difficulty concentrating, and communicated less at 3½ years.

Parental Functioning and History

The Brief Symptom Inventory (BSI) (Derogatis, 1993) is a 53-item questionnaire that takes approximately 5 to 10 minutes to complete. It was developed from a longer 90-item scale, the Symptom Checklist–90 (SCL90). The inventory reflects psychological symptom patterns found in psychiatric patients as well as in community samples. Each item is rated on a 5-point scale and is scored for nine primary symptoms: Somatization, obsessive-compulsive, interpersonal sensitivity, depression, anxiety, hostility, phobic anxiety, paranoid ideation, and psychoticism. Two week test-retest reliability coefficients for the standardization sample ranged from .68 for somatization to .91 for phobic anxiety. It showed very high convergence with the SCL90, the Minnesota Multiphasic Personality Inventory (MMPI), and psychiatric evaluations.

The Centre for Epidemiologic Studies Depression Scale (CES–D) (Myers & Weissman, 1980) is a self-report state measure of depressive symptomatology. It has two major practical applications: Initial screening and research. As an initial screening device, the instrument can sig-

nal a need for further clinical intervention, although it cannot be used to diagnose. It is a 20-item questionnaire assessing the frequency/duration of symptoms associated with depression in the preceding week. Test-retest reliabilities are between .48 and .50, and convergent validities of .3 and .8 have been found with other tests of depression.

The Mother-Father-Peer Scale (Ricks, 1985) includes dimensions of acceptance-rejection (by mother and father) and defensive idealization (of mother and father). Examples of items on the scale include, "When I was a child, my mother could always be depended on when I really needed her help and trust" (mother acceptance); "When I was a child my mother often said she wished I'd never been born" (mother rejection); and "Mother was close to a perfect parent" (defensive idealization). Ricks (1983) found that the relationship between mothers' reports of childhood relationships on this scale and the quality of infant attachment are highly related. In other words, mothers of anxious infants felt less accepted by their parents than did mothers of securely attached infants.

Sociodemographic and Societal Factors

The Family Assessment Device: General Functioning Subscale (FAD) (Byles, Byrne, Boyle, & Offord, 1988) a 12-item scale with scores of 1 to 4. All items are added together to generate a scale score. Higher scores indicate dysfunction, and a score of 27 has been used to classify families as dysfunctional. The model used includes six dimensions of family functioning: Problem-solving, communication, roles, affective responsiveness, and behavioral control. Test-retest reliabilities range from r = .66 (problem-solving) to r = .76 (affective involvement). It has been reported that scores from this scale showed a higher relationship to mental disorders in children four to 16 years of age than any other demographic or risk variable in the Ontario Child Health Study.

The Social Support Inventory (Cutrona & Russell, 1989) assesses reliable alliances, social integration opportunity for nurturance, and sense of support from family and friends. There are six items assessed on a 4-point scale. Test-retest reliability is r = .92, and the test correlates with other social support measures and measures of the individual's personal relationships.

The Neighborhood Cohesion Instrument (Buckner, 1988) estimates the sense of support within the community. It is an 18-item scale with a test-retest reliability of .95 and coefficient alpha reliability of .95. Evidence for the scale's validity comes from the fact that it discriminated well among three neighborhoods that had been selected a priori as differing in cohesion.

The Life Experience Survey (LES) (Sarason, Johnson, & Siegel, 1978) is a 57-item self-report that quantifies stress associated with changes in life circumstances over the previous 12 months. The format has subjects rate separately the desirability and impact of events they have experienced. The test yields a positive and a negative change score, as well as a total change score. This has been shown to be a powerful method of assessing the stress experienced in association with changes in life circumstances.

The Family Resource Scale (FRS) (Dunst & Leet, 1987) is a scale consisting of 31 items and measuring the adequacy of a variety of resources in the homes of young children. Split-half reliability was .95, and short-term stability over two to three months was r = .52 (p < .001). A factor analysis identified eight factors, financial support, health, necessities, nutrition, communication, physical shelter, employment, and child care. Criterion validity found personal well-being of parents (r = .57) and maternal commitment to carry out professional programs (r = .63) were significantly related to the total score on the test.

Using Assessment in a Community-Based Setting

In this section, two examples of the use of assessment in community-based settings from the author's own work are presented. In the first project, Staying on Track, assessment was used primarily as an intervention strategy, as well as a way to identify the need for further visits or other interventions. With the Growing Together project, assessment currently is primarily used clinically in order to help identify the needs of families for various types of interventions.

The Staying on Track Project

Staying on Track operated in a low-risk, relatively stable community of 20,000 in

Brockville, Ontario. There was very little cultural diversity. The program was a joint project between a public health unit and children's mental health center with the goal of promoting healthy development in the young children in the area. The program was designed to reach all children in the area in order to track their development, identify problems, and provide immediate services or refer them to other agencies in the area. A cohort design was used, and different cohorts were assessed by public health nurses. Cohort 1 received services from birth to 18 months, Cohort 2 from 18 months to 3½ years, and Cohort 3 from 3½ to 5½ years. This allowed comparison at 18 months, 3½ years, and 5½ years of children who had participated in the program with a group who had not. When difficulties were identified by the nurses or parents, on-the-spot counseling was provided, or families were referred to other agencies. Nurses also provided telephone counseling and sent out printed information as needed. On average, 70 percent of families in the area agreed to participate in the program, and few families dropped out unless they moved out of the area. Results of the study showed that children who had received services from birth to 18 months did better on a large proportion of tests than those who had not been in the tracking system. The effect of participation was less strong at 3½ years for Cohort 2 and least strong at 5½ years for Cohort 3 compared to a comparison group (see Landy et al., 1998, for further information on the project).

Intervention was provided in the home or at the clinic, and there was no set curriculum as it was seen as important to allow flexibility to respond to parents' questions, as well as to follow up on the assessments. The assessments were central to the visits and were used to provide information on normal growth and development and answer questions about the child's particular developmental pattern. Apart from the improvement in development for children involved in the tracking system, an important finding was the number of families who had three or more risk factors which were identified in the initial assessment. Over 30 percent needed and received some kind of follow-up, a finding which was unexpected due to the comparatively "low-risk" nature of the area in which the study took place. It was also clear that families in Cohort 2, who did not receive any intervention until their child was 18 months old, experienced more anxiety about their toddler than parents of children who had received visits and follow-up from birth until 18 months. With some families, an intensive intervention was needed that could be provided immediately without having to place children on a waiting list.

Growing Together

The Growing Together project is a prevention and early intervention program operating in the St. James Town area in Toronto, Ontario, Canada. The goal of the program is to enhance the health, well-being, and development of infants, young children, and their families living in the area. A number of principles and objectives for service guide the program. The major broad objectives are as follows:

- To enable children by five years of age to have adequate physical and mental health, cognitive ability, social skills, and motivation to allow them to adjust to and learn from the school, home environment, and other experiences they encounter in the future.
- To establish sound parental functioning so that parents have the knowledge, health, and emotional stability to provide optimal experiences after their children enter school and as they pass through subsequent developmental phases.
- To assist parents to make greater use of available services and work toward a sense of belonging, ownership, and control over their community, so that in St. James Town they can have access to the basic prerequisites for health and safety.

The project is jointly sponsored by a children's mental health care center and the Department of Public Health. The project also has strong links with other agencies through joint sponsorship of various parts of the program and the Advisory Committee. These agencies include a large hospital, the Board of Education, a youth center, Child Protection Services, and local day cares. Funding is provided by a variety of sources from government departments, special government grants, research funding agencies, and private foundations. There are currently 14 staff members with a wide range of training and experience in the program. A number of volunteers and students also contribute their time and expertise.

ST. JAMES TOWN

A number of factors in St. James Town place the development of children at risk. The area is the most densely populated in Canada, with 22,000 people living in a very small area and with 350 to 400 babies born there each year. Poverty in the area is linked to unemployment, low educational level, and the receipt of financial assistance. The family income of the residents is 41 percent below the Toronto average, and currently, more than 50 percent of families are unemployed. Poverty can bring a downward spiral and in St. James Town is associated with the highest rates of low birth weight infants and hospital admissions for young children in Ontario. Rates of abuse and neglect are high. Suicide rates are increasing, and the stressful life circumstances and absence of social supports for many families contribute to a multiplicity of physical and mental health problems. The area is extremely culturally diverse with only 35 percent of families speaking English in the home. Tamil, Tagalog (Filipino), and Chinese make up the largest language groups. These statistics do not recognize the large number of the population who are recent refugees. Many of these families are dealing with post-traumatic stress with few supports or services to help them cope with the distressing symptoms that result. Moreover, compared to similar areas of the city, St. James Town has been neglected with regard to the provision of community services and resources. Parents in the area are concerned about the high crime rate, drug and alcohol abuse, and lack of safe areas where their children can play.

Principles of the Growing Together Program

The basic principles of the program were developed on the basis of a needs assessment of families with infants and young children in the area, experience from the "Staying on Track" project, and research on the effects of multigenerational, multidimensional programs. Results on the effectiveness of these types of programs have tended to show few improvements in child development, modest changes in parenting capacity, but more significant improvements in parents' sense of competence and use of services (St. Pierre et al., 1995). Given the level of problems at risk identified in Brockville, it was anticipated that in the inner city neighborhood a number of families exhibiting serious dysfunction would be identified, necessitating that staff be able to provide complex clinical services. With the multiethnic community, it was necessary to employ a number of lay or paraprofessional home visitors of the same ethnic backgrounds as the parents. Lastly, if the program was to be successful in meeting the goals of improving child development, it was clear that some services needed to be provided that could focus on the child and particularly on any delays or emotional or social difficulties that might be identified.

The most important principle of the project is that services are provided on a population-wide basis with efforts to reach the whole community. Assessment and intervention are guided by a transactional model that acknowledges the influence of multiple interdependent systems on development of the child, parent-child interactions and parenting, parent functioning and history, and the family, community, and society. Special strategies are designed to meet the needs of highly challenged families. Outreach through home-visiting relationships and provision of a supportive and consistent environment at the center are seen as crucial to the success of treatment. The child's development remains an important focus and efforts are made to have periodic assessment of the child and parent(s), so that services can be offered when necessary. If delays are identified, the parents are offered the services of a speech pathologist, preschool program, and in-home developmental guidance and stimulation activities for the child. The program has a commitment to community development and advocacy, and parents are involved in the planning and provision of various program components. The program also has an evaluation component and has completed a process evaluation and short-term outcome study and will be carrying out a long-term impact study of the program's effectiveness.

Entry into the program happens for about 56 percent of the families with newborns with a home visit after they come home from the hospital. Other families are referred from outside agencies, join during the prenatal period, or choose various program components such as the toy-lending library, infant monitoring system, advocacy services, community kitchens, or community organization groups. As can be seen, there are multiple entry points into the program with many specially designed to offer incentives to meet the needs of families facing unemployment, poverty, and isolation. Many families only make use of these programs while others quickly avail themselves of assessment for their children, parenting groups, and, if eligible, having a home visitor or counselor. See Figure 10.2 for an explanation of the various entry points into the program and the tracking system.

Certain core components of the program are offered at all times. These include:

- Screening of families by public health nurses by telephone from the birth registration notices.
- Home visits to families immediately after baby comes home from the hospital for families who request it.
- A prenatal program which provides information and food coupons.

- A variety of parenting groups, for example, When Baby Comes Home (in English and Tamil), Nobody's Perfect, Fathers' Group, Filipino Mothers' Group.
- Groups to enhance parents' sense of competence, for example, computer skills, arts and crafts, community organizing group, and anger management.
- Infant monitoring system mailed to and completed by parents. If delays are suspected, the child is referred to the Developmental Clinic.
- Toy-lending library.
- Risk identified interventions for families most at risk provided by clinical staff and community home visitors that can include teaching, support, health promotion, counseling, referral, therapy, and child stimulation.
- Community development initiatives

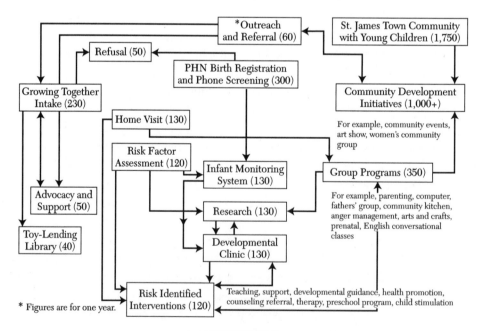

FIGURE 10.2
Growing Together Referral and Tracking System

that include community mobilization efforts by parents and a number of community events.

- Risk identifications at entry into the program.

The Process of Assessment or Risk Identification

At Growing Together, assessment of risk takes place at the center in a clinical setting, at the Developmental Clinic or through the Infant Monitoring System, or most frequently, in the home. Whenever possible, assessment of risk takes place in the home which offers a unique opportunity to begin to build trust with the family and to understand the unique distresses or strengths that a family brings to parenting their infant and young child. How otherwise could the worker know that a mother keeps all her possessions in shopping carts "in case she has to run away quickly" from her abusive, unpredictable boyfriend or about the wonderfully warm nurturing environment of family and neighbors who are available to support a very young, anxious mother as she hesitantly learns about how best to provide care for her medically fragile baby? Assessments that are done in the home take place as soon as possible after a new baby is brought home from the hospital and can be carried out by a public health nurse, clinician, or community home visitor. The choice will usually depend on information that is available about the family, either from a public health nurse screening or information from the hospital. Sometimes the choice depends on the ethnic background of the family,

and a staff member sharing the same cultural background and language would complete the assessment. Given the cultural diversity of the population, this is not always possible, and then a clinician would complete the first visits with an interpreter. If there are known breast-feeding or medical issues, a public health nurse would complete the assessment, or if psychiatric issues are suspected, a psychiatrist might be involved. In other cases, a social worker or psychologist would carry out the visit. At times, parents reject having a home visit but will come to the center where the same procedure is followed. Some families do not want to have an assessment of this kind but do agree to be part of the Infant Monitoring System or bring their infant to the Developmental Clinic. Overall, 35 percent of families assessed are identified as moderate to extreme risk and are offered in-home services. In these assessments, the majority carried out soon after a baby is born have found the highest levels of risk with the categories of parental history and current functioning and sociodemographic and societal issues. The fewest problems are usually identified with interactional or parenting variables, although this is usually reversed with older children. It is likely that the early postpartum visits are less likely to reveal difficulties in the parenting area unless they are extreme.

Assessment of risk and protective factors which takes place in the home or clinic follows a risk and protective factor assessment protocol that has been developed for the project and is clinically meaningful for staff. The assessment requests that staff collect data in the following areas: (1) infant development and functioning, (2) parental history in family of origin, (3) parental functioning past and present, (4) family and sociodemographic characteristics, and (5) interaction between mother and child. A number of questions are provided in order to elicit information, but the visit also follows the agenda of the family. In this way, much of the required information is provided without any formal assessment procedures or questions being asked. It is often impossible to collect accurate information on sensitive issues in the initial visits, either because the interviewer sees them as not appropriate to ask or information is not revealed until much later, either when the parent(s) become aware of it or feel comfortable to talk about the situation. These areas are usually about parental history and certain sociodemographic information such as socioeconomic status, violence in the home, previous abuse or neglect of child, or drug or alcohol abuse. Because the information collected is used for research purposes, questions from the Postpartum Inventory, Dysfunctional Parenting Scale (Larson et al., 1987) are also collected so that an assessment with known reliability and validity is included and the scores considered in assigning risk. In addition, because it is sometimes difficult to assess the interaction and the mother's mental functioning, the Centre for Epidemiologic Studies Depression Scale (CES–D), Family Assessment Device (FAS), and the Massie-Campbell Scale of Mother-Infant Attachment Indicators During Stress (ADS) are also used. For research purposes, some of the other measures outlined previously may be utilized. After the risk assessment has been completed, it is presented at a multidisciplinary team meeting. The family and infant or child are described, and after considering the risk and protective factors and the requests of the family for support and services, decisions are made about the level of risk to be assigned and appropriate services that can be offered to the family. If the family is considered to be at moderate, high, or extreme risk, a home visiting program is usually offered, while families at mild or very little risk are encouraged to attend the variety of groups and programs available at the center. After a moderate to high risk family has received ongoing intervention for about two months, the case is then formulated and ongoing services and the therapeutic approaches being used are explored. All families are reviewed at least once a year and offered attendance at the Developmental Clinic for a full assessment of their child. Similar assessments are also carried out when families self-refer or are referred from inside or outside the program when the child is older. In this case, some parts of the assessment may not be appropriate.

Tracking and monitoring of infants and young children is seen as essential in order to determine if children rated at low risk initially continue to do well and assess the progress of children initially considered at risk for developmental, emotional, behavioral, or social difficulties. When infants or young children are enrolled in the infant monitoring system, they are regularly sent the Ages and Stages Questionnaire at the appropriate age. If the questionnaire is not returned, a follow-up telephone call is made. Once received, the questionnaire is scored. The parents are informed that their child is doing well, or if there appear to be delays, they are offered an assessment at the Developmental Clinic. The clinic is offered one afternoon per week. Infants and young children are seen by a public health nurse who takes information and provides parenting, nutrition, feeding, and other health promotion information, the pediatrician and developmental psychologist when appropriate, and referred to the speech pathologist, if necessary. Developmental screening is carried out by the developmental psychologist using the Developmental Inventory for Screening Children (DISC) and at times, using more in-depth, norm-referenced tests such as the Bayley Scales of Infant Development. If a child cannot be assessed using standardized tests, a play-based assessment may be used. Referrals are also made for physiotherapy and occupational therapy assessments and neurological assessment when necessary. The program is working toward carrying out a Brazelton Neonatal Behavioral Assessment Scale within one month of the infant's birth, using the format of the Mother's Assessment of the Behavior of her Infant (MABI) (Fields, Dempsey, Hallock, & Shuman, 1978) items. This allows the mother to administer parts of the examination and assesses the mother's attributions of her baby and the mother-infant interaction at the same time. Currently, cutbacks at the Public Health Department and early hospital discharges have made this difficult to achieve.

Case examples are presented in this section in order to illustrate the use and process of the assessment procedures.

Margarita (23 years old) and Jody (3 months old)

Margarita and Jody were referred to the Growing Together program after Margarita phoned the Public Health Department about accessing resources for herself and her baby. An assessment in the home was begun as soon as the referral was received. It was known that Margarita was a new refugee from Guyana who spoke only French and had a three-month-old baby. Because of the language, one of the therapists who speaks French fluently carried out the assessment. Margarita agreed to having the assessment in the home but also expressed interest in coming to see the center. During the assessment Jody, the three-month-old baby, was found to be doing well. He appeared to be an alert, responsive, and very strong infant who was meeting or surpassing developmental milestones. No biological or temperament issues were identified by the mother or the clinician. Margarita was breast-feeding him and was very content and satisfied with the feeding and sleeping schedule that had been established. Family history revealed that Margarita's natural mother had died when she was young and she had been raised in a large family by her aunt and uncle. She described the family as warm and caring and when possible maintained contact with them. She reported no incidences of past abuse or neglect, only the separation and loss of her natural mother. She had also had little contact with her natural father. It was the recent history that was obviously extremely traumatic for Margarita, and she talked about flashbacks and nightmares that she had continued to experience. She had become separated from her husband during the political unrest in Guyana and had fled to Canada alone not long before the birth of her baby. She had no indication of whether her husband was alive or dead or information of his whereabouts. Margarita appeared to be very intelligent and have good coping strategies. She had completed high school at home and had been employed as a secretary. She was very interested in using available services and in learning to speak English. No signs of psychopathology or criminal activities were evident. Although obviously under extreme stress and grieving the loss of her husband and family, Margarita did not appear to show signs of clinical depression and was able to provide very nurturing, affectively positive, sensitive, and age-appropriate interactions for her baby. She had a good knowledge of infant development and seemed confident about caring for her baby, having shared the caregiving of some of her younger "siblings" with her aunt. It was clear that she saw her son as a promise for a new life and was excited about his very positive development. The apartment that Margarita lived in was cold, cockroach- and mice-infested, and without any furniture or furnishings except a crib and a few toys for her baby. Margarita was feeling extremely isolated without her husband and extended family and could not converse with anyone in English. As a result of the assessment and the balance of risk and protective factors that the family presented, Margarita was assessed as moderate risk and offered and accepted the following services: A home visitor, who was French-speaking and could help her with issues of trauma and loss and post-traumatic stress symptoms, an advocacy worker to assist in areas she identified such as housing, immigration, learning English, and employment, assessment of Jody at the Developmental Clinic, attendance at a

specially formed group for mothers who only speak French about infant care and maternal postpartum adjustment, and attendance at English language classes. Many of these programs were able to reduce Margarita's isolation as she was able to meet other recent refugees from her own country. Table 10.3 shows the risk and protective factors identified in this family and the services chosen.

Christine (22 years old) and Michael (one month old)

Christine and Michael were referred to the program by the hospital after Michael's birth because of her father's unusual behavior in the delivery room and suspected incest. Christine was pleased to have a home visit, saying that the baby was doing well but her three-year-old was "driving her crazy." She also told the psychologist that she had moved out of her father's home and was enjoying being in her own place. At the home visit that followed, assessment was carried out and as much information gathered as possible. It was clear, however, that Christine was either unwilling or unable to give accurate information about some of the questions. At first glance, it was clear that there was very little structure and routine in the home. The apartment was filthy and strewn with empty beer bottles and cigarette butts, which had either been accumulating for some time or were left over from a recent party. The baby was sleeping soundly on the couch, but Rick, the three-year-old, was screaming inconsolably, inadequately dressed for the cold temperature, and unsafely climbing on bookcases and the kitchen cupboard throughout the visit. Christine reported no problems with Michael at birth. He weighed 8 pounds, 3 ounces and was able to leave the hospital

TABLE 10.3
Margarita and Jody

Risk Factors	Protective Factors	Services Offered
Infant	*Infant* • Feeding and sleeping pattern established • No biological or genetic difficulties • Mother interested in developmental information	*Infant* • Assessment at Developmental Clinic
Interactional or Parenting Variables • Missing support of extended family in parenting	*Interactional or Parenting Variables* • Positive attribution of infant • Sensitive, affectively positive, and attuned interactions with infant • Knowledge and parenting competence adequate	*Interactional or Parenting Variables* • Group about infant caregiving and postpartum adjustment
Parental History and Current Functioning • Loss of natural mother and little contact with natural father • Separation from husband • Trauma experienced during political unrest	*Parental History and Current Functioning* • No history of abuse/neglect • Well-educated and intelligent • Good employment history • No history of medical condition, mental health problems, alcohol or drug abuse, or criminality • No clinical depression but positive attitude	*Parental History and Current Functioning* • Home visitor to deal with resolution of past history
Sociodemographic and Societal Issues • Inadequate housing • Refugee issues • No English • On welfare/unemployed • Isolation and lack of family support • Recent stressful life events	*Sociodemographic and Societal Issues* • Interest in using range of services • Only one child	*Sociodemographic and Societal Issues* • Advocacy services to help locate housing and other services • English conversation classes

Overall Risk Level = (3) Moderate risk, need for intervention expected to be of short duration.

363

with his mother after 24 hours. Christine said he was already sleeping through the night and fed well when he was awake. When Michael woke up for feeding, he appeared to be alert and responsive. Christine noted that she was disappointed he was "another" boy, as she had four boys now, with the two oldest children being in foster care. Christine expressed extreme frustration about the behavior of Rick. She described him as "bad and hitting all the time" and expressed concern that he was "stupid, like his father" because he could not speak yet. When Michael woke up for feeding, Christine tried to prop a bottle for him so he "could learn to do it himself." Little eye-to-eye contact or vocalization was noted, and Christine only spoke in order to scream at Rick or to tell me about his behavior. As soon as Michael was fed, he was put down on the couch again to sleep. Although Christine did not present as depressed, she did describe difficulties with sleeping and eating and wanting to sleep all day. Christine described her parents in very black and white terms. Her mother was described as rejecting and very physically abusive. She was also alcoholic and had serious medical conditions. Christine ran away when she was 12 years of age and ended up in a home for runaways "because no foster home could deal with me." On the other hand, Christine described her father as "perfect and wonderful." He gave her everything she wanted and had always done so. Sexual abuse by anyone was denied. Although Christine seemed to be of average intelligence, she had only a Grade 10 education and had never been employed. She described a number of borderline symptoms such as extreme rage reactions and the need for relationships with men, but great difficulty in dealing with the closeness and intimacy of living with anyone.

"All the boys have a different father, and they're all no good, and I don't want anything to do with any of them," she explained. During the visit Christine went from lying on the couch, seemingly exhausted, to chatting on the phone in an animated way on what appeared to be a "sex line." When told about the Growing Together services, Christine was excited about them but showed some ambivalence. On the one hand, she wanted Rick in day care but at the same time wondered how she would get up in time to get him on the bus or walk him there. As a result of the assessment, a rating of extreme risk was assigned. Christine was offered ongoing home visits and help with finding day care for Rick. A development assessment to "see the reasons" for Rick's lack of speech was offered. Christine also agreed to attend a parenting class that could help her with Rick and computer classes so that she could "get a job." Table 10.4 lists the risk and protective factors and the services offered.

The Katana Family: Rostina (mother, 32 years old), Luksam (father, 35 years old), and Delicia (daughter, 1 month old)

Delicia and her parents were referred to Growing Together after an initial telephone screening by the public health nurse indicated that the family was very interested in services. It was also noted that Delicia had been born with a chromosomal disorder and that the parents were finding it very difficult to adjust to the disability. Both mother and father enthusiastically agreed to a home visit. As soon as the Tamil community home visitor arrived at the house, she was shown a picture of the parents' first baby, who had died at birth. Shortly after Rostina shared her fear about caring for Delicia and concerns that she, too, might die. It was clear that because of her anxiety, Rostina found it

TABLE 10.4
Christine and Michael

Risk Factors	Protective Factors	Services Offered
Infant	*Infant*	*Infant*
• Mother disappointed in sex of child	• Feeding and sleeping well • No biological or genetic difficulties	
Interactional or Parenting Variables	*Interactional or Parenting Variables*	*Interactional or Parenting Variables*
• Very negative and nonnurturing interaction • Older child has behavioral difficulties • Two eldest children in foster care	• Indicates some interest in learning about dealing with Rick's behavior problems	• Assessment at Developmental Clinic for Rick • Parenting class, Helping Encourage Affect Regulation (HEAR) to learn to deal with discipline and aggression of child
Parental History and Current Functioning	*Parental History and Current Functioning*	*Parental History and Current Functioning*
• Abuse and neglect by mother • Suspected sexual abuse by father • Separation into foster care and group home • Grade 10 education • Borderline symptoms including rage reactions • Lack of structure/routine • Some alcohol abuse • Possible prostitution	• Average intellectual level	• Home visitor to provide support and therapy
Sociodemographic and Societal Issues	*Sociodemographic and Societal Issues*	*Sociodemographic and Societal Issues*
• On welfare/unemployed • Subsidized housing • Ambivalent about using services • Single mother • Lack of support from mother		• Advocacy worker to access day care for Rick • Attendance at computer skills class

Overall Risk Level = (1) Extreme risk.

365

very difficult to hold and care for her infant in an involved way. The baby was obviously clean and well cared for, but it was Luksam who spent time with her and was able to encourage and coach her into warm interactions. Both parents reported that they came from warm, loving homes with many family members who took care of them as they were growing up. They also explained that their parents now lived in Canada and the whole family were very involved in the Tamil community. At this point, Rostina cried again about the shame she felt about Delicia's problems and how it was hard for her to attend family and community events with her. Both parents talked about their first baby's loss at this time indicating that they still felt very sad and did not understand the reason for his death. Both parents appeared to be intelligent and educated, had college educations, and although Luksam was underemployed performing factory work, he was attending classes and saw this only as a temporary situation. The home was well-organized, and a structure and routine were observed. Luksam spoke excellent English and Rostina was attending English as a Second Language classes when possible. The couple had a very supportive relationship and showed appropriate affection toward one another. In fact, one had the feeling that the couple had the ability to parent Delicia well, if they could be helped to provide interactions to encourage a secure attachment and enhance her development as much as possible. In view of the infant's biological difficulties and her mother's problems with bonding to the baby, a level of moderate risk was assigned. Mr. and Mrs. Katana were offered a variety of services. Two Tamil home visitors worked with the family, one in a more supportive role and the other to help them to enhance Delicia's development. It was particularly important to accompany the parents to the many medical visits that Delicia needed and even more important, to help the parents understand, assimilate, and use the information that was provided. Rostina attended a Tamil mothers' group where her worker was able to gradually help her share her concerns about Delicia with the other participants. Both parents were invited to join a parenting group where they could learn to provide stimulating activities for their daughter. See Table 10.5 for a list of the risk and protective factors and programs proposed for the family.

Conclusion

Assessment of infants, young children and their families in community-based settings presents a number of challenges and opportunities. Moreover, a program that is population-based and tries to reach all the families with young children in a particular high-risk area must be flexible and adapt regularly to be able to meet the needs identified by parents and respond to an ever-changing ethnic and cultural diversity. These realities create a number of challenges not encountered to the same extent by clinics that families choose to attend or by researchers who evaluate selected samples of the total population over a period of time. A balance constantly has to be found between offering and persuading parents in moderate to extreme risk situations to accept services and becoming too intrusive or threatening when they refuse to accept services. When services are refused, workers often feel they have failed the child and

TABLE 10.5
The Katana Family

Risk Factors	Protective Factors	Services Offered
Infant • Infant has chromosomal disorder • Intellectual delays and physical handicaps	*Infant* • Feeding and sleeping well • Infant responsive when alert	*Infant* • Full assessment at Developmental Clinic • Tracking of infant's development at clinic
Interactional or Parenting Variables • Mother concerned about attaching to infant • Mother feeling deep shame about infant's disabilities • Keeps infant at home so she will not be seen	*Interactional or Parenting Variables* • Infant physically well cared for • Committed father who provides sensitive, affectively warm interactions with baby	*Interactional or Parenting Variables* • Attend Tamil mother's group • Attend parent stimulation class
Parenting History and Current Functioning • Loss of first child • Grieving loss of "perfect" child	*Parental History and Current Functioning* • Warm marital relationship • Intelligent, well-educated parents • Father employed • Neither parent has medical condition or mental health problem	*Parental History and Current Functioning* • Home visitor to help parents deal with grief and losses • Support around attending and interpreting medical visits and information • Ideas to help them stimulate Delicia's development
Sociodemographic and Societal Issues • Recent life stresses of loss of baby and birth of handicapped baby	*Sociodemographic and Societal Issues* • Father employed • Upgrading and learning English	*Sociodemographic and Societal Issues*

Overall Risk Level = (3) Moderate risk.

have to be supported in understanding that the program cannot be meaningful to all families.

Nevertheless, the kind of assessment and program components discussed allow a unique opportunity to provide services within an ecological or transactional framework, integrating a variety of philosophies and approaches to intervention to the benefit of families. Although understanding and accepting the different perspectives on intervention of various workers has been difficult, it has allowed staff to increase both their understanding and expertise in providing a much broader range of services. Those who have tended to look only for risk and pathology are more open to seeing strengths and resiliency, while workers who emphasize health promotion are becoming more aware of symptoms and ways to work with very high-risk families.

Perhaps the most important lesson from these types of assessments has been that understanding both the strengths and risks within families allows us to continually strive to provide a variety of services. These aim to both enhance the strengths of families while at the same time designing and using proven approaches to deal with parental pathology, enhance rejecting or nonsensitive interactions, and provide families with support while reducing their isolation. This kind of approach, taking into account the problems but using strengths, allows the program to bring understanding to staff and through that understanding, a sense of optimism and a new purpose to families.

References

Aber, J. L., Allen, J. P., & Carlson, V. (1989). The effects of maltreatment on development during early childhood: Recent studies and their theoretical, clinical and policy implications. In D. Cicchetti & V. Carlson (Eds.), *Child maltreatment: Theory and research on the causes and consequences of child abuse and neglect* (pp. 579–619). Cambridge: Cambridge University Press.

Ainsworth, M. D. S., Blehar, M. C., Waters, E., & Wall, S. (1978). *Patterns of attachment: A psychological study of the strange situation.* Hillsdale, NJ: Erlbaum.

Allen, M. C., Brown, P., & Finlay, B. (1992). *Helping children by strengthening families: A look at family support programs.* Washington, DC: Children's Defense Fund.

Allen, M. C., Donohue, P. K., & Dusman, K. (1993). The limit of viability: Neonatal outcome of infants born at 22 to 25 weeks gestation. *New England Journal of Medicine, 329,* 1597–1601.

Andur, J. R., Mainland, M. K., & Parker, K. (1988). Diagnostic Inventory for Screening Children: Manual Kitchener. Kitchener Waterloo Hospital.

Anthony, E. J. (1982). The preventive approach to children at high risk for psychopathology and psychosis. *Journal of Children of Contemporary Society, 15*(1), 67–72.

Ards, S., & Harrell, A. (1993). Reporting of child maltreatment: A secondary analysis of the national incidence surveys. *Child Abuse and Neglect, 17*(3), 337–344.

Beardslee, W. R., Bemporad, J. V., Keller,

M. B., & Klerman, G. L. (1983). Children of parents with major affective disorders: A review. *American Journal of Psychiatry, 140*(7), 825–832.

Bell, R. Q., & Pearl, D. (1982). Psychosocial changes in risk groups: Implications for early intervention. *Prevention in Human Services, 1*(4), 45–59.

Benoit, D., & Parker, K. C. H. (1994). Stability and transmission of attachment across three generations. *Child Development, 65*(5), 1444–1456.

Bradley, R. H., Whiteside, L., Mundfrom, D. J., & Casey, P. H. (1994). Early indications of resilience and their relation to experiences in the home environments of low birth weight premature children living in poverty. *Child Development, 65*(2), 346–360.

Bricker, J., Potter, L. W., & Bricker, D. (1995). *The ages and stages questionnaire-(ASQ) User's guide.* Baltimore, MD: Brookes.

Brickman, P., Kidder, L. H., Coates, D., Rabinowitz, V., Cohn, E., & Karuza, J. (1983). The dilemmas of helping: Making aid fair and effective. In J. D. Fisher, A. Nadler, & B. M. DePaulo (Eds.), *New directions in helping: Vol. 1. Recipient reactions to aid* (pp. 18–51). New York: Academic.

Buckner, J. C. (1987). The development of an instrument to measure neighbourhood cohesion. *American Journal of Community Psychology, 16*(6), 771–791.

Byles, J., Byrne, C., Boyle, M. H., & Offord, D. R. (1988). Ontario child health study: Reliability and validity of the general functioning subscale of the McMaster family assessment device. *Family Process, 27*, 97–104.

Caldwell, B., & Bradley, R. (1984). *Home ob-servation for measurement of the environment.* Arkansas: University of Arkansas.

Canadian Centre for Justice. (1992). *Family violence in Canada.* Ottawa, Ontario: Author.

Carnegie Task Force on Meeting the Needs of Young Children. (1994). *Starting points: Meeting the needs of our youngest children.* New York: Carnegie Corporation of New York.

Carro, M. G., Grant, K. E., Gotlib, I. H., & Compass, B. E. (1993). Postpartum depression and child development: An investigation of mothers and fathers as sources of risk and resilience. *Development and Psychopathology, 5*(4), 567–579.

Casey, P. H., Bradley, R. H., Nelson, J. Y., & Whaley, S. A. (1988). The clinical assessment of a child's social and physical environment during health visits. *Developmental and Behavioral Pediatrics, 9*(6), 333–338.

Cicchetti, D., & Rizley, R. (1981). Developmental perspectives on the etiology, intergenerational transmission and sequelae of child maltreatment. In R. Rizley & D. Cicchetti (Eds.), *New directions for child development: Developmental perspectives on child maltreatment* (pp. 31–55). San Francisco: Jossey-Bass.

Cicchetti, D., & Rogosch, F. A. (1996). Equifinality and multifinality in developmental psychopathology. *Development and Psychopathology, 8*(4), 597–600.

Coll, G. C., Kagan, J., & Resnick, J. S. (1984). Behavioral inhibition in young children. *Child Development, 55*, 1005–1019.

Crnic, K. A., Greenberg, M. T., & Slough, N. M. (1986). Early stress and social support influences on mothers and high-risk infants' functioning in late infancy. *Infant Mental Health Journal, 7*(1), 19–33.

Crnic, K. A., & Stormshak, E. (1997). The effectiveness of providing social support for families of children at risk. In M. J. Guralnick (Ed.), *The effectiveness of early intervention* (pp. 209–225). Baltimore, MD: Brookes.

Crockenberg, S., & Litman, C. (1990). Autonomy as competence in 2-year-olds: Maternal correlates of child defiance, compliance and self-assertion. *Developmental Psychology, 26*(6), 961–971.

Cutrona, C., & Russell, D. (1989). The provision of social relationships and adaptation to stress. *Advances in Personal Relationships, 1*, 37–67.

Dail, P. W. (1990). The psychosocial context of homeless mothers with young children: Program and policy implications. *Child Welfare, 69*(4), 291–308.

Davies, P. T., & Cummings, E. M. (1994). Marital conflict and child adjustment: An emotional security hypothesis. *Psychological Bulletin, 116*(3), 387–411.

Derogatis, L. R. (1993). *Brief symptom inventory: Administration, scoring and procedures manual.* Minneapolis, MN: National Computer Systems, Inc.

Doherty, G. (1997). *Zero to six: The basis for school readiness.* Hull, Quebec: Applied Research Branch, Human Resources Development Canada.

Dubrow, N. F., & Garbarino, J. (1989). Living in the war zone: Mothers and young children in a public housing development. *Child Welfare, 68*(1), 3–20.

Dumas, J. E. (1986). Indirect influence of maternal social contacts on mother-child interactions: A setting event analysis. *Journal of Abnormal Child Psychology, 14*(2), 205–216.

Dunst, C., Trivette, C., & Deal, A. (1988). *Enabling and empowering families: Principles and guidelines for practice.* Cambridge, MA: Brookline Books.

Dunst, C. J., & Leet, H. E. (1987). Measuring the adequacy of resources in households with young children. *Child: Care Health and Development, 13*, 111–125.

Dunst, C. J., & Trivette, C. M. (1987). Enabling and empowering families: Conceptual and intervention issues. *School Psychology Review, 16*(4), 443–456.

Egeland, B., & Sroufe, A. (1981). Developmental sequelae of maltreatment in infancy. In R. Rizley & D. Cicchetti (Eds.), *New directions for child development: Developmental perspectives on child maltreatment* (pp. 77–92). San Francisco: Jossey-Bass.

Egeland, B., & Erickson, M. F. (1990). Rising above the past: Strategies for helping new mothers break the cycle of abuse and neglect. *Zero to Three, 11*(2), 29–35.

Fergusson, D. M., Horwood, L. J., & Lynskey, M. T. (1992). Family change, parental discord, and early offending: Neuropsychological deficits. *Journal of Child Psychology and Psychiatry and Allied Disciplines, 33*(6), 1059–1075.

Fields, T. M., Dempsey, J. R., Hallock, N. H., & Shuman, H. H. (1978). The mother's assessment of the behavior of her infant. *Infant Behavior and Development, 1*, 156–167.

Finkelhor, D., & Dziuba-Leatherman, J. (1994). Victimization of children. *American Psychologist, 49*(3), 173–183.

Fisher, D. G. (1985). *Family relationship variables and programs influencing juvenile delinquency.* Ottawa, Ontario: Solicitor General of Canada.

Garbarino, J. (1992). *Children and families in the social environment.* New York: Aldine de Gruyter.

Garbarino, J., Kostelny, K., & Dubrow, N. (1991). *No place to be a child: Growing up in a war zone.* Lexington, MA: Lexington Books.

Glick, P. C. (1988). The role of divorce in the changing family structure: Trends and variations. In S. A. Wolchick & P. Karoly (Eds.), *Children of divorce* (pp. 3–34). New York: Gardiner Press.

Gobel, S., & Shindledecker, R. (1993). Characteristics of children whose parents have been incarcerated. *Hospital and Community Psychology, 44*(7), 656–660.

Gomby, D. S., Larson, C. S., Lewit, E. M., & Behrman, R. E. (1993). Home visiting: Analysis and recommendations. *The Future of Children, 3*(3), 6–22.

Greenspan, S. I., Wieder, S., Nover, R. A., Lieberman, A. F., Lourie, R. S., & Robinson, M. D. (Eds.). (1987). *Infants in multirisk families: Case studies in preventive intervention.* Madison, CT: International Universities Press.

Hack, M., Taylor, G., & Klein, N. (1994). School outcomes in children with birth weights under 750 g. *New England Journal of Medicine, 331,* 753–759.

Hanvey, L., Avard, D., & Graham, I. (1994). *The health of Canada's children* (2nd ed.). Ottawa, Ontario: Canadian Institute of Child Health.

Hart, B., & Risley, T. R. (1995). *Meaningful differences in everyday experiences of young children.* Baltimore, MD: Brookes.

Hechtman, L. (1989). Teenage mothers and their children: Risks and problems. A review. *Canadian Journal of Psychiatry, 34*(6), 569–575.

Helfer, R., Hoffmeister, J., & Schneider, C. (1978). *Michigan Screening Profile of Parenting (MSPP) Manual.* Boulder, CO: Test Analysis and Development Corp.

Hewlett, S. A. (1991). Mainstream kids and the time deficit. In S. Hewlett (Ed.), *When the bough breaks: The cost of neglecting our children* (pp. 62–100). New York: Basic Books.

Ireton, H. (1992). *Manual of the child development inventory.* Minneapolis, MI: Behavior Science Systems.

Jouriles, E., Murphy, C., & O'Leary, D. (1989). Interspousal aggression, marital discord, and child problems. *Journal of Consulting and Clinical Psychology, 57*(3), 453–455.

Lalonde, R. N., Majumder, S., & Parris, R. D. (1995). Preferred response to situations of housing and employment discrimination. *Journal of Applied Social Psychology, 25,* 1105–1119.

Landy, S. (1996). *Research on home visiting in early intervention programs.* Paper prepared for the Infant Mental Health Project, Toronto, Ontario.

Landy, S. (In press). *Pathways to competence: A program to encourage healthy social and emotional development in young children.* Baltimore, MD: Brookes.

Landy, S., Peters, Dev. R., Arnold, R., Allen, A. B., Brookes, F., & Jewell, S. (1998). Evaluation of "Staying on Track": An early identification, tracking and referral system. *Infant Mental Health Journal, 19*(1), 34–58.

Larson, C. P., Collet, J. P., & Hanley, J. A. (1987). The predicture accuracy of prenatal and post-partum high risk identification. *Canadian Journal of Public Health, 78,* 188–192.

Lero, D. S., Goelman, H., Pence, A. R., Brockman, L. M., & Nuttall, S. (1992). *Parental work patterns and child care needs.* Ottawa, Ontario: Statistics Canada.

Lewis, D. O. (1992). From abuse to violence: Psychophysiological consequences of maltreatment. *Journal of American Academy of Child and Adolescent Psychiatry, 31*(3), 383–391.

Lung, C. T., & Daro, N. (1996). *Current trends in child abuse reporting and fatalities: The results of the 1995 Annual Fifty State Survey.* Chicago, IL: National Committee for the Prevention of Child Abuse.

Luthar, S. S., & Zigler, E. (1992). Intelligence and social competence among high-risk adolescents. *Development and Psychopathology, 4,* 287–299.

MacMillan, H. L., Fleming, J. E., & Trocme, N. (1997). Prevalence of child physical and sexual abuse in the community: Results from the Ontario Health Supplement. *Journal of the American Medical Association, 278,* 131–135.

Magura, S., Moses, B. S., & Jones, M. A. (1987). *Assessing risk and measuring change in families: The Family Risk Scales.* Washington, DC, Child Welfare League of America.

Main, M., & Goldwyn, R. (1984). Predicting rejection of her infant from mother's representation of her own experiences: Implications for the abused-abusing intergenerational cycle. *Child Abuse and Neglect, 8*(2), 203–217.

Malinosky-Rummell, R., & Hansen, D. J. (1993). Long-term consequences of childhood physical abuse. *Psychological Bulletin, 114*(1), 68–79.

Mantini-Atkinson, T. (1993). *Competence and adaptation in developmentally delayed children: The moderating effects of child and family qualities.* Unpublished doctoral dissertation, University of Toronto, Canada.

Massie, H. N., & Campbell, B. K. (1984). The Massie Campbell Scale of Mother Infant Attachment Indicators During Stress. In H. N. Massie & J. Rosenthal (Eds.), *Childhood psychosis in the first four years of life* (pp. 253–282). New York: McGraw-Hill.

McLoyd, V. C., & Wilson, L. (1991). The strain of living poor: Parenting, social support, and child mental health. In A. C. Huston (Ed.), *Children in poverty* (pp. 105–135). New York: Cambridge University Press.

Miller, J. S., Williams, K. M., English, D. J., & Olmstead, J. (1987). *Risk assessment in child protection: A review of the literature.* Washington, DC, American Public Welfare Association.

Milner, J. S., Gold, R. G., Ayoub, C., & Jacewitz, M. M. (1984). Predictive validity of the Child Abuse Potential Inventory. *Journal of Consulting and Clinical Psychology, 52,* 879–884.

Moroney, R. M. (1992). Social support systems: Families and social policies. In S. L. Kagan, D. R. Powell, B. Weissbourd, & E. Zigler (Eds.), *America's family support programs: Perspectives and prospects* (pp. 31–37). London: Yale University Press.

Murphy, S., Orkow, B., & Nicola, R. M. (1985). Prenatal prediction of child abuse and neglect: A prospective study. *Child Abuse and Neglect, 9,* 225–235.

Myers, J. K., & Weissman, M. M. (1980). Use of a self-report symptom scale to detect depression in a community sample. *American Journal of Psychiatry, 37,* 1081–1084.

New York State Department of Social Services. (1991). *New York State Risk Assessment: An overview.* Albany, New York: Author.

Offord, D. R., Boyle, M. H., Fleming, J. E., & Blum, H. M. (1989). The Ontario Child Health Study: Summary of selected results. *Canadian Journal of Psychiatry, 34*(6), 483–491.

Offord, D. R., & Lipman, E. L. (1996). Emotional and behavioural problems. National Longitudinal Study of Children and Youth. In Statistics Canada, *Growing up in Canada*. Ottawa, Ontario: Statistics Canada.

O'Leary, K. D. (1987). *Prevalence, etiology, and treatment of spousal abuse*. Address at the National Institute of Mental Health, Washington, DC.

Pape, B., Byrne, C., & Ivask, A. (1996). *Analysis of the impact of affective disorders on families and children*. Submitted to the Strategic Fund for Children's Mental Health, Health Canada, Ottawa.

Pedersen, W. (1994). Parental relations, mental health, and delinquency in adolescence. *Adolescence, 29*(116), 975–990.

Pence, A. R., & Goelman, H. (1991). The relationship of regulation, training and motivation to quality of care in family day care. *Child and Youth Care Forum, 20*(2), 83–101.

Pepper, S., & Stuart, B. (1992). Quality of family day care in licensed and unlicensed homes. *Canadian Journal of Research in Early Childhood Education, 3*(2), 109–118.

Phares, V., & Compas, B. E. (1993). The role of fathers in child and adolescent psychopathology: Make way for Daddies. In M. E. Hertzig & E. A. Faber (Eds.), *Annual progress in child psychiatry and child development* (pp. 344–401). New York: Brunner/Mazel.

Rabkin, J. G. (1979). Ethnic density and psychiatric hospitalization: Hazards of minority status. *American Journal of Psychiatry, 136*(12), 1562–1566.

Ramey, C. T., Ramey, S. L., Gaines, R., & Blair, C. (1994). *Two-generation early interventions: A child development perspective*. Article prepared for the Foundation of Child Development.

Reich, W., Earls, F., Frankel, O., & Shayka, J. J. (1993). Psychopathology in children of alcoholics. *Journal of the American Academy of Child and Adolescent Psychiatry, 32*(5), 995–1002.

Ricks, M. H. (1983). *Individual differences in the preschoolers' competence: Contributions of attachment history and concurrent environmental support*. Unpublished doctoral dissertation, University of Massachusetts at Amherst.

Ricks, M. H. (1985). The social transmission of parental behaviour: Attachment across generations. In I. Bretherton & E. Waters (Eds.), Growing points of attachment theory and research (pp. 211–227). *Monographs of the Society for Research in Child Development, 50* (1–2, Serial No. 209).

Rutter, M. (1979). Protective factors in children's responses to stress and disadvantage. In M. W. Kent & J. E. Rolf (Eds.), *Social competence in children* (pp. 49–74). Hanover, NH: University Press of New England.

Rutter, M. (1989). Intergenerational continuities and discontinuities in serious parenting difficulties. In D. Cicchetti & V. Carlson (Eds.), *Child maltreatment: Theory and research on the causes and consequences of child abuse and neglect* (pp. 317–348). Cambridge: Cambridge University Press.

Rutter, M. (1990). Psychosocial resilience and protective mechanisms. In J. Rolf, A. S. Masten, D. Cicchetti, K. H. Niechterlein & S. Weintraub (Eds.), *Risk and protective factors in the development of psychopathology* (pp. 181–214). New York: Cambridge University Press.

Sameroff, A. J., & Fiese, B. H. (1990). Transactional regulation and early intervention. In S. J. Meisels & J. P. Shonkoff (Eds.), *Handbook of early childhood interven-*

tion (pp. 119–149). Cambridge: Cambridge University Press.

Sameroff, J. J., Seifer, R., Barocas, R., Zax, M., & Greenspan, S. I. (1987). Intelligence quotient scores of 4-year-old children: Social environmental risk factors. *Pediatrics, 79*(3), 343–350.

Sanson, A., Oberklaid, F., Pedlow, R., & Prior, M. (1991). Risk indicators: Assessment of infancy predictors of pre-school behavioral adjustment. *Journal of Child Psychology and Psychiatry and Allied Disciplines, 32*(4), 609–626.

Sarason, I. G., Johnson, J. H., & Siegel, J. M. (1978). Assessing the impact of life changes: The development of the Life Experiences Survey. *Journal of Consulting and Clinical Psychology, 46*(5), 932–946.

Schteingart, J. S., Molnar, J., Klein, T. P., & Lowe, C. B. (1995). Homelessness and child functioning in the context of risk and protective factors moderating child outcomes. *Journal of Clinical Child Psychology, 24*(3), 320–331.

Schultz-Jøgensen, P., Kyng, B., Maar, V., Rasmussen, L., & Højlund, L. (1987). Is prevention possible in the preschool years? A longitudinal study of a group of preschool children in a local community. *Nordic Psychology, 39*, 255–267.

Shaw, D. S., & Vondra, J. I. (1993). Chronic family adversity and infant attachment security. *Journal of Child Psychology and Psychiatry and Allied Disciplines, 34*(7), 1205–1215.

Shaw, D. S., Vondra, J. I., Hammerding, K. D., Keenan, K., & Dunn, M. (1994). Chronic family adversity and early child behavior problems: A longitudinal study of low income families. *Journal of Child Psychology and Psychiatry and Allied Disciplines, 35*(6), 1109–1122.

Sims-Jones, N., Stewart, P., Hanvey, L., &

McDonald, J. (1997). *Screening and assessment of pregnant women and postpartum families: The Healthy Babies/Healthy Children Program*. Ottawa, Ontario: Ottawa-Carleton Health Department.

Sluzki, C. E. (1979). Migration and family conflict. *Family Process, 18*(4), 379–390.

St. Pierre, R. G., Layzer, J. I., & Barnes, H. V. (1995). Two-generation programs: Design, cost and short-term effectiveness. *The Future of Children, 5*(3), 76–93.

Steinhauer, P. D. (1996). *Developing resiliency in children from disadvantaged populations*. Toronto, Ontario: University of Toronto.

Strauss, M. A., Gelles, R. J., & Steinmetz, S. K. (1980). *Behind closed doors: Violence in the American family*. New York: Anchor Books.

Thomas, A., Chess, S., & Birch, H. G. (1968). *Temperament and behavior disorders in children*. New York: New York University Press.

Trocme, N., McPhee, D., Tam, K. K., & Hay, T. (1994). *Ontario incidence study of reported child abuse and neglect*. Toronto, Ontario: Institute for the Prevention of Child Abuse.

Wasik, B. H., Ramey, C. T., Bryant, D. M., & Sparling, J. J. (1990). A longitudinal study of two early intervention strategies: Project CARE. *Child Development, 61*(6), 1682–1696.

Weinman, M., Robinson, M., Simmons, J., Schreiber, N., & Stafford, B. (1989). Pregnant teens: Differential pregnancy resolution and treatment implications. *Child Welfare, 68*, 45–55.

Weiss, H. B. (1993). Home visits: Necessary but not sufficient. *The Future of Children, 3*(3), 113–128.

Werner, E. E. (1989). High-risk children in young adulthood: A longitudinal study from birth to 32 years. *American Journal of Orthopsychiatry, 59*(1), 72–81.

Werner, E. E. (1993). Risk, resilience, and recovery: Perspectives from the Kauai Longitudinal Study. *Development and Psychopathology, 5,* 503–515.

Werner, E. E. (1995). Resilience in development. *Current Directions in Psychological Science, 4*(3), 81–85.

White, K. (1984). *The different and legitimate roles of advocacy and science.* Paper presented at the CEC/DBC conference, Greely, CO.

Wieder, S., Jasnow, M., Greenspan, S. I., & Strauss, M. (1983). Identifying the multirisk family prenatally: Antecedent psychosocial factors and infant development trends. *Infant Mental Health Journal, 4*(3), 165–201.

Wolfner, G. D., & Gelles, R. J. (1993). A profile of violence towards children: A national study. *Child Abuse and Neglect, 17*(2), 197–212.

Zeanah, C. H., Boris, N. W., & Larrieu, J. A. (1997). Infant development and developmental risk: A review of the past 10 years. *Journal of the American Academy of Child and Adolescent Psychiatry, 36*(2), 165–178.

Zigler, E., & Weiss, H. (1985). Family support systems: An ecological approach to child development. In R. N. Rapoport (Ed.), *Children, youth and families: The action-research relationship* (pp. 166–205). Cambridge: Cambridge University Press.

Zyblock, M. (1996). *Child poverty trends in Canada: Exploring depth and incidence from a total money perspective, 1975–1992.* Ottawa, Ontario: Human Resources Development Canada.

11

Training Mental Health and Other Professionals in Infant Mental Health: Conversations with Trainees

Jeree H. Pawl, Maria St. John, and Judith H. Pekarsky

11

Introduction

From 1973 until mid-1979, Selma Fraiberg directed an infant mental health program, the Child Development Project at the University of Michigan. It was a program funded by the National Institutes of Mental Health and the Grant Foundation to explore and demonstrate the efficacy of working therapeutically with relationships between babies and/or toddlers and their parents. Fraiberg's work in this area is commonly recognized as a founding force in the field of infant mental health.

In 1979, Fraiberg and two colleagues from the University of Michigan began a similar program, the Infant-Parent Program, at the University of California, San Francisco. Since that time the Infant-Parent Program has provided services to families with troubled relationships with their infants and toddlers and, over time, has focused on ever more seriously troubled families. An urban population in 1998, is more beset by chaos, stressors of all kinds, mental health problems, chemical dependence, violence, despair, and hopelessness than was the population of a small university town, however distressed, in 1973. Nonetheless, the basic understanding of why intervention at this time of life is crucial and why the parameters of the therapeutic relationship between parent, child, and therapist are critical remain unchanged.

Since its inception in 1979, the Infant-Parent Program has been involved continuously and increasingly in the training of various mental health professionals and other professionals from different disciplines in in-

fant mental health. The arduous effort involved in the work with these increasingly stressed families (visible and palpable) over 19 years has sharpened the awareness of what trainees need to learn, why they need to learn it, and how such learning might occur.

The Challenges of Working with Infants and Parents

Working with infants and toddlers is provocative and evocative. Many child therapists find that a child's feelings can be more disturbing to the therapist than the feelings of an adult. Children engage the therapist at a lesser distance from the therapist's childhood experience. So too, people experience the abuse of a child as far more enraging than adult abuse though this too is certainly distressing. The special quality of the rage of most adults in response to the maltreatment of a child stems from the fact that a parent or caregiver, someone entrusted and possibly trusted, has violated a basic cohering expectation of ongoing civilization: The expectation of the nurturance and protection of the young. Simultaneously, the abuse of a child engages in adults whatever resentments, antagonisms, anxieties, and even terrors that their own childhood relationships held.

An experienced social worker in a hospital pediatric setting knows how challenging it is to modulate and reframe the outrage that staff who suspect parental abuse or neglect feel toward the parents. The expression of that rage will need to be contained so that it does not complicate an already complex parental response to what has occurred and become, in effect, a further interference.

The challenges increase exponentially when a therapist relates to a relationship—that of a parent and a child. As an aspect of training, many programs including the Child Development Project and at times the Infant-Parent Program have used observation of volunteer mothers in their homes to learn about infant-parent interaction. The reported power of the observer's experience underscores the potency simply of standing wholly outside of a parent-child relationship and watching. When people become parents and enter a parent-child relationship in this way, it, of course, is even more powerfully engaging. As parents, however, they do not expect of themselves the balanced, nonjudgmental, self-reflective awareness of their responses necessary for an infant-parent therapist to achieve. It is with awareness of this challenging context that we have thought about what the goals of training need to be.

Training Goals: What We Most Want People to Learn

General Description

Many kinds of knowledge may be usefully accumulated and applied in infant-parent psychotherapy, but what we seek primarily to cultivate with trainees is a set of sensibilities integrated with a particular body of knowledge. These include an appreciation of early development in all its complexity, an appreciation of adult development with some special areas of emphasis, and an ability to think in terms of the interplay between the internal experience of a small child and the internal experience of his or her parents.

These abilities must be embedded in an increasing self-awareness on the part of the trainees of their own internal processes, awareness of their own impact on the parents and child, and ultimately the continual striving for a balanced and comfortable sense of their therapeutic place in the interpersonal system into which they enter. The fact that this experience within our program is embedded in a home-visiting model also has many important influences on the trainee, the parent and child, and the process of treatment. While the staff of the Infant-Parent Program have varied disciplinary identities, areas of expertise, and theoretical approaches, we share a commitment to thinking with trainees about these related realms of experience in the context of conveying knowledge infant development, adult development, and the internal experiences of infant and parent. These are the areas in which we wish to affect the development of our trainees. Indeed, we have learned from annual evaluation conversations with trainees about the work and the training program that these are the areas in which they feel their development is affected. The formal didactic part of the program evolves over the years partly in response to what we learn from trainees. These conversations with trainees have also influenced this chapter and are referred to as they seem particularly relevant to the issues discussed.

Infant Development

We understand infant development as an interactive phenomenon. We see the infant-parent system as driven in part by the rapidly emerging cognitive, motor, and social-emotional capacities of the infant. When these unfold without undue environmental impingement, the pace of development is at the same time gradual and breakneck. Infant development demands astounding levels of responsivity and flexibility on the part of parents and at the same time it teaches these. It unfolds along predictable lines in ways that are in every instance absolutely unique.

Trainees rarely enter the program with extensive academic or experiential backgrounds in early childhood development. With some important exceptions, trainees from all disciplines report having received very little training in infant development, and few have worked clinically with infants and toddlers. Those trainees who do enter the program with more experience with infants and toddlers tend to have worked in childcare, early childhood education, or early intervention settings. Sometimes these trainees report that these backgrounds are a liability in the early months of the training program, because they provide structures of thought, ways of mentally and emotionally organizing material about infants and toddlers, and, most forcefully, ways of interacting with them that have to be unlearned or at least loosened, in order that the new sensibilities in question may be developed.

At base, attention to development in the Infant-Parent Program means viewing the infant as an active participant in the relationships in which he or she is embedded, a participant whose methods, patterns, and qualities of interaction expand rapidly and both shape and are shaped by their experiences in the world. It means identifying the existence in a parent-child dyad or triad of those aspects of the relationship that can offer the possibility of change and growth. One attempts with the family to acknowledge and appreciate both these positive aspects and their impediments. It implies a unique position for the therapist and a special orientation for the treatment, since the central focus is not on explicating the therapist-patient relationship, but on the *infant-parent* relationship and on the relationship of the therapist to that context. Hope for positive change rests less with the traditional therapeutic process than with the healing and generative potential of the infant-parent relationship itself. Central, however, is the experience of the parent within the therapist-patient relationship.

Adult Development

The Infant-Parent Program is uniquely able to assist trainees in thinking about two particular aspects of adult development. These are adult patients' experiences of being parents and, more broadly, the minutiae of parents' daily lives. Clearly these two areas of experience are intimately related, but they may be considered separately.

Most trainees enter the program with some level of understanding of individual psychopathology, whether their prior training has involved primarily children or adults. While diagnostic skills are clearly indispensable, we find that most trainees have had little help in considering and factoring in the material conditions or concrete circumstances, particularly, as literally observed, of people's lives. This ability must be cultivated in order for a diagnostic profile or psychodynamic formulation to be meaningful and useful. Trainees must learn to observe the ways in which a parent's concrete circumstances both reflect and affect his or her personality, emotional experience, patterns of thought, preoccupations, commitments, and characteristic modes of relating, including style as a parent.

This process of observation is a delicate one. Because our primary mode of intervention is home-visiting, trainees receive an enormous amount of information about the external realities of parents' lives. Often during the first months of the training year, the most urgent project for trainees involves managing and organizing the dizzying wealth of information and impressions they are absorbing. Often many of the painful aspects of this material surpass the individual family to which the therapist is there to attend and reflect as well a whole way of existing in the world that is very new to the trainee. It takes time for trainees to be able to distinguish between their responses to an individual family and a set of social and historical realities. It is crucial that they be assisted in sorting through their own internal experiences so that they are able to make such distinctions. Serious dangers adhere in trainees remaining either hyper- or hypoimpressed by the social conditions with which patients contend.

Trainees are able to assist parents in thinking about and identifying their feelings about their class, race, or ethnic position only if the trainees are capable of conducting such an analysis of themselves and clearly identifying their own responses to the class, race, and ethnic presentation of the patient. Any or all of these realms of experience may or may not be central to a given treatment, and to impose an inquiry into any one of these, when it is a remote or irrelevant matter to a patient, is as injurious as ignoring it when it is central. These three are only the crudest of the categories which a trainee must take in and be prepared to take up or not, according to the desire and needs of a family. Immigration histories and generational histories, ideas of community and social roles, political and intellectual identities, positions in relation to institutions, sexual and gender experiences, experiences of time, expectations regarding age, relationships to language, and senses of bodily reality are among the many realms of experience about which trainees must be prepared to abandon their expectations. The same tattoo on two different forearms, the same word on two different pairs of lips, or the same game of pretend-dropping a child played by two different fathers may have meanings which are vastly divergent and may or may not be something that needs or invites therapeutic discussion. With respect to the way the parent interacts with his infant or toddler, therapists must strive for a similar radical suspension of expectations, accompanied by exquisite attention and infinite curiosity. There are an infinite number of ways to raise a child, and it is not the role of the infant-parent therapist to prescribe one. Instead, the infant-parent therapist uses all of his or her skills, ability to think and feel, and personal style to collaboratively define with the parent his or her experience of being a parent and experience and understanding of his or her child.

The Internal Experiences of Infant and Parent

Professional recognition that infants have internal experiences which are complex, yet coherent, has been bestowed only fairly recently. The ideas that infants and toddlers do not understand much, do not think or feel much, and cannot participate in things much persist with appalling tenacity. An emergency room doctor at a leading pediatric hospital recently prepared to perform a painful procedure on the 18-month-old son of one of our mothers. This woman had come to understand enough to ask the doctor to tell her what he was going to do so that she could explain it to the child. The doctor responded by saying, "There's no use telling him. He's too young to understand."

Infant-parent psychotherapy works because infants do understand. From their earliest hours and days, they recognize what is familiar, register deviations from the norm, respond to particular people above almost all else, and attempt actively to influence their world. Infants do what they do and behave as they do not randomly, but for internal reasons, and this is true even in the face of any degree of physiological or environmental impingements. Perhaps the most important thing trainees learn at the Infant-Parent Program is to credit and attempt to understand the specific logic of each infant's internal experience. This is a perception that must be

conveyed to (if it is not initially shared with) a parent, and it is a process that can only be carried out in collaboration with the parent.

This assumption of the intelligibility of the infant's internal experience is extended also to the infant that the parent once was. A central tenet of infant-parent psychotherapy holds that for many parents, confusions and strange convictions remain regarding their own earliest experience. These confusions and convictions exert a powerful influence throughout one's life and frequently come to bear in problematic ways when one finds oneself in the position of caring for an infant of one's own. It is often the task of an infant-parent psychotherapist to reconstruct with a parent the logic of his or her own internal experience as an infant or small child in order to understand how this history is living on in the parent's present relationship with his or her child.

This process of reconstruction may not be overt, however. Some treatments do pivot around a parent's becoming conscious, for example, of a previously unconscious feeling or belief which lingers from his or her early childhood and gradually articulating this verbally in order to release himself or herself from a painful repetition with the child. Many other treatments progress, however, in more oblique relation to a parent's historical troubles or even traumas, and conversations remain at an overt level faithful to the present relationship between parent and child. Change is possible in these instances when a parent is able, with assistance, to think about the relationship between his or her own ideas and feelings and his or her child's. This present understanding can reverberate within the parent in such a way that historical constrictions and convictions are loosened and losses are mourned even without historical events being specifically discussed or consciously remembered or identified by the parent. Concomitantly, as well, a relationship between the parent and the therapist, when the therapist is consistently geared to understanding, respecting, and showing genuine curiosity and concern, may also work in the same way to loosen parental expectations about relationships, in general. Parental expectations that narrow the possibilities of a parent perceiving anything other than what he or she expects may be challenged such that a parent can experience contemporary interpersonal transactions for their own specific qualities.

The tendency for both infants and therapists to represent for parents images from their own infancies is thus as much of an asset as it is a liability. It allows for painful repetitions, but it also enables powerful transformations. When trainees develop a sense of the intergenerational significance of early experience and the potentially intergenerational resonance of therapeutic intervention, this has an effect on their clinical work regardless of the mode of treatment they go on to practice.

Home Visiting

All of the things that trainees learn about infant development, adult development, and the internal experience of infants and parents occur in the context of their experience in making home visits. The basic reason for providing mental health services through a home-visiting model is to be able to offer those services to people who, for whatever reason, would not otherwise be able to receive them. Whether because of serious disturbance, lack of motivation, general hopelessness, utter inconvenience, or even impossibility, these people would be unable to arrive at an office at a given time with any regularity or at all.

This possibility of services being delivered in the home will be perceived by the recipients with delight, curiosity, relief, dismay, suspicion, rage, boredom, acquiescence, and a variety of other interesting affects. In effect, the therapist becomes the activist in this essential role reversal, offering, seeking, pursuing, and possibly even feeling uncomfortably seductive. From the beginning, this creates a very different dynamic than the usual therapeutic arrangement, instantly raising the issue of how this offer and oneself are perceived and resulting in encounters that have a unique meaning to each particular person.

Almost always, the offer itself is embedded in a series of precipitating events, requests, suggestions, or even mandates, and these further define it. As it happens, the home-visited are rarely individuals who are actively seeking or trying to arrange for mental health treatment. Again, this is a reversal. Imagine someone sophisticated about mental health (you, for example) who was seeking mental health treatment for himself or herself and being told that the therapist prefers to see his or her patients in their homes. The response to that scenario casts into relief the fact that the population likely to be home-visited tends to be unsophisticated regarding mental health treatment, perhaps even hostile toward it, but at the same time, they are rarely distressed by the offer being contradictory to what they imagine mental health treatment to be. There are exceptions to this, but it is generally true. It illuminates as well the reversal the mental health professional experiences.

The special issues raised by home-visiting are interesting, challenging, and endless, and our trainees continue to confront them throughout their training. The treatment efforts of most mental health professionals, including our trainees, have been confined to offices, often with a display of door plaques that suggest their expertise. The therapist sits in a designated seat. The patients all sit in the seat indicated to them. There are no unexpected interruptions, and it is clear that the person seeking help will arrive at a particular time and leave at a designated time. Those who seek professional help expect all of this, anticipate that the therapist will be helpful and that the therapist will be in charge. Therapists often oblige.

None of the preceding is true within the home-visiting model. The framework for the treatment will have to be created each time with each patient, and this reality too must be learned. The great virtue of home visiting for the development of a professional is that one's professionalism becomes internalized and not tethered to an environment, a predictable format, or anything but the continual understanding of this unique professional therapeutic process—a process of which the professional is the careful, attentive, respectful shepherd.

Many trainees express concerns initially about making home visits. Some people are worried about their physical safety or the safety of their cars in high-crime neighborhoods. Many are properly worried about the integrity of their professional sense of themselves outside of the "frame" of the clinical office. Indeed, while trainees have very rarely in the history of the program felt their physical safety was actually threatened, all report that their sense of themselves as therapists was seriously challenged in the context of home visiting.

Home visiting means many things even prior to the individual meanings any particular hour of contact has for any particular family and trainee. "Home" means that this is the place where this family lives. It is an intimate place, even if it is not wholly private in the sense that it may be owned by someone else, and/or the family may feel or may perhaps be obliged to admit social workers who come, public health nurses, or infant-parent psychotherapists regardless of their own preferences on these matters.

This home may or may not be the place a parent thinks of as home. A Mexican woman was referred to our program under the auspices of "medical neglect" of her two-year-old daughter. In the course of treatment, it became clear that this woman's "home" was not the small urban apartment in which she and her daughter dwelled, but the village in which she herself had grown. She could imagine her daughter healing only there, at "home," and if her daughter were to recover in the United States, this mother's idea of home would be radically challenged.

For most very young children, home is the place where everything that means anything happens. For some children it represents the absolute limits of their world. One mother in our program was severely depressed, such that it was extremely difficult for her to take her toddler daughter even to the park more than a couple of times per week. This little girl watched the comings and goings of the pigeons outside her window with steady interest as they, her neighbors, and the infant-parent therapist represented the only reminder she had of a world beyond her mother and their apartment. To be a regular visitor in a small child's home is to be a figure in his or her inner world.

Recently, a therapist was working with a father and stepmother in a situation where the father shared physical custody of his 16-month-old daughter with her biological mother. The court had requested that the biological mother and daughter also be seen so that the child's constantly transitory care might feel less disruptive to her as possible. Initially, the biological mother refused to participate. Then, after three months of the therapist's meeting weekly in the father's home with the father, his daughter, and the stepmother, the biological mother agreed to be visited by the therapist in her home as well. The therapist arranged the visit on a day when the child would be with her mother. The child's responses to seeing the therapist now with her mother and then again a few days later with her father and stepmother provided a dramatic external view of how children construct their internal worlds and who belongs in them. In the presence of her mother, this child was very shy and troubled toward the therapist with whom she had become very relaxed and friendly in the father's household. Only gradually was the little girl able to accept the presence of the therapist in this new context.

This child's existence was bifurcated in an unusual way. She was the only palpable bridge between her two worlds, and this reaction is a demonstration of her experience of that. But it also demonstrates more broadly the importance of the home-visiting therapist as a member of the complex, interconnected matrix of relationships a child weaves. There is a need to be aware of the occurrence of this level of inclusion as an effect of home visiting.

Visiting is a unique mode of meeting. It implies a special kind of impermanence, with respect to the duration of the immediate contact if not the relationship as a whole. One is dropping by, passing through, or looking in. It also implies a particular social contract. One party is the visitor or guest, while the other is the host. Patients express their concepts and feelings about the social contract involved in home visiting in more or less direct ways. Not infrequently, they think and feel complex and even contradictory things about it. A person might, for example, feel harassed, courted, beholden, exposed, valued, monitored, looked after, remembered, checked up on, intruded upon, taken care of, or any combination of these things in response to being visited at home by a therapist. "I didn't clean up" could mean "I am worried that you will think my place is or I am a mess," "Things feel out of control to me,"

"I'm not sure what the etiquette is around a home visit by a therapist," or "I feel comfortable enough with you to let you see me as I am right now," among other possibilities. An offer of food could reflect a patient's gratitude in response to the therapist's efforts, a form of hospitality it would be unthinkable to forego with anyone, a wish that the visit were more social than professional, concern for the therapist's well-being, curiosity about the therapist, concern about a feeding problem that the baby is exhibiting, conviction that the patient is worthless and a wish to make the therapist's trip worthwhile, or pride regarding her culinary skills. It rarely reflects any single idea, but instead usually means a number of things at the same time.

Uniformly, however, home visiting creates a situation in which the visited feels little control over the information revealed about herself. An office speaks to a prearranged environment designed for the visitor and designed to convey what its occupant chooses to convey. The visitor in that office will present herself and convey the details of her life as she chooses. But when this same person is home-visited, her life is on display and information is everywhere. She cannot arrange her space to convey a limited and preferred image of herself as a therapist can his or her own.

Trainees in any setting in which the orientation is psychodynamic will be asked to think of the minute exchanges between themselves and their patients in terms of many possible meanings. A psychotherapy conducted in the context of home visits is, however, unique in that such speculation and exploration must take into considera-

tion the fact that it is the therapist, rather than the patient, who is a guest. This fact must be accommodated for when making initial arrangements for meeting and throughout the treatment. At a practical level, the therapist must defer to the patient regarding the circumstances of their meeting.

A therapist was greeted at the door by a patient with whom she had been meeting for nearly a year. To the therapist's surprise, the patient announced that this was "not a good time." The therapist spent the next week pouring over the details of the previous session in search of an explanation for the canceled session. But when she saw the patient the following week, the patient explained that there had been a drug deal involving a new boyfriend going on in her kitchen and she had wanted to protect the therapist from walking in on that. Certainly, there were many things for patient and therapist to discuss as a result of this incident, but it was the therapist's strong sense that had she challenged her patient's decision at the time not to meet, events would have taken place which would have made it much more difficult for patient and therapist to think together about the problems which the drug-dealing incident presented and reflected.

In addition to offering an example of the importance of deferring to the patient as host in a home visit, this vignette also raises the more general issue of surprises in home visits. Home visiting can be a radically disorienting practice for the therapist. There can be people or things present or absent, interruptions, disruptions, or events all out of keeping with the therapist's expectations. Even a therapist with a most unflappable personality has a story to tell about being taken by surprise in the course of a home visit.

The ability to be surprised is a valuable thing in a psychotherapist. It goes hand in hand with the ability to be curious about other people and to inspire in patients curiosity about themselves. It ought not be a goal of home visitors to be less surpriseable, but rather to have as many choices as possible regarding what to do when surprised. There are times when it is best for a therapist to note privately his or her sense of surprise and to proceed with something of a poker face. On the other hand, there are times when expressing and even amplifying one's sense of surprise is valuable. There are many times when registering one's surprise at a moderate level (even if it is experienced more strongly) is the most helpful course or indeed, when to fail to register it out loud would be an absurdity or a lost opportunity. Home visiting provides trainees with ample practice in the area of registering and making use of their own responses of surprise.

The ability to be straightforward is also a valuable thing in a psychotherapist. Often trainees come to the program feeling that they should know and figure out everything and never have to ask. The extremes of this tendency may be sorely tested as they once were, for example, when one particular day a man's feet protruded beyond a door jamb in the home of a single mother and child, and the therapist pretended not to notice. What happens in patients' homes is a natural happening—simply the flow of their lives. In this setting, one must learn what it would be bizarre to overlook and what is reasonable simply to note silently. It is ut-terly parallel to knowing when to inquire regarding a sense that a patient seems somehow "different" on this day and when simply to wait. The home-visiting context highlights the need to be aware of one's choices and why one is making them and deepens the process of being aware of that at every level. If home visiting is at first challenging, bewildering, and overwhelming, it ultimately becomes challenging, rich, and rewarding.

As one trainee expressed it in an interview regarding her experience at the Infant-Parent Program,

The thing that had the biggest impact on me personally and professionally was really the families. It took me by surprise. It was really moving. I was apprehensive about going into the Tenderloin, and it turned out to be the very best part—to be let into people's homes. It changed my perspective as a human being and my way of walking through the city. One woman lived with her little boy. We would walk through the Tenderloin together, and all of these people who seemed so unlikely to me would greet them. You end up as a therapist feeling empathic toward everyone you work with, but here there were people where from the outside you would think, "Don't even try."

The Structure of the Infant-Parent Program

Selection of Trainees

Each year the Infant-Parent Program receives from 60 to 65 requests for training at the program. Approximately 35 of these applicants are granted interviews. Those applying from mental health fields are social workers, psychiatrists, and clinical psychologists. Professionals from other disciplines include nurses, developmental psychologists, and special educators. These latter have been in the minority, and have always represented special instances where individuals have particular and persuasive reasons for seeking this specific training because it fits both their experience and their professional career goals. In some ways, the specificity of interests and intentions for this group are far clearer than those of the mental health professionals who apply.

The trainees are selected in order to create a diverse, well-qualified group of individuals who show evidence of genuine interest (if not dedication), relevant experience in some capacity, and relevant language capacity. The program also values trainees who represent perspectives on particular cultures, subcultures, ethnicity, and race. Because many trainees stay longer than the initially agreed upon time, the number of trainees accepted each year must vary according to the supervisory hours that remain available to accommodate them. The average number of new trainees accepted is eight.

The Clinical Experience

Trainees at the Infant-Parent Program commit themselves for a period from early September through July of the following year during which each follows four or five infant-parent cases at a time. As much as possible, cases are assigned to utilize the trainees' skills, experience, and interests. Some families are seen by the trainee for the entire training year. They may continue beyond this if the trainee extends his or her involvement with the program into a second year and if the needs of the family demand this continuing work. Such a family would be transferred to a new therapist if the first therapist did not continue. Trainees also follow infants and parents for briefer periods depending on the preferences and circumstances of the family. When clinical cases finish, the trainee is assigned another infant-parent case so that the clinical experience of any one trainee may include up to six or eight families over the training year.

The clinical cases seen all involve some kind of difficulty between parent(s) and infant or toddler. The nature of these troubles is exceedingly diverse—ranging from a mother whose bipolar disorder interferes pervasively with her ability to sustain attention on and empathize with her small child to a teenager facing the complex task of pursuing her own needs and interests while being responsible for nurturing her infant.

As the clinical work of the program is largely supported by public health funds, the families are drawn from the population dependent on publicly-supported services. This means that most live in circumstances of economic hardship, with public housing or single room apartments being the typical living arrangement. Forty percent of the families seen are African-American, 40 percent are Caucasian, 15 percent are Latino, and 5 percent represent other ethnicities. They are referred by the range of professionals who deal with infants, toddlers, and parents—including pediatric and public health providers, public health nurses, social workers from hospitals and the social welfare system, mental health professionals working with adults, and a variety of parent support programs. The trainee's clinical work includes collaborative contact with any of these other service providers who remain involved in the family's life or any representative of involved institutions such as the Department of Human Services or legal professionals.

Formal Training

The formal components of the Infant-Parent Program training are comprised of 90 minute weekly case review which continues throughout the year, a weekly year-long seminar on infant and toddler development, a one-semester seminar on home visiting, observation, treatment, and related issues, and a one-semester seminar on infant-parent psychotherapy and psychoanalytic theory.

A single case is presented each week at case review. For the most part, cases are presented by trainees, although presentations are also occasionally made by senior clinical staff. There is no strict formula for presenting an infant-parent case, but it is the responsibility of the presenter to convey a sense of the child, the parent(s), the known history of each, the quality of the interaction between them, the family's circumstances, the way the therapist fits into the parent-child system, and the foci and spirit of the treatment. Often trainees find it helpful to include numerous specific

small vignettes from their observations of and interactions with the family and also one or two lengthy excerpts from case notes. When a trainee has used the first 45 minutes of case review to convey this information, staff and trainees are in a good position to think collectively about the family and the treatment for the remaining half of the meeting time.

Trainees often report finding the case review conversations to be among the most useful aspects of their training experience. They account for this in a number of ways. The senior staff at the Infant-Parent Program have a long history of intelligently disagreeing with one another about specific approaches to and understanding of small children, parents, and the role of the clinician. These disagreements or differences occur in the context of overarching shared commitments and convictions and deep and genuine mutual respect. When trainees observe staff understanding families in different ways, they develop new levels of appreciation for the complexity of the issues involved, find themselves considering alternative ways of being as clinicians, and practice suspending the urge to "know" in favor of sustaining an openness to a multiplicity of meanings.

Case review is also a time when trainees have the opportunity to hear one another think clinically, share information regarding resources such as useful community organizations, and learn about experiences other trainees have with particular agencies and figures. Perhaps most importantly, trainees are exposed at the case review to many more families than they have an opportunity to meet personally in the course of their training year. Trainees and staff alike find it inspiring that families are so infinitely unique. Even families facing very similar psychosocial stressors, perhaps living in the same housing complex and having infants the same age, present with troubles and with strengths that are completely their own. While many things about a family are necessarily neglected in a 90-minute conversation, trainees report feeling that the uniqueness of individual experience is never lost sight of in the Infant-Parent Program case review.

The seminar on development is cotaught by a developmental neuropsychologist and a clinical psychologist. Its purpose is to provide trainees with a sense of what might be expected in the typical development of children from prenatal development through preschool. A primary goal is to understand the child's contribution to interactions with others and how various factors including biological/physiological factors shape this contribution. Weekly reading assignments address developmental issues in chronological sequence throughout the year, and although the seminar leaders introduce and embed the didactic material in its relevance to the potential for relationships, the seminar is primarily organized as a discussion of the issues. While examples from trainees' caseloads are certainly welcomed, trainees are also encouraged to draw from their experiences with their own children, children they know, or children they notice in the world in order to develop together not a clinical, diagnosis-oriented, abstract idea of development, but a robust, practical, well-informed ability to see children as developing beings.

The seminar on home visiting and related issues is taught serially by senior staff. The foci of these meetings include practical and clinical considerations in home visiting such as the issues raised by that setting, evaluation of infant-parent relationships including perspectives from attachment theory, cultural issues in local communities and in the therapist-client relationship, perspectives regarding treatment, and the intricacies of the social welfare system. This seminar is also discussion oriented and is geared toward assisting trainees with a myriad of practical challenges encountered in infant-parent work.

The final seminar addresses the theory and practice of infant-parent psychotherapy as it is informed by psychoanalytic theory. It is taught by a clinical psychologist who is also a psychoanalyst. The format is an informal combination of lecture and discussions. The goals of the seminar include familiarizing trainees with psychoanalytic concepts, articulating what it can mean to assume an analytic stance with a family, and assisting trainees in constructing psychodynamic formulations of infant-parent relationships. This means enabling trainees to identify the distorted ways that parents perceive infants and the coercive ways that parents interact with children, as well as the costly ways that children use to adapt to the internal and external demands that are placed on them. Trainees are encouraged to form hypotheses about these patterns and to consider effective interventions. Trainees read and discuss seminal papers by Selma Fraiberg and papers by program staff, as well as many other clinicians and theoreticians who contribute so richly to the field. The seminar reflects the Infant-Parent Program's commitment to thinking about the internal worlds of patients in careful ways despite the considerable social pressure which public therapists are under to address only circumstantial and behavioral issues.

Supervision

All of the seminars as well as the case review contribute to the achievement of the goals we hold for our trainees' development. But supervision, in our view, embodies the heart of the matter. It provides the place where the most learning about the trainee's role in the process of treatment occurs. In part, that is true because it is intended to provide the trainee with the place for reflection, focusing on and understanding one's particular impact in relation to a particular family, as well as understanding one's own responses as one seeks to understand the patient. But, it is also true because supervision is itself, of course, a relationship, and relationships are what the therapeutic endeavor intends to understand and influence.

Because this supervisory process is held to be so important, new trainees in this 20 hours per week placement are assigned only four home-visiting cases and are typically supervised on each case for one hour per week. Second year trainees working eight to ten hours per week receive one hour per case every other week. Despite the obvious pressures to increase caseloads and decrease supervisory hours, there is a reluctance to forego the time needed by beginning trainees for the relaxed mutual exploration that is so valuable. The trainees make explicit how much they value the devotion of this time to their development and, in effect, to the families with whom they work.

The primary patient in infant-parent psychotherapy is the relationship between the parent(s) and child. Although each family member is, in a sense, understood and supported as an individual, it is what happens between them that is the central focus. Thus, the supervision of this work includes issues of parallel process on three transacting levels: The relationship between supervisor and supervisee, between supervisee (therapist) and parent and child, and between parent and child. This series of mutually influencing relationships is challenging to encompass.

It is the supervisee who possesses all of the data which the supervisor will use, just as the parent and child possess all of the data the supervisee will use. It is helpful to think of the essential effort toward understanding all along the line as the mutual construction of meaning with one another and the avoidance of the unilateral imposition of meaning.

A parent and child are always engaged in constructing meaning. The crucial questions are how does each understand the other and how mutual is the process of that understanding. Meaning constructed in dialogue creates a context for mutual interaction which reflects and contains each person's intentions and impressions of the other. This is, in fact, a useful way to understand the impediments to adequate intersubjective communication and productive transaction. It is the unilateral ascription or assignment of meaning by a parent, for example, that distorts or negates the meaning of the behavioral expressions of a baby or a toddler. This preemption of meaning whether by projection, misapprehension, or any other process is problematic because one of the partners is essentially unheard.

It is the task of a parent to seek to understand the intentions and meaning of the expressive behaviors of his or her infant or small child. It is, therefore, useful to think of the major task of the infant-parent psychotherapist working with a family for whom this process has gone awry as creating and making a space—holding a space—such that the infant or toddler's voice can be heard. This is, in a sense, equally true of any therapist who assumes complex subjectivity on the part of any patient and holds a space for the patient's various and perhaps conflicting internal voices to be heard. In the case of infant and parent, however, it is not simply that meaning may be ascribed inaccurately or that an impulse or belief may go unrecognized but that the infant's or toddler's meanings, feelings, and intentions are sometimes unheard and lost to the parent. When this happens, those meanings and intentions are also lost to the child. Other constructs take their place within the child and represent enduring limitations on the child's ability to experience the world. These constructs are intended to manage their experiences of being unheard or inaccurately perceived and most often include that lack of mutuality as an important aspect.

The supervisor ensures the space for the supervisee's voices (and the voices he or she reports) to be heard. The supervisor's task is multiple in this regard, but it begins by knowing that the supervisee is a true partner in constructing all the many meanings toward which they will struggle together. As part of the three-level parallel process, the supervisory relationship must contain continued movement toward mutual understanding. The parameters of interaction we wish to see between parent and child must be firmly adhered to in the supervisory process. Greater experience and theoretical knowledge are not a license for preemption of the right of the less experienced (whether child or supervisee) to make meaning. In fact, in the best of all worlds, it is a license to listen, understand, and include.

In this regard, the supervisor is ever alert to whose voice seems absent. Often, trainees, whose primary experience has been the individual treatment of adults, concentrate almost exclusively on the adult's compelling narrative. In fact, the previous professional experiences of all trainees lead them to drift toward the familiar and comfortable in the face of this most jarring, odd, and murky endeavor. It is the supervisor who holds the space for whomever is missing and inquires or comments. Who is being listened to? Who is being seen? Who is absent? Who is being accounted for? Who is being thought about? These are some of the first issues to be explored with supervisees new to the field. Often this space-holding function is as concrete as a supervisor becoming aware that, although the trainee has been describing observations, conversations, and thoughts for some time, the baby has yet to be mentioned except, perhaps, in passing. In effect, it is as if the baby had not been present at all. In this stark example, the baby is in a crucial way *not* there, either for the parent or for the trainee. The baby must be brought into the conversation at every level.

In such an instance, understanding why the baby is "absent," not spoken to, about, or for may be one of the first mutual tasks that supervisor and supervisee undertake. The reasons are always multiple, but efforts begin to conceptualize who the baby is for the parent. This involves thinking about the environment, the stressors, the speech, dress, appearance, affect, and attitudes of the parent, and the baby's personhood, as well as the reactions, impressions, hesitations, discomforts, excitements, and amazements evoked in the supervisee. As part of this process, images and ideas are generated regarding the possible experiences of the infant or toddler. This array of content in the supervisory conversation encompasses most of the areas of focus and curiosity that will continue over the time that the supervisor and supervisee spend together.

Supervisory explorations of the responses of the supervisee, while important, are not to be confused with treatment. Prolonged, extensive joint examinations of the sources of feelings are well beyond the purview of supervision. There is a fine but usually discernible line between a gradual mutual awareness of a source of sensitivity for a trainee and pursuing it beyond relevance to the case at hand. As one trainee reported, "People at the Infant-Parent Program are really interested in my process, but not my 'stuff'." One danger of failing to

heed that line is that, in parallel fashion, the supervisee will probe with his or her patients beyond the tolerance of the therapeutic relationship, violating the patient's readiness to productively entertain particular ideas, feelings, or pieces of information.

Just as there is no permission to conduct "therapy" in supervision, there is no initial permission to conduct "therapy" with the patients whom we visit. The process and framework must be constructed with them, and a more or less explicit therapeutic contract must be agreed upon as they make known their tolerances, desires, and wishes and as the process unfolds as a mutual endeavor undertaken by the patient and the therapist. It is always therapeutic but can evolve only gradually into a permissioned "therapy."

The great majority of the patients we see rarely expect or encounter such mutuality in intimate relationships, let alone professional or institutionally mediated ones. Many of these patients enter treatment reluctantly, ignorantly, or without much hope that it will be helpful to them. Many feel coerced or are, in fact, either coerced or mandated to pursue treatment. This necessitates a far greater caution than usual regarding the degree to which a therapist may provoke perturbations. It also speaks to the necessity for an easy forthrightness, for clear concern, and for clearer interest and curiosity. Overcaution can be as useless as not being cautious is destructive, and these are the other issues with which supervisee and supervisor frequently struggle.

The supervisor brings a great deal of experience to the endeavor. Many of the dilemmas are familiar to the supervisor, and this familiarity can be readily shared. The supervisor's own reported experiences of dismay, shock, deep sadness, and confusion may humanize and temper both the supervisee's similar experiences and need to control and know.

It is essential that the supervisor maintain a welcoming, flexible center of calm. There is almost always a storm, and the supervisor must be the eye of it. If the supervisee is to achieve such a stance of calm in relation to the patient in the overwhelming internal and external environment he or she encounters, that stance must be continuously available to him or her through the person of the supervisor. The supervisor is the stable, reliable, flexible anchor which the supervisee organizes around in order to explore and reflect on whatever is demanded. The lives of the majority of the families and the supervisee's experience will often be painful and difficult. Without that reflective space, the supervisee will all too readily be drawn into the chaos he encounters and will feel and act overly responsible, empowered to fix, angry, resentful, too pleased, too impassioned, or any number of ways which will not inform but interfere with the enhancing of the parent-child relationship.

While the supervisor's receptivity and collaboration with the supervisee is crucial, the importance of assertiveness and of having and stating opinions and needs is equally crucial. The supervisor is by virtue of his or her greater experience and training the bearer of a certain authority, and it must be appropriately and clearly exer-

cised as necessary. In parallel, the supervisee must forthrightly assert his or her ideas and needs both to supervisor and patients when appropriate and necessary. The parent often will need to learn to be appropriately assertive as well, including asserting his or her needs and assuming appropriate authority with the child. The child, in turn, must have an equal invitation to assert his or her own needs and ideas. The issue here is that everyone is trying to listen to everyone, trying to be heard, and trying to create mutual meaning. The same parameters reverberate throughout all the levels of this system.

Thinking with someone very hard about something important is in itself an intrinsic pleasure. Being useful as a therapist to a family also has its obvious rewards. The supervisory situation provides yet an additional pleasure to each participant, that of coming to know another person by this process. No supervision is like any other. The mix of family, supervisor, and supervisee makes each experience triply unique. It is the coming together of two sets of sensibilities, two histories, two world views, and two sets of values around those of yet another set of people (parents and child) that makes the process so rich and so personal. Bits of history, surprising and unique perspectives, all in surrounding respect and trust create a very unusual interpersonal experience. Some supervisions are more compelling and interesting than others, and some are more difficult or feel less satisfying. But all are utterly engaging. The process is a very special privilege for both participants and simply having the time to engage in such an undertaking is mutually appreciated.

Because the experience of supervision is intense and because there is a strong tendency for a supervisee to identify with a supervisor, the decision was made early in the program's development to provide different supervisors to the same supervisee for different cases. One of the major things one wishes for a supervisee is that he or she find his or her own unique way of being as a therapist. Having a number of supervisors both sharpens the need for and expands the possibilities of learning about how the supervisee chooses to be. Although trainees report that, at first, working with as many as three or four supervisors is confusing and sometimes uncomfortable, they all report that midway through the year they have come to truly appreciate being exposed to the supervisors' different perspectives and styles. Learning what does and does not fit them from each supervisor no longer seems confusing, but enriching. They will, after all, in the course of their professional lives see many families and in working with each one will need to adapt themselves to shifting and ever changing expectations of them. They will always be experienced differently and will need anew, each time, to understand their unique place and impact in each new situation and its effect on them.

Finally, within all of these crucial processes, the supervisee is simultaneously learning how categories of pathology and theories of psychological functioning and treatment are both heuristically valuable and never complex enough to encompass unique human experience. The supervisee also becomes aware that learning about the experiences of others both humanizes and informs theory in an endless cycle of discovery and rediscovery.

The Culture of the Program

Every year in the early summer the Infant-Parent Program holds a picnic on Angel Island, a small island in the middle of San Francisco Bay belonging to the California State Park System. Angel Island is accessible only by boat, and the program convenes there by ferry from various directions, because we are committed to a tradition of making sure we get to see each other and be together. If they want to, people bring their friends and/or families. Trainees from years past call the office to find out which Sunday the annual picnic falls on and join us. Some people arrive on the early ferry and depart in the late afternoon, while others spend only 1½ hours on the island. Some people spend most of their time walking the perimeter of the island deep in conversation with a well-known colleague, some have serial conversations with people with whom they have rarely spoken in the course of the year, some play ball, some loll on the grass, and all eat. Everyone brings their own picnic plus something to share.

Some people do not attend the picnic because they do not want to or because life intervenes. This does not mean that they have missed their graduation. On the contrary, while the daily work of conducting infant-parent psychotherapy is certainly no picnic, the spirit of this tradition extends throughout the year and is reflected in the fact that there is a 4′ × 6′ kitchen at the Infant-Parent Program into which as many as five people frequently crowd making use of sink, microwave, coffee pots, and dishes. In December, there is a potluck lunch which is famous for the delicacies it inspires.

On a practical level, the shared use of our single playroom for developmental assessments and occasional on-site family sessions requires clear communication and generosity of spirit. In spite of increasing limitations of space, every trainee is provided with a desk and a telephone so that all literally have a place to be when they are at the program.

We believe these things to be important to include in this discussion of training, simply because they reflect something about how we attempt to manage and influence our working environment. Psychotherapy in general in the context of home visiting in particular with families facing dire circumstances even more emphatically, can leave a person feeling isolated if not existentially shaken. It is not possible to perform the work effectively unless one is provided with an environment conducive to making sense of everything up to the brink of the unthinkable. Beyond that point a sense of community and commonality of purpose is the only sustenance or balm a training program can provide.

References

Cherniss, D., Pawl, J., & Fraiberg, S. (1980). Nina: Developmental guidance and supportive treatment for a failure to thrive infant and her adolescent mother. In S. Fraiberg (Ed.), *Clinical studies in in-fant mental health: The first year of life* (pp. 103–140). New York: Basic Books.

Fraiberg, L. (Ed.). (1987). *Selected writings of Selma Fraiberg*. Columbus, OH: Ohio State University Press.

Fraiberg, S. (1974a). Billy: Psychological intervention for a failure-to-thrive infant. In M. Klaus, T. Leger, & M. Trause (Eds.), *Maternal attachment and mothering disorders: A round table sponsored by Johnson and Johnson Baby Products Co.* (pp. 13–19). Sausalito, CA.

Fraiberg, S. (1974b). The clinical dimension of baby games. *The Journal of American Child Psychiatry, 13,* 202–220.

Fraiberg, S. (1978). Future care of mothering disorders. *Birth and Family Journal, 5,* 239–241.

Fraiberg, S. (1982a). The adolescent mother and her infant. In S. C. Feinstein, J. G. Looney, A. Z. Schwartzberg, & A. D. Sorosky (Eds.), *Annals of the American Society for Adolescent Psychiatry: Vol. 10. Adolescent psychiatry: Developmental and clinical studies* (pp. 7–23). Chicago: University of Chicago Press.

Fraiberg, S. (1982b). Pathological defenses in infancy. *Psychoanalysis Quarterly, 51,* 612–635.

Fraiberg, S., & Adelson, E. (1977). An abandoned mother, an abandoned baby. *Bulletin Menninger Clinic, 41,* 162–180.

Fraiberg, S., Adelson, E., & Shapiro, V. (1975). Ghosts in the nursery: A psychoanalytic approach to the problems of impaired infant-mother relationships. *Journal of the American Academy of Child Psychiatry, 14,* 387–421.

Fraiberg, S., Aradine, C., & Shapiro, V. (1978a). Collaborating to foster family attachment. *American Journal of Maternity Child Nursing, 3,* 92–98.

Fraiberg, S., & Bennett, J. (1978b). Intervention and failure to thrive: A psychiatric outpatient treatment program. *Birth and Family Journal, 5,* 227–230.

Fraiberg, S., & Fraiberg, L. (Eds.). (1980). *Clinical studies in infant mental health: The first year of life.* New York: Basic Books.

Fraiberg, S., Lieberman, A. F., Pekarsky, J., & Pawl, J. (1981). Treatment and outcome in an infant psychiatry program: Parts 1 and 2. *Preventative Psychiatry, 1*(1), 89–111, (2), 143–165.

Fraiberg, S., Shapiro, V., & Adelson, E. (1976). Infant-parent psychotherapy on behalf of a child in a critical nutritional state. *Psychoanalytic Study of the Child, 31,* 461–491.

Fraiberg, S., Shapiro, V., Bennett, J., & Pawl, J. (1980). Brief crisis intervention. In S. Fraiberg (Ed.), *Clinical studies in infant mental health: The first year of life* (pp. 79–102). New York: Basic Books.

Glasser, M. E., & Lieberman, A. F. (1984). Failure to thrive: An interactional developmental approach. In C. VanDyke, L. Temoshok & L. Zegans (Eds.), *Emotions in health and illness: Applications to clinical practice* (pp. 199–207). San Diego: Grune & Stratton.

Harris, E., Weston, D., & Lieberman, A. F. (1989). The quality of mother-infant attachment and pediatric health care use. *Pediatrics, 84*(2), 248–254.

Kalmanson, B. (1992). Diagnosis and treatment of infants and young children with pervasive developmental disorders. *Zero to Three: Bulletin of the National Center for Clinical Infant Programs, 4*(4), 46–52.

Kalmanson, B., & Lieberman, A. F. (1982). Removing obstacles to attachment: Infant-parent psychotherapy with an adolescent mother and her baby. *Zero to Three: Bulletin of the National Center for Clinical Infant Programs, 3*(1), 10–13.

Kalmanson, B., & Pekarsky, J. (1987, Winter). Infant-parent psychotherapy with an autistic toddler. *Infant Mental Health Journal, 8*(4).

Kalmanson, B., & Pekarsky, J. (1987, February). Infant-parent psychotherapy with an autistic toddler. *Zero to Three: Bulletin of the National Center for Clinical Infant Programs, 7*(3), 1–6.

Lieberman, A. F. (1983). Infant-parent psychotherapy during pregnancy: A case illustration. In S. Provence (Ed.), *Infants and parents: Clinical case reports* (pp. 85–142). New York: International Universities Press.

Lieberman, A. F. (1985). Infant mental health: A model for service delivery. *Journal of Clinical Child Psychology, 14*(3), 196–201.

Lieberman, A. F. (1987). Psychoanalytic and ethological perspectives in separation and development. In J. & S. Bloom-Feshback (Eds.), *The psychology of separation through the life span* (pp. 109–135). New York: Jossey-Bass.

Lieberman, A. F. (1989). What is culturally sensitive intervention? *Early Child Development and Care, 50,* 190–204.

Lieberman, A. F. (1990a). Culturally sensitive intervention with children and families. *Child and Adolescent Social Work Journal, 7*(2), 101–120.

Lieberman, A. F. (1990b). Infant-parent intervention with recent immigrants: Reflections on a study with Latino families. *Zero to Three: Bulletin of the National Center for Clinical Infant Programs, 4,* 8–11.

Lieberman, A. F. (1991). Attachment theory and infant-parent psychotherapy: Some conceptual, clinical and research considerations. In D. Cicchetti & S. Toth (Eds.), *Rochester Symposium on Developmental*

Psychopathology: Vol. 3 (pp. 261–287). Hillsdale, NJ: Erlbaum.

Lieberman, A. F. (1992). Infant-parent psychotherapy with toddlers. *Development and Psychopathology, 4*(4), 559–574.

Lieberman, A. F. (1993). *The emotional life of the toddler.* New York: Free Press.

Lieberman, A. F. (1996). Aggression and sexuality in relation to toddler attachment. *Infant Mental Health Journal, 17*(3), 276–292.

Lieberman, A. F. (1997). Toddlers' internalization of maternal attributions as a factor in quality of attachment. In L. Atkinson & K. Zucker (Eds.), *Attachment and Psychopathology* (pp. 277–291). New York: Guilford.

Lieberman, A. F., & Birch, M. (1985). The etiology of failure to thrive: An interactional developmental approach. In D. Drotar (Ed.), *New directions in failure to thrive: Research and clinical practice* (pp. 259–279). New York: Plenum.

Lieberman, A. F., & Blos, P. (1980). Make room for Paulie: Building attachment before birth. In S. Fraiberg (Ed.), *Clinical studies in infant mental health: The first year of life* (pp. 242–259). New York: Basic Books.

Lieberman, A. F., & Pawl, J. H. (1984). Searching for the best interests of the child: Intervention with an abusive mother and her toddler. *The Psychoanalytic Study of the Child, 39,* 527–548.

Lieberman, A. F., & Pawl, J. H. (1988). Clinical applications of attachment. In J. Belsky & T. Nezworski (Eds.), *Clinical Implications of Attachment* (pp. 327–351). New York: Erlbaum.

Lieberman, A. F., & Pawl, J. H. (1990). Attachment and secure base behavior in the second year of life: Conceptual issues and clinical intervention. In M. Greenberg, D. Cicchetti, & M. Cummings (Eds.), *Attachment in the preschool years* (pp. 375–397). Chicago: University of Chicago Press.

Lieberman, A. F., & Pawl, J. H. (1993). Infant-parent psychotherapy. In C. Zeanah (Ed.), *Handbook of infant mental health* (pp. 427–442). New York: Guilford.

Lieberman, A. F., Pekarsky, J. H., & Pawl, J. H. (1988). Toward a comprehensive infant mental health program for a community. In J. Anthony & C. Chiland (Eds.), *The child in his family: Child raising and identity formation under stress: Vol. 8* (pp. 263–289). New York: Wiley.

Lieberman, A. F., & Slade, A. (1997a). The first year of life. In J. Noshpitz (Ed.), *Comprehensive textbook of child psychiatry.* New York: Basic Books.

Lieberman, A. F., & Slade, A. (1998b). The second year of life. In J. Noshpitz (Ed.), *Comprehensive textbook of child psychiatry.* New York: Basic Books.

Lieberman, A. F., VanHorn, P., Grandison, C. M., & Pekarsky, J. H. (1997). Mental health assessment of infants, toddlers and preschoolers in a service program and a treatment outcome research program. *Infant Mental Health Journal, 18*(2), 158–170.

Lieberman, A. F., Weston, D. R., & Pawl, J. H. (1991). Preventive intervention and outcome with anxiously attached dyads. *Child Development, 62,* 199–209.

Lieberman, A. F., & Zeanah, C. H. (1995). Disorders of attachment in infancy. In K. Minde (Ed.), *Infant psychiatry: Child and adolescent psychiatric clinics of America, 4*(3), 579–588.

McCune, L., Kalmanson, B., Glazewski, M., & Sillari, J. (1990). An interdisciplinary model of infant assessment. In S. Meisels

& J. Shonkoff (Eds.), *Handbook of early childhood intervention*. New York: Cambridge University Press.

Pawl, J. H. (1984). Strategies of intervention. *International Journal of Child Abuse and Neglect, 8*, 261–270.

Pawl, J. H. (1992). Interventions to strengthen relationships between infants and drug-abusing or recovering parents. *Zero to Three: Bulletin of the National Center for Clinical Infant Programs, 13*(1), 6–10.

Pawl, J. H. (1993). A stitch in time: Using emotional support, developmental guidance, and infant-parent psychotherapy in a brief intervention. In E. Fenichel & S. Provence (Eds.), *Development in jeopardy* (pp. 203–229). New York: International Universities Press.

Pawl, J. H. (1994). On supervision. In L. Eggbeer & E. Fenichel (Eds.), *Educating and supporting the infant/family workforce: Models, methods and materials*.

Pawl, J. H. (1995). The therapeutic relationship as human connectedness: Being held in another's mind. *Zero to Three: Bulletin of the National Center for Clinical Infant Programs, 15*(4), 1–5.

Pawl, J. H., & Bennet, J. (1980). Martha: A focused clinical use of the Bayley in consultation. In S. Fraiberg (Ed.), *Clinical studies in infant mental health: The first year of life* (pp. 260–269). New York: Basic Books.

Pawl, J. H., & Lieberman, A. F. (1997). Infant-parent psychotherapy. In J. Noshpitz (Ed.), *Comprehensive textbook of child psychiatry* (pp. 339–350). New York: Basic Books.

Pawl, J. H., & Pekarsky, J. H. (1983). Infant-parent psychotherapy: A family in crisis. In S. Provence (Ed.), *Infants and parents:*

Clinical case reports: Vol. 2 (pp. 39–84). New York: International Universities Press.

Pekarsky, J. (1981). Infant mental health consultation in a well-baby clinic. *Zero to Three: Bulletin of the National Center for Clinical Infant Programs, 1*(4), 6–9.

Pekarsky, J. (1992). Supervision and mentorship of students: Scenes from supervision. *Learning through supervision and mentorship* (pp. 53–55). Zero to Three: National Center for Clinical Infant Programs.

Seligman, S. (1989). Emotional and social development in infancy and early childhood: An overview. *Early Childhood Update, 5*(4), 1–2.

Seligman, S. (Ed.). (1989). Special Issue on Emotional Development in Infancy. *Early Childhood Update, 5*(4).

Seligman, S. (1993). Infant observation and psychoanalytic theory. *The Psychoanalytic Quarterly, 62*(2), 274–278.

Seligman, S. (1994). Applying psychoanalysis in an unconventional context: Adapting infant-parent psychotherapy to a changing population. In A. J. Solnit, P. B. Neubauer, S. Abrams, & A. S. Dowling (Eds.), *The psychoanalytic study of the child: Vol. 49* (pp. 487–510). New Haven and London: Yale University Press.

Seligman, S. (1994). Le programme enfant-parent: Le developpment d'un programme pilote de sate mentale infantile. *Devenir: Revue Europeenne du Developpement de L'Enfant, 6*(1), 7–29.

Seligman, S., & Pawl, J. (1984). Impediments to the formation of the therapeutic alliance in infant-parent psychotherapy. In J. Call, E. Galenson, & R. Tyson (Eds.), *Frontiers of infant Psychiatry: Vol. II* (pp. 232–237). New York: Basic Books.

Seligman, S., & St. John, M. (1995). No space

for baby: Pseudomaturity in an urban little girl. In E. G. Corrigan & P. E. Gordon (Eds.), *The mind object: Precocity and pathology of self-sufficiency* (pp. 155–176). Jason Aronson, Inc.

Slade, A., & Lieberman, A. F. (1997). Infant-parent psychotherapy. In J. Noshpitz (Ed.), *Comprehensive textbook of child psychiatry* (pp. 112–122). New York: Basic Books.

12

Intervention-Centered Assessment: Opportunity for Early and Preventive Intervention

Jean M. Thomas, Anne Benham, and Karen A. Guskin

12

Introduction

Intervention-centered assessment conceptualizes and structures mental health assessment of children ages birth to four years and their families to maximize the opportunity for early and preventive intervention in developmental, emotional, behavioral, and relational domains. Identification of risk and intervention before the appearance of disorder are both central to the field (Emde, Bingham, & Harmon, 1993) and the "prevention of mental disorder throughout the lifespan" (Fonagy, 1996, p. 1). Intervention-centered assessment is anchored in the transactional biopsychosocial model of development that defines a matrix of mutually influencing biological and social factors which shape the child's development (Sameroff & Chandler, 1975). Constitutional/maturational and social/contextual influences mutually contribute to the regulation of physiology, emotion, and behavior. Relationships provide the context and the power for healthy development and for change within the family and the therapeutic process. For this reason, intervention-centered assessment creates a family-centered mutual process of learning about the child and building on the child's and the family's strengths within the extended caregiving context. Collaborative, interdisciplinary efforts are necessary to facilitate the integration of biological, developmental, and psychological research, theory, and clinical experience (American Academy of Child and Adolescent Psychiatry, 1997, 1998; Thomas, Guskin, & Klass, 1997).

A recent overview of early childhood mental health assessment purposes, aims, and process is provided by the "Practice Parameters for the Psychiatric Assessment of Infants and Toddlers (0–36 months)" (American Academy of Child and Adolescent Psychiatry, 1997) for which two of us were central contributors (JT & AB). This chapter reiterates and elaborates central aspects of the Academy's Practice Parameters, including the Infant and Toddler Mental Status Exam (ITMSE) and the integration of standard diagnostic systems with the new *Diagnostic Classification 0–3* (DC: 0–3) (Zero to Three, 1994).

We focus on three ways in which assessment is intervention. Firstly, information (biological and psychosocial) is intervention when the parents increase their understanding of the child based on clinical interview and observation or formal interdisciplinary assessment. When this information changes the way a family feels about their child, behaves toward their child, or facilitates the "goodness of fit" (Chess & Thomas, 1989) between the parents' expectation and who the child is, assessment becomes intervention. Secondly, empathy and support provided within the therapeutic alliance are intervention when they increase parental empathy, patience, and hope. Finally, facilitation of the family's knowledge and use of services and their advocacy for their child is also intervention.

In this chapter, we bring together current advances in brain and social sciences, theory, and clinical practice which emphasize and provide strategies for implementing the urgent need to intervene early and preventively. First, we focus on the transactional biopsychosocial model of development that defines the mutual influence of nature and nurture on development. Within this framework, we discuss the contribution of individual differences and the power of relationships in the regulation of emotions and behavior. Second, we focus on creating a family-centered assessment process. Third, we focus on pragmatic assessment strategies for listening, observing, and understanding the child in four domains of his or her functioning: Developmental, emotional, behavioral, and relational.

Transactional Biopsychosocial Model of Development

The transactional model of development (Sameroff & Chandler, 1975), now well accepted, defines how biology and psychosocial experiences, especially within the primary caregiving environment, mutually influence the child's development. Development is the unfolding of the child's biological potential as it is influenced by the specific caregiving environment. "Children inherit parent's genes, their parents, their peers, and the communities they inhabit. . . . Nature and nurture stand in reciprocity, not opposition . . . [and] mind/brain . . . is jointly constructed by both" (Eisenberg, 1995).

We are beginning to understand how the human brain is shaped by experience (Eisenberg, 1995), and more specifically, how early experience, especially early rela-

tionships, help define brain substrate on which later brain development is established. During the earliest years of life, neuronal patterns are rapidly developing and organizing brain structures which lay the foundation for future development. Underutilized neurons are eliminated to make way for neurons and neuronal patterns which are frequently utilized. This process continues until senility but is most rapid during early development when the foundation of future development, either healthy or disordered, is established by the brain's "use-dependent" selection of healthy or disordered neuronal patterns (Perry, Pollard, Blakely, Baker, & Vigilante, 1995). This new knowledge about the human brain magnifies the urgency of early and preventive intervention (American Academy of Child and Adolescent Psychiatry, 1997, 1998; Eisenberg, 1995).

Constitutional and Maturational Influences

Constitutional and maturational influences central to development cannot be easily separated from environmental influences. Biobehavioral shifts at 2 to 3 months, 7 to 9 months, 12 to 13 months, and 18 to 20 months are characterized by qualitative reorganization of social, cognitive, motoric, and symbolic capacities (American Academy of Child and Adolescent Psychiatry, 1997; Emde, 1985; Emde, Gaensbauer, & Harmon, 1976; Kagan, 1984; McCall, Eichorn, & Hogarty, 1977; Stern, 1985; Zeanah, Anders, Seifer, & Stern, 1989). This rapid developmental change facilitates therapeutic change. According to

Fraiberg (1980), it is "like having God on your side." The impact of individual differences in physiology (Mayes, 1995; Mrazek, 1993), sensory-motor and cognitive functions (Degangi, DiPietro, Greenspan, & Porges, 1991; Degangi, Porges, Sickel, & Greenspan, 1993), and temperament are well appreciated but may be difficult to separate from environmental influence. Rothbart and Ahadi (1994) help clarify the mutual influences on temperament that they define as "constitutionally based individual differences in reactivity and self-regulation, influenced over time by heredity, maturation, and experience."

Relationships and Broader Contextual Factors

The centrality of relationships was the first of two major themes that emerged from the October 1997, National Institute of Mental Health (NIMH) meeting, "Assessment of Infant and Toddler Mental Health." The recognition of context as central is the most significant advance in developmental research over the last 25 years, according to Sameroff (1992). It is well known that the number of risk factors appears more predictive than any specific risk factor (Sameroff, Seifer, Zax, & Barocas, 1987; Zero to Three, 1994). Although biological risk, including developmental delays and deviance, low birth weight, and prematurity are known risk factors for subsequent psychopathology, there is evidence that environmental risk is a better predictor of later psychopathology (Minde et al., 1989; Sameroff, 1997). It appears that, when studied together, environmen-

tal factors that directly compromise the quality of parenting are most likely to be associated with greater risk (Shaw, Vondra, Hommerding, Keenan, & Dunn, 1994; Zeanah, Boris, & Scheeringa, 1997).

It is axiomatic that the child must be understood and treated in the context of the caregiving environment including the parent(s) or foster parent(s), the family, extended family, and friends, the community and community agencies that support children and families, and the specific culture with its unique expectations and cultural ideals (American Academy of Child and Adolescent Psychiatry, 1997, 1998; Thomas et al., 1997; Winnicott, 1965).

Centrality of the parent-child relationship in shaping and regulating the emotional and behavioral development of the infant was first conceptualized by Bowlby. The "attachment behavior system" creates the infant's sense of security which facilitates exploration of the environment (Bowlby, 1982; Ainsworth, Blehar, Waters, & Wall, 1978). The emotional scaffolding that supports a child's emerging capacities (Clark, Paulson, & Conlin, 1993; Vygotsky, 1978) has been variously described by multiple theorists. Winnicott (1965) describes parent-child relationships as a "holding environment." Ainsworth describes secure attachments as facilitated by "sensitive" and "responsive" parent-child relationships (Ainsworth et al., 1978). Emde describes reciprocity in the parent-child relationship—the attachment of the child to the parent and the bonding of the parents with the child. For example, the infant's ability to share and regulate affect is facilitated by the parents' empathic responsiveness (Sameroff & Emde, 1989). The importance of parent-infant relationships has been expanded to include the nuclear and extended family and community caregiving relationships (Zeanah & Lyons-Ruth, 1993; Crockenberg, Dickstein, & Lyons-Ruth, 1993; Sameroff, 1989).

Regulation of Physiology, Emotion, and Behavior

Regulation of physiology, emotion, and behavior, including related issues of temperament, relationships as regulators, and self-regulation, was the second of two major themes that emerged from the October 1997, NIMH meeting. The evolution of human beings and other higher organisms has favored a biology that prescribes both internal (neurological) and external (social) regulatory mechanisms for the developing organism to establish physiologic homeostasis, safety in exploring, and adaptive socialization to a specific environment (Amini et al., 1996; Barrett & Campos, 1987; Bowlby, 1969; Eisenberg, 1995; Hofer, 1987; Kraemer, 1992; Lyons-Ruth & Zeanah, 1993; Suomi, 1997; Vygotsky, 1987; Zeanah et al., 1989; Zeanah et al., 1997). Kraemer (1992) sees these biologically programmed social homeostatic mechanisms as *the* central organizing system in the brain of higher social mammals. These external homeostatic mechanisms have been variously described as the "attachment system" (Bowlby, 1982), "affect attunement" (Stern, 1984), and "multiple regulators woven into the fabric of relationship, at the biological as well as psychological level" (Hofer, 1987, p. 645).

Psychodynamic and Systems Models

Both psychodynamic and systems models guide clinical work. Representation of relationships, a central construct in the field, borrows from psychodynamic theories that view "transference" as the unconscious imposition of expectations and qualities of central relationships in the past onto relationships in the present. Fraiberg describes how "ghosts" of unresolved feelings about past relationships shape the parents' expectations of their relationship with their infant or young child (Fraiberg, 1980). Bowlby's concept of "internal working models" elaborates how unconscious models of parenting from the past shape parents' expectations and experience of their parenting role (Bowlby, 1980). Main and colleagues describe intergenerational patterns of attachment and show how the attachment pattern of the child is predicted by the nature and quality of a mother's representations of her own mother (Main & Goldwyn, 1984; Main, Kaplan, & Cassidy, 1985). Stern (1985, 1989) describes ways in which representation may emerge in the child's unconscious and how family narratives or conscious representations mingle with unconscious representations to form a child's evolving world view.

The practicing family as defined by Reiss (1989) focuses on the contribution of systems theorists and is contrasted with representational models of the family. Reiss and colleagues suggest that models in the minds of individuals are created and sustained by common group practice. Reiss advocates careful assessment of the mechanisms of change that may depend on a combination of alterations in internal working models and alterations in the common practice of important social groups, especially families. Robert-Tissot and colleagues (1996) demonstrate that there is equal therapeutic advantage in approaches that target family representations and those that target interactions of the practicing family.

Creating a Family-Centered Assessment Process

The process of building a therapeutic alliance begins during the first telephone contact (Fraiberg, 1980) with an initial inquiry about parental concerns and an explication of the aims and format of the assessment. Preparing families as fully as possible facilitates the family's sense of competence and increased assertiveness in their central role in the assessment (Meisels & Fenichel, 1996). When parents are actively involved in the process, assessment is more likely to have therapeutic value according to Clark, Paulson, and Conlin (1993) and others. All primary caregivers are strongly encouraged to participate. Extended family and community caregivers and siblings are sometimes included initially and often included later.

The process of intervention-centered assessment must focus on concerns and *strengths,* risk factors and *protective factors,* and vulnerability and *resilience.* The clinician understands that parents' concerns often reflect their own vulnerabilities, their fears that their child is damaged

and that they themselves are to blame. "The clinician will be trusted only if he or she represents more hope for the child than fear and guilt for the parents" (Guedeney & Lebovici, 1997, p. 174). Expecting and looking for the child's and the parents' best, what the parents hope for and want for their child, creates an atmosphere that builds on the child's and family's biopsychosocial strengths. A family-centered process focuses on the child's experience, the parents' experience, the family's experience, and building on the strengths of the child, parents, and family.

The Child's Experience

The experience of the very young child, how he or she is feeling and understanding both the context in which he or she lives and the assessment process, is difficult to elicit. Because these very young children often cannot tell us their experiences in words, we attempt to understand them through their behaviors, play, affect, and interactions. Emde (1989) focuses the clinician on the child's experience, especially the role of affect in organizing the child's experience. Social referencing is one example of how the parent's affect is transmitted to and organizes the young child's behavior. When a child of six months or older encounters a novel experience, the child will look toward the parent and adjust behavior in response to the parent's affective communication of danger or safety (Emde, 1989; Sorce, Emde, Campos, & Klinnert, 1985).

The child's experience of himself or herself and of relationships emerges from the unconscious blending of composite experiences of his or her relationship with each caregiver (Stern, 1989, 1985, 1994). Child-caregiver interactions guide the child's expectations of or "schema of being with" each important caregiver, in accord with Bowlby's theory of attachment and the research of Ainsworth, Main, and many others (Ainsworth et al., 1978; Bowlby, 1973; Fonagy, Steele, & Steele, 1991; Main & Goldwyn, 1984; Sroufe, 1989; Stern, 1995).

The Parents' Experience

The parents' experiences of loving their child, wanting the best for their child, and worrying about their adequacy as parents are important to understand in establishing a family-centered therapeutic process. In a nationwide survey of 1,022 parents of zero-to three-year-olds, only a few parents felt completely prepared for their first child, but a large majority of parents felt "'in love' with their baby and happier than ever before" (Zero to Three, 1997, p. iii). Most first-time parents felt "stressed and worn out" and "afraid of doing something wrong" (Zero to Three, 1997, p. 5). Parents felt "two fundamental barriers stand in the way of better parenting . . . they don't spend as much quality time with their child as they would like . . . and they have an 'information deficit' . . . [especially with regard to] babies' and toddlers' emotional, social, and intellectual development" (Zero to Three, 1997, p. 12–14).

The Family's Experience

The family's experience is both represented in their mutually shared internal working models and created and sustained in the family's common practices. These internal working models and common practices include and are elucidated by family stories about the child, siblings, parents, or extended family and friends, family rituals, family genograms, family photographs or videotapes, and family interactions within the assessment process. In addition, 60 percent of the children ages zero to three are cared for regularly by someone other than their parents (Zero to Three, 1997). Information from a variety of individuals increases the clinician's sense of the family as a context within the greater contexts of the community and culture (AACAP, 1997; Emde, 1994; Lyons-Ruth & Zeanah, 1993; Reiss, 1989).

The family's experience of learning about the child and building on strengths, accomplished through the clinician's working alliance with the family, is "built on respect for the parents' knowing their child, being a central influence in their child's life, wanting to make a better life for their child (Fraiberg, 1980), and having unique values, preferences, and cultural ideals" (American Academy of Child and Adolescent Psychiatry, 1997, p. 22S). The clinician's "supportive and empathic attitude toward the client in the process of gathering information is the crucial factor in obtaining accurate, valid, and clinically relevant data in preparation for treatment regardless of the specific instruments or methodology involved" (Lieberman, Van Horn, Grandison, & Pekarsky, 1997, p. 169). Flexibility in approach allows focus on the parents' and child's needs and concerns (Guedeney & Lebovici, 1997).

Family Interview

The goal of assessment is "history making, not history taking" (Hirschberg, 1993, 1996). The family and clinician together develop a mutual understanding of the parents' concerns, child's difficulties, and impact of these on the child, parents, and family. The family-centered team's mutual effort is to gather information in the service of understanding the challenges and successes of the child and the family and to support the healthy development of the child. The goals of this mutual effort to understand and help the child include: To determine whether disorder or conditions leading to risk or vulnerability are present in the child, family relationships, or broader context, to establish a developmentally-based differential working diagnosis, and to collaborate in an ongoing process of discovery, formulation, and treatment planning. "History making" reframes and narrates a new, hopeful, mutual understanding. It is ongoing and evolves throughout the interview and intervention process (American Academy of Child and Adolescent Psychiatry, 1997, 1998; Hirschberg, 1993, 1996; Thomas et al., 1997).

The parents may be interviewed initially with or without the child. When the parents are interviewed with the child, parents may initially feel more comfortable with the focus on the child and may feel their concerns about the child are more understandable because the clinician has first-hand knowledge of the child. The clinician explains in advance that private time is available and encourages the parents to respond as they would at home to the needs of the child during the interview. Clinicians often find that "history making" is facilitated by observing the child's interactions with the family during the interview. When the parents are interviewed alone first, they may feel freer to talk about the child, their own histories and relationships, and their feelings toward the child and his or her difficulties, without feeling constrained to edit for the child's ears. With both strategies, the primary goal is the most rapid development of a therapeutic alliance with the family which will allow for an open, complete exploration of all issues and will engage the family on the child's behalf. The age of the child and the parents' needs, wishes, and cultural patterns also guide the choice of format.

Parents' Explicit and Implicit Concerns, Motivations, and Expectations

THE PARENTS' EXPLICIT CONCERNS
The family interview begins with the parents' description of their concerns about the child including the child's baseline, recent changes, what makes the things better or worse, and the impact of the child's difficulties on the child and the family. Parents' presenting concerns may be physiological, emotional, behavioral, developmental, relational, or a complex combination of these. For infants, the most frequent concerns are disturbances in the regulation of physiological function, such as irritable or colicky behaviors and sleeping or feeding difficulties, including failure-to-thrive. For

toddlers or preschool age children, the most frequent concerns are disruptive behaviors including aggression, temper tantrums, impulsivity, and hyperactivity. Other parent concerns focus on fearful or withdrawn behaviors, such as withdrawal from peers or separation anxiety focused on going to sleep or separations at child care. Parents or professionals may also present concerns that the child has been physically or sexually abused. Parental concerns may detail or suggest constitutional and maturational difficulties including developmental delays or more subtle physiologic, sensory, or sensory-motor processing difficulties. Concerns often reflect the fact that the parents' expectations of their child differ from the child's actual constitution or developmental status. These mismatches or problems with "goodness of fit" (Chess & Thomas, 1989) may create relationship disturbances that lead to referral (American Academy of Child and Adolescent Psychiatry, 1997, 1998).

Concerns for which the parents brought the child are the natural focus of clinical attention. It is also essential to focus on questions about the child's strengths and areas of good adjustment and protective factors within the child and within the family, extended family, and community contexts. In looking for strengths, it is important to remain empathic and not to minimize the parents' experienced frustrations and concerns.

THE PARENTS' IMPLICIT CONCERNS
The parents' implicit, as well as explicit concerns, motivations, and expectations, are central to the intervention-centered assessment process. Open-ended questions facilitate the parents' spontaneity. In eliciting the parents' concerns, the clinician is listening to understand, "What do the parents feel? What do the parents need? How will they feel heard and understood? How can I help them understand what the child needs? How will I help them hear what they need to hear?" Queries about the parents' hopes and fears for the child often provide significant clues to the parents' internal working models. The clinician also listens for the parents' expectable perceptual biases which are embedded in the narrative and provide clues to motivations, expectations, suffering, and reenactment of the past in the present (American Academy of Child and Adolescent Psychiatry, 1997, 1998). This can be especially important when caregivers have been traumatized. The child often provides a catalytic connection for the parents into their past and their own experience of being parented as a child (Fraiberg, 1980).

Details and Specifics

"Most of what we are looking for in a comprehensive evaluation process comes from details, and repetition, 'terrible and exacting details'" (Fraiberg, 1980, p. 165; Guedeney & Lebovici, 1997, p. 179). Detailed, systematic questions to explicate recent examples of specific behaviors both clarify what is meant (Cox & Rutter, 1985; Stern, 1995) and communicate to parents that their concerns merit careful listening. Details flesh out the parents' account of their concerns: Why now? What is the frequency, intensity, and duration of the problem? What makes it better or worse? When were you first concerned? How was the child developing up until and beyond that point? Were there medical problems? Were there increased stressors in the family or at work during this time? Details of specific examples, including the who, what, why, when, and how of symptoms or behaviors are most helpful.

Specific questions about how the parents felt about the pregnancy, the first few weeks, developmental milestones, new siblings, and changes in work or relationships elicit important verbal and affective clues from the parents and the child. Specific questions about what the child does on a typical day, including rising, getting dressed, mealtimes, caregiving arrangements at home and beyond, and bedtime, help to structure detail gathering (Provence, 1977). It is essential to detail the impact of the child's difficulties on the child, parents, and family.

Developmental History

Developmental history includes details of the unfolding of the child's biological potential within the child's specific social environment. Many of these details will have been addressed or at least touched on when discussing the parents' presenting concerns. Important details about the perinatal history include the adequacy of prenatal care and complications of pregnancy including preeclampsia, bleeding, gestational diabetes, maternal illness, and maternal drug or alcohol use. The duration of labor, type of delivery, apgar scores, and complications of delivery or the immediate

postpartum period should be documented. The perinatal course for premature babies is especially relevant. Clinicians should obtain details about the child's medical, feeding/eating, and sleep history, separation and individuation, and age at which stage-specific milestones and capacities were reached, including language and communication, gross and fine motor skills, self-help skills, play, curiosity, preferences for active versus passive learning, activity level, and attention to shared and individual activities. In addition, parents must be asked explicitly about the possibility of the child's exposure to trauma, abuse, or neglect (American Academy of Child and Adolescent Psychiatry, 1997, 1998; Boris, Fueyo, & Zeanah, 1997; DeGangi et al., 1991; Emde, 1989; Greenspan & Wieder, 1997).

Regulation of Emotion and Behavior

Regulation of emotion and behavior provides a framework for collection of interview and observational data that facilitates the team's understanding of contributing biological and social risk and protective factors and facilitates intervention. Emotion and behavior are regulated by a combination of internal biological and external social processes that are so well integrated that they cannot easily be separated. Internal regulators include temperament, that is, individual differences in reactivity and self-regulation that are known to be influenced by environmental factors (Rothbart & Ahadi, 1994) and are related to sensory, sensory-motor, and organizational processing styles. External regulators include environmental factors, especially primary caregiving attachments and "affect attunement" (Stern, 1994).

Emotional and behavioral symptoms "often stem from underlying problems in sensory modulation and processing, motor planning, and affective integration" (Greenspan & Weider, 1997). To elicit information from parents about the child's individual differences in sensory, motor, and affective regulation, the clinician looks for the child's hypersensitivities and hyposensitivities to various sensory experiences. Special attention is focused on self-regulation, attention, sleep, touch, movement, listening, language, looking, and attachment (DeGangi, Poisson, Sickel, & Wiener, 1995). Hyper- or hypo-aroused patterns can be elicited with specific details about how the child responds to feeding, bathing, dressing, and other routines (Williamson & Anzalone, 1997).

Family relationships are the primary vehicle for regulating emotion and behavior and intervening with all children, including those with individual differences that include processing difficulties (Greenspan & Wieder, 1997). Questions about interpersonal connections, especially mutual attention, mutual engagement, and early communication (Weider, 1997), are helpful to elicit information about the child's early behavioral organization, ability to regulate affect, and relational capacities. Family regulatory styles are embedded in internal working models, family rituals, and disciplinary measures. Thus, it is helpful to ask the parents about the meaning of a child's specific behavior. Eliciting details about the family's evening meal and bed-time rituals provides information about the regulatory processes that families use to structure their daily activities and transitions. In addition, asking, "What discipline works or sometimes works?" is a supportive, nonjudgmental approach that frequently yields openness about disciplinary efforts that have helped or not helped (Clark et al., 1993; Greenspan & Wieder, 1997; Reiss, 1989; Thomas et al., 1993; Weider, 1997). These family relationship patterns that regulate children's behavior provide a window into the family experiences that guide the child's development.

Family Relational and Parents' Histories

Understanding the family and external caregiving arrangements and the child's responses to daily and prolonged separations is a crucial part of intervention-centered assessment. Creating a genogram of the extended family may facilitate exploration of current and previous parental relationships, caregiving arrangements including nuclear family, external caregivers, and special attachment figures, and who the parents depend on for help.

It is important to provide the parents with an understanding of how their own histories are linked to their child's. The parents' educational and work histories, psychiatric and legal histories, and early histories of being parented are best explored using specific verbal linkages in the context of gathering information about the child. For example, it is helpful to explain to parents that most parents first learn about parenting from their own parents and that how we are parented often influences how we parent our children. Creating this bridge of understanding is one way assessment naturally leads to family relational intervention and change.

Hypothesizing or "Wondering Along" with the Family

Hypothesizing or "wondering along" (Clark et al., 1993) with the family is a process of listening, observing, and thinking together. This process is an opportunity to elicit representations (Who does he or she remind you of?) and observe and understand the meaning of behaviors and how the family system regulates emotion and behavior (Why is the child doing this? What works to reinforce or stop the behavior?). "Looking together becomes the motto, without jumping too quickly to conclusions, despite the parents' often urgent need for reassurance and advise" (Guedeney & Libovici, 1997, p. 177). Looking together becomes intervention as the team understands, "co-constructs" (Emde, 1994) new narratives, and explores the parents' alternative solutions together.

Clinical Observation

Observation of the Child and Family Interactions

Many settings are appropriate for observation, including the child's home, child care setting, and the clinician's office. A playroom with age-appropriate toys such as a doll house, animals, baby doll and bottle, blocks, easy puzzles, shape boxes, cars, dress-up clothes, and a kitchen area is ideal but not necessary. Too many toys can be overstimulating. Carpeting facilitates children's, parents', and clinicians' floor play. Assessments may also be done with a few toys, for example, animals, a baby doll, and some small blocks. Paper and pens are useful for young preschoolers.

A free play session serves an important function in allowing parents to interact with their child as they might at home. Family and parent-child dyadic play is often videotaped and/or observed from behind a one-way mirror to facilitate the review of observational data and synthesis of history and observations. A videotaped play session may also be used to create a focus for hypothesizing or "wondering along" with the parents during subsequent assessment or intervention sessions.

Ideally, the child is seen at some point with all of the most important people in his or her life, including both parents and other regular caregivers such as grandparents or a nanny, who care for him or her a significant part of the day. It is often helpful to see the child with the whole family and alone with each parent or primary caregiver, as the interactions may vary considerably. Observation in the child care setting is helpful if the child is experiencing difficulties there or if he or she seems particularly upset upon returning home. It is helpful to see the child on at least two different days to access a range of the child's functioning and behavior that may be highly state-dependant. A tired, hungry, or ill child looks very different when he or she is rested and physically comfortable. Both states yield important data about the child and the family interactions.

The clinician wishes to see the widest possible range of the child's behavior to assess strengths, vulnerabilities, developmental status, and clear symptomatology in both the child and the child-parent dyads. Entry into a new situation can provoke both anxiety and interest/stimulation. The clinician seeks to observe the child's range of responses to "newness," to both stress and the exciting stimulation inherent in a new situation. The clinician also wants to observe how the parents help the child modulate stress and anxiety (or aggravate it), support the child's curiosity and exploration (or discourage it), and cope with their own emotional responses.

Observation is the clinician's most important tool in the evaluation of young children. Quiet watching in the waiting room and in the assessment process precedes attempts to interact with the young child, so as to minimally disturb the child and family's own patterns. The parents' comfort is facilitated by input from the clinician such as, "We would like you to play with your child as you would at home to help him feel comfortable here." As the child feels more comfortable, he or she will begin to behave more as he or she does at home. In some children, this means a "blossoming" into talking, interacting, full affective display, and intense play. For others, greater comfort means "blossoming" into more provocative, negativistic behavior with a parent or more risk taking or aggression. After the observation period, parents are asked how the child, as observed, was similar to or different from the way he or she is typically at home.

Regulation of Emotion and Behavior Provides an Observational Framework

Regulation of emotion and behavior provides a conceptual framework that can structure observation of the child's coping style or internal regulation and family relationships that are the primary vehicle for external regulation. By evolutionary design, the child's self-regulatory capacities are supplemented and augmented by the parents. Difficulties in emotional and behavioral regulation occur when the match between the child's ability to self-regulate and the parents' emotion regulation strategies is less than optimal. This mismatch may be due to constitutional/maturational factors in the child and/or the parents' lack of knowledge about or sensitivity to their child's cues.

Difficulties with regulation of emotion and behavior frequently present to our early childhood psychiatry clinics after the age of two years, when the developmental push toward autonomy and the emotional lability of toddlerhood result in increased acting out behavior and subsequent decreased parental ability to cope effectively. Although toddler temper tantrums and aggressive behavior are not indicators in themselves of psychopathology or risk for psychopathology, when the intensity is such that parents fear for their child's safety and feel angry, scared, helpless, and unable to gain control, the child is at risk for ongoing behavior problems. An emotion regulation framework enables the clinician to intervene in a nonblaming manner and reframe patterns between parent and child.

Infant and Toddler Mental Status Exam

The Infant and Toddler Mental Status Exam (ITMSE) was developed to help clinicians organize their observations of both infant and dyad across a variety of settings, sessions, and changes in the child's behavior, emotional state, and levels of interaction. The focus is on describing the child in clinical, descriptive, and specific terms. The ITMSE is not a rating scale, nor a coding system for behavior, nor a test with norms. This examination is a reference tool which describes the ways in which traditional categories of the mental status examination for adults and children may be adapted for use with infants and toddlers. It may be used to describe observations from a brief session or piece of videotape or to pool data from many contacts, perhaps including a home visit, play session, behavior during testing, observation at day care, and the child's response to a separation from the parent.

Categories have been added to the ITMSE, including sensory regulation and state regulation, which reflect important facets of infant development and disorders in young children. Developmental status in young children (both constitutional and maturational factors) may be characterized by age-expected skills, precociousness, delays, and deviations from the norm. The following sections of the ITMSE provide information most relevant to developmental status: III. Self-regulation, IV. Motor, V. Speech and Language, VIII. Play, and IX. Cognition.

The clinician must be sufficiently famil- iar with early child development to use this examination as a mental checklist in deciding whether a given child needs specific testing in any of these aspects of development. Many children will not need such testing. In certain locations, finding specialists qualified to perform such evaluations in young children is difficult or impossible. Observations from the ITMSE, coupled with developmental questionnaires, will aid the clinician in making decisions about further evaluation.

Further Uses of Specific Parts of the ITMSE

The following are examples of the use of observations from the ITMSE (see Table 12.1) to generate differential diagnoses or diagnostic hypotheses. These examples are in no way exhaustive or complete.

I. APPEARANCE.

The child's appearance may suggest certain syndromes. Some genetic anomalies (trisomy 21) or syndromes related to prenatal toxins (Fetal Alcohol Syndrome) have well known, easily observable, characteristic physical features. Unusual shape or positioning of the eyes, ears, nose, mouth, or tongue, micro- or macrocephaly or unusual head shape, and skin abnormalities may suggest congenital or chromosomal disorders. The child can then be referred to a geneticist for further evaluation. Small size and/or disproportionately low weight to height should alert the clinician to rule out failure-to-thrive or other medical conditions, usually in consultation with the child's pediatrician.

TABLE 12.1
Infant and Toddler Mental Status Exam

I. Appearance.

Size; level of nourishment; dress and hygiene; apparent maturity compared with age; dysmorphic features, for example, facies, eye and ear shape and placement, epican-thal folds, digits, and so on; abnormal head size; cutaneous lesions.

II. Apparent Reaction to Situation.

Note where evaluation takes place and with whom.

A. Initial reaction to setting and to strangers: Explores; freezes; cries; hides face; acts curious, excited, apathetic, or anxious (describe).

B. Adaptation.

1. Exploration: When and how child begins exploring faces, toys, strangers.
2. Reaction to transitions: From unstructured to structured activity; when exam-iner begins to play with infant; cleaning up; leaving.

III. Self-Regulation.

A. State regulation: An infant's state of consciousness ranges from deep sleep through alert stages to intense crying. Predominant state and range of states ob-served during session; patterns of transition, for example, smooth versus abrupt; capacity for being soothed and self-soothing; capacity for quiet alert state. (Some of these categories also apply to toddlers.)

B. Sensory regulation: Reaction to sounds, sights, smells, light and firm touch; hy-perresponsiveness or hyporesponsiveness (if observed) and type of response, in-cluding apathy, withdrawal, avoidance, fearfulness, excitability, aggression or marked behavioral change; excessive seeking of particular sensory input.

C. Unusual behaviors: Mouthing after one year of age; head banging; smelling ob-jects, spinning; twirling; hand-flapping; finger-flicking; rocking; toe-walking; staring at lights or spinning objects; repetitive, perseverative, or bizarre verbalizations or behaviors with objects or people; hair-pulling; ruminating; or breath-holding.

D. Activity level: Overall level and variability (note that toddlers are often incor-rectly called hyperactive). Describe behavior, for example, squirming constantly in parent's arms; sitting quietly on floor or in infant seat; constantly on the go; climbing on desk and cabinets; exploring the room; pausing to play with each of six to eight toys.

E. Attention span: Capacity to maintain attentiveness to an activity or interaction; longest and average length of sustained attention to a given toy or activity; dis-tractibility. Infants: Visual fixing and following at one month; tracking at two to three months; attention to own hands or feet and faces; duration of exploration of object with hands or mouth.

F. Frustration tolerance: Ability to persist in a difficult task, despite failure; capacity to delay reaction if easily frustrated, for example, aggression, crying, tantrums, withdrawal, avoidance.

G. Aggression: Modes of expression; degree of control of or preoccupation with ag-gression; appropriate assertiveness.

TABLE 12.1 Continued

IV. Motor.

Muscle tone and strength; mobility in different positions; unusual motor pattern, for example, tics, seizure activity; intactness of cranial nerves, for example, movement of face, mouth, tongue, and eyes, including feeding, swallowing, and gaze (note excessive drooling).

   A. Gross motor coordination. Infants: Pushing up; head control; rolling; sitting; standing. Toddlers: Walking; running; jumping; climbing; hopping; kicking; throwing and catching a ball. (It is useful to have something for the child to climb on such as a chair.)

   B. Fine motor coordination. Infants: Grasping and releasing; transferring from hand to hand; using pincer grasp; banging; throwing. Toddlers: Using pincer grasp; stacking; scribbling; cutting. Both fine motor and visual-motor coordination can be screened by observing how the child handles puzzles, shape boxes, a ball and hammer toy, small cars, and toys with connecting parts.

V. Speech and Language.

   A. Vocalization and speech production: Quality; rate; rhythm; intonation; articulation; volume.

   B. Receptive language: comprehension of others' speech as seen in verbal or behavioral response, for example, follows commands; points in response to "where is" questions; understands prepositions and pronouns (include estimate of hearing, especially in child with language delay, for example, response to loud sounds and voice; ability to localize sound).

   C. Expressive language: Level of complexity, for example, vocalization, jargon, number of single words, short phrases, full sentences; overgeneralization, for example, uses "kitty" to refer to all animals; pronoun use including reversal; echolalia, either immediate or delayed; unusual or bizarre verbalizations. Preverbal children: Communicative intent, for example, vocalizations, babbling, imitation, gestures, such as head shaking and pointing; caregiver's ability to understand infant's communication; child's effectiveness in communication.

VI. Thought.

The usual categories for thought disorder almost never apply to young children. Primary process thinking, as evidenced in verbalizations or play, is expected in this age group. The line between fantasy and reality is often blurred. Bizarre ideation, perseveration, apparent loose associations, and the persistence of pronoun reversals, jargon, and echolalia in an older toddler or preschooler may be noted in a variety of psychiatric disorders, including pervasive developmental disorders.

   A. Specific fears: Feared object; worry about being lost or separated from parent.

   B. Dreams and nightmares: Content is sometimes obtainable in children 2 to 3 years old. Child does not always perceive it as a dream, for example, "A monster came in the front door."

   C. Dissociative state: Sudden episodes of withdrawal and inattention; eyes glazed; "tuned out"; failure to track ongoing social interaction. Dissociative state may be difficult to differentiate from an absence seizure, depression, autism, or deafness. The context may be helpful, for example, child with a history of neglect freezes in a dissociative state as mother leaves room. Neurologic or audiologic evaluation may be warranted.

TABLE 12.1   Continued

    D. Hallucinations: Extremely rare, except in the context of a toxic or organic disorder, then usually visual or tactile.

VII. Affect and Mood.

The assessment of mood and affect may be more difficult in young children because of limited language, lack of vocabulary for emotions, and use of withdrawal in response to a variety of emotions from shyness and boredom to anxiety and depression.

    A. Modes of expression: Facial; verbal; body tone and positioning.

    B. Range of expressed emotions: Affect, especially in parent-child relationship.

    C. Responsiveness: To situation, content of discussion, play, and interpersonal engagement.

    D. Duration of emotional state: Need history or multiple observations.

    E. Intensity of expressed emotions: Affect, especially in parent-child relationship.

VIII. Play.

Play is a primary mode of information gathering for all sections of the ITMSE. In very young children, play is especially useful in the evaluation of the child's cognitive and symbolic functioning, relatedness, and expression of affect. Themes of play are helpful in assessing older toddlers. The management and expression of aggression are assessed in play as in other areas of behavior. Play may be with toys or with child's own or another's body, for example, peek-a-boo, roughhousing; verbal, for example, sound imitation games between mother and infant; interactional or solitary. It is important to note how the child's play varies with different familiar caregivers and with parents versus the examiner.

    A. Structure of play (age-approximate).

        1. Sensorimotor play.

            a. 0–12 months: Mouthing, banging, dropping and throwing toys or other objects.

            b. 6–12 months: Exploring characteristics of objects, for example, moving parts, poking, pulling.

        2. Functional play.

            a. 12–18 months: Child's use of objects shows understanding and exploration of their use or function, for example, pushes car, touches comb to hair, puts telephone to ear.

        3. Early symbolic play.

            a. 18 months and older: Child pretends with increasing complexity; pretends with own body to eat or sleep; pretends with objects or other people, for example, "feeds" mother; child uses one object to represent another, for example, a block becomes a car; child pretends a sequence of activities, for example, cooking and eating.

        4. Complex symbolic play.

            a. 30 months and older: Child plans and acts out dramatic play sequences, uses imaginary objects. Later, child incorporates others into play with assigned roles.

        5. Imitation, turn-taking, and problem-solving as part of play.

TABLE 12.1   Continued

B. Content of Play. The toddler's choice and use of toy often reflect emotional themes. It is desirable to have on hand toys that tap different developmental and emotional domains. An overfull playroom may be overwhelming or overstimulating and reduce meaningful observations. Young toddlers of both sexes often gravitate to dolls, dishes, animals, and moving toys, such as cars. The examiner's choice of specific materials may facilitate the expression of pertinent emotional themes. For example, a child traumatized by a dog bite may more likely reenact the trauma if a dog and doll figures are available. The child's reaction to scary toys, such as sharks, dinosaurs, or guns, should be noted, especially if they are avoided or dominate the session. Does aggressive pretend play become "real" and physically harmful? By 2½ to 3 years old, a child's animal or doll play can reveal important themes about family life, including reactions to separation, parent-child and sibling relationships, experiences at day care, quality of nurturance and discipline, and physical or sexual abuse. The examiner must use caution in interpreting play, viewing it as a possible combination of reenactment, fears, and fantasy.

IX. Cognition.
Using information from all preceding areas, especially play, verbal and symbolic functioning, and problem-solving, roughly assess child's cognitive level in terms of developmental intactness, delays, or precocity.

X. Relatedness.
A. To parents: How "in tune" do the child and parent seem? Does the child make and maintain eye, verbal, or physical contact? Is there active avoidance by child? Note infant's level of comfort and relaxation being held and fed, "molding" into caregiver's body. Does toddler move away from caregiver and check back or bring toys to show, put into his or her lap, or play with together or near caregiver? Comment on physical or verbal affection, hostility, reaction to separation and reunion, and use of transitional objects (blanket, toy, caregiver's possession). Describe differences in relating if more than one caregiver is present.

B. To examiner: Young children normally show some hesitancy to engage with a stranger, especially after six to eight months of age. Appropriate wariness in young children may result in a period of watching the examiner, staying physically close to a familiar caregiver before engaging, or showing some constriction of affect, vocalization, or play. After initial wariness, does the child relate? Does the child engage too soon or not at all? How does relatedness with a stranger compare to that with a parent? Is the child friendly versus indiscriminately attention-seeking or guarded versus overanxious? Can examiner engage the child in play or structured activities to a degree not seen with caregiver? Does the child show pleasure in successes if the examiner shows approval?

C. Attachment behaviors: Observe for showing affection, comfort-seeking, asking for and accepting help, cooperating, exploring, controlling behavior, and reunion responses. Describe age-related disturbances in these normative behaviors. Disturbances often are seen in abused and neglected children, for example, fearfulness, clinginess, overcompliance, hypervigilance, impulsive overactivity, and defiance; restricted or hyperactive and distractible exploratory behavior; and restricted or indiscriminate affection and comfort-seeking.

II. APPARENT REACTION TO SITUATION.

Clues to the child's temperament may be seen in his or her initial behavior. The slow to warm up child will initially cling to the parent and do little exploring. Such infants often explore with visual scanning but may fuss and require soothing. Toddlers often hide in their parent's clothing or hide their faces. The infant or toddler who continues to be distressed, crying or fussing, and trying to leave, could be: (1) overtired (purely situational), (2) physically ill, (3) slow to adapt to change/newness/stimulation (suggesting a temperament or constitutional/maturational factor), (4) in a distressed relationship with the parent or caregiver present (evaluate for a disorder in the relationship), and so on. Zeanah, Mamman, & Lieberman (1993) describe the balance between attachment behaviors and exploration in toddlers as key to understanding the child's ability to use the attachment figure as a secure base (for exploration) and safe haven (for comfort and reassurance).

III. SELF-REGULATION.

State Regulation and Sensory Regulation

This category is of importance in exploring many presenting concerns in infants, toddlers, and young preschoolers. In infants, poor state regulation can alert the clinician to questions about the infant's neurologic intactness and maturity. Certain infants, by temperament or because of a specific genetic or perinatal influence such as cocaine exposure, may have difficulty with sensory regulation. Such infants are easily overstimulated, so that holding, feeding, making eye contact, and cooing to them simul-

taneously is so overwhelming that the infant cannot feed and may fuss instead. For many fussy infants, lowering the lights, talking very softly, or moving them very slowly or not at all may facilitate calming and turn an irritable infant into a quiet, observing one in the evaluation session. DC: 0–3 has identified a diverse group of Regulatory Disorders, which reflect constitutional/maturational difficulties associated with specific behavioral patterns (Zero to Three, 1994). Hypersensitive children with difficulties in sensory regulation in a busy child care setting or home may try to shield themselves from bright lights, loud noises, or high emotional tone by withdrawal, covering their eyes or ears, or angry or aggressive pushing away of peers or adults. Hyposensitive children may crave sensory input, seen in hyperactive or inattentive behaviors such as repeated jumping on furniture or flitting from toy to toy with little engagement.

Activity Level, Attention Span, and Frustration Tolerance

The triad of activity level, attention span, and frustration tolerance should be carefully observed, as a many parents describe their normal toddlers as "hyperactive." True "hyperactivity" may represent an early form of Attention Deficit Hyperactivity Disorder (ADHD) (American Psychiatric Association, 1994) or a Regulatory Disorder (Zero to Three, 1994). Young traumatized children with Post-Traumatic Stress Disorder (American Psychiatric Association, 1994) or Traumatic Stress Disorder (Zero to Three, 1994) may show difficulties in this triad of behaviors including high arousal with hyperactivity, poor attention span and concentration, and irritability with low frustration tolerance or impulsivity (Thomas, 1995; Thomas & Tidmarsh, 1997). Low frustration tolerance with frequent irritability and tantrums may be temporally linked to a child's inability to communicate his or her wishes or needs to a caregiver. This may be caused by unrecognized delays in receptive or productive language or the parent's difficulty "reading" the child, which is often due to the parent's lack of information about what the child needs.

The setting may greatly influence the child's behavior. Large playrooms with a dazzling array of toys can elicit "flitting," distractible behavior from many normal children, especially those who do not have access to many toys. The child who is reacting to this novelty and stimulation often calms down in the course of one session or two sessions. A less stimulating assessment setting may elicit a wider range of behavior in the child, more meaningful interaction with the clinician and parent, and more sustained play sequences.

Aggression

It is useful to note spontaneous aggression in children (e.g., hitting the parent, sibling, or examiner) as well as preoccupation with aggressive themes in play (from banging everything or crashing cars to monsters and dinosaurs killing all the people). Some children avoid all aggressive-looking toys and may become very fearful if a wolf puppet or toy dinosaur is presented. It is helpful to test a child's reactions to such "scary" toys if this has not happened sponta-

neously. The child's use of the parent for safety may be triggered, and reactions of both child and parents' can be observed.

IV. MOTOR.

Most infant mental health assessments do not include a formal neurological examination. However, every young child should be observed for basic intactness of motor strength or weakness, left-right symmetry of body appearance and movement, and impaired function or actual paralysis. The clinician should watch the way the child moves, sits, gets up from sitting or lying, runs, climbs, and so on. The parent should be queried about unexpected observations. Any previously undiagnosed motor or coordination problems should be referred to a neurologist or back to the pediatrician for evaluation. The same is true if minor motor seizures, also known as absence seizures or staring spells, are seen during the evaluation. (Clues from context help differentiate staring spells associated with anxiety or dissociation from absence seizures.) Gross and fine motor coordination are screened by observing the child (as outlined in ITMSE). Coordination and balance problems are often further evaluated by an occupational or physical therapist.

Communicating the Clinician's Observations

Clinicians have many styles of organizing their observations into written reports. Some clinicians have used the ITMSE outline structure to collate and communicate their observations of the child. Others prefer to describe each session, focusing more on the process of the parent-child interaction and incorporating observations of the child into that description. The ITMSE reminds the clinician to observe the infant through multiple lenses, including constitutional/maturational and interpersonal. In the formulation, the clinician integrates history, observations, and structured evaluations or questionnaires (if used) into a description of the child's developmental, emotional, behavioral, and interpersonal functioning and symptomatology. This can then be integrated with the assessment of the environment, including the child's family, current caregivers, and wider social risk or protective factors, to generate the clinician's best formulation of diagnoses, etiology, and recommended intervention strategies. The observations section should be detailed enough that another clinician can use the data to say "I would agree with his or her conclusions" or "I would understand it differently, especially since I have also seen the child in another setting with the following observations."

Questionnaires and Standardized Instruments

Questionnaires and standardized instruments help structure clinical data collection and save time. Questionnaires about demographic information, pregnancy, birth, neonatal period, areas of development, family, social, and medical history, and specific symptom checklists are often sent to parents before the first visit so that they can review these issues at home, consult other family members or medical records, and be prepared with information pertinent to the evaluation. When parents return the forms already completed, the clinician can review these records prior to the assessment.

How Many Questionnaires Are Too Many?

Many clinicians are concerned that too much written material will overwhelm a family. This is especially a concern when the family speaks a different language or has a limited educational background. If difficulty filling out forms is anticipated, the clinician can include a note or ask the family to think about the questions and offer help from staff immediately prior to the assessment. Some clinicians prefer to establish rapport with the family in person first, before asking parents to complete some or all of the questionnaires or inventories. Questionnaires are particularly critical when the child is in foster care or will be brought by a social worker or nonfamily member. The relevant agency must be informed that the infant specialist needs important background information that may be buried in files which a judge must release. Allowing for sufficient time to obtain records may be a necessary part of the intake structure in such cases.

Which Standardized Instruments Are Helpful In Our Clinics?

In addition to the Infant and Toddler Mental Status Exam, other structured assessments may be used to assess developmental, emotional, behavioral, and relational domains. The following section provides a brief overview of some of the assessment tools that may prove useful in understanding a child's difficulties. Clinicians are urged to select those which fit the child's needs and parents' understanding of the problem, in conjunction with the clinician's own hypotheses about the case. Clearly, some structured assessments are more appropriate than others for particular cases. We describe the standardized instruments that have been most helpful in our clinics. These measures streamline the collection of clinical data about the child, parent, and relationship between parent and child.

Parental Report Measures

Children's developmental status can be assessed by having the parents completed the *Child Development Inventory* (CDI) (Ireton & Thwing, 1992). This 300-item questionnaire is designed to assess children from age 15 months to 6 years. The inventory includes questions about general developmental issues, language development, motor development, social skills, and self-help skills. It also includes behavioral problem and symptom items. It takes approximately 30 minutes for parents to complete. Its strength is the wide age range with which it can be used, as well as the focus on developmental issues.

Young children's behavior problems and symptoms can be assessed using the Child Behavior Checklist 2–3 (CBCL 2–3) (Achenbach, Edelbrock, & Howell, 1987). This 100-item questionnaire is a parental report

of the child's symptoms and is appropriate for children ages two through three. It typically takes parents 15 minutes to complete the measure. Although it does not focus on the child's strengths or assessment of development, it provides a standardized way to collect information on the magnitude and variety of specific externalizing and internalizing symptoms, as well as somatic and sleep complaints.

The *Infant/Toddler Symptom Checklist* (DeGangi et al., 1995) is a screening and diagnostic tool that assesses 7-to 30-month-old infants and toddlers for the presence of regulatory disorder symptoms. This measure is comprised of five separate checklists for different age groups and one general checklist that covers the entire age range. The checklist is completed by parents and assesses infants' and toddlers' self-regulation, attention, sleep, eating or feeding, dressing, bathing, and touch, movement, listening and language, looking and sight, and attachment/emotional functioning. The checklist provides cutoff scores based on normative data that allow clinicians to determine children are at risk for regulatory disorders.

The *Parenting Stress Index* (PSI) (Abidin, 1995a, 1995b) is a questionnaire that asks parents to report on the stress associated with being a parent. The full PSI has 120 items and measures child factors, parent factors, and parent-child interaction factors. The short form of the PSI has 36 items and measures parental sense of competence and parenting isolation, child adaptability and demandingness, and life stress. Both can be used to identify areas where families may be particularly at risk.

Observational Measures

The *Parent-Child Early Relational Assessment* (PCERA) (Clark, 1985) is a standardized protocol for observing the quality of young children's interaction with their parents. It includes an opportunity for clinicians to observe parents and children in a free play session, structured teaching task, feeding interaction, and separation/reunion situation. The interaction is videotaped and can be coded for the quality of affect and behavior, including infant positive and negative affect, dyadic mutuality and tension, and parental sensitivity and responsiveness. Although specialized training is required to use the coding system in a standardized empirical way, the assessment protocol can also be used without this training as a clinical tool that provides multiple contexts for viewing parent-child interaction and guides the clinicians' observations.

The Crowell Clinical Problem-Solving Procedure (Crowell, Feldman, & Ginsberg, 1988) assesses interaction between mother and child across varied situations: Free play, cleanup, separation-reunion, and four tasks using common toys. The tasks are developmentally graded, and the pair is presented with tasks of increasing difficulty from easy to too hard for the child. The mother's behavior toward the child is observed in areas such as support and quality of assistance, while the child is observed for interactive behaviors such as affection, negativity, and reliance on the mother. The assessment is designed for children whose chronological or developmental age falls in the range of 24 to 54 months.

In addition, specific clinical and research assessment tools that may be useful have focused on children's coping (Early Coping Inventory, Zeitlin, Williamson, & Szczepanski, 1988), family-focused team assessments of young children (Connecticut Infant Toddler Developmental Assessment, Erikson & Vater, 1988), and adult representations of attachment relationships (Adult Attachment Interview, Main & Goldwyn, 1984). Helpful overviews of assessment instruments and strategies for the assessment of young children can be found in several recent works (American Academy of Child and Adolescent Psychiatry, 1997; California Infant Mental Health Work Group, 1996; Fenichel & Meisels, 1996; Shonkoff & Meisels, 1990; Zeanah, 1993).

Ongoing Mutual Formulation and Diagnosis

Ongoing Mutual Formulation

Throughout the assessment, the clinician is listening and observing on multiple levels: Development, emotion, behavior, and relationships. The parent presents a concern in a particular domain, which may appear developmental (he or she is not talking yet), emotional (he or she seems really upset and cranky since the new baby was born), behavioral (he or she is really aggressive in the child care center and they are threatening to kick him out), or relational (he or she seems really uncomfortable with his or her father since the parents separation, and the mother does not know how much to push or allow visitation). For each of these presenting concerns, the clinician should have immediate questions about the other domains. The following represent one or two examples in each domain of the dozens of questions which might be pursued.

Not talking:

Developmental	At what level is the child's development in other areas?
Emotional	Is the child withdrawn in other ways?
Behavioral	How does the child communicate wishes and needs? How does the child deal with frustration?
Relational	Has the child been in a stable, nurturing environment?

Upset and cranky with new baby:

Developmental	What does the child understand about the baby? Can the child talk or play out his or her feelings?
Emotional	Is the child happy and playful for the part of the day or is the child's range of moods narrowed?
Behavioral	Is the child acting-up or aggressive with baby or mother?
Relational	How was and is the child's relationship with his or her mother? Is the child getting increased time/attention/love from others?

Aggressive in day care:

Developmental	Is the child at age level in developmental skills? Is the child placed with peers he or she can relate to or are they much older or younger?
Emotional	How is the child's mood at home? Is the child stressed by significant changes occurring there? Is the child angry or only impulsive?
Behavioral	Is the child's aggression directed at selected children or adults or at everyone? Are peers picking on the child? Is the child always blamed for any disruption in the group?
Relational	What is the nature of the child's primary relationships at home and with the caregivers at the child care setting? Does the child turn to anyone for help and nurturing there?

Uncomfortable with father:

Developmental	At what level is the child's emotional development, for example, separation anxiety, object permanence? Is the child's language adequate to communicate about experiences?
Emotional	What is the child's predominant mood, range of

	affect? Can the child have fun? Is this a drastic change or intensification of the child's usual temperament?
Behavioral	Is the child showing discomfort suggestive of traumatic experiences with the father for example, change in behavior around feeding, diapering, being scolded?
Relational	Have other relationships changed, especially the relationship with the child's mother?

Some parents are eager to pursue with the clinician these other related avenues of inquiry. When such inquiry supports the need for a widening scope of assessments, both clinician and parents must stop and discuss *why* this seems relevant to the clinician. When the clinician presents a rationale for collecting data, whether by questionnaires, further history about or direct testing of the child, further history about the parents' feelings about the child, relationships, or symptomatology, many parents eagerly join the clinician in this pursuit of greater understanding.

The clinician's and family's mutual formulation of the problems is ongoing throughout the assessment process and formally summarized periodically, sometimes at the end of each session. The biopsychosocial formulation summary is a mutual effort to understand the long-term and recent biological and social risk and protective factors as they affect the child and the family.

Diagnosis

Diagnostic thinking provides a frame to organize the family interview, observations of the family interactions and relationships, and ongoing formulation and treatment planning with the family. Diagnosis provides a common language for communication among clinicians and between clinicians and caregivers. Diagnostic systems are evolving rapidly for the field of infant and toddler mental health. The *Diagnostic and Statistical Manual of Mental Disorders,* 4th edition (DSM–IV) (American Psychiatric Association, 1994) and *International Classification of Diseases* (ICD–10) (World Health Organization, 1992) offer diagnoses specifically helpful in this age group, including Motor Skills and Communication Disorders, Pervasive Developmental Disorders, and Mental Retardation. The newest system, the *Diagnostic Classification of Mental Health and Developmental Disorders of Infancy and Early Childhood* (DC: 0–3), also known as *Diagnostic Classification: 0–3* (Zero to Three, 1994), describes many disorders similar to other diagnoses in the DSM–IV (such as Posttraumatic Stress Disorder, Reactive Attachment Disorder of Infancy or Early Childhood, Sleep Disorders, and Eating Disorders) and some arising from new constructs. DC: 0–3 extends the DSM–IV system downward to describe disorders as they arise in infancy and disorders that may change with time. For example, DC: 0–3's Regulatory Disorders, a new construct, address constitutional/maturational difficulties which may improve with maturation or may be described later as DSM–IV's

Attention-Deficit Hyperactivity Disorder (ADHD). In addition, DC: 0–3 includes a decision tree that prioritizes certain diagnoses over others. For example, if a child is exposed to a clear traumatic event or series of events, Traumatic Stress Disorder is considered before other diagnoses. The Zero to Three/National Center for Clinical Infant Programs' Diagnostic Classification Task Force collected preliminary data from 1987 to 1994 in their development of the DC: 0–3. The Task Force is currently planning standardized training, field testing, and ongoing data collection toward further development of the DC: 0–3 (AACAP, 1997; Zero to Three, 1994).

DC: 0–3's multiaxial system describes key aspects of the child's experience, context, and development. Axis I, Primary Diagnosis, describes the disorder within the child, that is, the child's internal experience of distress or his or her dysfunctional behavioral expression. Axis II, Relationship Classification, describes the child's relationship with each primary caregiver. The PIR–GAS provides a 90-point scale that rates the strength and vulnerability within each primary relationship. A relationship disorder is specified on Axis II when the PIR–GAS score falls below 40 (Zero to Three, 1994).

DC: 0–3 Axis I disorders identify specific risk factors. For example, Traumatic Stress Disorder and Adjustment Disorder are associated, respectively, with severe or lessor environmental risk factors, Regulatory Disorders, a new construct which describes the child's constitutional/maturational and related specific behavioral difficulties, are primarily associated with constitutional/maturational risk factors, and Disorders of Affect, frequently related to loss or some difficulty in a primary relationship which has generalized beyond that relationship, are often associated with interactional risk factors (Zero to Three, 1994). DSM–IV and DC: 0–3 complement and augment each other. As these diagnostic frameworks continue to evolve, the clinician may draw from both systems.

Treatment Planning with the Family

The process of intervention begins with the clinician and family's first contact. The clinician must be assessing, from the outset, the family's capacity to change for the sake of the child. This may involve a change in outlook toward the child (e.g., from blaming to understanding), change in handling the child and his behavior, or change in the family environment when it is marked by high stress, interpersonal tension, chaos, or violence. Can the family cope emotionally and financially with taking the child for sessions of whatever intervention may be needed? If the clinician takes a collaborative stance with the family, "wondering along" with them and sharing hypotheses, change may be seen even within the first session and certainly over the course of an extended evaluation.

The clinician must be attuned to several issues in making treatment recommendations. What do the parents want addressed versus what does the evaluator feel is necessary or ideal for the child? If the child has

431

multiple needs, should they all be addressed now or should they be prioritized with a sequential approach to intervention (to respond to parent issues of financial impact, time, emotional economy, or the needs of the rest of the family)? When should one recommend intervention versus waiting? Some major environmental changes, such as placement in foster care (or return home), change in child care from poor to good fit, or a parent decreasing work and spending more time with the child, may have a powerful effect and may move the child's problematic behavior, affective state, relationships, or developmental status toward the norm.

A brief and/or single discipline evaluation may result first in referral for further evaluations. Such referrals may precede or coexist with psychotherapy recommendations. Such referrals include referrals to other medical specialists, such as neurology, genetics, ophthalmology, audiology, or primary pediatric screening. These are usually made through or in consultation with the child's pediatrician. Children may be referred for developmental testing by psychologists, speech and language pathologists, or occupational therapists, either within one's own clinic or team or to colleagues in the community. It is helpful to develop regular relationships with such specialists to form your own 'team' if you are a private practitioner. The family will be best served if someone, usually the infant mental health specialist, coordinates all of the evaluations into a coherent diagnostic formulation and treatment approach. Another common referral for children with developmental delays is to a re-

gional center and/or local school district for further evaluation and services.

Treatment Planning for a Child With Emotional, Behavioral, and/or Relational Difficulties

The child, parents, family, and child's wider social ecosystem should all be considered in treatment planning. The clinician must first be sure that the child is safe (physically and emotionally, including protection from abuse and neglect). If not, the clinician's first responsibility is referral to the appropriate child protective agency. Even this step can be used therapeutically if the parent can be enlisted to join the clinician in calling for help in service of his or her child. A parent requesting assistance from a child protective service is more likely to be viewed positively by that agency.

The next challenge is to help the parents understand more fully "Who is my baby?", then, "Why is he acting and feeling the way he does?", and finally, "Why am I feeling the way I do about parenting him?" The assessment begins that process. Treatment may be needed to pursue these questions in their many implications for day-to-day care of the child. The range of interventions may include:

1. Dyadic treatments of the parent-child unit.
2. Information for the parents, including classes, reading, and parent guidance (with or without the baby present).
3. Treatment of individual parent psychopathology or marital/relationship discord.

4. Therapist interventions with the child, including play therapy (usually with a parent present except in a few pre-schoolers).
5. Specific therapies for developmental delays or disturbances.
6. Assisting the parents in seeking more appropriate child care, home care, pre-school or special programs.
7. Direct intervention (usually educational in nature) with the child care or preschool providers, nannies, grand-mothers, or other extended caregivers.
8. Referral for social services including income support, housing, medical care, Parents as Teachers, Early Head Start, and Head Start.

Additional planning for the child with developmental/constitutional differences and needs. When an interdisciplinary team assessment or an individual clinician's assessment identifies clear developmental delays or disabilities, the clinician may assist the parents in obtaining services. Depending on the child's age and local funding and service providers, referral may be to individual speech and language, occupational or physical therapists, Federally-funded programs or local school districts.

Family support is crucial for the child with multiple special needs. The infant specialist is often the first one to confirm the parents' worry that something is "wrong" with their child. The clinician making such a diagnosis needs to help the parents both cognitively with information and psychologically with support and empathy. Some families need ongoing support from a mental health professional. Any of the therapies noted in the previous section may be applicable to the family and child with developmental delays or disorders, from mild to severe. A period of dyadic treatment to help the parent support the child's development may be useful.

Assessment as Successful Intervention

The assessment initiates a process in which the parents may perceive and interact with the child in new ways. Enhanced understanding of the child's temperament, sensitivities, and strengths may lead the parent to change the child's daily activities or setting or for example, introduce a slow-to-warm-up child much more slowly to transitions and new experiences. Even in the first session, a clinician may demonstrate that a very irritable baby is calmed by decreasing stimulation (lowering the sound, lights, or physical stimulation) that may lead quickly to the parents' increased effectiveness and pleasure with their baby. Parents may see their child's unrecognized capacities and new ways of interacting when the clinician reviews with the parents a videotaped parent-child play session or the clinician draws the toddler into reciprocal or early symbolic play. The evaluation itself may initiate a healing process. Dramatic examples of this may occur with the elucidation of previously unrecognized trauma.

Case Example: A 3½-year-old boy presented with aggression toward peers and marked oppositionality toward his parents at home and in the clinician's office. The history revealed that his father had broken his pelvic

433

bone in a motorcycle accident when Steven was two years old. The father required a 2-week hospitalization and months of recovery at home in a bed. He was later wheelchair bound but had a full recovery after nine months. Direct questioning and play stories revealed that Steven believed, "Daddy got hurt in the woods. He died. He hurt his pee pee. The doctor fixed his pee pee." Steven lowered his pants to show that *his* pee pee was okay. He held strongly to this understanding of his father's absence and broken pelvis. His mother was able to explain what had really happened, that Daddy had *not* died and was now fine. She realized no one had ever explained events fully to Steven as a two-year-old, and he had worried profoundly over these events. Her empathy and his resulting flood of questions and reenactment of the accident in play led to a much improved parent-child relationship with dramatically decreased aggression and oppositionality.

"Assessment as successful intervention" often represents a nudge of the child back into the path of normal development. However, the clinician must bear in mind that the phenomenon of "transference cure" or "flight into health" can be transitory. It is important to provide a mechanism for the parents to check back in a few weeks or months and return, if necessary, without a sense of failure.

Consultation Model of Assessment and Treatment

The consultation model of infant assessment (usually one session of 60 to 90 minutes) has a role in our clinical practice, but one which should be exercised with cau-

tion and only by clinicians experienced with young children. It is virtually impossible to examine all four domains (developmental, emotional, behavioral, and relational) adequately in one contact. Some situations where this may be necessary include: (1) Managed care practices which will only authorize one session at first, forcing triage and justification for further assessment sessions, (2) Parents who are "not sure if this is really a problem" and want to come with or without the child for a consultation, and (3) Parents who view an infant mental health assessment as similar to a visit to the pediatrician. Parents may be skeptical about seeing a mental health professional for what they see as a typical problem of babies (sleeping, eating, fussiness). Usually such families have been referred because the typical problem is extreme in degree, duration, or parent response. It may take great tact to persuade such parents to explore the emotional or relational domains.

Case Example: Mrs. M, a high-pressure professional, was referred with her four-month-old son by their pediatrician because "Brian won't look at me and I am worried he is autistic." The pediatrician noted that Mrs. M did a lot of professional travel and was terrified of being told that might affect her baby. The baby was developing normally in all other domains but did gaze avert from the mother although not from the pediatrician. In a 90-minute session, the clinician observed an alert, comfortable baby who molded well and fed easily with his mother. When she tried to interact with him, she spoke loudly and quickly. As he averted his gaze, she lifted him over her head, moving him up and down and talking more animatedly to get his attention. He avoided more actively. The clinician suggested "an experiment." She turned off the overhead lights and spoke very quietly to the baby, who turned to her voice with interest. Establishing the sensory hypersensitivity of this baby, the clinician coached the mother on a calm, quiet approach, noting how counterintuitive this seemed for the mother, whose usual style worked well in other settings. As Mrs. M experienced success with the baby, she and the clinician explored how she could create such quiet moments for contact when she came home from work to Brian and his high energy three-year-old brother.

Mrs. M was reassured that Brian did not seem autistic but showed sensory hypersensitivity, that he was demonstrating a preferential turning to her (attachment behavior) in the office setting by nestling in, even though not gazing. She was encouraged to try this new approach for one week, keep notes (which engaged her intellectual approach), and return. Some of her fears about autism, damage, and so on could be explored, but in one session the primary goal was to engage her, as she was highly ambivalent and anxious about the referral. Marital problems, work/mothering conflicts, and the effect of her own very active and somewhat abrasive style had to wait to see if she could tolerate further assessment. The "autism" was cured in one week, but the mother continued to use the clinician in an intermittent approach/avoidance style for the next three years, never completing a full assessment but deriving considerable clinical benefit from very infrequent sessions.

This consultation was facilitated by a good history from the pediatrician about the baby, his parents, and his sibling so that developmental concerns were low and the cli-

nician could feel comfortable with a simple consultation, a session with an alert baby who was observed to eat, play, be comforted when distressed, and showed a range of behavior with mother and the clinician, and a healthy enough mother to maintain this relationship and view the clinician as a resource. When Mrs. M returned at 18 months with a concern about "hyperactivity" (not clinically substantiated), the clinician was able to raise concern about Brian's expressive language development and eventually persuaded Mrs. M to have this assessed. The challenges of this case were the mother's unwillingness to explore her own issues more than superficially and father's complete lack of participation, despite the therapist's urging. Mrs. M eventually disclosed that she had her own therapist and thus, purposely kept her own issues out of her contact with the infant specialist (to the clinician's frustration). This, coupled with the father's lack of involvement, meant that marital issues and the relative absence of the father were sensed but could not be explored. This is clearly not an ideal assessment or treatment. However, because of the mother's skittishness, the clinician had to settle for "half a loaf." Intermittent consultation contacts over time continued to suggest the child's basically healthy development.

Conclusion

In this chapter we have brought together current advances in brain and social sciences, theory, and clinical practice. We have focused on the transactional biopsychosocial model of development and discussed the contribution of individual differences and the power of relationships in the regulation of emotions and behavior. We have focused on pragmatic assessment strategies for listening, observing, and understanding the child in four domains of his or her functioning: Developmental, emotional, behavioral, and relational. It is the clinician's role to synthesize information from history, observation, and interactional and structured assessments in these four domains into a multidimensional understanding of the child. Intervention-centered assessment creates a therapeutic alliance which values and validates the family's knowledge of their child, shares information that facilitates the "goodness of fit" between the family's expectations of their child and who the child is, increases the family's empathy, hope, and enjoyment, and facilitates the family's use of services and advocacy for their child. The process of looking carefully at the child together mobilizes the clinician's and family's collaborative attention to the child's strengths, needs, and potential and provides an opportunity to intervene early and preventively.

References

Abidin, R. R. (1995a). *Parenting stress index*. Odessa, FL: Psychological Assessment Resources, Inc.

Abidin, R. R. (1995b). *Parenting stress index: Short form*. Odessa, FL: Psychological Assessment Resources, Inc.

Achenbach, T. M., Edelbrock, C., & Howell, C. T. (1987). Empirically based assessment of behavioral and emotional problems of 2-, 3-year-old children. *Journal of Abnormal Child Psychology, 15*, 629–650.

Ainsworth, M. D. S., Blehar, M. C., Waters, E., & Wall, S. (1978). *Patterns of attachment: A psychological study of the strange situation*. Hillsdale, NJ: Erlbaum.

American Academy of Child and Adolescent Psychiatry. (1997). Practice parameters for the psychiatric assessment of infants and toddlers (0–36 months). *Journal of the American Academy of Child and Adolescent Psychiatry, 36*, 21S–36S.

American Psychiatric Association. (1994). *Diagnostic and statistical manual of mental disorders* (4th ed.). Washington, DC: Author.

Amini, F., Lewis, T., Lannon, R., Louie, A., Baumbacher, G., McGuinness, T., & Zierker-Schiff, E. (1996). Affect, attachment, memory: Contributions toward psychobiologic integration. *Psychiatry, 59*, 213–239.

Barrett, K. C., & Campos, J. J. (1987). Perspectives on emotional development II. In J. D. Osofsky (Ed.), *Handbook of infant development*. New York: Wiley.

Boris, N., Fueyo, M., & Zeanah, C. (1997). The clinical assessment of attachment in children under five. *Journal of the American Academy of Child and Adolescent Psychiatry, 36*(2), 291–293.

Bowlby, J. (1973). *Attachment and loss: Vol. 2. Separation, anxiety and anger*. New York: Basic Books.

Bowlby, J. (1982). *Attachment and loss: Vol. 1. Attachment* (2nd ed.). New York: Basic Books.

Chess, S., & Thomas, A. (1989). Issues in the clinical application of temperament. In G. A. Kohnstamm, J. E. Bates, & M. D. Rothbart (Eds.), *Temperament in childhood* (pp. 377–386). New York: Wiley.

Clark, R. (1985). *The Parent-Child Early Relational Assessment.* Madison, WI: Department of Psychiatry, University of Wisconsin Medical School.

Clark, R., Paulson, A., & Conlin, S. (1993). Assessment of developmental status and parent-infant relationships: The therapeutic process of evaluation. In C. H. Zeanah (Ed.), *Handbook of infant mental health* (pp. 191–209). New York: Guilford.

Cox, A., & Rutter, M. (1985). Diagnostic appraisal and interviewing. In M. Rutter & L. Hersov (Eds.), *Child and adolescent psychiatry: Modern approaches* (2nd ed., pp. 233–248). Boston: Blackwell Scientific.

Crockenberg, S., Dickstein, S., & Lyons-Ruth, K. (1993). The family context of infant mental health: II. Infant development in multiple family relationships. In C. H. Zeanah (Ed.), *Handbook of infant mental health* (pp. 38–55). New York: Guilford.

Crowell, J. A., Feldman, S. S., & Ginsberg, N. (1988). Assessment of mother-child interaction in preschoolers with behavior problems. *Journal of the American Academy of Child and Adolescent Psychiatry, 27,* 303–311.

DeGangi, G. A., DiPietro, J. A., Greenspan, S. I., & Porges, S. W. (1991). Psychophysiological characteristics of the regulatory disordered infant. *Infant Behavior and Development, 14,* 37–50.

DeGangi, G. A., Poisson, S., Sickel, R. Z., & Wiener, A. S. (1995). *Infant/toddler symptom checklist: A screening tool for parents.* Tucson, AZ: Therapy Skill Builders.

DeGangi, G. A., Porges, S. W., Sickel, R. Z., & Greenspan, S. I. (1993). Four-year follow-up of a sample of regulatory disordered infants. *Infant Mental Health Journal, 14,* 330–343.

Eisenberg, L. (1995). The social construction of the human brain. *American Journal of Psychiatry, 152,* 1563–1575.

Emde, R. N. (1985). The affective self: Continuities and transformations from infancy. In J. Call, E. Galenson, & R. Stinson (Eds.), *Frontiers of infant psychiatry* (Vol. 2). New York: Basic Books.

Emde, R. N. (1989). The infant's relationship experience: Developmental and affective aspects. In A. J. Sameroff & R. N. Emde (Eds.), *Relationship disturbances in early childhood: A developmental approach* (pp. 33–51). New York: Basic Books.

Emde, R. N. (1994). Developing psychoanalytic representations of experience. *Infant Mental Health Journal, 15*(1), 42–49.

Emde, R. N., Bingham, R., & Harmon, R. (1993). Classification and the diagnostic process in infancy. In C. H. Zeanah (Ed.), *Handbook of infant mental health* (pp. 225–235). New York: Guilford.

Emde, R. N., Gaensbauer, T. J., & Harmon, R. J. (1976). Emotional expression in infancy: A behavioral study. *Psychological Issues: A Monograph Series, 10,* 1–198.

Erikson, J., & Vater, S. (1988). *Connecticut Infant-Toddler Developmental Assessment Program (IDA): Report of a four year demonstration project.* New Haven, CT: Child Study Center, Yale University.

Fonagy, P. (1998). Prevention, the appropriate target of infant psychotherapy: *Infant Mental Health Journal, 19*(1), 24–150.

Fonagy, P., Steele, H., & Steele, M. (1991). Maternal representations of attachment during pregnancy predict the organization of infant-mother attachment at one year of age. *Child Development, 62,* 891–905.

Fraiberg, S. (1980). *Clinical studies in infant mental health.* New York: Basic Books.

Greenspan, S. I., & Wieder, S. (1997). An integrated developmental approach to interventions for young children with severe difficulties in relating and communicating. *Zero to Three, 17*(5), 5–18.

Guedeney, A., & Lebovici, S. (1997). Evaluation into the relationship: Reflections on new trends in evaluation, assessment, and classification. *Infant Mental Health Journal, 18*(2), 171–181.

Hirshberg, L. M. (1993). Clinical interviews with infants and their families. In C. H. Zeanah (Ed.), *Handbook of infant mental health* (pp. 173–190). New York: Guilford.

Hirshberg, L. M. (1996). History-making, not history-taking: Clinical interviews with infants and their families. In S. J. Meisels & E. Fenichel (Eds.), *New visions for the developmental assessment of infants and young children* (pp. 85–124). Washington, DC: Zero to Three/National Center for Infants, Toddlers and Families.

Hofer, M. A. (1987). Early social relationships: A psychobiologist's view. *Child Development, 58,* 663–647.

Ireton, H., & Thwing, E. (1992). *Child Development Inventory.* Circle Pines, MN: American Guidance Service.

Kagan, J. (1984). *The nature of the child.* New York: Basic Books.

Kraemer, G. W. (1992). A psychobiological theory of attachment. *Behavioral and Brain Sciences, 15,* 493–541.

Lieberman, A. F., & Pawl, J. H. (1993). Infant-parent psychotherapy. In C. H. Zeanah (Ed.), *Handbook of infant mental health* (pp. 427–442). New York: Guilford.

Lieberman, A. F., Van Horn, P., Grandison, C. M., & Pekarsky, J. H. (1997). Mental health assessment of infants, toddlers and preschoolers in a service program and a treatment outcome research program. *Infant Mental Health Journal, 18*(2), 158–170.

Lyons-Ruth, K., & Zeanah, C. (1993). The family context of infant mental health: I. Affective development in the primary caregiving relationship. In C. H. Zeanah (Ed.), *Handbook of infant mental health* (pp. 14–37). New York: Guilford.

Main, M., & Cassidy, J. (1988). Categories of response to reunion with the parent at age 6: Predictable from infant attachment classifications and stable over a 1-month period. *Developmental Psychology, 24,* 415–426.

Main, M., & Goldwyn, R. (1984). Predicting rejection of her infant from mother's representation of her own experience: Implications for the abused-abusing intergenerational cycle. *Child Abuse and Neglect, 8,* 203–217.

Mayes, L. C. (1995). The assessment and treatment of the psychiatric needs of medically compromised infants: Consultation with preterm infants and their families. In K. Minde (Ed.), *Infant Psychiatry: Child and Adolescent Psychiatry Clinics of North America* (pp. 555–570). Philadelphia: W.B. Saunders and Company.

McCall, R. B., Eichorn, D., & Hogarty, P. (1977). Transitions on early mental development. *Monographs of the Society for Research in Child Development, 42,* 1177.

Meisels, S. J., & Fenichel, E. (1996). *New visions for the developmental assessment of infants and young children.* Washington DC: Zero to Three/National Center for Infants, Toddlers, and Families.

Meisels, S. J., & Shonkoff, J. P. (1990). *Handbook of early childhood intervention.* New York: Cambridge University Press.

Minde, K. K., Goldberg, S., Perotta, M., Washington, J., Lojkasek, M., Corter, C., & Parker, K. (1989). Continuities and discontinuities in the development of 64 very small premature infants to 4 years of age. *Journal of Child Psychology, Psychiatry and Allied Disciplines, 30,* 391–404.

Mrazek, D. A. (1993). Psychosomatic processes and physical illnesses. In C. H. Zeanah (Ed.), *Handbook of infant mental health* (pp. 350–358). New York: Guilford.

Perry, B. D., Pollard, R. A., Blakley, T. L., Baker, W. L., & Vigilante, D. (1995). Childhood trauma the neurobiology of adaptation, and "use-dependent" development of the brain: How "states" become "traits." *Infant Mental Health Journal, 16,* 271–291.

Reiss, D. (1989). The represented and practicing family: Contrasting visions of family continuity. In A. J. Sameroff & R. N. Emde (Eds.), *Relationship disturbances in early childhood: A developmental approach* (pp. 191–220). New York: Basic Books.

Robert-Tissot, C., Cramer, B., Stern, D. N., Serpa, S. R., Bachmann, J. P., Palacio-Espasa, F., Kanuer, D., De-Muralt, M., Berney, C., & Mendiguren, G. (1996). Outcome evaluation in brief mother infant therapies: Report on 75 cases. *Infant Mental Health Journal, 17*(2), 97–114.

Rothbart, M. K., & Ahadi, S. A. (1994). Temperament and the development of personality. *Journal of Abnormal Psychology, 103,* 55–66.

Sameroff, A. J. (1989). Principles of development and psychopathology. In A. J. Sameroff & R. N. Emde (Eds.), *Relationship disturbances in early childhood: A developmental approach* (pp. 17–32). New York: Basic Books.

Sameroff, A. J. (1992). Systems, development and early intervention. Commentary in J. Shonkoff, P. Hauser-Cram, M. W. Krauss, & C. C. Upshur, Development of infants with disabilities and their families (pp. 154–163). *Monographs of the Society for Research in Child Development, 57* (6, Serial No. 230).

Sameroff, A. J. (1997). Social context of early psychopathology. In J. Noshpitz (Ed.), *Handbook of Child and Adolescent Psychiatry*. New York: Wiley.

Sameroff, A. J., & Chandler, M. J. (1975). Reproductive risk and the continuum of caretaking casualty. In F. D. Horowitz, E. M. Hetherington, S. Scarr-Salapatek, & G. Siegel (Eds.), *A Review of Child Development Research,* Vol. 4. Chicago: University of Chicago.

Sameroff, A. J., & Emde, R. N. (1989). *Relationship disturbances in early childhood: A developmental approach.* New York: Basic Books.

Sameroff, A. J., Seifer, R., Zax, M., & Barocas, R. (1987). Early indicators of developmental risk: Rochester longitudinal study. *Schizophrenia Bulletin, 13,* 383–394.

Shaw, D. S., Vondra, J. I., Hommerding, D., Kennan, K., & Dunn, M. (1994). Chronic family adversity and early child behavior problems: A longitudinal study of low income families. *Journal of Child Psychology, Psychiatry and Allied Disciplines, 35,* 1109–1122.

Sorce, J. F., Emde, R. N., Campos, J. J., & Klinnert, M. D. (1985). Maternal emotional signaling: Its effect on the visual cliff behavior of one-year-olds. *Developmental Psychology, 21,* 195–200.

Sroufe, L. A. (1989). Relationships, self, and individual adaptation. In A. J. Sameroff & R. N. Emde (Eds.), *Relationship disturbances in early childhood: A developmental approach* (pp. 70–94). New York: Basic Books.

Stern, D. N. (1984). Affect attunement. *Frontiers of Infant Psychiatry, 2,* 3–14.

Stern, D. N. (1985). *The interpersonal world of the infant.* New York: Basic Books.

Stern, D. N. (1989). The representation of relational patterns: Developmental considerations. In A. J. Sameroff & R. N. Emde (Eds.), *Relationship disturbances in early childhood: A developmental approach* (pp. 52–69). New York: Basic Books.

Stern, D. N. (1994). One way to build a clinically relevant baby. *Infant Mental Health Journal, 15*(1), 9–25.

Stern, D. N. (1995). *The motherhood constellation: A unified view of parent-infant psychotherapy.* New York: Basic Books.

Suomi, S. J. (1997). Early determinants of behaviour: Evidence from primate studies. *British Medical Bulletin, 53*(1), 170–184.

Thomas, J. M. (1995). Traumatic stress disorder presents as hyperactivity and disruptive behavior: Case presentation, diagnosis, and treatment. *Infant Mental Health Journal, 16,* 306–317.

Thomas, J. M., Guskin, K. A., & Klass, C. S. (1997). Early development program: Collaborative structures and processes. *Infant Mental Health Journal, 18*(2), 198–208.

Thomas, J. M., & Tidmarsh, L. (1997). Hyperactive and disruptive behaviors in very young children: Diagnosis and intervention. *Infants and Young Children, 9,* 46–55.

Vygotsky, L. S. (1978). *Mind in Society.* Cambridge, MA: Harvard University Press.

Wieder, S. (1997). Creating connections: Intervention guidelines for increasing interaction with children with multisystem developmental disorder (MSDD). *Zero to Three, 17*(5), 19–27.

Williamson, G., & Anzalone, M. (1997). Sensory integration: A key component of the evaluation and treatment of young children with severe difficulties in relating and communicating. *Zero to Three, 17*(5), 29–36.

Winnicott, D. W. (1965). The theory of the parent-infant relationship. In D. W. Winnicott (Ed.), *The maturational processes and the facilitating environment* (pp. 37–55). New York: International Universities Press.

World Health Organization. (1992). *International statistical classification of diseases and related health problems* (ICD–10), (10th rev.). Geneva: Author.

Zeanah, C. H., Anders, T. F., Seifer, R., & Stern, D. N. (1989). Implications of research on infant development for psychodynamic theory and practice. *Journal of the American Academy of Child and Adolescent Psychiatry, 28,* 657–668.

Zeanah, C., Boris, N., & Scheeringa, M. (1997). Psychopathology in infancy. *Journal of Child Psychology and Psychiatry, 38*(1), 81–99.

Zeitlin, S., Williamson, G. G., & Szczepanski, M. (1988). *Manual for the Early Coping Inventory: A measure of adaptive behavior.* Bensenville, IL: Scholastic Testing Service.

Zero to Three/National Center for Clinical Infant Programs. (1994). *Diagnostic classification of mental health and developmental disorders of infancy and early childhood.* Arlington, VA: Author.

Zero to Three. (1997). Key findings from a nationwide survey among parents of zero-to three-year-olds.

13

Observation, Reflection, and Understanding: The Importance of Play in Clinical Assessment of Infants and Their Families

Elizabeth Tuters and Sally Doulis

13

"Playing and cultural experience can be given location if one uses the concept of the potential space between the mother and the baby. . . . " (Winnicott, 1971, p. 53)

"It is in playing and only in playing that the individual child or adult is able to be creative and to use the whole personality and it is only in being creative that the individual discovers the self . . . "(Winnicott, 1971, p. 54).

Rationale

We understand potential space to be the subjective play space created between a mother and her infant, where creativity, thought, and imagination converge. Using Winnicott's compelling idea of "potential space" as background, we describe how we use observation, play, and reflection of play and the relational systems in the process of data gathering in the assessment and evaluation of infants (0 through 4) and their families in the presence of a clinician. We also describe how the clinician uses the concept of reflective "potential space" created between the mother and baby and oneself and the family in the presence of the observing clinical team to understand the problem and formulate the intervention strategy. Case illustrations are provided to show the efficacy of this approach and model of assessment.

Policy

The policy of the Infant and Family Assessment and Treatment Team (IFATT) of the Hincks Dellcrest Children's Mental Health Centre (a publicly-funded center) is to offer a comprehensive assessment to any family, within the catchment area of the inner city, who self-refers for help with a regulatory or psychosocial problem with an infant age zero to four years. All assessments conducted at the center use a multidisciplinary team approach: (1) The training component—the center is a teaching resource for pre- and postprofessional mental health workers represented by psychiatry, psychology, social work, child psychotherapy, and early childhood education and (2) The belief system—a more comprehensive assessment is provided to the family if a team of multidisciplinary professionals is involved since from a multiperspective approach offer broader insights and understanding and minimize countertransference issues.

Philosophy

Recent infant observational and attachment research emphasizes the importance of the earliest infant-caregiver relationship for the development of optimal human

We thank the Infant and Family Assessment and Treatment Team for their support and collaboration, in particular those who provided case illustrations: Susan Eadie, Ph.D., Valerie Iles, B.A., and Judith Coates, M.S.W. All contributors are child psychotherapists trained in the Toronto Child Psychoanalytic Program and members of the IFATT. We are grateful to the families for the privilege of working together.

functioning. The infant's development must always be considered within the context and quality of the caregiving relationship and caregiving environment (Bretherton, 1985, 1990; Emde, 1988, 1991; Fraiberg, 1980; Main & Goldwyn, 1984; Stern, 1985, 1995; Beebe & Lachman, 1988; Sanders, 1988).

The theoretical orientation of the Infant and Family Assessment and Treatment Team uses psychoanalytic principles. The team attempts to understand each infant and family in terms of the interplay between past and present, actuality and fantasy, self and other, internal and external, and conscious and unconscious (Mitchell & Black, 1995). The range of thinking is from classical to contemporary psychoanalytic theory. The major sources of influence are Bion (1961), Bowlby (1969, 1973, 1979, 1980), Emde (1991), Fraiberg (1980), A. Freud (1936, 1965), S. Freud (1914–1921), M. Klein (1952), Kohut (1959, 1971, 1977, 1985), Cramer (1990, 1992), Mitchell and Black (1995), Stern (1985, 1995), and Winnicott (1969, 1971). The subsequent attachment theory work of Mary Ainsworth (Goldberg, 1991), who developed the Strange Situation protocol to measure the nature of the child's tie to its mother through a detailed paradigm of the introduction of a stranger, separation from, and reunion with the parents, has been adapted to be used in clinical assessment.

Kohut's contributions to the theory of psychoanalysis have affected the team's ethos. We are particularly concerned with the feeling states of the mothers and fathers who seek our help with their infants. We suspend our organizing frames of reference and preconceived ideas, based on other psychoanalytic theories and theories of child development, and attempt to understand the experience of the parents from their points of view. Kohut (1959) described this approach as "empathic immersion and vicarious introspection" (Mitchell, 1995, p. 157).

Ways of Thinking: Implications for Technique

Infant research has affected the way we think about infants and their families. In particular, we have been influenced by the work of Daniel Stern (1985), who cites his own and others' evidence that a sense of self is present from birth, if not before. He and others postulate that the development of a cohesive sense of self depends on the infant accomplishing the tasks of the various senses of self in relation to the infant's center of initiative performed against the background of the parents' empathic immersion in the child's needs (Basch, 1991).

According to Basch (1991), psychic structure is formed through the action and interaction of the infant within the caregiving environment. This article cites contributions by Lachman and Beebe (1983, p. 8), who suggest there are four processes to structure formation "1) the process of ongoing mutual and self-regulation between mother and infant . . . 2) the process of frustration and gratification [important to Freud] . . . 3) the process of rupture and repair [Kohut's optimal frustration] . . . 4) the structure-forming effects of heightened affective moments" [Pine]. These four processes are held in mind as we observe and assess infants and their families.

In our clinical work, we are dealing with the essentials of intersubjectivity, between the family and clinician and the clinician and the observing team. The concept of intersubjectivity is outlined in the passage which originally appeared in *Structures of Subjectivity* (Atwood & Stolorow, 1984):

"In its most general form, our thesis . . . is that psychoanalysis seeks to illuminate phenomena that emerge within a specific psychological field constituted by the intersection of two subjectivities—that of the patient and that of the analyst . . . Psychoanalysis is pictured here as a science of the intersubjective, focused on the interplay between the differently organized subjective worlds of the observer and the observed. The observational stance is always one within, rather than outside, the intersubjective field . . . Being observed, a fact that guarantees the centrality of introspection and empathy as the method of observation . . . Psychoanalysis is unique among the sciences in that the observer is also the observed . . ." (pp. 1–2)

This theorizing can apply directly to assessment and treatment of infants and their families. The clinician is always affected by the observed and is affecting the field of observation (see C and S cases). We agree with Kohut's often quoted comment, "If there is one lesson I have learned during my life as an analyst, it is the lesson that what my patients tell me is likely to be true . . . but many times when I believed I was right and my patients were wrong, it turned out, though only after a prolonged search,

that my rightness was superficial whereas their rightness was profound" (Kohut, 1984, pp. 93–94). The clinical examples that follow illustrate the wisdom of this statement.

During the IFATT assessment, we attempt to keep these recent theoretical contributions in mind. We look for the strengths and vulnerabilities—how the infant and family impact upon us as a team and upon the individual clinician in the room. We believe mothers come to us for help wanting to be understood in a way they have longed for but not experienced.

The clinicians and team understand each infant, mother, and family in terms of the parents' background and the infant's development and the current expressed problem in relation to the whole system. The IFATT assessments are careful and thorough in terms of observation and data gathering and in collaboration with the parents. If a rupture occurs, which at times may happen, we examine where we have failed in our understanding of the problem (see J and V cases). The cases discussed show the clinician, team, and family at work.

Observation as a Model of Training

We base our concept of observations on the model developed in 1949 by Esther Bick (Tuters, 1988), psychoanalyst at the British Psychoanalytic Society. This model has been used subsequently in the training of all psychoanalysts and child psychotherapists in Britain and other parts of the world, including the training of child psychotherapists in Canada.

Infant observation is an emotional learning experience where trainees experience the impact upon themselves of observing a developing infant through understanding the feelings aroused in themselves. For mental health workers, this means becoming able to see what in the past they have been unable to recognize: That is, the pain and distress of an infant and his or her parents working out a relationship together, being separated from each other, and the effect of this experience on the developing infant and on the parents and how they all cope.

Infant observation seminars involve the students in weekly in-home observation of the developing infant in the family from birth over a period of one to two years. Observations last for one hour with the observer behaving as naturally as possible and interacting minimally with the infant and family. Note-taking is discouraged. Narrative descriptions of the observations are subsequently written from memory and discussed in weekly seminar groups. The observations that have been described and the feelings that have been evoked are shared with other group members and worked through in discussions. The IFATT discussions follow a similar format.

The model used in infant observation seminars is of exploration, where the leader encourages the participants to present their observations in such a manner that other group members can begin to develop a mental picture of the infant and parents and have affective resonance with the observer. This method of observing and sharing observations within a seminar group enhances the development of the reflective self in the observer (Fonagy, 1991). Each observer presents his or her observed material in terms of what is remembered, what is seen, and what is not seen. The leader helps the observer and the group work in such a way as to produce a collective picture of the infant in the developing relationship with the caregiving parent. The observational experience exposes the observer to many and varied opportunities to know about infant-parent development in a different way and how infants and their families relate and impact upon one another. The observer is not there in a professional role and does not need to take action. Rather, the observer is there to look afresh at the infant-caregiver system, which develops sensitivity to the system, as it unfolds.

The observer becomes aware of the impact upon the self of observing a new infant-mother pair find their way and their fit together. The observer is affected at many levels by what is being observed. Infant and child developmental theories provide a direction, however, at a deeper level, the observer is dealing with his or her conscious and unconscious issues that are impacted upon by observation of the field. The observation group offers a containment to the observer to share the observations as written narratives, within the seminar group. The clinical observation discussion follows a similar format and offers the same containment to the clinician and team members.

Application of Method and Observation to Clinical Team Observation

The method of learning in Infant Observation Seminars is adapted and used in the clinical observation approach by the clinical team. The majority of team members have been trained in programs using observation. These members have developed a reflective stance that can be used to relate meaningfully to others. Those with the experience of observation seem to have an easier time observing, tracking observations, holding in mind what they see, making sense of the observed material, and sequencing it as a part of the assessment and therapeutic process (see B case).

Play

In a clinical assessment of infants and their families, play is regarded as a way of informing us about the infant's struggles with self-regulation and self-development and the nature and quality of the infant's relationship with each parent.

"In playing, and perhaps only in playing, the child or adult is free to be creative. This consideration arises in my mind as a development of the concept of transitional phenomena and it takes into account the difficult part of the theory of the transitional object, which is that a paradox is involved which needs to be accepted, tolerated, and not resolved ... Playing and cultural experience can be given a location if one uses the concept of the potential space between the mother and the baby . . . " (Winnicott, 1971, p. 53)

This potential space between the mother and baby is examined by observing play sequences. We are in agreement with Melanie Klein (1975) that through the analysis of play the inner conflicts of the infant can be observed and understood. However, we use a relational model in our thinking rather than an individual drive defense model. We use a set of toys (named following) in our play exploration. These same toys are used throughout the assessment and subsequent intervention.

TOYS

(1) Doll bed (large enough for infant into which to climb); (2) Anatomically-correct boy and girl baby dolls, with diapers; (3) Two bottles (one milk, one juice); (4) Two plastic telephones; (5) A set of mixing bowls with plastic spoons; (6) A container of wild and domestic plastic animals; (7) A container of various shaped wooden blocks; (8) Large, colored plastic blocks; (9) Doctor's kit with contents; (10) Small plastic families (black and white); (11) Train track and train; (12) Blue plastic mat on which to play; and (13) Large pillow or bean bag.

The toys are always placed in the same way on the mat prior to the beginning of each session. The toys and mat offer a safe play space for the infant and parents. The toys and the mat are treated similar to an analytic frame to contain the work to be done through the play. We observe: (1) what toys the infant chooses and how the infant uses the toys; (2) whether the infant plays alone or tries to engage the parents; (3) how the parents respond; (4) how the parents are affected by the play; (5) whether the play is the same or varied (from session to session); (6) the affective moments observed during the play; and (7) the gaze of infant and parents (see B case).

As part of our assessment procedure, we use a free play session with parent and infant. No instruction is given, and the parent is asked to play with the child as they naturally would at home. This play session gives us a baseline to see how the infant and parent interact. We look for the role the parent is assuming. Is the parent leading the play? (see S and B cases.) Is the parent instructing? (see S case.) Is the parent bored? (see J case.) Is the parent unable to play? (see V case.)

Following the free play session, the parent discusses the play with the clinician in terms of what it was like for the parent, how the parent understood the child's play, and what the parent made of it. We attempt to understand how the parent regards the child. Within the paradox what is created needs to be accepted, tolerated, and not resolved. We attempt to understand how the parent regards play with the child, and we attempt to create a space in the parent's mind to think about the child's communication through play (see B and C cases). (For a detailed clinical example of the use of the observational method in the initial assessment phase, see the B case.)

Following the initial assessment, we often choose to extend our assessment through the use of a variation of an intervention, a series of six play sessions called "Watching, Waiting, Wondering" (Muir, 1992), where the parent(s) is asked to follow the lead of the child and play for 20 minutes, after which the parent and clinician discuss the play and the meaning of the play together.

The play of a child is the child's way of communicating to the other what the child is struggling with and thinking. We treat the play of the child with the seriousness of adult free associations. We explain, when necessary, the conflicts we think are revealed through the play. We ask the parent to engage with the clinician in wondering what the play means. If the parent or clinician is able to engage with the child and enter the child's world through play, themes are developed and narratives played out. We treat play much like Sigmund Freud wrote about conflict resolution in his 1914 paper, Remembering, Repeating, and Working Through. We find the infant will reveal through play with the parent, the nature of the problem. The parent's ability to attune to the infant's inner world is enhanced through the presence of the clinician. This process affords rich opportunities for change in the dyadic system.

Assessment of Mother and Father

An essential part of the IFATT assessment is to evaluate the individual development of the mother and father as a means of determining the part of the parents' personality which functions as a parent and manifests itself in the parent-infant/child relationship and evaluate the parenting capacity of each parent. The process of evaluation begins by meeting with each parent individually and encouraging the parent to join with the clinician in relating their individual story from birth onward.

Although a free flowing approach is desirable in this interview, it is important to cover pertinent data in the interview by finding an appropriate time to introduce areas for discussion which are not mentioned by the parent. Of importance is the parent's relationships with others throughout their lifetime, especially with their own mothers, fathers, and siblings. The clinician encourages the parent to give a picture of his or her personality so the clinician can form a real, live impression of the parent. The clinician encourages the parent to relate a story about himself or herself that reflects their childhood relationship with mother and/or father. How did mother and/or father express affection, handle discipline, and balance the needs of more than one child? What were parental roles in the family? What was the nature of the communication patterns in the family? Determine relationship with siblings, past and present, and whether anyone else lived with the family and if so, explore the nature of those relationships, too. Determine relationships with grandparents or any other person with whom the person had an important, close relationship. It is important to know about attachments and separations, at what age they occurred, why they occurred, and the effect of the separation on the development of self.

It is necessary to meet with the parents together to explore their relationship as a married couple, to determine how they made and kept connections (attachments) and explore the development of the family, that is, the developmental history of the infant or child: The anticipatory fantasy and pregnancy history, attachment and early adaptation, separation and individuation, self-regulation and latency, and adolescence. During the interview, the clinician will vigilantly scan for the affect reexperienced by the mother or father as they relate the early developmental data and/or look for repressions and denials against reexperiencing unpleasant affects associated with difficult periods in the infant or child's development (Doulis, 1997).

These interviews, along with the material from family interviews and observations of the infant or child interactions with each parent, will enable the clinician and team to develop a comprehensive view of the infant or child in context with the experience of the family. Once the data is collected, the IFATT will evaluate the parental capacities with respect to the seven domains of functioning presented by Emde (1989) where there is agreement among theorists about important areas of observation: Attachment relationship, safety and protection, physiological regulation, play, teaching and learning, power and control, and regulation of emotion (Hirshberg, 1993).

The Clinical Team: The Potential Space

The clinical team is composed of multidisciplinary members—psychoanalytic child therapists, psychoanalysts, early childhood educators, and students in psychology, psychiatry, social work, and child psychotherapy trainees. The team leader has been trained at the Tavistock Clinic in Infant

Observation Seminar Groups as a psychoanalytic child psychotherapist at the Toronto Child Psychoanalytic Program, and as an adult psychoanalyst at the Canadian Institute of Psychoanalysis.

The aim of the team is to use a case study method, where all members are encouraged to free associate applying their professional knowledge base to the observation of the case dynamics in terms of objective and subjective data, relational systems, and understanding the play interactions between the infant and parents. Tentative hypotheses are generated before the case is seen and undergo revision for the duration of the assessment, culminating in a formulation of the case and intervention strategies following the assessment process.

A primary clinician (sometimes a secondary) is assigned and responsible for the clinical work of the case, while the team leader functions as supervisor and case manager. The clinician quickly develops comfort working with the team approach behind a two-way mirror. The purpose of the team is to develop understanding about the nature of the infant and parents' difficulties with each other. The team members explore thinking and expand ideas in a creative fashion, thus creating a potential space through reflection to complement the clinician's understanding.

Summary: Process of Assessment and Evaluation

The IFATT's approach to the assessment process is to conduct as comprehensive an investigation as possible. This investigation includes exploring the reason(s) for referral, history of current and previous difficulty, history of development of the infant or child, evaluating the family (relationships, interactions, and functioning), and evaluating the developmental status of the infant or child.

1. The first interview is with all of the family members. The team and clinician observe the relationships and the interactions of the parents with the child, the parents with each other, the child with the other children and the parents, the child's verbal and nonverbal communications with the parents, and how the infant or child plays with the toys and what toys are used (see toys, preceding).

2. The clinician leaves the room toward the end of each session to discuss with the team their observations, what to feed back to the parents, and the expected direction of the next session.

3. The parents are seen together as a couple and alone, for the purpose of exploring history, marital and parental relationships, and individual development of the infant or child.

4. If the infant is over 12 months, the infant is seen separately to observe the effect on the infant of separation from the parent(s), the way the child relates through play to a clinician who is a stranger, and the reunion behavior of the child with the parent upon return.

5. Separate free play sessions are conducted between infant and each parent in the presence of the clinician. No instruction is given. The parent is asked to

play as he or she would at home. The aim is to observe how the parent and infant play together. Following a play sequence, the parent and clinician discuss the play and the parent's feelings about the play.

6. The assessment continues for approximately six weeks. Following each session, the team meets for one hour with the clinician to discuss the observations and impressions. This discussion includes the impact of the family upon the clinician and team and the clinician and team upon the family. The clinician always keeps in mind the importance of involving the parents in the process of assessment in order to build a working alliance and empower them to know, understand, and correct the difficulty.

7. When the team has gathered all the data necessary, the clinician and team meet for the purpose of synthesizing and integrating the material into a formulation of the core conflict and dynamics to be shared with the family, which attempts to explain how and why the infant or child has developed in the specific way he or she did, utilizing the biological, psychological, and environmental factors which have contributed. We involve the family in the process so that the formulation and the first intervention make sense to the family.

8. Often the next step is to offer a six-session intervention with review and reformulation, as we attempt to determine whether an intervention into the relational system between the parents and infant will be sufficient to resolve the difficulty or whether more intensive ther-

apy will be indicated (see J case). The purpose of this step is to determine the family's response to the intervention.

Case Illustrations

The following case studies show our method of assessment and treatment intervention: Case Study 1. Detailed Assessment Process and Case Studies 2 through 5 Condensed Assessment and Intervention Process. The cases have been written by the primary clinicians and reflect the working alliance between the family, the clinician, and the team.

Case Study 1

B Case: Billy—Age 2 Years, 8 Months—Sally Doulis

The case illustrates the use of data gathering to formulate details of a comprehensive assessment process.

Billy, 2 years, 8 months old, living with his father, mother, and 8-month-old brother, was referred by the family physician. The parents' concerns were that Billy cried constantly, was never relaxed, demanded his mother's attention, was impatient, perfectionistic, demonstrated aggression toward his mother and brother, and had sleep problems. Mother worried about her feelings of frustration with him, and father wondered if his absences from the family due to his work were contributing to his son's difficulties.

HISTORY AND DEVELOPMENT
OF THE FAMILY

Father was the middle child of three with middle-class traditional European parents. His father was described as a serious, ambitious man who was a good teacher and devoted family man. He did not show emotion, nor did he display affection. There was little cause for discipline as the children were obedient. He described his mother as devoted to her children, dependable, and loving, but not physically demonstrative. Family ties were strong.

Mother was the youngest of two girls of working-class traditional parents. Mother had no recall about her relationship with her mother, rather her memories were crystalized around family activities and her father. She described her mother as caring and perfectionistic, but calm, loving, and helpful. They were an active family. She had a "great" relationship with her father whom she described as patient and fun loving. She was more involved with her father since he coached her sports teams. As a couple, they shared a satisfying ten-year relationship prior to marriage.

Billy was a planned baby. Both parents were excited about the pregnancy, but mother was anxious and unsure what the future would be like with a child. Her vision was of an easy time where she and her child would go for peaceful walks together. She did not enjoy being pregnant. She was uncomfortable with the changes in her body and her slower pace. The couple planned for a natural childbirth, and they attended prenatal classes. However, Billy was delivered unexpectedly by caesarean section, since the umbilical cord was wrapped around his neck. Both parents were emotionally unprepared for the complications they encountered. Mother and baby were separated after delivery until mother recovered from surgery. The parents were thrilled with a male baby. Although mother was certain she did not want to breast-feed, she was talked into it and attempted breast-feeding. Baby and mother were unhappy, and with the encouragement of her mother and doctor, she gave up after three weeks. Billy adapted to the bottle yet he remained a difficult baby who cried and could not be comforted. Mother insisted she was not depressed, only anxious and upset about her baby. Complicating the family's stress over a difficult birth experience and a child with a difficult temperament, at the time of Billy's birth, father received a promotion, which meant he often worked late at the office, leaving mother alone to attend to their son's needs. She received help from her mother. She returned to her work three days a week when Billy was six-months-old, and Billy stayed with a nanny. The situation began to settle. When Billy was two years, one month old his brother was born. The pregnancy and delivery were uneventful. The second boy, Max, was a healthy, easy, placid baby. Around the third week, mother began to notice that Billy was discontent. His routines were changed, and he showed negative feelings toward his brother.

At the time of the assessment, Billy's unhappiness and stress over simple things being out of place was the identified problem. Although father and mother were perfectionistic themselves, they were exasperated and angry to see perfectionism in their small child. While their own relationship was strong, it was under stress due to their frustrations with Billy and father's relative unavailability to share the parenting. Mother had few outlets for herself. The couple did nothing alone. The emphasis was on family activities.

The following interviews demonstrate the interactions between mother, father, and child and the child's play, as well as the observation and reflection of the play.

SUMMARY OF PLAY IN THE FAMILY INTERVIEW

In the first family interview, Billy's play was varied and organized, but aggressive when he lost his parents' attention. He played independently while his parents talked to the clinician. He put together the train tracks while he sat close to his mother. When he asked for attention, his father responded visually. He became interested in the two doll babies, the bottles, and the blankets. He wrapped one doll in the blanket and asked his father to open it. Then he moved to the building materials and the medical kit. He asked his father to hold the doll while he became the doctor. Billy gave his father a shot, hit his father hard on the head with the medical hammer, and father protested. Billy dumped the blocks. Mother had been holding Max in her arms, and she handed Max to father. Max cried, and father rocked him. Billy got up and grabbed his mother's hand and got the doll's blanket. Mother related her disappointment in Billy, having wanted a peaceful, easy, happy child. Billy put the naked doll on the pillow and threw a few toys and

took Max's bottle and pushed it at mother. She pushed his hand away. Billy then pushed the bottle at Max, and he cried. Father told Billy "No." Mother tried to distract Billy. Mother became somewhat disorganized for a moment as the clinician addressed Billy's aggression and mother explained that Billy does this when they are with other children, too. Billy dumped the blocks into the bowls and then threw them out. He put the baby doll underneath the pillow, kicked it, moved the doll and pillow closer to father, and lay on his back and sucked his thumb. Billy said he wanted to leave. Max screamed. Father handed Billy an animal, and he threw it at his mother's face. Billy paced the room, grabbed his mother's hand, and took her to the chalk board. Max cried, and mother took him and fed him while father engaged with Billy. Father followed Billy's lead. Billy told his father what to draw. Mother rocked Max and kissed his hand. Billy and father returned to the play materials—animals. Billy played with the tiger, and father asked questions about the animals. Billy asked for the cow, and father handed him the tiger. Billy asked his father if he liked monkeys. Father asked Billy to build a tower. Billy did not respond.

SUMMARY OF PLAY WITH THE MOTHER

The family was separated with mother and Billy remaining in the room while father and Max went into a separate room. Billy had a strong reaction to his father's departure, and it took him some time to settle. The clinician and mother talked about his upset, and mother tried to distract Billy. She was dismissive in her explanation to

Billy. Finally, she held him on her lap with his back to her, but Billy was not comforted. The clinician suggested that mother be with Billy as she would at home, She focused her attention on Billy, and he settled. Billy chose the medical kit and invited the clinician to join him in putting a bandage on his mother's finger. Billy put a bandage on his finger too, and mother asked if he felt better. Billy did not answer. Mother asked Billy (the doctor) if she was okay? He said no. Billy put together the train tracks, and he asked the adults for help. Mother explained that when they were in the car Billy would drop his toys and cry for his parents to get them. Now they listen to music instead and told him they would talk to him only when he stopped crying. Mother felt she needed strategies to deal with Billy. The best times were when they were outside together being active. Mother and the day care viewed him as bright and quick. In day care, he was not a problem. Billy interrupted and gave his mother a lion and became aggressive with the tiger when she did not respond to him. Mother identified this, and Billy said the tiger needed a daddy. Mother confirmed this is how things usually go. She never gets a break. Mother began to teach Billy about the animals and asked him to line up the animals in a straight line. When asked how this session was for her, mother said she was not sure it was helpful. She felt she needed to learn how to talk to Billy. When father returned to the room, Billy greeted him by running to him, and father picked him up. As it was time to end, Billy began to pick up the toys and began to pick up without any prompting from his parents.

SUMMARY OF PLAY WITH FATHER

The session started all together. Billy was shy, and he sat in his own chair and asked his mother to sit next to him. Mother told him he would be staying in the room today to play with his father. When mother and Max left the room, Billy did not react. Father directed Billy to the train tracks, but Billy preferred to play with the animals. Father tried to get Billy to name and then count the animals, and Billy complied. Billy was interested in the baby dolls. Billy gave a doll to father and directed him to remove the diaper as he did the same with the other doll. Billy carefully put the blanket and the diaper by his side and told father to do the same. Billy held and fed his doll with its back to him. Billy noticed his father held his baby differently and imitated his father's approach. Father asked if they should put the blankets back on, and Billy said no. Billy was interested in the sexual differences of the male and female dolls. Father identified the vagina as a "bellybutton" and said "it's different." Father looked uncomfortable and again asked Billy if they should diaper the dolls. Billy said, "No." Billy took the doctor kit and explored the other toys in the room. He chose the tiger and involved his father in his play with the animals. As the clinician asked father his thoughts about his son's play, Billy selected the train tracks and asked his father's help in building a bridge. Father said Billy could play like this all day long, but he prefers to do outdoor activities.

FORMULATION

Billy was an attractive, bright, curious, anxious, insecure, obsessional almost three-year-old boy being investigated for crying, sleeplessness, attention seeking, demanding, impatient, perfectionistic, and aggressive behavior, the latter toward his mother and others. Both parents wanted children, and Billy was planned. Mother was uncomfortable with the changes in her body during her pregnancy and her inactivity as a result. She was also anxious about the transition to parenthood and the changes and responsibilities that accompanied it. Complications in the delivery were unexpected. An emergency caesarean section was performed. Billy was a normal, healthy baby who was temperamentally active, restless, irritable, and unsoothable, and his sleep patterns were erratic and short. Both mother and infant appeared to have been affected by the unexpected and traumatic birth experience. Billy's state-regulation difficulties had an impact on the formation of a mutual regulating relationship between mother and baby. Mother could not attune to his needs. Billy may have been an unclear cuegiver given his internal distress, and mother may have been too anxious and distressed to read his cues carefully, setting up what appeared to be an anxious, insecure attachment. Mother and child have had a difficult time with the nature of their "fit" together and negative interactions have evolved when attachment issues were activated. To complicate matters, the parenting partnership was altered by a change in father's workplace which necessitated his absence from the home. Thus, mother was the sole caregiver for this distressed infant except on the weekends and when she received help from her parents. Given these difficult circumstances, Billy's birth

may have been experienced as a loss rather than a gain, combined with the couple's loss of their active, enjoyable lifestyle. Once entering parenthood, "family" pursuits were advanced to the exclusion of individual needs and the needs of the couple, which created stress and unhappiness in the family. Into this situation, Max was born when Billy was two years old, after which Billy's aggressive and obsessional behavior developed. Mother's pregnancy and birth experience with her second son were more positive. Given the couple's previous experience, preparedness for a surgical delivery and parenthood and Max's easy, placid temperament culminated in a secure attachment pattern between mother and Max.

Billy's symptoms express anxiety and insecurity in his attachment to his mother. These are exacerbated by Max's more secure attachment pattern which activates Billy's attachment needs. He feels he loses his mother and parents' attention, which he experiences as rejection. He becomes angry and behaves aggressively toward Max or his mother and displaces his angry feelings onto objects. Thus, he unwittingly contributes to triggering his parents' anger and disapproval and he, therefore, defeats what he wants the most, that is love, security, and closeness with his mother and parents. Billy's obsessionality and perfectionism (the need for things to be in order and in the right place) can be viewed as partly psychological, representing a defense against anxieties that he cannot find his place where he "fits" in his family, and partly social, as he has accommodated to his parents' perfectionism in order to please them.

Perpetuating factors: Mother and father's instrumental and instructive approach to Billy. They were not reflective and had little knowledge about affective development. Both families of origin were similar, where affective communication was not prominent and involvement with their parents revolved around activities. With mother, a negative cycle had evolved where she responded to Billy's emotional needs in a dismissive manner using distraction, redirection, and teaching.

Protective factors: Mother and father were both high functioning, responsible, parents who provided a stable environment for their children. Billy was a bright, precocious, likeable child. The relationship between father and Billy appeared more secure, and although father engaged with his son in an instrumental manner, he was warm and caring. When father was present and the couple parented their children together, they seemed to read each other's cues as they shifted back and forth from child to child. The marital relationship appeared strong, and they had close relationships with their extended families.

TREATMENT RECOMMENDATIONS

Dynamic Mother-Child Play Intervention is recommended to effect mutual regulation and strengthen the relationship, to be provided by a clinician who is cognizant of principles of child development and dynamics and will interact with the mother-child dyad. The technique utilized by the clinician will be an adaptation of the "Watching, Waiting, and Wondering" (Muir, 1992). There will be a set time (20 minutes) for the infant-mother dyad to engage without the clinician's involvement. In this approach, the mother will be instructed to get down on the floor with the child, *watching* (observing) what he does *without initiating* activity, *waiting* for the child to initiate, and *wondering* (becoming curious about the activity) with the goal in mind of understanding the child's view of himself and his world at that moment and the child's feelings about it. Through this activity, with the clinician's input, both mother and child will come to know each other's temperament better, thus enhancing their attachment and enjoyment of each other. Mother will learn to attend to her son's emotional needs and respond in an affective manner rather than avoiding, distracting, or teaching. As mother observes Billy's activities, the clinician will also observe mother's style of tracking her son and their style of interaction. As issues become clear to the clinician through the interaction in the sessions, an additional emphasis will be placed on bringing to the mother's awareness a perspective on what she may be reliving from her past through interaction with and the development of her child.

Case Study 2

S Case: Sari—Age 1½ to 3 Years—Elizabeth Tuters

The case illustrates the clinician, mother, and infant working together to find the best intervention. Sari and mother were unable to experience themselves as separate from each other.

Sari and her mother were referred by the father for help with the mother-infant relationship. Father was a physician who spent long hours away from the home. He felt worried about the relationship between his wife and infant. His wife was experiencing their infant as aggressive. The infant preferred to be with the father. In the team discussion prior to seeing the family, we speculated that the mother's felt aggression by the infant was probably due to the conflict originating in the mother's past relationship with her own mother. We asked all family members to attend our initial meeting. We observed a close marital relationship between the couple. Father sat close to the mother throughout the sessions, holding her hand and stroking her arm when she became upset. The infant played alone with baby dolls, dressing and undressing and feeding and putting them to bed. The parents shared their background of moving temporarily from Scotland so that father could pursue his training. Sari interrupted her doll play when the mother became upset. She went to mother, handed her the doll, and put her head on mother's lap. Mother stopped crying, commented on the doll, and asked Sari if she wanted the doll to be held. Sari indicated no, took the doll back, and continued her play.

The IFATT began to hypothesize that mother was attuned to her infant daughter, and Sari to her mother. However, we felt we were observing a child who was sensitive to the affective states of the mother and who reacted to mother's upset, much as the father did by trying to soothe her. Mother told us a story of being lonely without friends. They had recently moved to the city, and mother felt isolated. She spent all day with her much loved daughter. Both parents revealed difficulties since Sari's birth, who was born three months premature and of low birth weight. Mother felt throughout her pregnancy that her baby was well, however, when labor commenced, mother felt that she and her baby might die. Mother and baby were separated from each other for several weeks due to their medical conditions. Soon after discharge from the hospital, father left the country to take up a residency position. Mother felt abandoned. She did not have a good relationship with her own mother, who was angry at her for having a premature baby. Mother feared her own mother would harm her. Without resolving the conflict, she left to join her husband. Together in a new place, they were very much alone with their worries about their premature baby. They sought advice from specialists as Sari had problems with self-regulation, feeding, and sleeping. The relationship between the parents became strained. Mother was with her infant. Her world revolved around the baby, trying to meet all of the infant's needs and expecting the infant to meet her needs as well.

PLAY SESSION WITH MOTHER

In the play session with mother and infant, we observed a play sequence where mother took the lead and the infant followed compliantly. The theme of the play was bathing and feeding the babies. Sari watched her mother carefully and imitated her play. She repeated her mother's words and joined in the mother's story. We observed Sari being watchful of her mother, needing her mother's imagination and playfulness to engage her in play. As a team, we felt concerned that Sari had not been given an opportunity to develop her own sense of initiative and agency and was dependent upon her mother to make sense of her world. The mother complained that Sari could not play alone and always needed mother to be present and playing with her. We thought Sari had not developed her own separate sense of self in the presence of her mother.

PLAY SESSION WITH FATHER

The free play session with father revealed a different scene. Sari quickly told father they would play with the dolls. She handed father one doll, and she kept the other. She told father they were riding together on the subway. She indicated that the couch was the subway and you could tell if a train was approaching by the wind in your face. Father followed Sari's play with interest, enthusiasm, and humor. We felt we had observed a father and child in mutual play. Father allowed Sari to communicate her story to him. Sari seemed to feel she could engage with him as a separate person.

Following a team discussion, our focus of intervention was with the mother-infant pair. We suggested to the parents a series of play sessions with the mother and the daughter. Both parents agreed with the focus of intervention.

The first play session revealed the problem more clearly. The infant and mother continued the themes of washing and feeding the baby dolls. However, we observed that mother could not follow the lead of the infant because the infant was dependent upon mother to take the lead. In the discussion that followed the play, mother expressed dissatisfaction with the focus of the intervention. She felt she was doing the same thing she did all day, and nothing was improving. Sensitive to the mother's distress, I asked if she had something in mind she felt would be more helpful. Mother said she felt she needed to talk about the feelings she had, but she knew this was a problem because she could not leave Sari with anyone to create a space for herself, since Sari would not leave her. The team agreed that mother needed an opportunity to talk about her overwhelming feelings, but knew she would be unable to tolerate a separation from her daughter. Thus, one of the team members joined us to play with Sari in the presence of mother, while the mother and I talked together.

This change of intervention, at the mother's initiative, began immediately to change the dynamics between the mother and daughter. The team hypothesized that Sari had been thwarted in her development, due to mother's inability to let her be separate. We felt we were observing a reversal and a displacement in the relationship. Mother needed Sari to be a narcissistic object for her, to meet her own needs. Mother seemed to be caring for herself in her relationship with her daughter. There was no differentiation in the mother's mind between herself and her daughter. Sari quickly began to engage with the child therapist in play who followed her lead. Play themes began to become elaborate.

Mother talked in a free associative way, remembering events from her past that had been haunting her. She told me about her abusive relationship with her mother from the time she was a little girl. She never understood while growing up why she was always the bad one, but kept holding on to the notion that her mother really loved her. She knew her mother preferred her brothers. Her mother abused her verbally and physically, but she never told her father. She idealized her father, and she felt ashamed. At eleven she developed an eating disorder which she hid from everyone until she met her husband. She was certain once he knew, he would leave her. So, she left him. He came after her, which proved his love. Soon after they married, she became pregnant with Sari. As mother was sharing her past history and difficulties, we noticed a marked development in Sari's play. Sari was more autonomous and showed more initiative. It was as if she had been allowed to separate and individuate as a person in her own right from her mother, with mother being present as a secure base. The team wondered if mother felt the loss of the symbiotic relationship would result in her becoming pregnant, and indeed, she did. We worked together for the duration of the pregnancy. Mother continued to share her past conflicts, and Sari continued to develop and showed a marked improvement. When the second baby was born, mother reported a very different experience. She felt bonded to the new baby from the beginning and was surprised she could feel love for two infants at the same time. Mother felt pleased with herself as a mother of two infants.

The family planned to return to their home country when the new baby was three months old. Termination was painful as mother felt they had benefited from our work together. In the final session, mother was deeply moved to tears and said how much she had been helped. We too were moved—the only ones who did not cry were the infants. Sari stood at the door saying, "Come on, we're ready to go, we're leaving now, goodbye." We all admired this little girl who was now so autonomous that she could experience her own feeling states, separate from the others.

The positive outcome of this case was due to the careful assessment of the problem between the mother and infant and the clinician and team's sensitivity to following the lead of the mother in letting her effect an intervention that would work for her in the presence of her infant.

Case Study 3

V Case: Vita—16 Months— Valerie Iles

The case illustrates unresolved mourning in a mother and father who tragically lost their five-year-old daughter in a car accident and had a replacement child. Mother felt unable to create a space in her mind for her infant.

ASSESSMENT

The D family was referred by their family doctor. Ms. D had not been able to mourn the loss of her five-year-old daughter, who had been killed by a car while traveling abroad with her maternal grandparents two years earlier. Since the death of their

461

first child, they had a replacement child, Vita, who was 16 months old when we first met them. During the assessment, Vita, a quiet child, small and fragile, seemed younger than her age. She kept close to her mother most of the time. The mother admitted she was overprotective of Vita for fear of something happening to her. Over the period of the assessment, Vita appeared detached, languishing in her own world. At times, she would wander around the room, rarely showing interest in the toys provided. She would move between her parents trying to engage them. Her mother would then pick her up but not really focus on her. Her father, engrossed in his own needs, never seemed to notice she was there. At these times, Vita seemed more fragile and withdrawn.

Ms. D appeared to be a quiet, timid woman. She spoke very little, letting her husband dominate most of the session. When she did express her feelings about her daughter's death, her husband would always interrupt with his opinions. Ms. D would then immediately withdraw and remain quiet. In her individual session, Ms. D was more relaxed and able to express herself. She told the clinician that she found it difficult to let her daughter explore around their home, for fear that the child would get hurt and they might lose her. Ms. D also spoke about her mother pressuring her to quickly have another child. She was close to her parents, but ambivalent in her feelings about them. She complained that when they came to visit, they were always critical about things, especially relating to her husband. She kept her feelings to herself. She became depressed and often wept.

During the assessment, Vita's father disclosed a history of physical and emotional abuse by his parents and the death of his eighteen-year-old sister when he was fifteen. Mr. D dominated the assessment process with his own needs and concerns. He wanted his wife to deal with their daughter's death, but always interjected when his wife made any attempt to express herself. He would turn the conversation to the issue of his attention deficit disorder (ADD) or the fact that no one seemed to understand his needs. He insisted had dealt with his own feelings about his daughter's death, and it was his wife who needed to change. He thought she needed to become more independent from her parents, to speak up for herself. It was clear that Mr. D was deflecting and displacing his own psychic pain.

FORMULATION

The team thought both parents had unresolved feelings of loss and guilt over the trauma of their daughter's death. They were in a continual state of helplessness and vulnerability. There was no space in which they could begin to work through their pain. They could not give psychic life to their live infant, Vita. We chose to extend the assessment period to explore further the relationships within the family. The parents agreed with our decision.

My experience as the clinician in the room with this family was like being in a frozen space. I felt that Vita was in a state of suspended animation, that her inability to play and explore was because she was being held in this dead empty space. At one point, Vita came over and handed me her personal doll staring at me intently. Then she moved around behind my chair and began to push me. I understood this as Vita's telling me that I was to find a way to release her and her parents from this dead space.

Over the next several sessions, it became clear to the team that the father's overriding needs made it impossible to begin exploring the relationships within the family. I felt trapped, unable to find entry into a therapeutic relationship with the family. I empathized with Vita. There seemed no place, no space, and no skill. Aware of my countertransference, I reached the conclusion with the team that there had to be a change in the therapeutic approach. We felt that father's needs would have to be attended to before anything could begin to change. Father had asked us to find an individual therapist for him, which we did. With this in place, we felt a change in the focus of the therapy was now possible. We recognized the father's strength to bring his family for treatment, yet he could not let his wife engage. It was important that both parents be part of the process and decision-making. To lose the father's participation would jeopardize the treatment. Now an entry point was possible, and the therapeutic process could begin. We brought the father alongside the team by asking him to join with the clinician observing the mother and child at play.

INTERVENTION

The intervention consisted of a six week parent-infant play therapy, where the mother and child played together, after which the mother and clinician would discuss how the mother experienced the play.

The father was asked to sit quietly. Just as the sessions were to begin, Ms. D broke her arm and injured her foot while getting out of a taxi. She identified her pain with the pain her dead daughter must have felt when she was struck, with the result that she became depressed, feeling she should be with her in death. At this time, Vita had a seizure brought on by a high fever. The thought of losing her living child terrified her. For the first time, Vita became real to her. By being able to talk about her mixed feelings of wanting to be with her dead daughter and needing to protect her live daughter, Vita, Ms. D made space for the work to continue. Initially, Ms. D and Vita were finding it difficult to create their play together. They were both very quiet, whispering together. Vita used the two baby dolls that had been provided. She gave one (the dead baby) to me, and she took the other doll (herself) to her mother, likely asking mother "to take care of me." Very little happened between them during the twenty minutes. Their interaction seemed strained and disjointed.

In the discussion, Ms. D said she found the process difficult and felt self-conscious. She said it brought back memories of the daughter she lost. These memories kept her from being in the present with Vita. I felt the purpose of the treatment was to help the mother return to the past, to help her mourn. I thought we needed to help the mother go through her pain so she could emerge in the present and relate to her present live daughter, Vita. I felt to be able to do this, we would have to adapt the therapy. Vita's looks to me were a plea for me to help, to become more involved. I

463

needed to be on the floor with her and her mother. I felt that Ms. D needed the freedom and space to begin to mourn the loss of her dead daughter and at the same time, begin to attach with Vita. Using the reflective self in the potential space that had been created, the clinician could support them both. I would be able to help the mother connect with Vita's attempts to engage her and be with the mother as she began to work through her loss.

I presented my thoughts to the team, and they agreed to my entering the mother's and daughter's space on the floor. Ms. D agreed to the change, and said she would be more relaxed with me on the floor with them. Over the next several sessions before the summer break, the therapy changed dramatically. Vita was much more demonstrative in her play, showing us it was time to move things along. The baby doll play continued as before. By giving me the dead baby and her mother the live baby, the play became more alive. Vita and her mother were more interactive and verbal together. They seemed to enjoy each other more. Their space was no longer static. The mother began to talk more openly about the death of her first daughter. As she spoke about her, she had an insight. She realized that her first daughter had spent most of her time with her maternal grandmother and in a sense belonged to her. That was the reason she wanted to spend more time at home with Vita because she wanted Vita to be hers and not her mother's. In almost losing Vita to the seizure, she realized how much this child meant to her. Now that she was able to deal with her feelings about her lost daughter,

she could begin to look inward to a life with Vita.

As the anniversary of her daughter's death approached, Ms. D's mother again said it would be a good time to have another baby. Ms. D had just returned to work and was feeling good about how she and Vita were doing. She did not want another child at this time. As for Vita, she expressed her feeling about a new baby by using a toy doctor's mallet to hit the baby doll in the head. Vita's play became more active and constructive. At times, she would use blocks to make a seat between her mother and myself and sit between us listening quietly.

After the summer break, they decided to end. During the final session, Ms. D said she was happy and spoke about her work. She felt that Vita was doing well. Vita played as she had before, giving me the dead baby and busied herself taking care of her baby. She took off the doll's blanket and put the doll on her mother's chest facing forward. Several minutes later, as Ms. D and I continued talking, Vita went to her mother, removed the doll and took its place on her mother's chest facing forward. As we were saying our good-byes, Mr. D arrived. We briefly reviewed for him how well the treatment had gone. He talked about how well he was doing in his own therapy. We said our good-byes, with the door left open to return at any time.

CASE STUDY CONCLUSION

Our intervention became effective at the point where the family was able to tolerate the clinician entering their space. This nonintrusive stance made it possible for us to work together on the painful feelings.

Ms. D was able to release her daughter to the past and look toward the future with her daughter, Vita. Ms. D seemed able to become more autonomous in the relationships with her parents and her husband and become open to a real relationship—with her live daughter, Vita. As for Vita, at all levels, her life was just beginning.

Case Study 4

J Case: Joey—Age Four Years— Susan Eadie

The case illustrates a depressed mother and uninvolved father who were unable to deal with the aggression of their four-year-old son toward mother and the one-year-old son.

INITIAL ASSESSMENT PHASE

Joey, a four-year-old boy, was referred to the clinic by the mother who was concerned about his aggressive behavior toward her and his one-year-old baby brother. The assessment interviews were carried out by two clinicians. One met with the parents to take histories, and the other worked with the child in play to assess his ability to relate, play, and talk about his worries. The team observed behind a one-way mirror and worked with the clinicians in developing hypotheses and formulations.

In the formulation, the marital problems were considered to be the primary concern, and marital therapy was recommended. The assessment also indicated the mother was depressed. The mother was distressed with the feedback session. She felt that the family difficulties were being attributed to her, and the distress caused her by her husband's serious alleged aggression and lack of enthusiasm for parenting was not given enough emphasis. Therefore, to consider the mother's objection and the necessity to enable the mother to feel empowered in the process, an intervention to extend the assessment was proposed, to include each parent, one at a time, to play with Joey together in the presence of the clinician and the observing team. We were interested in the parents' input and staying with the potential space created between the child and themselves.

EXTENDED ASSESSMENT PHASE

The Dynamic Mother-Child Play Intervention technique was used (described earlier in Case Study 1, Treatment Recommendations). A variation of the "Watching, Waiting, and Wondering" (Muir, 1992) technique was used. The process of the parent-child interaction in play brought forward emotional themes that were important to the parent or the child. The effects of these emotional issues on the parent-child interaction were observed and discussed in the session. The team learned of the depths of the mother's depression and feeling of emptiness—the absence of representations of good caregiving objects in her internal world. In one play session, Joey made the toy animals die. Mother became tearful during this play and asked Joey if he could make the animals live because it made her too sad for them to die. He replied, "It's just a story," but complied with mother's request. In discussion, the mother related her experience in the play to her depression and her feelings of loneliness as a child. Her expression in and reflection on this play segment was an opportunity for the mother to visibly experience being listened to and understood by another. This allowed her to be reflective rather than attacking and feeling attacked as had been her response to the initial assessment feedback. In the discussion of this play sequence, the mother was first able to tolerate her pain, reflect on its origins (her own childhood with a mother who could not respond in a nurturing way), and even become aware of how her inner distress had impacted on her child. This enabled the team to better understand where this mother's feeling of being attacked in the initial assessment feedback came from—her persecuting and rejecting internal objects.

It also became evident, through the play series with the mother, that her overwhelming depression and sadness was affecting the child. When she cried, Joey became anxious and moved ambivalently as he tried to soothe her and seek comfort by soothing himself. He would hug her and curl up on her lap.

The father's play sessions with his son also provided opportunity to develop a fuller understanding of the impact of the father's early childhood experiences on the parental relationship and how his son responded. The father's disinterest in parenting young children was identified by the father himself in the initial assessment. The origins of his experience of boredom and its effect on his relationship with his son became better understood by the father and

the team during his discussions with the clinician in his play sessions with his son. He was able to access the origins of his feelings through reflection that came easily to him in the presence of a clinician. The following excerpts from the second session illustrate the father's growing awareness of his boredom, desire to lead the play with his son, and our mutual understanding of the origins of his feelings of boredom.

Joey moved blocks on a toy truck. Father suggested making a loading dock with the blocks. Father chose to introduce an animal, and asked Joey to name it. Joey continued moving blocks and asked father to, "Take those out (the animals) and we'll have more space . . . Dad, come on, get one of these blocks." Father introduced animals or new block constructions, but Joey reminded father to do as Joey suggested, "You follow me."

The father indicated he was able to use the reflection of his play with his son to track the origins of his boredom with parenting in interaction with his son. He realized he introduced activity into the play rather than follow his son's initiative, to make the experience more interesting to him. He recalled that when he was with his own parents, he was around them but did not play with them. He described how he complied with his mother's request, feigning interest in her topics in an attempt to please her.

The father's reflections enabled him and the team to see how his childhood experience of having to fit into an adult world to get attention led him to react with boredom when he viewed his son's repetitive exploratory play through adult eyes. Play with his young son also rekindled father's unmet childhood desires to have an important adult follow him with interest. This play with his son was like recapturing a lost opportunity. Thus, father seized the opportunity to create and explore his own ideas. The father became aware of his own "play" needs, what was emotionally absent in his childhood relationships, and that acting on his own needs restricted and interfered with his son's play. The play experience and the reflections with the clinician resulted in this father developing an interest in his own individual psychotherapy, an interest he did not have after the initial assessment.

In the initial assessment, the team had thought that marital and possibly individual psychotherapy for the parents might be sufficient to help the child get back on his developmental track. However, observation of the parent-child interaction over time in the play activity made evident that individual therapy for the child would also be important to help him resolve his internalized conflicts and anxieties about holding the marriage together and taking care of his mother. The parents responded positively to all these recommendations and supported Joey in his therapy.

Case Study 5

C Case: Caitlan—Age Three Years— Judith Coates

The case illustrates a depressed mother and father, who were unable to deal with the oral aggression of their three-year-old daughter toward their one-year-old daughter and themselves.

Caitlan and her family were referred by the family therapist at a day care center. Caitlan, who had entered the center at the age of eight months, now three years old, was reported to be engaging in aggressive behaviors, directed largely toward her one-year-old sister, Lucy, but also toward peers. Caitlan was biting, spitting, and hitting. Of particular concern to the day care was mother's passivity and failure to intervene when Caitlan attacked Lucy during a therapy session. Although Caitlan could sustain play and had positive relationships with some staff members, she was described as "not engaging" and having a "don't mess with me" look.

The M family consisted of father, mother, and the two girls. Mr. M was the only child of dysfunctional parents and was exposed to violence in the home. His father suffered from depression and committed suicide when Mr. M was in late adolescence. Mr. M had a history of psychiatric illness and of substance abuse. He worked intermittently.

Ms. M was the youngest of four children. Hers was a materially comfortable middle-class family. Her inability to supply much detail about her early childhood ultimately led the team to speculate that this was a family which maintained secrecy to protect itself from the outside world—a family in which there was little open discussion of feelings. Ms. M became anorectic at puberty, and her illness embarrassed and angered her family. She experienced her mother as emotionally unavailable to her. She felt misunderstood, rejected, and lonely. At the time of the assessment, she was taking medication for chronic depression. Ms. M had obtained a university degree and was working part-time. This family had little support from extended family members and appeared isolated within the community. Mother was seeing the family therapist at the day care center for individual therapy. Father was meeting with his family physician for individual counseling.

INITIAL ASSESSMENT PHASE

I first met the family in the waiting area. The parents appeared tired, harrassed, and guarded, although mother greeted me politely and pleasantly. They were burdened with stroller, bags, and children's clothing and, together with the children, struggled up to the therapy room.

Caitlan, age three, "the biter," looked like a sturdy and physically attractive little girl. Her face was fixed in an odd, tense grimace. Lucy, age 12 months, a round-faced cheerful baby just beginning to walk, was very engaging and easily able to monopolize attention. She smiled brightly throughout the first session, and with time, the team concluded that Caitlan's grimace represented an attempt to imitate Lucy's smile and, thereby, please others by smiling. I had been led to expect a fierce little girl, and noteworthy about the first observation of Caitlan's play was her lack of overt aggression. She was attacked several times by Lucy, who pulled her hair and grabbed toys from her. This Caitlan tolerated for the most part. Caitlan's speech was indistinct, and she was quiet during much of the first two sessions when parents and children

were together. I was often aware of being watched by her and felt that she was seeking approval—she had been identified as the "problem person" in the family. Periodically, Caitlan sought contact with her parents. In doing so, she was less persistent and assertive than her sister. While Lucy was successful in accessing her mother's lap and breast, Caitlan seldom was touched or even noticed by her parents. During the second session, the team observed Caitlan retiring to a corner of the room, having a bowel movement, and then fetching a diaper from a bag. The parents were unaware of all this until Caitlan placed the diaper on mother's lap. Even then, mother ignored the diaper, putting it elsewhere, and continued talking.

Mr. M, at first and for periods during succeeding sessions, was dour and reticent, slouching in his chair and regarding me enigmatically from behind tinted glasses. His removal of the spectacles came to indicate openness, a willingness to communicate. He rapidly used humor and shared stories as means to connect with me. Mr. M stated firmly at the outset that he was reluctant to explore his past because he had frequently given his history to various mental health professionals and was weary of repeating it. It was clear that he resisted being cast in the role of victim or damaged individual, and he was determined to persuade me and himself that his childhood had not been "all horrible."

Ms. M worked hard in reflecting upon and answering questions. She appeared a kind and compliant woman. At times, she was vague, and it felt as though she were occupying a different space and only with effort, could recall herself to the present situation. The impression was that, like Mr. M, she was turning away from herself and her past. This was reflected in my difficulty in maintaining eye contact with Ms. M during the earlier sessions. Clearly, it was painful for these parents to return to their childhoods. I remarked that their difficult childhood experiences had perhaps left them unsure of their abilities as parents. Ms. M was indeed concerned that she might be repeating with Caitlan her mother's treatment of herself.

Ms. M tended to reference her husband often and was afraid of annoying or upsetting him. When Mr. M was angry, he usually retreated from the situation, afraid of his anger and unwilling to discuss his feelings until he had calmed down. This resulted in Ms. M feeling distanced from him and lonely. I came to believe that she was actually afraid of his absence. This evoked the sense of despair she had experienced when her mother was "not there for her" when she was a young adolescent and attempting to speak of her feelings of depression.

For the remainder of the initial assessment, the children were seen separately while I continued to meet with the parents. The couple spoke of fears that their marital relationship could be damaged by parenting difficulties. Mr. M was disinclined to consider that there were marital problems stemming from issues other than Caitlan's behavior. He tended to pathologize Caitlan and characterized her as "a bully." The parents spoke of having different parenting styles. Mother was more inclined to try reasoning with the children and had difficulty intervening with firm words and actions in situations of sibling abuse and noncompliance. Father believed that firm limits should be placed on the children's behavior and blamed Ms. M for not following through with consequences—but he was unable to take action on a consistent basis. His misuse of antidepressant medication made him sleepy and moody and frequently prevented him from being of real assistance to her in coping with the children and the domestic work. Both parents were concerned that their anger was potentially destructive and were inclined to confuse discipline and the setting of firm limits with violence and punitive actions. Both described themselves as powerless in trying to manage Caitlan. Father spoke of feeling "emasculated."

FORMULATION

The team thought that Caitlan's biting signified failed contact with mother. It seemed that she had formed an insecure attachment with her mother reinforced by the birth of her sister. Both parents had undoubtedly experienced maternal deprivation. Both suffered from episodes of depression which at times must have been experienced by the children as emotional abandonment. We had witnessed Ms. M's psychic absences during sessions. The team was particularly concerned that the parents did not talk to one another or to Caitlan and that they often failed to notice her when she approached them. Caitlan sought attention in a manner bound to generate negative responses. It was observed that while away from her parents communication with the clinician enhanced Caitlan's verbalization.

INTERVENTION

We suggested a series of six family therapy sessions focussing on family relationships using play. On alternate weeks, one parent and the clinician would get down on the floor and play with the children, and the other parent would observe. The observing parent should reflect on what was going on in the play and in the interactions of family members. The focus within the play sessions was to be on the "here and now" and not on history. The parents were instructed to regard Caitlan as communicator and concentrate on understanding what she was communicating through her play.

It was quickly apparent that the children were delighted to have their parents on the floor playing with them. The parents were self-conscious but able to engage in play. There was some difficulty in playing with both girls without arousing resentment in one or the other. However, Ms. M managed to intervene when they appeared about to fight. She placed herself between them and redirected their play, giving special attention to Caitlan. Caitlan made frequent eye contact with me. She smiled and offered me the toy lion. I felt Caitlan sensed that I would be able to act as a container for the anxieties and burdens weighing on her and the family. Caitlan spent a good deal of each session playing with two baby dolls. She treated them with gentle care. I suggested that Caitlan was showing us that she wanted the same special and close attention she gave the babies. She smiled. Ms. M was able to respond to this by giving her closer attention. Mr. M's response was initially irritable. He contemplated gloomily the notion that he would

have to spend "twenty-four hours a day" with the children in order to make them feel secure.

Caitlan rapidly showed change. Her face relaxed, and the grimace disappeared within two family sessions. Her speech became much clearer, and I pointed out to the parents that this was in direct response to our addressing her and putting her feelings into words. The importance in keeping the focus on the present and on the children's activity in the room was illustrated during the second play session. When the parents and I discussed their childhood experiences, the children's play "fell apart." They became wild and aggressive behavior appeared. Mr. M made the creative suggestion that one or two of us remain on the floor for the entire session. We had been returning to our seats halfway through the session and discussing our observations. This tactic proved successful, and our adoption of it helped Mr. M to feel effective.

As the parents felt contained and safe, they could express their differences and feelings openly. In the third session, I provided complimentary feedback to them on their play with the children. Father rose abruptly and angrily left the room. Ms. M persuaded him to return, and he was able to verbalize his anger. He did not need me to tell him how well he played with his children, and he did not need to be taught to play. He readily agreed when I suggested he felt patronized. We clarified the difference between using the play to understand the children's communication and teaching parents "how to play." During this session, Mr. M criticized Ms. M's parenting. She reacted with unusual anger and complained that she was always blamed for the children's behavior and for most domestic problems. During these eruptions between the parents, the children's play ceased, Caitlan retreated into a corner, and Lucy cried. They clearly attuned to the affective tone of their parents' discord.

Mr. M became concerned about regressive tendencies on Caitlan's part. She was climbing into the carriage and was copying Lucy's baby talk. I suggested this was an effective way to get attention without using aggressive means and that perhaps Caitlan needed to go backward a little in order to go forward. Caitlan, listening to this exchange, made baby sounds and climbed onto her father's lap. Mother frequently stroked her hair and back.

Caitlan began each session by staking out her territory: The dolls' bed containing the two "babies." She cared for the babies with great devotion. At some point, Lucy would interfere in Caitlan's play and grab a baby or feeding bottle. The parents insisted that Caitlan share. Often Caitlan tolerated this, but sometimes she became angry. In the fifth session, I pointed out that Caitlan's game required the use of two dolls and that because of her age and stage, she needed to complete her play. Lucy could be redirected for the time being. "Taking turns" was a more appropriate concept in dealing with this situation than "sharing." I suggested that splitting up the dolls would be like taking a book away from someone when they were in the middle of a chapter and asking them to "share it." The parents immediately related to this, and Caitlan gave me a look of gratitude and crooned, "Baby, baby, baby."

In the sixth session, Caitlan climbed into the dolls' bed, and I commented that perhaps she was showing us she wanted sometimes to be a baby rather than a "big girl" looking after babies. Caitlan smiled her agreement, and mother covered her with the doll blankets. During the final part of this session, Caitlan lay sprawled on her father's lap with socks off and sucking on Lucy's bottle, the picture of contented regression. Although Mr. M was not wholly comfortable with this, he was able to tolerate it and to place his arms around Caitlan. Mother was holding Lucy on her lap—Lucy had reverted to the breast. The parents were side by side, each with a child on their lap, and the room felt very peaceful.

CASE STUDY CONCLUSION

Our focus in the intervention was on facilitation of exploration of family relationships by the family and the clinician through play. Our primary goal was to help Caitlan meet her needs through positive means, rather than having to resort to aggressive means such as biting and hitting. In order to realize this goal, the parents and clinician were to focus particularly on Caitlan and on what she was communicating through her play and indicate that her messages had been understood by putting what we thought her feeling states were into words. We believed that the parents did not communicate openly to one another and did not talk to Caitlan. It was essential that she receive positive attention from her parents and that she be talked to in order to enhance the attachment.

We learned from the intervention that

Caitlan was less disturbed than we had thought. Prompt intervention appeared to break through the family pattern of intergenerational deprivation. However, since it had taken the father some time to view the family play therapy as useful, it was thought that a further period of intervention was necessary. He had just become comfortable with the situation and both parents were speaking more openly to one another. We all wished to further enhance this progress. During the course of the intervention, through watching Caitlan play contentedly in the therapeutic space, both parents acquired some sense that good experiences of close attention in the present would ultimately enable her to play alone in the presence of her parents, leaving them to their own activities. They had also accepted that regression was a necessary prerequisite to Caitlan's moving forward. While they had come to us expecting very concrete, prescriptive advice, Mr. M and Ms. M had learned that by observing their children closely and reflecting upon what they observed, they could themselves arrive at solutions to their problems. The family planned to continue for a further six sessions. Father's playful comment was, "Don't change that dial. Same time, same place!"

volved in the problems the family brings by focusing on the uniqueness of the relationships between the infant and the family members as a way of understanding the problems through the use of observation, play, and reflection.

We look at the concept of *relational space* through the *existing space* to access the *potential space* between parents and infant or child, between clinician, parents, and infant or child, and between the observed and the observation team. To access the potential space leads to healthy development and healthier relationships. We attend to the inner experience and worlds of the participants as we explore, gather data, and reflect on the material as it unfolds in a creative way in our presence. Our aim is to understand the nature of the presenting problems, in terms of the present situation originating from the past experiences of parents in their growing up years and expectations for their children's future development. We have illustrated, by providing case studies, the importance of observation, reflection, and understanding, the importance of play in the assessment and evaluation of infants and their families, and the importance of the process of assessment to determine the most suitable intervention.

Conclusion

We have presented the model of assessment developed by the IFATT of the C. M. Hincks Dellcrest Children's Mental Health Centre, where we conduct a comprehensive assessment of the issues in-

References

Ainsworth, M., Blehar, M., Waters, E., & Wall, S. (1978). *Patterns of attachment: A psychological study of the strange situation.* Hillsdale, NJ: Erlbaum.

Ammaniti, M. (1991). Maternal representation during pregnancy: An early infant-mother interaction. *Infant Mental Health Journal, 12*(3), 246–256.

Bacal, H. (1994). The selfobject relationship in psychoanalytic treatment. In A. Goldberg (Ed.), *A decade of progress: Progress in self psychology* (pp. 21–31). Hillsdale, NJ: Analytic.

Basch, M. (1991). Are selfobjects the only objects? Implications for psychoanalytic technique. In Goldberg (Ed.), *The evolution of self psychology: Progress in self psychology, 7* (pp. 3–17). Hillsdale, NJ: Analytic.

Beebe, B., & Lachman, F. (1988). Mother-infant mutual influence and precursors of psychic structure. In Goldberg (Ed.), *Frontiers in self psychology: Progress in self psychology, 3* (pp. 3–27). Hillsdale, NJ: Analytic.

Beebe, B., Lachman, F., & Jaffe, J. (1997a). Mother-infant interaction structures and presymbolic self and object representations. *Psychoanalytic Dialogues, 7*(2), 133–183.

Beebe, B., Lachman, F., & Jaffe, J. (1997b). A transformational model of presymbolic representations: Reply to commentaries. *Psychoanalytic Dialogues, 7*(2), 215–225.

Bibring, G., Dwyer, L., Huntington, D., & Valenstein, A. (1961). A study of the psychological processes in pregnancy and of the earliest mother-child relationship. *Psychoanalytic Study of the Child, 16,* 9–72.

Bick, E. (1964). Notes on infant observation in psychoanalytic training. *International Journal of Psycho-Analysis, 45,* 558–565.

Bion, W. (1961). *Experiences in groups.* London: Tavistock.

Bowlby, J. (1969). *Attachment and Loss: Vol. I. Attachment.* New York: Basic Books.

Bowlby, J. (1973). *Attachment and Loss: Vol. II. Separation.* New York: Basic Books.

Bowlby, J. (1979a). *The making and breaking of affectional bonds.* London: Tavistock.

Bowlby, J. (1979b). Knowing what you are not supposed to know and feeling what you are not supposed to feel. *Canadian Journal of Psychiatry, 24,* 403–408.

Bowlby, J. (1980). *Attachment and Loss: Vol. III. Loss, Sadness and Depression.* New York: Basic Books.

Brafman, A. H. (1997). Winnicott's therapeutic consultations revisited. *International Journal of Psycho-Analysis, 78*(4), 773–789.

Bretherton, I. (1985). Attachment theory: Retrospect and prospect. In I. Bretherton & E. Waters (Eds.), Growing points in attachment theory and research (pp. 3–35). *Monographs for the Society for Research in Child Development, 50* (1–2 Serial No. 209).

Bretherton, I. (1990). Communication patterns, internal working models, and the intergenerational transmission of attachment relationships. *Infant Mental Health Journal, 11*(3), 237–253.

Byng-Hall, J. (1990). Attachment theory and family therapy: Clinical view: *Infant Mental Health Journal, 11*(3), 228–237.

Byng-Hall, J. (1997). The secure family base: Some implications for family therapy. In Association for Child Psychology and Psychiatry, *Bonding and attachment: Current issues in research practice* (Occasional papers, No. 14, pp. 27–31).

Clulow, C. (1991). Partners becoming parents: A question of difference. *Infant Mental Health Journal, 12*(3), 256–267.

Cramer, B. (1992). *The importance of being baby.* Addison, NJ: Welsey.

Cramer, B., & Stern, D. (1988, Spring). Evaluation of changes in mother-infant brief psychotherapy: A single case study. *Journal of Infant Mental Health, 9*(1), 20–45.

Cramer, B., Robert-Tissot, C., Stern, D., Serpa Russconi, S., De Muralt, M., Besson, G., Palacio-Espasa, F., Bachmann, J.-P., Knauer, D., Berney, C., & D'Arcis, U. (1990, Fall). Outcome evaluation in brief mother-infant psychotherapy: A preliminary report. *Journal of Infant Mental Health, 11*(3), 278–300.

Demos, V. (1988). Affect and the development of the self: A new frontier. In A. Goldberg (Ed.), *Frontiers in self psychology: Progress in self psychology, 3* (pp. 27–55). Hillsdale, NJ: Analytic.

Doulis, S. (1997). *Manual for individual assessment of children and adolescents: A guide to conducting and reporting assessment.* Unpublished manuscript.

Emde, R. (1987). Infant mental health: Clinical dilemmas, the expansion of meaning and opportunities. In J. Osofsky (Ed.), *Handbook of infant development* (2nd ed., pp. 1297–1321). New York: Wiley.

Emde, R. (1991). The wonder of our complex enterprise: Steps enabled by attachment and the effects of relationships on relationships. *Infant Mental Health Journal, 12*(3), 164–174.

Fonagy, P., Steele, M., Steele, H., Moran, G., & Higgitt, A. (1991). The capacity for understanding mental states: The reflective self-parent in mother and child and its significance for security of attachment. *Infant Mental Health Journal, 12*(3), 201–219.

Fonagy, P. (1997). Can we use observations of infant-caregiver interactions as a basis for a model of the representational world? *Psychoanalytic Dialogues, 7*(2), 207–215.

Fraiberg, S. (1980). *Clinical studies in infant mental health.* New York: Basic Books.

Freud, A. (1936). *Ego and mechanisms of defense.* London: Hogarth.

Freud, A. (1965). *Normality and pathology in childhood.* New York: International Universities Press.

Freud, E. (1975). Infant observation: Its relevance to psychoanalytic training. *Psychoanalytic Study of the Child, 30,* 75–94.

Freud, S. (1914). *Remembering, repeating and working through* (Standard ed.). London: Hogarth.

Freud, S. (1929). *Inhibitions, symptoms and anxiety* (Standard ed.). London: Hogarth.

George, C., Kaplan, N., & Main, N. (1985). *An adult attachment interview.* Unpublished manuscript, Department of Psychology, University of California at Berkeley, California.

Goldberg, S. (1991, August). Recent developments in attachment theory and research. *Canadian Journal of Psychiatry, 36,* 393–400.

Hirshberg, L. M. (1993). Clinical interviews with infants and their families. In C. H. Zeanah (Ed.), *Handbook of infant mental health* (pp. 173–91). New York: Guilford.

Klein, M. (1975). *Love, guilt and reparation.* London: Hogarth.

Klein, M., Heimann, P., Isaacs, S., & Riviere, J. (1952). *Developments in psychoanalysis.* London: Hogarth.

Kohut, H. (1959). Introspection, empathy and psychoanalysis. *Journal of the American Psychiatric Association, 7,* 459–483.

Kohut, H. (1971). *The analysis of self.* New York: International Universities Press.

Kohut, H. (1977). *The Restoration of the Self.* New York: International Universities Press.

Kohut, H. (1984). *How does analysis cure?* Chicago: University of Chicago Press.

Kulka, R. (1997). Commentaries on paper by Beebe, Lachman and Jaffe: Quantum selfhood. *Psychoanalytic Dialogues, 7*(2), 183–189.

Main, M., & Goldwyn, R. (1984). Predicting rejection of her infant from mother's representation of her own experience: Implications for the abused-abusing intergenerational cycle. *Child Abuse and Neglect, 8*, 203–219.

Main, M., & Weston, D. (1982). Avoidance of the attachment figure in infancy: Descriptions and interpretations. In M. Parkes & J. Stevenson-Hinde (Eds.), *The place of attachment in human behaviour* (pp. 31–60). New York: Basic Books.

Mitchell, S., & Black, M. (1995). *Freud and beyond: A history of modern psychoanalytic thought.* New York: Basic Books.

Muir, E. (1992, Winter). Watching, waiting and wondering: Applying psychoanalytic principles to mother-infant intervention. *Infant Mental Health Journal, 13*(4), 319–329.

Muir, E., & Tuters, E. (1992). An infant mental health training model for day care professionals: The C. M. Hincks Institute National Day Care Training Project. In S. Provence, J. Pawl, & E. Fenichel (Eds.), *The Zero to Three child care anthology 1984–1992* (pp. 71–93). Arlington, VA: Zero to Three/NCCIP.

Murray, L. (1991). Intersubjectivity, object relations theory, and empirical evidence from mother-infant interactions. *Infant Mental Health Journal, 12*(3), 219–233.

Ogden, T. (1992). *The matrix of the mind.* London: Karnac.

Ornstein, A. (1974). The dread to repeat and the new beginning: A contribution to the psychoanalysis of narcissistic personality disorder. *Annual of Psychoanalysis, 2,* 231–248.

Sandler, J., Kennedy, H., & Tyson, R. (1980). *The techniques of child psychoanalysis: Discussions with Anna Freud.* Cambridge, MA: Harvard University Press.

Sandler, L. (1988). The event-structure of regulation in the neonate-caregiver system as a biological background for early organization of psychic structure. In A. Goldberg (Ed.), *Frontiers in self psychology: Progress in self psychology* (pp. 64–81). Hillsdale, NJ: Analytic.

Schwaber, E. (1984). Empathy: A mode of analytic listening. In J. Lichtenberg (Ed.), *Empathy II* (pp. 143–172). Hillsdale, NJ: Analytic.

Stern, D. (1984). Affect attunement. In J. Call, E. Galenson, & R. Tyson (Eds.), *Frontiers of infant psychiatry* (pp. 3–15). New York: Basic Books.

Stern, D. (1985). *The interpersonal world of the infant: A view from psychoanalysis and developmental psychology.* New York: Basic Books.

Stern, D. (1991). Maternal representations: A clinical and subjective phenomenological view. *Infant Mental Health Journal, 12*(3), 174–187.

Stern, D. (1995). *Motherhood constellation.* New York: Basic Books.

Stern-Bruschweiler, N., & Stern, D. (1989, Fall). A model for conceptualizing the role of the mother's representational world in various mother-infant therapies. *Infant Mental Health Journal, 3,* 142–56.

Stevenson-Hinde, J. (1990). Attachment within family systems: An overview. *Infant Mental Health Journal, 11*(3), 218–228.

Stolorow, R. (1988). Transference and the therapeutic process. *The Psychoanalytic Review, 75*(2), 245–254.

Thomson, P. (1991). Countertransference in an intersubjective perspective: An experiment. In A. Goldberg (Ed.), *The evolution of self psychology: Progress in self psychology* (pp. 75–93). Hillsdale, NJ: Analytic.

Tuters, E. (1988, Spring). The relevance of

infant observation to clinical training and practice: An interpretation. *Journal of Infant Mental Health,* 9(1), 94–104.

Tuters, E. (1996). Dyadic circularity in the mother-infant relationship. In B. Abosh & A. Collins (Eds.), *Mental illness in the family* (pp. 154–161). Toronto: University of Toronto Press.

Tuters, E., Muir, E., Huntley, M., & Rustin, M. (1989). *Workshop presentation on infant observation.* 4th Congress, World Association of Infant Psychiatry and Allied Disciplines, Lugano, Switzerland.

Wesner, D., Dowling, J., & Johnson, F. (1982). What is maternal infant intervention? The role of infant psychotherapy. *Psychiatry, 45,* 307–315.

Williams, M. H. (1987). *Collected papers of Martha Harris and Ester Bick.* Perthshire, Scotland: Clunie.

Winnicott, D. W. (1972). The capacity to be alone. In J. Sutherland (Ed.), *The maturational processes and the facilitating environment* (pp. 29–37). London: Hogarth.

Winnicott, D. W. (1971). The use of an object in relating through identifications. *Playing and reality* (pp. 86–95). London: Tavistock.

Winnnicott, D. W. (1971a). Transitional objects and transitional phenomenon. *Playing and reality* (pp. 1–26). London: Tavistock.

Winnicott, D. W. (1971b). Playing: A theoretical statement. *Playing and reality* (pp. 38–53). London: Tavistock.

Winnicott, D. W. (1971c). Playing: Creative activity and the search for the self. *Playing and reality* (pp. 53–65). London: Tavistock.

Winnicott, D. W. (1971d). The location of cultural experience. *Playing and reality* (pp. 95–104). London: Tavistock.

14

Assessment of Temperament in Infancy

John Worobey

14

Introduction

The concept of temperament, as applied to normal development in human infancy, refers to individual differences in early behavioral style. The inclusion of a chapter on temperament in a volume such as this is more than appropriate, as the increased interest in issues that surround infant mental health over the past 20 years has been paralleled by a veritable explosion of research on the behavioral style of infants. As the numerous books (Buss & Plomin, 1984; Thomas & Chess, 1977), edited volumes (Porter & Collins, 1992; Strelau & Angleitner, 1991), empirical reviews (Rothbart & Bates, 1998; Seifer & Sameroff, 1986), and

Work on this chapter was facilitated by an Academic Study Leave from Rutgers University during the Fall of 1997, which allowed the author to spend a semester as a visiting faculty member at the Institute for the Study of Child Development at the University of Medicine and Dentistry of New Jersey. The support of Dr. Michael Lewis and the faculty and staff of the Institute is gratefully acknowledged.

scholarly discussions (Goldsmith et al., 1987; Kohnstamm, 1986) attest, the concept of temperament has been embraced by developmental psychologists, practicing pediatricians, clinical psychiatrists, behavioral geneticists, personality theorists, and early interventionists, with contributions from all of their respective disciplines. To appreciate the rapid growth of the literature in this area, consider that the first edition of the *Handbook of Infant Development* (Osofsky, 1979) did not even list the word "temperament" in its index, while the second edition (Osofsky, 1987) included a chapter that focused entirely on the topic (Bates, 1987), as does the most recent *Handbook of Child Psychology* (Damon & Eisenberg, 1998). As some have lamented, the paucity of clinical research on temperament as it relates to childhood psychopathology (Carey, 1989a; Maziade, 1994), reserving an entire chapter for the subject of temperament signifies that sufficient applied research now exists to warrant its coverage in a handbook devoted to the field of infant mental health.

The present chapter attempts to summarize some of the major themes that characterize the study of temperament as currently portrayed in the early human development literature. As a sizable number of comprehensive reviews of the concept of temperament (Rothbart & Bates, 1998; Goldsmith et al., 1987) as well as critical reviews of strategies for its assessment (Slabach, Morrow, & Wachs, 1991; Windle, 1988) even specific to infancy (Bornstein, Gaughran, & Homel, 1986; Goldsmith, & Rieser-Danner, 1990) are now available, no more than an overview is provided for some of the issues that are arguably better addressed by the aforementioned authors. Rather, particular attention is directed to areas that pertain to the practical considerations of measuring temperament in infancy and the clinical applications of the concept, topics that are of greater relevance to the infant mental health specialist. The reader is encouraged to consult any of the reviews that are cited within this chapter, whose full citations appear in the reference section.

Historical Perspective on the Concept of Temperament

The concept of temperament, if taken to mean that personality differences are related to physiological factors, has both an ancient and more modern interpretation. Some 2,000 years ago, the physicians Hippocrates and Galen linked the individual's blood or preponderance of black bile, for example, to a sanguine or melancholic personality type, respectively. With a predominance of either, the individual would be characterized as affiliative or instead prone to sadness (Diamond, 1957). As opposed to this typology that attributed personality differences to the individual's bodily humors, the twentieth century work of Sheldon served to place the word temperament into the psychological lexicon, albeit briefly (Sheldon & Stevens, 1942). Stated simply, the individual's body type or morphology predicted personality. For example, an endomorphic (i.e., heavy set) individual would display the characteristic of sociability. These concepts were most often applied to adults and generally, only to adult males (Huntington, 1989). While somewhat amusing from today's perspective, neither of these "theories" are taken seriously by current researchers in temperament or personality.

In stark contrast to these relatively crude body temperament associations, current approaches to the understanding of individual differences in normal development are quite elaborate in terms of their premises, components, and processes of influence. Indeed, the widespread interest in temperament by researchers and clinicians today, especially in its expression during infancy, may itself be explained by a confluence of factors that defy simplicity. Rothbart and Bates (1998), in their excellent review, delineate three modes of inquiry that may help to explain the rapid growth of contemporary research on temperament. First, the normative studies of large samples of children in the early part of this century showcased the variability of early personality (Gesell, 1925; Shirley, 1933). Second, behavioral geneticists and comparative psychologists investigated motivational and approach-withdrawal systems (Loehlin & Nichols, 1976; Schneirla, 1959). Finally, research by more biologically-oriented clinicians identified individual differences in children's reactivity and resiliency (Escalona, 1968; Murphy & Moriarty, 1976). This line of research is exemplified by the writings of Thomas and Chess (Thomas, Chess, Birch, Hertzig, & Korn, 1963), whose pioneering efforts in describing behavioral style may be credited as both an inspirational source and influential force

in terms of moving the field of temperament forward (McDevitt, 1994; Rutter, 1994). Despite the several hundred papers that have been published on the topic over the last 25 years, however, questions such as "What is temperament?" or "Which dimensions of temperament are worthy of study?" continue to persist (Strelau, 1994).

Theoretical Approaches to Temperament

Theories of temperament are as varied as the subcategories that comprise the concept. One may be as likely to run across a research paper that stresses the biological foundations of temperament, with some consideration of environmental factors, as they are to locate a paper that presents an environmental orientation, yet manages to address biological factors (Bates, 1987). Before describing the differing perspectives, however, some commonalties across theoretical positions can be identified. In a thoughtful overview to a roundtable discussion he convened, Goldsmith has synthesized points of consensus as well as disagreement between contemporary temperament theorists (Goldsmith et al., 1987). In terms of agreement, most theorists appear to accept the following: (1) temperament is a label for a body of related traits, rather than a trait itself, and encompasses phenomena such as irritability, sociability, and activity level, (2) temperament dimensions reflect tendencies rather than discrete actions, (3) temperament has some biological basis and displays some continuity, (4) temperament and behavior connections are most direct during infancy in comparison to the increasing complexity of such linkages with increasing age, (5) temperament refers to individual differences rather than species-general traits, and (6) temperament is modifiable. Points of contention include: (1) differing criteria for what constitutes behavioral style, (2) differing views of the relation of temperament to emotional behavior, (3) differing emphases on the importance of inheritance, (4) differing views on the boundaries between temperament and personality, (5) differing views on the utility of the concept of temperamental "difficulty," and (6) differing numbers of dimensions that are considered to comprise temperament.

Since no single definition of temperament or agreed upon list of dimensions exists, it may be instructive to present the more widely accepted approaches to infant temperament by the theorists who have formulated these varying positions. While scores of individuals have contributed to this growing literature through their research and writings, treatment in this chapter is limited to those theorists who have articulated a specific viewpoint on temperament through their published works, have additionally contributed to the field by developing one or more instruments for measuring temperament, and have evaluated their formulation through the study of infants.

A Clinical Perspective—
Thomas and Chess

The contribution of Thomas and Chess and their collaborators to the modern study of temperament and behavioral individuality cannot be overestimated. Through interviews with mothers of infants as young as three months, these investigators devised a coding system to identify "primary reaction patterns" as expressed at home and in other everyday contexts (Thomas et al., 1963). Adopting the word "temperament" to describe how the infant behaved, they further distinguished this construct from motivation (the why of behavior) and abilities (the what of behavior). As their work evolved into the New York Longitudinal Study (NYLS), results of which were widely disseminated (Thomas, Chess, & Birch, 1968; Thomas & Chess, 1977), their taxonomy of temperament dimensions, along with the related concepts of difficulty and goodness of fit (addressed later in this chapter), were operationalized and investigated by dozens of clinical and basic researchers. The NYLS group originally posited nine dimensions of temperament, and despite a number of studies that indicate overlap or low discriminant validity across dimensions (Bohlin, Hagekull, & Lindhagen, 1981; Sanson, Prior, Garino, Oberklaid, & Sewell, 1987), the originators are still committed to the full list. The nine dimensions are activity level, regularity (of biological functions such as hunger, sleep and wake cycles, and bowel elimination), approach/withdrawal (positive or negative response to a new situation, person, or environmental demand), adaptability (to a required change in an established behavior pattern), sensory threshold, quality of mood (preponderance of positive versus negative mood expression), intensity (of mood expression, irrespective of whether it is positive or negative), distractibility (ease or difficulty with respect to an ongoing activity by an extraneous stimulus), and attention span/persistence (length and degree of, respectively) (Chess & Thomas, 1991).

One of the more intriguing aspects of temperament in the NYLS framework that has generated considerable debate is the issue of temperamental difficulty. Consider the lively exchange that resulted when Bates (1980) published his thoughts on the issue (Bates, 1983; Kagan, 1982; Plomin, 1982; Rothbart, 1982; Thomas, Chess, & Korn, 1982). For Thomas and Chess the constellation of "difficult" temperament refers to an attribute of the individual infant, comprised of an irregularity of biological functions, tendency to withdraw from new situations and stimuli, slow adaptability to change, tendency for intensity in expressiveness, and negative mood (Thomas et al., 1968). An infant deemed "easy," in contrast, would show the opposite constellation, being highly regular, approaching, and so on. A third special pattern, known by the cumbersome title of "slow to warm up," refers to negative responses of mild intensity to anything new, with slow adaptability after repeated contact (Chess & Thomas, 1991). Although clinicians understandably place great store in the difficult-easy constellation (Carey, 1986; Turecki & Tonner, 1985), theorists are mixed in how they treat the concept (Goldsmith et al., 1987). The implications of the difficult pattern and "temperament risk factors" (Carey, 1989b) are addressed later in the chapter.

A Developmental/Contextual Perspective—Lerner and Windle

Building on the NYLS framework, Lerner and Windle have taken what may be termed a developmental/contextual approach to study temperament across the lifespan (Lerner, Palermo, Spiro, & Nesselroade, 1982; Windle, 1988). With a focus on examining the goodness of fit model from the NYLS, they believe that temperament's meaning lies in the extent to which the child's attributes coincide with the contextual demands regarding behavioral style and not in the attributes themselves (Lerner & Lerner, 1983). Unlike other temperament theorists, they are interested in temperament dimensions that are age-continuous and can be used from the early years through young adulthood. This bears directly on the issue of measurement, since the items they devised for tapping each dimension must also meet this criteria. Although they began with the nine dimensions defined by Thomas and Chess, their item development, factor analyses, and ultimate scale construction made for a different set of variables applicable over a relatively wide age range. Their dimensions are activity (general and during sleep), approach, flexibility, mood, rhythmicity (in sleeping, eating, and daily habits), and task orientation (Windle & Lerner, 1986).

A Personality Perspective— Buss and Plomin

Buss and Plomin view temperament as a subclass of personality traits, specifically, inherited personality traits that appear during the first year of life and persist later in life (Buss, 1991; Buss & Plomin, 1984). Operating from a behavior-genetic position, they are most interested in traits that they believe are genetic in origin, rather than erupting through environmental events, and that provide a foundation for later personality. As such, their list of dimensions is much shorter than other temperament researchers. Indeed, based on their own further research on heritability, they reduced their four dimensional catalog to three, deleting impulsivity from their original formulation (Buss & Plomin, 1975). Acknowledging that other individual differences are observable in infants and that other personality traits may be inherited, the three dimensions that satisfy both of these criteria are emotionality, activity, and sociability, which they represent with the acronym EAS (Buss, 1991). It is noteworthy that these dimensions are the very three that have been deemed most applicable to the study of behavioral style in newborns (Worobey, 1990) and of parent-infant interaction (Bates, 1989a).

A Psychobiological Perspective— Rothbart and Derryberry

In the psychobiological approach of Rothbart and Derryberry, temperament is defined as individual differences in reactivity and self-regulation that are relatively stable and are assumed to be biologically-based (Derryberry & Rothbart, 1984; Rothbart & Derryberry, 1982). Reactivity means the arousability of physiological and behavioral systems of the organism, as assessed

through response parameters of threshold, latency, intensity, rise time, and recovery time. Self-regulation refers to processes that serve to modulate reactivity, such as attention and avoidance. Drawing on the work of their predecessors who explored individual differences (Diamond, 1957; Escalona, 1968; Thomas et al., 1963), these researchers first generated a list of eleven temperament variables that they viewed as having a strong biological base and could be identified in infants. With an eye toward the time course of their expression, as well as their outcomes in adulthood, Rothbart has since reduced the field to four or possibly five dimensions that can be observed across the first year of life. These are negative reactivity (irritability or distress threshold), positive reactivity (expressed and felt positive affect), behavioral inhibition (to novel or intense stimulation), duration of orienting (attention span), and the beginnings of effortful control (Rothbart, 1991).

An Emotional Perspective— Goldsmith and Campos

To Goldsmith and Campos, temperament may be described in terms of structures that organize the expression of primary emotions and arousal in infancy (Goldsmith & Campos, 1982). Their inclusion criteria specify that temperament is emotional in nature, pertains to individual differences, and refers to behavioral tendencies rather than actual occurrences of behavior (Goldsmith et al., 1987). Although they have researched physiological and genetic-based determinants of temperament (Goldsmith

& Campos, 1986; Goldsmith & Gottesman, 1981), they confine their definition to the behavioral level since they believe it to be most meaningful in a social context. Unlike the other theorists discussed previously, Goldsmith and Campos do not propose their own list of temperament dimensions. But since they define temperament as individual differences in the expression of primary emotions, they consider those that are agreed upon by emotion theorists (Ekman, 1982; Izard, 1977). In terms of emotions they have studied to date, they list anger, fear, joy and pleasure, interest (the durational component of which corresponds to persistence), and activity level (because motor activity may partially reflect arousal that is not differentiated into another primary emotion) (Goldsmith et al., 1987).

Questionnaire Approaches for Assessing Temperament

The theoretical positions outlined previously have inspired a generation of infant researchers to work at describing the concept of temperament and its components, its interactions with other constructs and implications for later development. This next section describes some of the instruments that have derived from these theoretical positions, so that reference to any tools or methods in a later section are better understood in the context of the findings of a particular study that is mentioned. As Bates (1989b; Rothbart & Goldsmith, 1985) has outlined, there are four main ways that temperament concepts are operationalized in order to measure individual differences among infants. The first way is by parental report, including both questionnaires and structured interviews that rely on the caregiver's observations. The second approach is the use of naturalistic observations, most likely in the infant's home where presumably representative behavior can be displayed to an objective observer. The third method is the laboratory situation, where a number of challenges presented to the infant may promote the expression of temperament-like behavior. The fourth technique is the use of psychophysiological measures that involve the presentation of a particular stimulus to elicit behavior representing a specific temperamental dimension.

Although all of these methods are discussed in the present chapter, most of the coverage addresses the use of parental reports, more specifically, the utility of temperament questionnaires for a number of practical reasons. Parent questionnaires have been the most widely used approach for measuring temperament, and as a component of future multimethod investigations, will likely remain so. All of the theorists whose frameworks were described in the previous section have relied and continue to rely on parent questionnaires. Indeed, questionnaires that embody each of their theoretical approaches have been developed, if not by them, by investigators partial to their theory, and are described later. Today's questionnaires are much improved from the earlier versions, with adequate reliability and validity evidence available in most cases (see reviews by Hubert, Wachs, Peters-Martin, & Gandour, 1982; Slabach, Morrow, & Wachs, 1991).

Despite critics who condemn the use of parental reports in general (Kagan, 1994), even basic researchers acknowledge the useful contribution that the caregiver's perspective can provide (Rothbart & Bates, 1998; Goldsmith & Rieser-Danner, 1990). For the clinician, the very idea that parental reports would be of no worth, even in scientific studies of temperament, is unthinkable. To paraphrase Carey (1989b), while a physician does not have to believe everything that he or she is told by the parents, it would be quite impossible to function as a clinician only on the basis of what may be observed directly. For the pediatrician, the child's history, physical exam, and indicated laboratory tests are what makes for a diagnostic impression. For the infant mental health specialist, the caregiver's report along with observed parent-infant interaction may be all that realistically is obtainable. In other words, the myriad of approaches to assessing temperament, despite their critical importance in helping to advance our understanding of the concept, are not likely to be employed by the practitioner who is working with infants and their families in a clinical context. In light of these reasons, a detailed description of the temperament questionnaires deemed most suitable for infant and toddlers is provided next.

The Clinical Perspective

A number of questionnaires derived from the NYLS framework are currently available. The pioneer in this approach to assessing temperament is Carey, whose initial questionnaire predated the instruments that were later devised by Thomas and Chess themselves. After analyzing protocols from the NYLS, he developed a 70-item inventory that assessed all nine of the NYLS dimensions on a 3-point rating scale and included an additional nine items that allowed the caregiver to globally rate each of the NYLS dimensions. Norming the device on 200 infants from his private practice who ranged in age from 3½ to 8½ months, Carey (1970) dubbed the instrument the Infant Temperament Questionnaire (ITQ). Despite the attractiveness of this shorthand approach to measuring temperament, early use of the questionnaire indicated a number of psychometric limitations.

Sensitive to the instrument's weaknesses, Carey and McDevitt (1978) undertook a substantial revision of the ITQ, modifying certain items, adding new items, and changing the response format to a 6-point scale to indicate the frequency of behavior. The questionnaire was normed on 203 infants from middle-class families. Similar to its predecessor, the Revised Infant Temperament Questionnaire (RITQ) measures the nine NYLS dimensions, namely activity, rhythmicity, approach, adaptability, intensity, mood, persistence, distractibility, and threshold, with 95 items and nine global ratings. An example of an item reflecting approach is:

	almost never				almost always
45. The infant's initial reaction at home approach by strangers is acceptance.					
	1	2	3	4	5	6

On the 6-point scale, 1 = Almost never, 2 = Rarely, 3 = Variable usually does not, 4 = Variable usually does, 5 = Frequently, and 6 = Almost always.

As the RITQ was normed for 4 to 8-month-old infants, Carey and his colleagues subsequently developed parallel forms of the questionnaire for the toddler, preschool, and middle childhood periods, with their most recent efforts aimed at extending the infant scales downward. All follow the NYLS framework and the 6-point scale format, though the numbers of questions differ across questionnaires. Of relevance to infant workers, the relatively new Early Infancy Temperament Questionnaire (EITQ) (Medoff-Cooper, Carey, & McDevitt, 1993), normed on 404 infants from 1 to 4 months of age and applicable for that range, is 76 items long and again, includes the nine global ratings. An item that roughly corresponds to the preceding approach (withdrawal) item from the RITQ is:

	almost never				almost always	
30. The infant turns head away and looks for mother when held by new person.	1	2	3	4	5	6

The Toddler Temperament Scale (TTS) (Fullard, McDevitt, & Carey, 1984) was normed on 309 infants and toddlers from 12 to 36 months and extends the NYLS framework beyond the first year limit of the RITQ. Many of the 97 items differ from those of the RITQ, reflecting the older capacities and situations encountered by a toddler. But some do resemble items that

appear on the RITQ. For example, question 45 from the RITQ for approach appears on the TTS as:

	almost never				almost always	
76. The child's initial reaction at home to approach by strangers is acceptance (looks at, reaches out)	1	2	3	4	5	6

In addition to scoresheets that allow for hand calculations of summary scores for each of the nine NYLS dimensions, the various Carey Temperament Scales include profile guidelines for determining if the infant's scores are in excess of one standard deviation above or below the normative value for each dimension. This is of great use to the clinician who may be interested in classifying the infant's temperament as easy, intermediate low/easy, difficult, intermediate high/difficult, or slow-to-warm-up. For example, difficulty is determined by high scores on activity, intensity, and negative mood, and low scores on rhythmicity, approach, and adaptability.

Although the Carey Scales are probably the most often used questionnaires for measuring temperament, they are not without criticism. For example, concerns have been raised about low levels of internal consistency for a few of the subscales, namely sensory threshold, adaptability, and intensity (Slabach et al., 1991), while others have noted the high degree of overlap across the subscales (Rothbart & Mauro, 1990), a criticism that has been levied against the NYLS framework in general (Bates, 1987; Goldsmith & Rieser-Danner, 1990). Indeed, a number of investigators, quite partial to the NYLS framework, have nonetheless further revised or reduced the RITQ through item reformulation and factor analysis.

For example, Bohlin and colleagues (1981) began by translating the RITQ into Swedish, and after rewording, deleting, and generating additional items, developed two NYLS-based instruments. The Baby Behavior Questionnaire, a 54-item instrument that is suitable for 4 to 6-month-olds, produces factor scores for intensity/activity, regularity, approach/withdrawal, sensory sensitivity, attentiveness, manageability, and sensitivity to new foods (Bohlin et al., 1981), though a more recent report suggests that they have dropped the foods factor (Hagekull & Bohlin, 1989). The Toddler Behavior Questionnaire includes an additional 6 items for a total of 60 and measures adaptability as well (Hagekull, Lindhagen, & Bohlin, 1980). Sanson et al. (1987), working in Australia, factor-analyzed the RITQ and developed a short form of the RITQ that they term the SITQ. Aside from minor revisions to conform to Australian language forms (Oberklaid, Prior, Golvan, Clements, & Williamson, 1984), the SITQ resembles the RITQ but is only 30 items long and measures five factors, namely approach, rhythmicity, cooperation-manageability, activity-reactivity, and irritability. It also lends itself to an easy-difficult summation, where low approach, low cooperation-manageability, and high irritability would suggest difficulty.

Some mention should also be made of the instruments that are more loosely based on the Thomas and Chess (1977) dimensions, finding their inspiration in some of the NYLS concepts but extending the field to measure dimensions that were not explicitly considered by Thomas and Chess (Bates, 1987). The theories articulated by Buss and Plomin, as well as Rothbart, and ultimately the instruments they developed owe much to the NYLS approach and are described shortly. The work of Bates, however, deserves special consideration, as he has devised a series of questionnaires that tap NYLS-like behavior but are particularly focused on parental perceptions of infant difficultness. The Infant Characteristics Questionnaire, with separate forms for 6 and 13 months (24 and 32 items, respectively), differentiates difficult temperament into the factors of fussy/difficult, dull, unadaptable, and unpredictable (Bates, Freeland, & Lounsbury, 1979). The response format for an item reflecting the unadaptable factor on the 13-month-old questionnaire is:

9. How does your baby typically respond to a new person?

1	2	3	4	5	6	7
always responds favorably			responds favorably about half the time, or is always neutral			always responds negatively or fearfully

The Child Characteristics Questionnaire, a 32-item instrument for 24-month-olds, revealed factors of difficult, negative adaptability, unstoppable/noncuddly, dependent, irregular, and sober (Lee & Bates, 1985). The Bates series of questionnaires may be most useful, then, for clinicians who are comfortable with the NYLS framework but are most interested in temperamental difficulty.

If not already obvious, it should be noted that all of these questionnaires that serve as alternatives to the RITQ, while NYLS-based, include factors that are somewhat different than the nine NYLS dimensions. Even in cases where the labels used are identical, the composition of the dimensions often are not (Goldsmith & Rieser-Danner, 1991). An exception is the work of Persson-Blennow and McNeil (1979, 1980) who developed a series of Swedish Temperament Questionnaires, the STQ–6, STQ–12, and STQ–24 (for 6-, 12-, and 24-month-old infants, respectively), that are true to the nine NYLS dimensions but were derived independently of the Carey Scales.

Despite the criticisms that have been voiced against the Carey Scales, they have enjoyed widespread popularity. They are consonant with the nine NYLS dimensions, they allow for an easy versus difficult profile, parallel forms are available to track temperament from early infancy through middle childhood, and a formidable research base now exists that can serve as a frame of reference. Satisfactory test-retest reliability has been shown for the RITQ and TTS (Sanson et al., 1987; Gibbs, Reeves, & Cunningham, 1987), with published data available on their internal consistency (Carey & McDevitt, 1978; Fullard et al., 1984) and convergence with other temperament questionnaires (Goldsmith, Rieser-Danner, & Briggs, 1991). The EITQ has similar reliability data available (Medoff-Cooper et al., 1993), as well as displaying interinstrument agreement

in a recent study (Worobey, 1997). Besides its adoption by other English-speaking researchers, the RITQ has been translated effectively into at least two other languages (Chinese, by Hsu, Soong, Stigler, Hong, & Liang, 1981, and French, by Maziade, Boudreault, Thivierge, Caperaa, & Cote, 1984), and with the commercial availability of a computer-based scoring system (Carey et al., 1995), the continued use of all the Carey Scales is likely to remain stable, if not increase.

The Developmental / Contextual Perspective

Consonant with their life span emphasis, Lerner and his colleagues began with a questionnaire that could be used for different age groups, validating the instrument on nursery school, elementary school, and college-age subjects (Lerner et al., 1982). The Dimensions of Temperament Survey (DOTS) had 89 and later 42 items in its preliminary versions. After an impressive series of validation efforts, the authors presented a 34-item survey that measured five factors in a true-false format. Some efforts were even directed at developing a special version of the DOTS for infants (Busch-Rossnagel & McArdle, 1983; Lerner, Belsky, & Windle, 1983), however, this instrument is no longer in use.

Further refinement of the DOTS led to a revised version, the DOTS–R (Windle & Lerner, 1986). Beginning with a pool of 106 items, the authors conducted content-, item-, and factor-analytic procedures to derive a nine factor model of temperament (Windle, 1988). The final version is comprised of 54 items, scored on a 4-choice format, and measuring the dimensions of activity level—general, activity level—sleep, approach-withdrawal, flexibility-rigidity, mood, rhythmicity—sleep, rhythmicity—eating, rhythmicity—daily habits, and task orientation (Windle & Lerner, 1986).

Moderate to high levels of internal consistency were shown for all nine dimensions across the validation samples of 4-year-olds (N = 114), 12-year-olds (N = 224), and 19-year-olds (N = 300). As the DOTS–R was designed to assess stability and change through cross-age administrations, it may prove to be extremely useful in a predictive sense (Windle et al., 1986). As with the DOTS, the DOTS–R is suitable for young children through young adults, with forms that allow parents to rate their children and children to rate themselves. The response format for a representative item from the approach dimension is as follows:

26. _____ On meeting a new person my child tends to move toward him or her.

In this case, A = Usually false, B = More false than true, C = More true than false, and D = Usually true.

The Personality Perspective

By and large, most questionnaires that are used to assess temperament in infancy rely on specific items that attempt to measure discrete behaviors in a particular situation, setting, or context. As Buss and Plomin (1984) view temperament as early developing personality traits that should display cross-situational consistency, their measurement approach is much more global. That is, emotionality, activity, and sociability are measured using items that broadly characterize behavior. The EAS, which represents the most recent incarnation of the evolving EASI–I, EASI–II, and EAS–III series (Buss & Plomin, 1975, 1984; Buss, Plomin, & Willerman, 1973), has been validated by its authors in its formative stages on 274 pairs of twins from one to nine years of age, as well as with 547 college students. Using questions from the NYLS interview protocols and what may be termed the EASI system, Rowe and Plomin (1977) developed the Colorado Child Temperament Inventory (CCTI). The instrument was validated on an additional 91 pairs of twins and, as reported by the authors, has considerable internal consistency and moderately high test-retest reliability. The normative sample ranged from five months to nine years, with a mean age of 3.6 years. In contrast to the EAS, but reflecting the NYLS influence, the six factor-analytically derived dimensions are sociability, emotionality, activity, attention span-persistence, reaction to food, and soothability. Each scale is determined through five questions for a total of 30 items. A sample item that measures sociability is:

	not at all like my child				a lot like my child
2. Child is very friendly with strangers.	1	2	3	4	5

As with the DOTS–R described previously, the CCTI provides a psychometrically-sound alternative to the more clinically-oriented Carey Scales that nevertheless owes much to the NYLS.

The Psychobiological Perspective

After reviewing the work of other researchers in early personality, notably Shirley (1933) and Thomas et al. (1963), Rothbart conducted interviews with new parents and added her own questions to an item pool. Based on conceptual and careful item analysis, she formulated the Infant Behavior Questionnaire (IBQ). Despite its NYLS ancestry, however, the IBQ only contains one dimension that corresponds to the Thomas and Chess conceptualization, namely activity. The six IBQ dimensions are activity level, fear, distress to limitations, duration of orienting, smiling and laughter, and soothability (Rothbart, 1981). The 94-item instrument was validated on a cross-sectional sample of 463 infants, ages 3, 6, 9, and 12 months, though it has also been used successfully with younger (Worobey, 1986a) and older ages (Thompson & Lamb, 1984). Extensive work by Rothbart and others has demonstrated substantial test-retest reliability for the IBQ (Rothbart, 1986; Worobey & Blajda, 1989), with additional reports confirming its interinstrument (Goldsmith, Rieser-Donner, & Briggs, 1991) and external validity (Worobey, 1986b). In sharp contrast to the global approach taken by Buss and Plomin, the instructions for the IBQ ask the caregiver to respond to each item using the previous week as a frame of reference and further estimate the frequency of the stated behavior in a particular context such as play or feeding. The following example illustrates the format for item 79 from the fear dimension:

When introduced to a strange person, how often did the baby:
1 2 3 4 5 X . . . (79) approach the stranger at once?

In this scale, 1 = Never, 2 = Very rarely, 3 = Less than half the time, 4 = About half the time, 5 = More than half the time, 6 = Almost always, 7 = Always, and X = Does not apply.

The IBQ does not lend itself to a difficulty score, and Goldsmith and Rothbart (1991) caution against its appropriateness in clinical settings, stressing its use for research purposes only. However, the procedure of extracting a negative emotionality factor by combining the infant's scores on the fear and distress to limitations dimensions has been tried with some success (Rothbart, 1986; Worobey & Blajda, 1989). Perhaps because of their reservations regarding this approach to assessing temperamental difficulty, O'Boyle and Rothbart (1990) devised a 45-item questionnaire to identify negative reactivity to sensory stimulation. As opposed to parental perceptions of infant difficultness, the Infant Reactions Inventory (IRI) was developed to measure irritability in infants from 12 to 20 weeks of age. The IRI was normed on 89 families with 4-month-old infants and found to correlate significantly with the two negative reactivity scales of the IBQ.

Rothbart and her colleagues have also developed a number of companion instruments that extend her reactivity framework to older individuals. To date, a parent report form for children's behavior and separate self-report scales for adolescents and adults are now available. While both a motor activity and fear dimension are contained in each of these questionnaires, the remaining dimensions, of which there are ten or so for each instrument, serve to explicitly differentiate positive and negative emotionality. Despite a different nomenclature for each segment of the life span, the set of measures will undoubtedly be useful in longitudinal work.

The Emotional Perspective

Although Goldsmith and Campos did not choose to specify actual dimensions when articulating their theory of temperament, instead defaulting to others' listings of primary emotions, a parent-report instrument that nevertheless operationalizes their approach does exist. Goldsmith, Elliott, and Jaco (1986) developed the Toddler Behavior Assessment Questionnaire (TBAQ), in order to extend the applicability of the IBQ to their infant sample that had grown into toddlerhood. Goldsmith (1996) constructed the scale through a three-part, iterated process involving item writing, item testing, and item rewriting and retesting. The process continued over four waves of data collection, using seven samples of subjects ages 16 to 36 months, and totaling 1,012 behavioral records. This procedure resulted in a 108-item questionnaire that measures activity level, pleasure, social fearfulness, anger proneness, and interest/persistence. The format is very much like that of the IBQ, as can be seen in the following item from the social fear category:

When first meeting a stranger coming to visit in the home, how often did your child:
1 2 3 4 5 6 7 NA (104) abandon the parent to go the stranger?

In this scale, 1 to 7 are identical to the IBQ definitions, but NA instead of X refers to "Does not apply."

Also in slight contrast to the IBQ, items are framed in terms of the last month instead of the last week. Since the TBAQ derives from the IBQ, it is the recommended instrument to use when following a sample that has been previously assessed with the IBQ (Goldsmith & Rothbart, 1991). The corresponding IBQ–TBAQ scales are distress to limitations-anger proneness, smiling and laughter-pleasure, fear-social fear, duration of orienting-interest/persistence, and activity level-activity level. (There is no TBAQ counterpart to IBQ soothability.) Internal consistency estimates for the TBAQ are quite impressive, around .80 for each scale, with longitudinal stability obtained as well (Goldsmith, 1996). Convergent validity with the TTS and EASI–III questionnaires has also been shown for the activity level and social fear dimensions (Goldsmith et al., 1991).

Other Questionnaire Formats

Before addressing the other methods that have been used in assessing temperament or its components, two variants of the questionnaire approach are worth mentioning. The Perception of Baby Temperament (PBT) scales, based on the nine NYLS temperament dimensions, employ a Q-sort format to obtain ratings that are meant to be free from social desirability and acquiescent tendencies of the caregiver (Pedersen, Zaslow, Cain, Anderson, & Thomas, 1980). Both mothers and fathers can independently sort a shuffled stack of 54 cards into response categories that represent the degree to which each statement is applicable to their infant. For example, the parent's perception of the baby's level of approach would be tapped with a card containing the statement:

When a visitor comes over and spends some time in our home, s/he shows a lot of interest in that person.

The caregiver would place the card onto a pile marked: "Very much like my baby, Sometimes or occasionally like my baby, Not at all like my baby," or "Have no experience with this."

Although the authors' validation sample of 26 families with 5-month-olds showed adequate split-half reliability for the PBT, interparental agreement was only achieved for five of the nine dimensions. A factor-analytic evaluation of the PBT raised some concerns about its psychometric properties (Huitt & Ashton, 1992), but a few studies support its continued use (Sirignano & Lachman, 1985; Sprunger, Boyce, & Gaines, 1985).

An alternate Q-sort measure of temperament is the recent effort by Goldsmith and Alansky (1987a). Their instrument is designed to assess positive emotionality, negative emotionality, interest/persistence, and activity level. The measure shows some promise as two of the four categories had good discriminant properties, and positive emotionality, in particular, was highly correlated with attachment security.

Finally, an instrument has recently been described that also qualifies as a questionnaire but represents a rather novel approach to evaluating the caregiver's perspective on the infant's temperament. Clarke-Stewart, Goldberg, and Fitzpatrick (1992) have developed a Pictorial Assessment of Temperament (PAT). The PAT consists of a set of 10 pictorial representations of infants' reactions in situations that evoke individual differences in behavioral style and was validated on a sample of 81 5-month-olds. For each situation, the caregiver chooses from three cartoons that represent an easy, a moderate/slow-to-warm-up, and a difficult infant, the one who is most like her baby. For example, their fourth situation portrays the mother's giving the baby to a stranger to hold while she is busy. The mother then chooses from Baby X, Y, or Z, whose captions range from an initial liking of the person with a later exclamation of enjoyment to an initial expression of dislike followed by a plea to get Mommy back. The pictures illustrate the infants as alternately smiling, neutral, or crying. Fitzpatrick, Goldberg, and Clarke-Stewart (1996) have recently reported that temperamental stability from 5 months to 30 months, as measured with the infant and a toddler version of the PAT, was linked to maternal sensitivity.

Naturalistic Approaches to Measuring Temperament

Although the sheer number of questionnaires just reviewed might seem to exhaust the possibilities for measuring temperament in the infancy and toddler period, the situation has drastically changed from the early years of research that followed the initial reports from the NYLS. Just ten years ago, for example, Bates (1987) concluded that the dominant type of temperament measure in infancy was the parent report, with the preferred measure of investigators being the questionnaire. In their recent review, however, Rothbart and Bates (1998) consider parent questionnaires as but one of three primary assessment methods, the others being home observation and laboratory measures. As the previous section illustrated, even within the category of parent questionnaires there exists tremendous variety—the variety among the other methods is no less complex. Rothbart and Bates (1998) have expertly summarized the advantages and disadvantages to each of these broad approaches, with other reviews from a methodological perspective also available (Rothbart & Goldsmith, 1985).

As already discussed, the clinician who may be interested in obtaining data on temperament from their case families will most likely utilize one or more of the questionnaires reviewed previously. Nevertheless, a brief treatment of the other methods that are currently being used to generate theory and data on early temperament is in order.

Interviews

The interview approach that served as the foundation for the NYLS framework of Thomas and Chess (1977; Thomas et al., 1963) was rapidly eclipsed by the wide-spread adoption of the questionnaire method. Despite the availability of scores of questionnaires, however, numerous investigators have on occasion relied on interviews in developing their own instruments (Rothbart, 1981), supplementing behavioral measures (Dunn & Kendrick, 1980; Wilson, Brown, & Matheny, 1971), or simply to avoid the difficulties that some mothers may have in completing a written instrument (Wolkind & DeSalis, 1982). Another instance where interviews are still extremely useful is with newborn samples, where standardized questionnaires that tap multiple dimensions of temperament have yet to be developed. For example, Wolke and St. James-Roberts (1986) employed interviews at five days postpartum to assess maternal perceptions of infant difficulty, while Worobey (1986a; Worobey & Anderson-Goetz, 1985) used the Thomas et al. (1968) interview protocol to assess convergence between IBQ ratings and an examiner-administered newborn assessment at four weeks.

The firsthand accounts that can be gleaned from an interview or a questionnaire, may be tempered by the biases inherent in parental reports (Vaughn, 1986). Rothbart and Goldsmith (1985) cite parental experience, personality, cognitive, and attitudinal characteristics, the interaction of these factors with their interpretation of the infant's behavior, and the chance that infant behavior may be elicited by idiosyncratic parental behavior. That an objective rating may be tainted by a caregiver who is emotionally attached to the infant is a possibility, but parents still provide a useful perspective on early temperament given their observations of the infant over a wide range of situations (Bates, 1994; Rothbart, 1995).

Naturalistic Observations

Observing the infant at home, under everyday conditions, is the obvious choice for assuring ecological validity. Using trained observers who should be less prone to personal biases serves to alleviate the concerns raised with parent reports (Rothbart & Goldsmith, 1985). However, the expense of such procedures, in terms of time and labor invested in data recording and coding, can prevent the investigator from sampling enough relevant behavior (Rothbart & Bates, 1998). Even if the researcher is armed with a reliable coding system, the mother may handle the infant in a manner that obscures temperamental variation or may alter her own behavior because of being observed (Rothbart & Goldsmith, 1985).

While hundreds of studies exist in the infancy literature that have employed naturalistic observations, most consider the infant as part of the mother-infant interactive system. Such a perspective has its merits, but if the infant's temperament is the construct of interest, it is necessary to ensure that sufficient temperamental behavior is displayed. Interestingly enough, a number of observational studies have focused precisely on temperamental differences and their association with caregiving behavior. As reviewed by Crockenberg (1986), most of these investigations relied on a temperament questionnaire to rate the infant's behavior with observations of mother-infant interaction to rate maternal responsive-

ness, though a few coded the infant's fussing behavior as well (Bates, Olson, Pettit, & Bayles, 1982; Fish & Crockenberg, 1981). Studies do exist, however, that have employed a coding scheme to rate observed infant behavior and have generally shown that maternal ratings on a temperament questionnaire can correspond to temperament-like behavior expressed at home (Rothbart, 1986; Worobey, 1986b, 1990).

Scripted Observations

The issue of sampling enough relevant behavior during an observational session to determine a temperamental profile has been addressed by investigators who have developed home-based instruments that increase the likelihood of relevant behavior being expressed. Bornstein and colleagues (1986) described a Baby Temperament Questionnaire–Observer Form (BTQ–O), wherein infant behaviors are observed in a combination of structured vignettes and free play periods that occur in an invariant sequence. Over the course of a 2-hour home visit, five dimensions of temperament are rated, namely positive affect, negative affect, persistence, motor responsivity, and soothability. In what would appear to be a revision of this instrument, Bornstein, Gaughran, and Segui (1991) further delineate an Infant Temperament Measure–Observer Form (ITM–O). Single items are scored in terms of their frequency over the course of a 30-minute home observation, structured by four vignettes, that are mother-infant play, free play, observer-infant play, and free play. The discrete behaviors consist of smiles and laughs (to mother, to the observer, and without eye contact), vocalizes, mouths, reaches, bangs, kicks, frowns, and fusses/cries.

With the Temperament Adjective Triad Assessment (TATA), Seifer, Sameroff, Barrett, and Krafchuk (1994) developed an instrument that would lend itself to repeated assessments in the home. To ensure the expression of temperament-like behaviors, the 1-hour session includes the recording of at least 10 minutes each of the infant with mother (with no caretaking), the infant alone, and the mother caretaking with the infant (e.g., feeding, diapering). Fourteen pairs of adjective triads are used to rate mood, approach, activity, intensity, and distractibility. For example, an approach item would be rated by assigning a score to the following:

5	4	3	2	1
Approaching/				Withdrawing/
moves toward/				avoidant/
contacting				ignoring

Suitable for families with infants in the first year of life, both the ITM–O and the TATA have parallel forms for mothers, so that observer-caregiver agreement can be determined. While laudable in terms of an effort to improve mother-observer convergence, results to date with the ITM–O and the TATA do not seem to indicate high interrater agreement (Rothbart & Bates, 1998).

Laboratory Approaches for Measuring Temperament

While most developmental psychologists may view the laboratory method as the most objective approach to the assessment of temperament, the benefits of this approach are not without cost (Rothbart & Goldsmith, 1985). The laboratory setting may inhibit the behavior of the mother and likely alter the infant's behavior, if only in terms of the novelty of the situation. While a laboratory observation allows the experimenter to control elicitors of the infant's behavior, the testing that may be necessary for measuring a complex trait can be impractical (Rothbart & Bates, 1998). Moreover, the need for multiple tests may result in carryover effects within sessions, the experimenter's sensitivity toward the infant may affect the baby's behavior, and the coder's abilities must be continually monitored (Bates, 1989b; Rothbart & Goldsmith, 1985).

Multidimensional Approaches

A number of investigators have attempted to measure behavioral style by structuring the events within a laboratory visit so as to elicit a variety of behaviors that characterize temperament. For the Louisville Twin Study, Matheny and Wilson (1981) developed a series of structured procedures, standardized by age so that each infant would experience a uniformity of treatment while in the laboratory. After a warm-up period with the mother, infant, and staff members, the mother leaves for a brief interview while an "interactionist" engages in specific activities with the infant that are videotaped. For example, for a 9-month-old, the interactionist instigates a repetitive imitative game (pat-a-cake, waving bye-bye, etc.) with gestures, expressions, and vocalizations for two minutes. A 12-month-old infant is picked up and held by the interactionist for two minutes to assess cuddling. At 24 months-old, the infant's interplay with a mechanical toy dog is observed for two minutes (Matheny, Riese, & Wilson, 1985; Riese, 1987; Wilson & Matheny, 1983). By refining the Bayley Infant Behavior Record (1969, a rating scale that measures temperament-like behavior which is completed by the examiner after administering the Bayley Scales), Matheny and Wilson (1981) created a rating scale to evaluate emotional tone, attentiveness, activity, and social orientation to staff.

Other laboratory approaches are also available, such as the Behavioral Assessment of Infant Temperament (BAIT; Garcia-Coll, Halpern, Vohr, Seifer, & Oh, 1992). In the BAIT, babies are presented with 17 stimuli at 3-months-old (e.g., experimenter brushes the infant's hair) and 14 stimuli at 7-months-old (e.g., the experimenter turns off the lights). The order of presentation is designed to gradually increase the number and intensity of sensory modalities involved and allows for scoring the temperament dimensions of sociability, irritability, approach, inhibition, soothability, and neutral.

By far, the most comprehensive package to date for the laboratory assessment of temperament has been developed by Goldsmith and Rothbart (1996). The Laboratory Temperament Assessment Battery (LAB–TAB) is an attempt by its authors to provide a standardized instrument that can be widely adopted, so that more accurate scores on large samples and comparison scores from different laboratories can be made available. Separate manuals exist for 6-month-olds (prelocomotor) and 12-month-olds (locomotor), but both describe approximately 20 episodes, at 3 to 4 per temperament dimension, to allow for scoring of fear, anger, joy pleasure, interest persistence, and activity level. An episode that assesses fear at 6 months, for example, involves presenting the infant with a series of scary masks. This episode is used again at 12 months, but fear of an approaching stranger is also assessed. Most helpful are the extremely detailed instructions that specify materials, setting, procedures, camera instructions, and scoring definitions. Despite the cohesive nature of LAB–TAB, Goldsmith and Rothbart (1996) encourage others to use just a few of the episodes in their own investigations if they so choose, depending on the specific goals of their own research.

Some investigators have employed laboratory procedures in just this way, assessing a particular temperament dimension of interest to examine its course or examining a single dimension in conjunction with another behavior or construct. The work by Kagan and his associates (Kagan, Reznick, Clark, Snidman, & Garcia-Coll, 1984; Kagan & Snidman, 1991) on behavioral inhibition is an example of the former, while Lewis and his colleagues (Lewis, Alessandri, & Sullivan, 1990; Sullivan & Lewis, 1989; Sullivan, Lewis, & Alessandri, 1992) exemplify the latter with their studies of early learning and emotional expression. Feeding influences on temperamental behaviors have also been studied in this way, using laboratory procedures to assess motor activity (Worobey, 1998).

Psychobiological Approaches

To infant researchers, one of the most exciting areas of current activity involves the groundbreaking work that examines the physiological bases of temperament. A far cry from the body temperament formulations of antiquity, the current model in psychobiology take a systems approach, that is, understanding physiology-temperament relations necessitates the study of dynamic interactions among systems (Gunnar, 1990). Rothbart and Bates (1998) succinctly review the recent efforts in this realm, treatment in this section is little more than an attempt to illustrate the wide array of current methods that are being used to explore temperamental variation.

The field of behavioral genetics has relevance here, as a number of studies have identified a genetic contribution to the development of temperament in infancy. Through an analysis of the major twin projects, Goldsmith, Buss, and Lemery (1997) indicate monozygotic twin correlations that range from .50 to .80 and dizygotic correlations from .00 to .50 in studies that employ parent report measures. Shared family influence was also shown for positive affect and approach, and activity level appears to show evidence of moderate genetic influence as well (Eaton, 1994; Goldsmith & Gottesman, 1981).

Hemispheric asymmetry and its relation to affect has been studied extensively by Fox and his associates. Based on their work with infants, they propose that the left hemisphere is associated with positive affect and approach and the right hemisphere with negative affect and avoidance (Fox & Davidson, 1984). For example, infants who were highly reactive and had negative affect at 4-months-old and displayed high right frontal activation at 9-months-old were most inhibited at 14-months-old (Calkins, Fox, & Marshall, 1996).

Heart rate and vagal tone have been linked by some investigators to temperament-related behavior. Kagan (Kagan & Snidman, 1991; Kagan, Snidman, & Arcus, 1992), for example, has found that infants who display a pattern of high irritability, high motor activity, and high heart rate constitute a behaviorally-inhibited temperamental profile. Vagal tone, which represents parasympathetic control of heart rate variability, has been associated with temperament through the programmatic research efforts of Porges (1986). Specifically, the measure has been related to reactivity (Porges, Doussard-Roosevelt, & Maiti, 1994), attention (Porges, 1991), and soothability (Huffman, Bryan, del Carmen, Petersen, & Porges, 1992).

Finally, adrenocortical activity, as measured by the secretion of salivary cortisol, has become a popular measure in temperament research. Typically obtained from the infant after undergoing a perturbation, a marked rise in cortisol output is generally a sign of a stressed response. Gunnar (1989; Gunnar, Connors, Isensee, & Wall, 1988), for example, has demonstrated that elevations in cortisol are associated with events that produce behavioral distress such as blood screening and circumcision, while Lewis (Lewis & Ramsay, 1995; Ramsay & Lewis, 1994) has shown this for inoculations.

Although these laboratory procedures for assessing temperament are unlikely tools for use by the clinician, they are mentioned here so that the reader is at least aware of the innovative approaches that are now being employed to add to our understanding of temperament. Future efforts will inevitably extend beyond these methods for that matter, as insights gleaned from neurology and biochemistry will be applied to the study of behavioral style in human infants (Kagan, 1998; Rothbart, Derryberry, & Posner, 1994).

Early Temperament and Psychological Adjustment

The wide array of methods for assessing temperament in infancy, whether by parental report or more direct observation or testing, would be of little use to the infant mental health worker if there were not, at least in theory, a link between individual differences in behavioral style and adjustment. Rothbart and Bates (1998; Bates, 1989a; Rothbart, Posner, & Hershey, 1995) have devoted a significant amount of effort to reviewing and synthesizing the extant literature on temperament as a predictor of adjustment, and a monograph by Carey and McDevitt (1989) that addresses the clinical applications of temperament research is also available. Therefore, the present section will only use examples to highlight the practical applications of a temperament perspective in working with families toward optimizing infant mental health.

Processes that Link Temperament and Adjustment

Given the complex nature of temperament itself and the large variety of markers that indicate psychopathology or even positive adjustment, there are numerous ways in which temperament may be related to mental health outcomes (Clark, Watson, & Mineka, 1994; Rothbart et al., 1995). Rothbart and Bates (1998) have separated these processes into four categories and review findings that illustrate such linkages from infancy through young adulthood. Their taxonomy has been slightly modified for the summary that follows, with an effort to simplify their framework for the studies that include infants and toddlers.

DIRECT LINEAR EFFECTS OF TEMPERAMENT

This category refers to a situation where a particular temperament trait contributes to the development of an adjustment pattern in a direct and linear manner. Additive effects of several dimensions are also conceivable but are considered following from an interactive perspective. To illustrate the process for a direct effect, however, Rothbart, Ahadi, and Hershey (1994) found that infant activity, as measured in the laboratory, predicted aggressiveness and negativity at age six while IBQ fear predicted lower levels of aggressiveness but higher levels of empathy, guilt, and shame at the later age. Hagekull (1994) found that parent reports of sociability/shyness as measured with the EASI scales at 28 to 36 months predicted parent's ratings of internalizing problems at 48 months, while early activity predicted later externalizing. Externalizing and internalizing problems in preschoolers have also been related to infant and toddler ICQ ratings of difficultness (Bates, Maslin, & Franke, 1985).

INDIRECT LINEAR EFFECTS
OF TEMPERAMENT

For an indirect, linear effect to be in place, a particular temperament trait would elicit a response from the immediate environment that subsequently directs the infant toward a positive or negative outcome. While the possibility of indirect effects of temperament on adjustment makes intuitive sense, the evidence for this model is less than substantive. However, the work of van den Boom (1989; van den Boom & Hoeksma, 1994) lends itself to this type of interpretation. Briefly, van den Boom found that highly irritable infants had mothers who ignored their crying, chose ineffective soothing strategies, and were unresponsive to the infants' social signals. In spite of an actual decrease in the infants' crying, the relatively insensitive care that the mothers gave to the infants was presumed to promote an insecure attachment, with over representation in the avoidant category.

TEMPERAMENT ×
TEMPERAMENT INTERACTIONS

Aside from their intercorrelations, a number of temperament traits that occur together raise the possibility that their interactive combination may have a magnified effect on adjustment outcomes. For example, the laboratory work of Kagan and his colleagues (Kagan et al., 1993) has demon-

strated that 4-month-old infants who are motorically active and highly irritable in response to novel stimuli, show high levels of fearfulness when tested again at 14 and 21 months. Such infants are called high reactive, and Kagan (1998) has reported that they become behaviorally inhibited 4-year-olds who in turn might be at higher risk for developing an anxiety disorder.

A more salient example for the clinician might be the "difficult" constellation of temperament dimensions described by Thomas and Chess (1977). Recall that five of the NYLS dimensions observed in infancy, namely low rhythmicity, withdrawal, slow adaptability, high intensity, and negative mood, were shown in combination to predispose the developing child to later behavioral problems. As Carey (1989b) notes, however, the widespread acceptance of this useful clinical concept was rapidly generalized to children of all ages, settings, and outcomes that consequently led to various problems in both practical and clinical areas. Based on their reviews of empirical tests of the difficult cluster, both Bates (1987) and Crockenberg (1986) concluded that infant difficultness does not invariably influence the social environment (i.e., mother-infant interaction) in a negative way. Yet more recent studies continue to link difficult temperaments with less supportive maternal care (Hannan & Luster, 1991) and emotional neglect (Harrington, Black, Starr, & Dubowitz, 1998). While some would recommend a dropping of the term "difficult" when discussing infants, since it may alter parental expectations for the baby whose temperament may be an asset at a later age or whose parents do not view the infant's individual expressions of behavior as problematic (Rothbart, 1982), the word "difficult" is not likely to disappear from the lexicon. Carey (1989b) has, therefore, suggested that it be restricted to its original usage, with "temperament risk factors" employed to describe behavioral characteristics that predispose a child to an incompatible relationship with the environment.

TEMPERAMENT ×
ENVIRONMENT INTERACTIONS

Temperament risk factors, as conceived of by Carey (1989b), exemplify the "goodness of fit" concept as put forth by Thomas and Chess (1977; Thomas et al., 1963). To paraphrase Super and Harkness (1994), different environments find some temperaments to be more suitable than others, and within any given environment, a particular temperament may elicit a different response. For example, high activity in an infant whose mother views such behavior as indicative of robustness and vitality would present a good fit between infant and environment, while high activity in an infant whose mother has little basis for comparison but a vague impression from the media that hyperactivity is a liability in childhood would make for a more defensive caregiving environment. Similarly, a highly irritable infant may drain one mother because of his or her need for attention and empower another because of her success in soothing the baby. Alternately, a baby low in approach might initially be perceived as cute because of his or her clinging behavior but later be perceived as annoying when his or her shyness interferes with adapting to a day care provider.

In this vein, it is interesting that Belsky (1997) has recently theorized that difficult infants may be the most susceptible to rearing influences. Crockenberg (1981), for example, found social support to be most important in facilitating attachment security for irritable infants. But an easy temperament may also interact with the environment. Hagekull and Bohlin (1995) found that 4-year-olds deemed easy (in terms of their TBQ manageability as toddlers) who were in high quality day care were less aggressive than the easy children in low quality care.

Research Linking Temperament to Psychosocial Outcomes

A sizable number of studies exist that have shown temperament in infancy to be a meaningful correlate of other areas of clinical relevance, if not a predictor of specific outcomes. Some have been alluded to already, for example, the work of Bates and colleagues (1985) or Goldsmith and Alansky (1987b) on temperament and attachment and the research of Kagan and his colleagues (Kagan et al., 1993) on early reactivity and behavioral inhibition. Engfer (1993) has shown that shyness in preschoolers may be linked to temperamental difficulty at 18 months. There are also studies of temperament that examine the evolution of particular traits over time, especially if they represent an extreme on the dimensions. Weissbluth's (1989) work on sleep disturbances that are traceable to temperament risk factors such as slow adaptability and stimulus sensitivity provides a salient illustration. Likewise, Sanson, Smart, Prior, and Oberklaid's (1993) study of difficult temperament in infancy as a predictor of hyperactivity and aggression makes a similar contribution.

Some rather interesting lines of research have focused on infant temperament as it relates to parental mental health. Aside from Wolkind and De Salis (1982), Cutrona and Troutman (1986) found an association between maternal depression and infant difficultness as measured with the RITQ at 3 months, while Murray, Stanley, Hooper, King, and Fiori-Cowley (1996) showed in a prospective study that either poor motor control or high irritability in newborns quadrupled the likelihood of subsequent postpartum depression in their mothers. Interestingly enough, Whiffen and Gotlib (1989) found that depressed mothers rated their 2-month-old infants as more difficult to care for than did their comparison group of nondepressed mothers, but they did not rate their infants as more difficult with the ICQ. Concerning adult personality, Sirignano and Lachman (1985) found that both parents, but especially fathers, increased in their sense of internal control if they rated their infant easy on the PBT and decreased on internal control if they perceived their infant as difficult.

Finally, some work has shown that infant temperament may be related not only to maladaptive behavior or disorders but to positive behaviors as well. For example, Worobey (1987) linked approach, adaptability, and low distractibility on the TTS to higher mental index scores on the Bayley Scales. Temperament may influence early coping ability through the modulation or

shaping of the infant's efforts to respond to the environment (Williamson & Zeitlin, 1990). In some of the most provocative work on temperament in recent years, Kochanska (1995) has investigated the role of inhibition to novelty by toddlers in the later development of conscience.

Implications of a Temperament Approach for the Infant Mental Health Specialist

As noted by Hannan and Luster (1991), infant mental health workers can assist families in a number of ways. In terms of providing resources, they can lend caregivers emotional support, add to their knowledge of infancy and parenting, and help families to identify essential services. But in terms of reducing stress, they can also help parents to better interpret and, thereby, cope with their infant's difficult behavior. While the subject of difficult temperament will never lack for an audience, the fact is that individual dimensions of temperament, as well as an appreciation for goodness of fit, are also of relevance to the infant mental health specialist.

Carey (1982, 1989b) has described in detail the three major ways that temperament data are useful to the clinician. At the most superficial level, the clinician and parent can engage in a general educational discussion about normal individual differences in the context of the infant's feeding, sleeping, and crying patterns. Through such a conversation, parents can appreciate their infant's behavioral predispositions from birth, absolve themselves of any guilt they may be feeling over what they have misperceived as outcomes of their caregiving, and be forewarned about what they may expect from their infant over time. At the second level, the infant's particular temperament profile may be identified to provide a more organized framework for viewing the infant. This may be very useful if the profile suggests difficulty, a number of temperament risk factors are present, or the mother's ratings of temperament do not coincide with her general perceptions of the baby. At the third level, the clinician may attempt to influence the temperament × environment interaction if a poor fit with resulting stress has led to reactive symptoms. The clinician can suggest alternate methods of parental management, in a sense reframing the infant's behavior in the context of the family environment (Bates, 1989a; Minuchin & Fishman, 1981).

Beyond the clinical assessment of behavioral style, the infant mental health specialist who works in a therapeutic setting may further benefit from adopting a temperament perspective. As Huntington and Simeonsson (1993) illustrate, recognizing the mediating role of temperament may be useful in designing an intervention that can better "fit" the individual characteristics of the infant or even serve as the focus of the intervention in its own right. For example, the infant whose difficultness stems from his or her high intensity and negative mood will warrant a different prescription for intervention than the infant whose extreme shyness is troubling to his or her caregivers.

We are not yet at the level of recommending that screening for temperament problems be made a routine part of a well-baby checkup. That is not to say that such assessments should be avoided. Indeed, Cameron and Rice (1986) have tested an anticipatory guidance program that used an RITQ-based intervention with some success, while others have suggested the use of a temperament approach in assessing developmental disabilities (Huntington & Simeonsson, 1993; McDevitt, 1988). However, more research with normal and clinical samples still needs to be conducted, with additional validation of our improved, yet ever evolving temperament instruments and further integration of differing frameworks and dimensions. In the meantime, the infant mental health worker may, nevertheless, wish to seize the opportunity to obtain information on the baby's temperament, given any indication on the part of the parents that some aspect of the infant's behavioral style or their expectations regarding the infant's behavioral style may be contributing to family stress, disharmony, or dysfunction.

References

Bates, J. E. (1980). The concept of difficult temperament. *Merrill-Palmer Quarterly*, 26, 299–319.

Bates, J. E. (1983). Issues in the assessment of difficult temperament: A reply to Thomas, Chess, and Korn. *Merrill-Palmer Quarterly*, 29(1), 89–97.

Bates, J. E. (1987). Temperament in infancy. In J. D. Osofsky (Ed.), *Handbook of infant development* (2nd ed., pp. 1101–1149). New York: Wiley.

Bates, J. E. (1989a). Applications of temperament concepts. In G. A. Kohnstamm,

J. E. Bates, & M. K. Rothbart (Eds.), *Temperament in childhood* (pp. 321–355). Chichester, England: Wiley.

Bates, J. E. (1989b). Concepts and measures of temperament. In G. A. Kohnstamm, J. E. Bates, & M. K. Rothbart (Eds.), *Temperament in childhood* (pp. 3–26). Chichester, England: Wiley.

Bates, J. E. (1994). Parents as scientific observers of their children's development. In S. L. Friedman & H. C. Haywood (Eds.), *Developmental follow-up: Concepts, domains and methods* (pp. 197–216). New York: Academic.

Bates, J. E., Freeland, C. A., & Lounsbury, M. L. (1979). Measurement of infant difficultness. *Child Development, 50,* 794–803.

Bates, J. E., Maslin, C. A., & Frankel, K. A. (1985). Attachment security, mother-child interaction, and temperament as predictors of behavior problem ratings at age three years. In I. Bretherton & E. Waters (Eds.), Growing points in attachment theory and research (pp. 67–193). *Monographs of the Society for Research in Child Development, 50*(1–2, Serial No. 209).

Bates, J. E., Olson, S. L., Pettit, G., & Bayles, K. (1982). Dimensions of individuality in the mother-infant relationship at 6 months of age. *Child Development, 53,* 446–461.

Bayley, N. (1969). *The Bayley Scales of Infant Development.* San Antonio, TX: The Psychological Corporation.

Belsky, J. (1997). Theory testing, effect-size evaluation, and differential susceptibility to rearing influence: The case of mothering and attachment. *Child Development, 64*(4), 598–600.

Bohlin, G., Hagekull, B., & Lindhagen, K. (1981). Dimensions of infant behavior. *Infant Behavior & Development, 4,* 83–96.

Bornstein, M. H., Gaughran, J. M., & Homel, P. (1986). Infant temperament: Theory, tradition, critique, and new assessments. In C. E. Izard & P. B. Read (Eds.), *Measuring emotions in infants and children* (Vol. 2, pp. 172–199). New York: Cambridge University Press.

Bornstein, M. H., Gaughran, J. M., & Segui, I. (1991). Multimethod assessment of infant temperament: Mother questionnaire and mother and observer reports evaluated and compared at five months using the Infant Temperament Measure. *International Journal of Behavioral Development, 14*(2), 131–151.

Busch-Rossnagel, N. A., & McArdle, J. J. (1983). *Exploration of the factor structure of the Dimensions of Temperament Survey for Infants.* Unpublished manuscript.

Buss, A. H. (1991). The EAS theory of temperament. In J. Strelau & A. Angleitner (Eds.), *Explorations in temperament: International perspectives on theory and measurement* (pp. 43–60). New York: Plenum.

Buss, A. H., & Plomin, R. (1975). *A temperament theory of personality.* New York: Wiley.

Buss, A. H., & Plomin, R. (1984). *Temperament: Early developing personality traits.* Hillsdale, NJ: Erlbaum.

Buss, A. H., Plomin, R., & Willerman, L. (1973). The inheritance of temperaments. *Journal of Personality, 41,* 513–524.

Calkins, S. D., Fox, N. A., & Marshall, T. R. (1996). Behavioral and physiological antecedents of inhibition in infancy. *Child Development, 67,* 525–40.

Cameron, J. R., & Rice, D. C. (1986). Developing anticipatory guidance programs based on early assessment of infant temperament: Two tests of a prevention model. *Journal of Pediatric Psychology, 11*(2), 221–234.

Carey, W. B. (1970). A simplified method for measuring infant temperament. *Journal of Pediatrics, 81,* 823–828.

Carey, W. B. (1982). Clinical use of temperament data in pediatrics. In R. Porter & G. M. Collins (Eds.), *Temperamental differences in infants and young children* (pp. 191–205). London: Pitman.

Carey, W. B. (1986). The difficult child. *Pediatrics in Review, 8,* 39–45.

Carey, W. B. (1989a). Introduction: Basic issues. In W. B. Carey & S. C. McDevitt (Eds.), *Clinical and educational applications of temperament research* (pp. 11–20). Berwyn, PA: Swets North America Inc.

Carey, W. B. (1989b). Practical implications in pediatrics. In G. A. Kohnstamm, J. E. Bates, & M. K. Rothbart (Eds.), *Temperament in childhood* (pp. 405–419). Chichester, England: Wiley.

Carey, W. B., & McDevitt, S. C. (1978). Revision of the Infant Temperament Questionnaire. *Pediatrics, 61,* 735–739.

Carey, W. B., & McDevitt, S. C. (Eds.). (1989). *Clinical and educational applications of temperament research.* Berwyn, PA: Swets North America Inc.

Carey, W. B., McDevitt, S. C., & Associates. (1995). *Carey Temperament Scales.* San Antonio, TX: The Psychological Corporation.

Chess, S., & Thomas, A. (1991). Temperament and the concept of goodness of fit. In J. Strelau & A. Angleitner (Eds.), *Explorations in temperament: International perspectives on theory and measurement* (pp. 15–28). New York: Plenum.

Clark, L. A., Watson, D., & Mineka, S. (1994). Temperament, personality, and the mood and anxiety disorders. *Journal of Abnormal Psychology, 103,* 103–116.

Clarke-Stewart, A., Goldberg, W., & Fitz-patrick, M. J. (1992). The great temperament race [Special ICIS Abstract Issue]. *Infant Behavior & Development, 15,* 349.

Crockenberg, S. B. (1981). Infant irritability, mother responsiveness, and social support influences on the security of infant attachment. *Child Development, 52,* 857–865.

Crockenberg, S. B. (1986). Are temperamental differences in babies associated with predictable differences in care giving? In J. V. Lerner & R. M. Lerner (Eds.), Temperament and social interaction in infants and children (pp. 53–73). *New directions for child development* (No. 31). San Francisco: Jossey-Bass.

Cutrona, C. E., & Troutman, B. R. (1986). Social support, infant temperament, and parenting self-efficacy: A mediational model of postpartum depression. *Child Development, 57,* 1507–1518.

Damon, W. (Series Ed.), & Eisenberg, N. (Vol. Ed.). *Handbook of child psychology: Vol. 3. Social, emotional and personality development* (5th ed.). New York: Wiley.

Derryberry, D., & Rothbart, M. K. (1984). Emotion, attention, and temperament. In C. Izard, J. Kagan, & R. Zajonc (Eds.), *Emotion, cognition and behavior* (pp. 132–66). Cambridge, England: Cambridge University Press.

Diamond, S. (1957). *Personality and temperament.* New York: Basic Books.

Dunn, J., & Kendrick, C. (1980). Studying temperament and parent-child interaction: A comparison of information from direct observation and from parental interview. *Developmental Medicine and Child Neurology, 22,* 484–496.

Eaton, W. O. (1994). Methodological implications of the impending engagement of temperament and biology. In J. E. Bates & T. D. Wachs (Eds.), *Temperament: In-*

dividual differences at the interface of biology and behavior (pp. 259–273). Washington, DC: American Psychological Association.

Engfer, A. (1991). Antecedents and consequences of shyness in boys and girls: A 6-year longitudinal study. In K. H. Rubin & J. Asendorpf (Eds.), *Social withdrawal, inhibition, and shyness in childhood* (pp. 49–79). Hillsdale, NJ: Erlbaum.

Ekman, P. (Ed.). (1982). *Emotion in the human face.* Cambridge, England: Cambridge University Press.

Escalona, S. K. (1968). *The roots of individuality: Normal patterns of development in infancy.* Chicago: Aldine.

Fish, M., & Crockenberg, S. B. (1981). Correlates and antecedents of nine-month infant behavior and mother-infant interaction. *Infant Behavior & Development, 4,* 69–81.

Fitzpatrick, M. J., Goldberg, W. A., & Clarke-Stewart, A. (1996). Maternal sensitivity and the stability of infant temperament [Special ICIS Abstract Issue]. *Infant Behavior & Development, 19,* 456.

Fox, N. A., & Davidson, R. J. (1984). Hemispheric substrates of affect: A developmental model. In N. A. Fox & R. J. Davidson (Eds.), *The psychology of affective development* (pp. 353–382). Hillsdale, NJ: Erlbaum.

Fullard, W., McDevitt, S. C., & Carey, W. B. (1984). Assessing temperament in one- to three-year-old children. *Journal of Pediatric Psychology, 9,* 205–217.

Garcia-Coll, C. T., Halpern, L. F., Vohr, B. R., Seifer, R., & Oh, W. (1992). Stability and correlates of change of early temperament in preterm and full-term infants. *Infant Behavior & Development, 15,* 137–153.

Gesell, A. (1925). *The mental growth of the pre-school child.* New York: Macmillan.

Gibbs, M. V., Reeves, D., & Cunningham, C. C. (1987). The application of temperament questionnaires to a British sample: Issues of reliability and validity. *Journal of Child Psychology and Psychiatry, 28,* 61–77.

Goldsmith, H. H. (1996). Studying temperament via construction of the Toddler Behavior Assessment Questionnaire. *Child Development, 67,* 218–235.

Goldsmith, H. H., & Alansky, J. A. (1987a). Construction of Q-Sort measures of temperament and their relation to security of attachment. *Abstracts of the Society for Research in Child Development, 6,* 445.

Goldsmith, H. H., & Alansky, J. A. (1987b). Maternal and infant temperamental predictors of attachment: A meta-analytic review. *Journal of Consulting and Clinical Psychology, 55,* 805–816.

Goldsmith, H. H., Buss, K. A., & Lemery, K. S. (1997). Toddler and childhood temperament: Expanded content, stronger genetic evidence, new evidence for the importance of environment. *Developmental Psychology, 33,* 891–905.

Goldsmith, H. H., Buss, A. H., Plomin, R., Rothbart, M. K., Thomas, A., Chess, S., Hinde, R. A., & McCall, R. R. (1987). Roundtable: What is temperament? Four approaches. *Child Development, 58,* 505–529.

Goldsmith, H. H., & Campos, J. J. (1982). Toward a theory of infant temperament. In R. Emde (Ed.), *Attachment and affiliative systems* (pp. 161–193). New York: Plenum.

Goldsmith, H. H., & Campos, J. J. (1986). Fundamental issues in the study of early temperament: The Denver Twin Temperament Study. In M. E. Lamb, A. L. Brown, & B. Rogoff (Eds.), *Advances in developmental psychology* (Vol. 4, pp. 231–283). Hillsdale, NJ: Erlbaum.

Goldsmith, H. H., Elliot, T., & Jaco, K. L. (1986). Construction and initial validation of a new temperament questionnaire [Special ICIS Abstract Issue]. *Infant Behavior & Development, 9,* 144.

Goldsmith, H. H., & Gottesman, I. I. (1981). Origins of variation in behavioral style: A longitudinal study of temperament in young twins. *Child Development, 52,* 91–103.

Goldsmith, H. H., & Rieser-Danner, L. A. (1990). Assessing early temperament. In C. R. Reynolds & R. W. Kamphaus (Eds.), *Handbook of psychological and educational assessment of children* (pp. 245–278). New York: Guilford.

Goldsmith, H. H., Rieser-Danner, L. A., & Briggs, S. (1991). Evaluating convergent and discriminant validity of temperament questionnaires for preschoolers, toddlers, and infants. *Developmental Psychology, 2(4),* 566–579.

Goldsmith, H. H., & Rothbart, M. K. (1991). Contemporary instruments for assessing early temperament by questionnaire and in the laboratory. In J. Strelau & A. Angleitner (Eds.), *Explorations in temperament: International perspectives on theory and measurement* (pp. 249–272). New York: Plenum.

Goldsmith, H. H., & Rothbart, M. K. (1996). *Laboratory Temperament Assessment Battery* (LAB-TAB): Prelocomotor and locomotor versions. Madison, WI: University of Wisconsin.

Gunnar, M. R. (1989). Studies of the human infant's adrenocortical response to potentially stressful events. In M. Lewis & J. Worobey (Eds.), Infant stress and coping (pp. 3–18). *New directions for child development* (No. 45). San Francisco: Jossey-Bass.

Gunnar, M. R. (1990). The psychobiology of infant temperament. In J. Colombo & J. Fagen (Eds.), *Individual differences in infancy: Reliability, stability, prediction* (pp. 387–409). Hillsdale, NJ: Erlbaum.

Gunnar, M. R., Connors, J., Isensee, J., & Wall, L. (1988). Adrenocortical activity and behavioral distress in newborns. *Developmental Psychobiology, 21,* 279–310.

Hagekull, B. (1994). Infant temperament and early childhood functioning: Possible relations to the five-factor model. In C. F. Halverson, G. A. Kohnstamm, & R. P. Martin (Eds.), *The developing structure of temperament and personality from infancy to adulthood* (pp. 227–240). Hillsdale, NJ: Erlbaum.

Hagekull, B., & Bohlin, G. (1989). Greater impact of infant temperament in multiparous mother's adaptation. In W. B. Carey & S. C. McDevitt (Eds.), *Clinical and educational applications of temperament research* (pp. 97–101). Berwyn, PA: Swets North America Inc.

Hagekull, B., & Bohlin, G. (1995). Day care quality, family and child characteristics, and socioemotional development. *Early Childhood Research Quarterly, 10,* 505–526.

Hagekull, B., Lindhagen, K., & Bohlin, G. (1980). Behavioral dimensions in one-year-olds and dimensional stability in infancy. *International Journal of Behavioral Development, 3,* 351–364.

Hannah, K., & Luster, T. (1991). Influence of parent, child, and contextual factors on the quality of the home environment. *Infant Mental Health Journal, 12,* 17–30.

Harrington, D., Black, M. M., Starr, R. H., & Dubowitz, H. (1998). Child neglect: Relation to child temperament and family context. *American Journal of Orthopsychiatry, 68,* 108–116.

Hsu, C. C., Soong, W. T., Stigler, J. W., Hong,

C. C., & Liang, C. C. (1981). The temperamental characteristics of Chinese babies. *Child Development, 52,* 1337–1340.

Hubert, N. C., Wachs, T. D., Peters-Martin, P., & Gandour, M. J. (1982). The study of early temperament: Measurement and conceptual issues. *Child Development, 53,* 571–600.

Huffman, L. C., Bryan, Y. E., del Carmen, R., Petersen, F. A., & Porges, S. W. (1992). *Autonomic correlates of reactivity and self-regulation at twelve weeks of age.* Unpublished manuscript. Rockville, MD: National Institute of Mental Health.

Huitt, W., & Ashton, P. (1982). Parent's perception of infant temperament: A psychometric study: *Merrill-Palmer Quarterly, 28,* 95–109.

Huntington, G. S. (1989). Assessing behavioral characteristics. In D. B. Bailey & M. Wolery (Eds.), *Assessing infants and preschoolers with handicaps* (pp. 225–248). Columbus, OH: Merrill.

Huntington, G. S., & Simeonsson, R. J. (1993). Temperament and adaptation in infants and young children with disabilities. *Infant Mental Health Journal, 14,* 49–60.

Izard, C. E. (1977). *Human emotions.* New York: Plenum.

Kagan, J. (1982). The construct of difficult temperament: A reply to Thomas, Chess, and Korn. *Merrill-Palmer Quarterly, 28*(1), 21–24.

Kagan, J. (1994). *Galen's prophecy: Temperament in human nature.* New York: Basic Books.

Kagan, J. (1998). Biology and the child. In W. Damon (Series Ed.) & N. Eisenberg (Vol. Ed.), *Handbook of child psychology: Vol. 3. Social, emotional and personality development* (5th ed., pp. 177–236). New York: Wiley.

Kagan, J., Reznick, J. S., Clarke, C., Snidman, N., & Carcia-Coll, C. (1984). Behavioral inhibition to the unfamiliar. *Child Development, 55,* 2212–2225.

Kagan, J., & Snidman, N. (1991). Infant predictors of inhibited and uninhibited profiles. *Psychological Science, 2,* 40–44.

Kagan, J., Snidman, N., & Arcus, D. (1992). Initial reactions to unfamiliarity. *Current Directions in Psychological Science, 1,* 171–173.

Kochanska, G. (1995). Children's temperament, mother's discipline, and security of attachment: Multiple pathways to emerging internalization. *Child Development, 66,* 597–615.

Kohnstamm, G. A. (Eds.). (1986). *Temperament discussed: Temperament and development in infancy and childhood.* Berwyn, PA: Swets North America Inc.

Lerner, J. V., & Lerner, R. M. (1983). Temperament and adaptation across life: Theoretical and empirical issues. In P. B. Baltes & O. G. Brim (Eds.), *Life-span development and behavior* (Vol. 5, pp. 197–231). New York: Academic.

Lerner, R. M., Belsky, J., & Windle, M. (1983). *The Dimensions of Temperament Survey for Infancy (DOTS-Infancy): Assessment of its psychometric properties.* Unpublished manuscript.

Lerner, R. M., Palermo, M., Spiro, A., & Nesselroade, J. R. (1982). Assessing the dimensions of temperamental individuality across the life-span: The Dimensions of Temperament Survey (DOTS). *Child Development, 53,* 149–159.

Lewis, M., Alessandri, S. M., & Sullivan, M. W. (1990). Violation of expectancy, loss of control, and anger expressions in young infants. *Developmental Psychology, 26,* 745–751.

Lewis, M., & Ramsay, D. S. (1995). Developmental change in infants' response to stress. *Child Development, 66,* 657–670.

Loehlin, J. C., & Nichols, R. C. (1976). *Heredity, environment, and personality.* Austin, TX: University of Texas Press.

Matheny, A. P., Reise, M. L., & Wilson, R. S. (1985). Rudiments of infant temperament: Newborn to nine months. *Developmental Psychology, 21,* 486–494.

Matheny, A. P., & Wilson, R. S. (1981). *Developmental tasks and rating scales for the laboratory assessment of infant temperament.* JSAS Catalog of Selected Documents in Psychology, 11 (Ms. 2367), 81–82.

Maziade, M. (1994). Temperament research and practical implications for clinicians. In W. B. Carey & S. C. McDevitt (Eds.), *Prevention and early intervention: Individual differences as risk factors for the mental health of children* (pp. 69–80). New York: Brunner/Mazel.

Maziade, M., Boudreault, M., Thivierge, J., Caperaà, P., & Cote, R. (1984). Infant temperament: SES and gender differences and reliability of measurement in a large Quebec sample. *Merrill-Palmer Quarterly, 30,* 213–216.

McDevitt, S. C. (1988). Assessment of temperament in developmentally disabled infants and preschoolers. In T. D. Wachs & R. Sheehan (Eds.), *Assessment of young developmentally disabled children* (pp. 255–265). New York: Plenum.

McDevitt, S. C. (1994). Introduction. In W. B. Carey & S. C. McDevitt (Eds.), *Prevention and early intervention: Individual differences as risk factors for the mental health of children* (pp. 3–11). New York: Brunner/Mazel.

Medoff-Cooper, B., Carey, W. B., & McDevitt, S. C. (1993). The Early Infancy Temperament Questionnaire. *Journal of Developmental and Behavioral Pediatrics, 14,* 230–235.

Minuchin, S., & Fishman, H. C. (1981). *Family therapy techniques.* Cambridge, MA: Harvard University Press.

Murray, L., Stanley, C., Hooper, R., King, F., & Fiori-Cowley, A. (1996). The role of infant factors in postnatal depression and mother-infant interactions. *Developmental Medicine & Child Neurology, 38,* 109–119.

Murphy, L. B., & Moriarty, A. E. (1976). *Vulnerability, coping, and growth: From infancy to adolescence.* New Haven, CT: Yale University Press.

Oberklaid, F., Prior, M., Golvan, D., Clements, A., & Williamson, A. (1984). Temperament in Australian infants. *Australian Pediatric Journal, 20,* 181–184.

O'Boyle, C., & Rothbart, M. K. (1990). Assessment of infant irritability through parental report [Special ICIS Abstract Issue] *Infant Behavior & Development, 13,* 554.

Osofsky, J. D. (Ed.). (1979). *Handbook of infant development.* New York: Wiley.

Osofsky, J. D. (Ed.). (1987). *Handbook of infant development* (2nd ed.). New York: Wiley.

Pedersen, F. A., Zaslow, M., Cain, R. L., Anderson, B. J., & Maureen, T. (1980). *A methodology for assessing parent perception of baby temperament.* JSAS Catalog of Selected Documents in Psychology, 10 (Ms. 1987), 10–11.

Persson-Blennow, I., & McNeil, T. (1979). A questionnaire for measurement of temperament in six-month-old infants: Development and standardization. *Journal of Child Psychology and Psychiatry and Allied Disciplines, 20,* 1–13.

Persson-Blennow, I., & McNeil, T. (1980). Questionnaire of measurement of temperament in one- and two-year-old children. *Journal of Child Psychology and Psychiatry, 21,* 37–46.

Plomin, R. (1982). The difficult concept of temperament: A response to Thomas, Chess, and Korn. *Merrill-Palmer Quarterly, 28*(1), 25–33.

Porges, S. W. (1986). Respiratory sinus arrhythmia: Physiological basis, quantitative methods, and clinical implications. In P. Grossman, K. Jannsen, & D. Valti (Eds.), *Cardiorespiratory and cardiosomatic psychophysiology* (pp. 101–115). New York: Plenum.

Porges, S. W. (1991). Autonomic regulation and attention. In B. A. Campbell, H. Hayne, & R. Richardson (Eds.), *Attention and information processing in infants and adults* (pp. 201–223). Hillsdale, NJ: Erlbaum.

Porges, S. W., Doussard-Roosevelt, J. A., & Maiti, A. K. (1994). Vagal tone and the physiological regulation of emotion. In N. A. Fox (Ed.), Emotion regulation: Behavioral and biological considerations (pp. 167–186). *Monographs of the Society for Research in Child Development, 59* (2–3, Serial No. 240).

Porter, R., & Collins, G. M. (Eds.). (1982). *Temperamental differences in infants and young children.* London: Pitman.

Ramsay, D. S., & Lewis, M. (1994). Developmental change in infant cortisol and behavioral response to inoculation. *Child Development, 65,* 1491–1502.

Riese, M. L. (1987). Temperament stability between the neonatal period and 24 months. *Developmental Psychology, 23*(2), 216–222.

Rothbart, M. K. (1981). Measurement of temperament in infancy. *Child Development, 52,* 569–578.

Rothbart, M. K. (1982). The concept of diffi-

cult temperament: Critical analysis of Thomas, Chess, and Korn. *Merrill-Palmer Quarterly, 28*(1), 35–40.

Rothbart, M. K. (1986). Longitudinal observation of infant temperament. *Developmental Psychology, 22,* 356–365.

Rothbart, M. K. (1991). Temperament: A developmental framework. In J. Strelau & A. Angleitner (Eds.), *Explorations in temperament: International perspectives on theory and measurement* (pp. 61–74). New York: Plenum.

Rothbart, M. K. (1995). Concept and method in contemporary temperament research: Review of J. Kagan's Galen's prophecy. *Psychological Inquiry, 6,* 334–348.

Rothbart, M. K., Ahadi, S. A., & Hershey, K. L. (1994). Temperament and social behavior in childhood. *Merrill-Palmer Quarterly, 40,* 21–39.

Rothbart, M. K., & Bates, J. E. (1998). Temperament. In W. Damon (Series Ed.) & N. Eisenberg (Vol. Ed.), *Handbook of child psychology Vol. 3. Social, emotional and personality development* (5th ed., pp. 105–176). New York: Wiley.

Rothbart, M. K., & Derryberry, D. (1981). Development of individual differences in temperament. In M. E. Lamb & A. L. Brown (Eds.), *Advances in developmental psychology* (Vol. 1, pp. 37–86). Hillsdale, NJ: Erlbaum.

Rothbart, M. K., Derryberry, D., & Posner, M. I. (1994). A psychobiological approach to the development of temperament. In J. E. Bates & T. D. Wachs (Eds.), *Temperament: Individual differences at the interface of biology and behavior* (pp. 83–116). Washington, DC: American Psychological Association.

Rothbart, M. K., & Goldsmith, H. H. (1985). Three approaches to the study of infant temperament. *Developmental Review, 5,* 237–260.

Rothbart, M. K., & Mauro, J. A. (1990). Questionnaire approaches to the study of infant temperament. In J. Colombo & J. Fagen (Eds.), *Individual differences in infancy: Reliability, stability, prediction* (pp. 411–429). Hillsdale, NJ: Erlbaum.

Rothbart, M. K., Posner, M. I., & Hershey, K. L. (1995). Temperament, attention, and developmental psychopathology. In D. Cicchetti & D. J. Cohen (Eds.), *Manual of developmental psychopathology* (Vol. 1, pp. 635–652). New York: Wiley.

Rowe, D. C., & Plomin, R. (1977). Temperament in early childhood. *Journal of Personality Assessment, 41*(2), 150–156.

Rutter, M. (1994). Temperament: Changing concepts and implications. In W. B. Carey & S. C. McDevitt (Eds.), *Prevention and early intervention: Individual differences as risk factors for the mental health of children* (pp. 23–34). New York: Brunner/ Mazel.

Sanson, A. V., Prior, M., Garino, E., Oberklaid, F., & Sewell, J. (1987). The structure of infant temperament: Factor analysis of the Revised Infant Temperament Questionnaire. *Infant Behavior & Development, 10,* 97–104.

Sanson, A. V., Smart, D., Prior, M., & Oberklaid, F. (1993). Precursors of hyperactivity and aggression. *Journal of American Academy of Child & Adolescent Psychiatry, 32,* 1207–1216.

Schneirla, T. C. (1959). An evolutionary and developmental theory of biphasic processes underlying approach and withdrawal. In M. R. Jones (Ed.), *Nebraska symposium on motivation* (Vol. 7, pp. 297–339). Lincoln, NE: University of Nebraska Press.

Seifer, R., & Sameroff, A. J. (1986). The concept, measurement, and interpretation of temperament in young children: A survey of research issues. In M. L. Wolraich & D. Routh (Eds.), *Advances in developmental and behavioral pediatrics* (pp. 1– 43). Greenwich, CT: JAI Press.

Seifer, R., Sameroff, A. J., Barrett, L. C., & Krafchuk, E. (1994). Infant temperament measured by multiple observations and mother report. *Child Development, 65,* 1478–1490.

Sheldon, W. H., & Stevens, S. S. (1942). *The varieties of human temperament.* New York: Harper Row.

Shirley, M. M. (1933). *The first two years: A study of 25 babies.* Minneapolis, MN: University of Minnesota Press.

Sirignano, S. W., & Lachman, M. E. (1985). Personality change during the transition to parenthood. *Developmental Psychology, 21*(3), 558–567.

Slabach, E. H., Morrow, J., & Wachs, T. D. (1991). In J. Strelau & A. Angleitner (Eds.), *Explorations in temperament: International perspectives on theory and measurement* (pp. 205–234). New York: Plenum.

Sprunger, L. W., Boyce, W. T., & Gaines, J. A. (1985). Family-infant congruence: Routines and rhythmicity in family adaptations to a young infant. *Child Development, 56,* 564–572.

Strelau, J. (1994). The concepts of arousal and arousability as used in temperament studies. In J. Bates & T. D. Wachs (Eds.), *Temperament: Individual differences at the interface of biology and behavior* (pp. 117–141). Washington, DC: American Psychological Association.

Strelau, J., & Angleitner, A. (Eds.). (1991). *Explorations in temperament: Interna-*

tional perspectives on theory and measurement. New York: Plenum.

Sullivan, M. W., & Lewis, M. (1989). Emotion and cognition in infancy: Facial expressions during contingency learning. *International Journal of Behavioral Development, 12,* 221–237.

Sullivan, M. W., Lewis, M., & Alessandri, S. (1992). Cross-age stability in emotional expressions during learning and extinction. *Developmental Psychology, 28*(1), 58–63.

Super, C. M., & Harkness, S. (1994). Temperament and the developmental niche. In W. B. Carey & S. C. McDevitt (Eds.), *Prevention and early intervention: Individual differences as risk factors for the mental health of children* (pp. 115–125). New York: Brunner/Mazel.

Thomas, A., & Chess, S. (1977). *Temperament and development.* New York: Brunner/Mazel.

Thomas, A., Chess, S., & Birch, H. G. (1968). *Temperament and behavior disorders in children.* New York: New York University Press.

Thomas, A., Chess, S., Birch, H. G., Herzig, M. E., & Korn, S. (1963). *Behavioral individuality in early childhood.* New York: New York University Press.

Thomas, A., Chess, S., & Korn, S. J. (1982). The reality of difficult temperament. *Merrill-Palmer Quarterly, 28*(1), 1–20.

Thompson, R. A., & Lamb, M. E. (1984). Assessing qualitative dimensions of emotional responsiveness in infants: Separation reactions in the strange situation. *Infant Behavior & Development, 7,* 423–445.

Turecki, S., & Tonner, L. (1985). *The difficult child.* New York: Basic Books.

van den Boom, D. C. (1989). Neonatal irritability and the development of attach-ment. In G. A. Kohnstamm, J. E. Bates, & M. K. Rothbart (Eds.), *Temperament in childhood* (pp. 299–318). Chichester, England: Wiley.

van den Boom, D. C., & Hoeksma, J. B. (1994). The effect of infant irritability on mother-infant interaction: A growth curve analysis. *Developmental Psychology, 30,* 581–590.

Vaughn, B. (1986). The doubtful validity of infant temperament assessments by means of questionnaires like the ITQ. In G. Kohnstamm (Ed.), *Temperament discussed: Temperament and development in infancy and childhood* (pp. 35–42). Berwyn, PA: Swets North America Inc.

Weissbluth, M. (1989). Sleep-loss stress and temperamental difficultness: Psychobiological processes and practical considerations. In G. A. Kohnstamm, J. E. Bates, & M. K. Rothbart (Eds.), *Temperament in childhood* (pp. 358–375). Chichester, England: Wiley.

Whiffen, V. E., & Gotlib, I. H. (1989). Infants of postpartum depressed mothers: Temperament and cognitive status. *Journal of Abnormal Psychology, 98*(3), 274–279.

Williamson, G. G., & Zeitlin, S. (1990). Assessment of coping and temperament: Contributions to adaptive functioning. In E. D. Gibbs & D. M. Teti (Eds.), *Interdisciplinary assessment of infants: A guide for early intervention professionals* (pp. 215–226). Baltimore, MD: Brookes.

Wilson, R. S., Brown, A. M., & Matheny, A. P. (1971). Emergence and persistence of behavioral differences in twins. *Child Development, 42*(5), 1381–1398.

Wilson, R. S., & Matheny, A. P. (1983). Assessment of temperament in infant twins. *Developmental Psychology, 19,* 172–183.

Windle, M. (1988). Psychometric strategies of measures of temperament: A methodological critique. *International Journal of Behavioral Development, 11,* 171–201.

Windle, M., Hooker, K., Lenerz, K., East, P. L., Lerner, J. V., & Lerner, R. M. (1986). Temperament, perceived competence, and depression in early- and late-adolescents. *Developmental Psychology, 22,* 384–392.

Windle, M., & Lerner, R. M. (1986). Reassessing the dimensions of temperamental individuality across the life span: The Revised Dimensions of Temperament Survey (DOTS-R). *Journal of Adolescent Research, 1*(2), 213–230.

Wolke, D., & St. James-Roberts, I. (1986). Maternal affective-cognitive processes in the perception of newborn difficultness. In G. Kohnstamm (Ed.), *Temperament discussed: Temperament and development in infancy and childhood* (pp. 27–34). Berwyn, PA: Swets North America Inc.

Wolkind, S. N., & DeSalis, W. (1982). Infant temperament, maternal state and child behavioral problems. In R. Porter & G. M. Collins (Eds.), *Temperamental differences in infants and young children* (pp. 221–239). London: Pitman.

Worobey, J. (1986a). Convergence among assessments of temperament in the first month. *Child Development, 57*(1), 47–55.

Worobey, J. (1986b). Neonatal stability and one-month behavior. *Infant Behavior & Development, 9*(1), 119–124.

Worobey, J. (1987). Temperament and sensorimotor intelligence. *Early Child Development and Care, 28,* 1–11.

Worobey, J. (1990). Behavioral assessment of the neonate. In J. Colombo & J. Fagen (Eds.), *Individual differences in infancy: Reliability, stability, prediction* (pp. 137–154). Hillsdale, NJ: Erlbaum.

Worobey, J. (1997). Convergence between temperament ratings in early infancy. *Journal of Developmental and Behavioral Pediatrics, 18*(4), 260–263.

Worobey, J. (1998). Feeding method and motor activity in 3-month-old human infants. *Perceptual and Motor Skills, 86,* 883–895.

Worobey, J., & Anderson-Goetz, D. (1985). Maternal ratings of newborn activity: Assessing convergence between instruments. *Infant Mental Health Journal, 6*(2), 68–75.

Worobey, J., & Blajda, V. M. (1989). Temperament ratings at 2-weeks, 2-months, and 1-year. *Developmental Psychology, 25,* 257–263.

15

Meeting a Desperate Need: One Man's Vision of Training for the Infant Family Field

Frances Stott and Linda Gilkerson

15

517

Introduction

Irving Harris understands that unless the people who care for, educate, and advocate for young children are well prepared for their jobs, programs designed to benefit young children and families will fail. Recognizing the importance of the early years for later human development and the creation of a stable society, Harris has advocated for decades for excellence in early care and education. More remarkably, he goes beyond those who simply support direct services for young children and families. He takes the long view, funding programs and institutions of higher education to ensure that formal knowledge will be applied specifically to the promotion of healthy development in the earliest years.

In Harris' view, increased training for early childhood development professionals constitutes an essential underpinning for implementing sound policy for children. More than a decade ago, he noted a desperate need for trained professionals:

We need specialists in early childhood development, in maternal and child health, and in clinical social work; and we need to increase the number of administrators and researchers as well as clinicians. At the undergraduate level in both universities and community colleges and in graduate programs,

Reprinted with permission of Zero to Three/National Center for Infants, Toddlers and Families, March 1999 we must rapidly increase the number of people professionally trained to serve as health care technicians, preschool teachers and child care specialists. (Harris, 1987, pp. 10–11)

Challenging the still-prevalent notion that higher education and training are unessential for the care of young children, Harris has established and supported schools and training programs to equip frontline service providers, administrators, and advocates with the intellectual and practical tools he believes they need to be effective.

This essay honors Harris' philosophical and practical commitment to the development of a workforce with the skills required to accomplish an ambitious agenda for children and families. We review historical trends and current dilemmas in practitioner preparation and by describing some of Irving Harris' major investments in training institutions and programs, offer a brief developmental profile of higher education in the emerging child/family field.

Toward an Integrated Approach to Practitioner Preparation

Historically, the care of young children has been guided by the conventions of child rearing beliefs in a particular community, with nuances of social class and caste accounting for different practices. Now we talk of more or less established fields of knowledge and professional practice— child development, early care and educa-

tion, or the "infant/family" field. What constitutes an appropriate base for practice in these areas? We suggest that academic, "local" (knowledge that is sensitive to context), and personal knowledge are essential to working with children and families.

Clearly, a knowledge base is necessary for working with and planning for other people's children and families, as basing practice solely on one's own history and experience has the potential for mischief. First, one's own experience can intrude in the form of transference and countertransference feelings and attitudes and stereotypical thinking. Second, firsthand experience of a familiar world can insulate one from the world that lies outside. To move the self from center depends on the ideas of others. The ideas provided by formal knowledge, along with a measure of selfknowledge, can keep us from being stuck in our own biases and narrow thinking and free us to consider what is possible and desirable and to develop transforming visions of action. Theories and research in child development can help us arrange our minds. They can give us greater ability to describe, illuminate, interpret, and translate our observations of children and families.

Indeed, during the past century, institutions of higher education, relying increasingly on theory and research, have begun to take a more active role in informing early care and education practice. Since the 1930s, advocates of child-centered pedagogical approaches have argued that care and education of young children should be oriented toward children's interests, needs, and developmental growth and informed by an understanding of child development.

Most recently, researchers and practitioners who study and work with young children have developed theoretical models that reveal the complex transactions between young children and their caregiving environments that shape development. Once we recognize that touching children's and families' lives is an inherently complicated business, we must also acknowledge the need to "embrace complexity" in the preparation of practitioners for the emerging infant/family field.

Yet, to base practitioner preparation on research and theories invites criticism. Soltis poses a crucial question: "To what degree does formal education make us more of a prisoner of that social world or on the other hand provide us with the means to achieve some measure of freedom to transcend it?" (Soltis, 1981, p. 100). Critics who have called into question the use of child development knowledge (theories and research) as a strict basis for practice make three chief arguments. First is their adherence to natural science methods and concepts, including the notion that knowledge is decontextualized and objective rather than anchored in relationships and experience. A second criticism of theories is their ethnocentric bias and assumptions of universality. A third criticism suggests that formal child development knowledge tends to be used to reinforce the status quo, thus further disenfranchising the poor and powerless by not including their experiences (Burman, 1994; Delpit, 1998, Jipson, 1991; Lubeck, 1996). While these criticisms need not lead to an abandonment of formal child development knowledge, they do suggest that it is a "slippery base

for practice"—necessary for practitioner preparation but not sufficient (Stott & Bowman, 1996).

We clearly need to understand and to teach the changing nature of theories. We need to temper our understanding about the source, characteristics, and limitations of theories and research and to subject them to the scrutiny of cultural relevance and personal reflection. While recognizing the limitations of personal experience as a guide to professional practice, we can accept the legitimacy of individuals' personal and cultural thinking and feeling and integrate these notions with a formal knowledge base.

The programs Irving Harris supports typically incorporate opportunities for reflective practice as essential to prepare professionals for work with young children and families. Practice in this field is an art that eludes technical description, analysis, and systematization. It is replete with important, complex, and messy problems that range from conflicting values, insecurities in the arena of practice, and differences in position and power to programs with ambiguous identity and sense of purpose as well as diffuse principles and methods. Donald Schon describes such a field as a "swamp" and contrasts it with the "high, hard ground," where problems may be less important but may be more amenable to technical understanding (Schon, 1987). Effective practice and leadership in the "swamp" cannot, by definition, be based only on the application of child development knowledge and clear rules developed on and for the high ground. It may be that more than any other skill, child and family practitioners and leaders need the capacity to make sense out of the mess and manage in the "swamp." Too many people fail at practice and leadership because they do not understand who they are, how to manage themselves, and how and when to compensate for what they can not do.

Intimate contact with the reality of the field and the ability to reflect on and learn from one's own and others' experiences can go a long way toward making sense of the problems. Practitioners need a process for reflection about dealing with the uncontrollable, the unexpected, and the contradictory. Perhaps the most important thing training institutions can do is help students begin the process of reflection, not only about the art of practice, but also about themselves. This, of course, is best accomplished in a context of mentorship and reflective supervision. Students need opportunities to reflect on practice and time to reflect on themselves with the same intensity and energy that is given to the study of others.

Preparing professionals to work with young children and their families is indeed a complex and tricky venture. Students need an educationally purposeful community where they are engaged and inspired. They need to learn the latest scientific and theoretical knowledge, not as isolated parcels of information but as a framework to hold information that they have already and will acquire in the future. While each student creates his or her own framework of knowledge, the educational community contributes to this framework a set of shared beliefs and values that include a disposition to understand, evaluate, and be

open to the ideas of others. Armed with formal knowledge and practical wisdom, students can use reasonably good judgment in their work and engage creatively and respectfully with children, families, and colleagues.

Irving Harris' Investments in Professional Education

A list of the educational institutions and programs that Irving Harris has supported in their efforts to prepare a skilled child and family workforce could constitute a table of contents for historical account of multidisciplinary professional education. The descriptions of Harris' major investments in education that follow are designed to highlight both crosscutting principles and program-specific approaches to professional training. Since descriptions are necessarily brief, readers are encouraged to contact individual programs for more information.

Erikson Institute

In the mid-1960s, scholars such as J. McVicker Hunt (1961) and Benjamin Bloom (1964) described the importance of the early years of life in human development and emphasized the powerful influence of experience on the development of competence in young children. Head Start, a key weapon in the War on Poverty, was based on this belief in the crucial impact of early experience on later development. During the same period, psychoanalysts Maria and Gerhardt Piers were convincing Irving Harris of the importance of the early years for later development and of the need to apply psychoanalytic and social science knowledge to the creation and staffing of new early childhood programs. Harris agreed to help start a graduate school in Chicago to educate Head Start and preschool teachers.

When Maria Piers and Harris met with Sargent Shriver, director of the Office of Economic Opportunity (OEO), the original home of Head Start, they discovered that OEO planned to train Head Start staff the way personnel had been trained in World War II. However, Harris and Piers' proposed graduate program was designed to be "anything but a six-week crash course" (Harris, 1996, p. 3). When, not surprisingly perhaps, OEO promises of support for the proposed graduate school proved illusory, Harris decided to provide the capital for a fully developed educational program himself. Irving Harris and Maria Piers along with Barbara Bowman and Lorraine Wallach founded the Chicago School for Early Education. The first class of students began in September 1966. By 1968, the school was affiliated with Loyola University Chicago and was renamed the Erikson Institute for Advanced Study in Child Development.

Erikson Institute's founders, including Irving Harris, had a profound concern—from the beginning—for the family, community, and culture that support the child. Located in downtown Chicago, Erikson Institute has a mission to recruit students from the culturally diverse urban population that it believes its graduates will serve. The Institute's research center and com-munity outreach program are particularly focused on issues of children and families at risk. Committed to a balance of theory and practice and an appreciation of development in context, Erikson Institute approaches children from a holistic and cross-disciplinary perspective. Its academic programs offer a relationship-based education with an emphasis on the latest knowledge on child development linked to reflective practice in the field. Since 1966, the Institute has graduated over 700 child development professionals from its Master's, Infant Studies, and Ph.D. programs.

Columbia College

In 1996, Erikson Institute partnered with Columbia College, an independent liberal arts college specializing in the arts, media, and communications, to begin an undergraduate program for early childhood teachers. Irving Harris and his wife, Joan Harris, a leading advocate for the arts, have been long-standing supporters of Columbia College. The Columbia/Erikson program will prepare students to teach kindergarten through third grade and to staff Head Start and child care programs in urban settings. A focus on the arts in education, an innovative two years of practice teaching, and a fifth year of professional consultation and mentoring establish the program as a model for undergraduate teacher education. Columbia College provides the liberal and fine arts studies in the first two years; Erikson provides courses in child development and schooling in a diverse society, as well as a mentorship approach to teaching practice and methods.

Studies in the visual and performing arts along with child development and methods of teaching prepare teachers to work in a creative interdisciplinary fashion with their students. New literature suggests that the joining of these domains strengthens the cognitive, social, and emotional development and academic achievement of young children as well as the creativity, problem-solving potential, and effectiveness of teachers in classrooms. In the program's third year, 80 students are currently enrolled in professional development courses at Erikson Institute.

Yale Child Study Center

Although Irving Harris is an alumnus of Yale University, it was through his connection with Zero-to-Three that he met Drs. Albert Solnit and Sally Provence of the Yale Child Study Center in the late 1970s. Invited to visit the Child Study Center, Harris watched Dr. Provence work with babies and toddlers and was captivated by her ability to understand the child's inner experience and to communicate this understanding to others. He later met Donald Cohen, current director of the Yale Child Study Center and Kyle Pruett, current President of Zero-to-Three. In 1987, honoring the many ideas and activities that emerged from relationships with Center researchers and clinicians, as well as his commitment to the Center's mission, Harris funded the Provence-Harris Child Development Unit of the Yale Child Study Center and the Center's continued work with young children.

The Yale Child Study Center has a tripartite mission: Research, training, and clinical service. Research efforts range from studies of typical development in infancy to studies of very young children with diagnosed psychiatric disorders. Methods range from psychoanalytically informed studies of the use of play therapy to the use of brain-imaging techniques to study how the brain processes emotions and regulates states of arousal. Clinical services also range from traditional long-term individual psychotherapy to on-site consultation at schools and early childhood centers.

Training efforts mirror the Center's clinical commitment to take services where children live. With recent new support from the Harris Foundation (see the following description of the Harris Professional Development Network), the Center has been able to expand opportunities for trainees from child psychiatry, social work, psychology, and pediatrics at the Yale Child Study Center to work in a variety of community-based child care and early intervention settings as part of their training experience. In March 1999, the opening of the Nissan and Irving Harris building at the Center will make possible the continuity and expansion of these early childhood and community programs.

The capacity for clinically based research and training to address urgent community problems is well illustrated by the Yale Child Study Center's efforts to study the impact of exposure to violence on young children and to implement preventive and treatment efforts in the community. The Child Study Center has pioneered the Child Development and Community Policing (CDCP) program with the

New Haven Police Department which, in addition to providing child development training to police officers, provides mobile psychiatric services at the scene of the crisis for children who witness or experience violence. Additionally, the Center now has mental health consultants in all of New Haven's Head Start programs and schools—another way the Center is extending its work with young children in the community.

The Irving B. Harris Graduate School of Public Policy Studies, University of Chicago

Beginning in the mid-1970s, Irving Harris advocated on a number of fronts to train individuals who could educate the public and policy makers about the importance of the earliest years of life and thereby, help to accomplish social change. As a trustee of the Bush Foundation, Harris successfully urged the Foundation to establish Centers in Child Development and Social Policy at Yale University, the University of Michigan, the University of North Carolina, and the University of California at Los Angeles. At the same time, Harris was serving on the Visiting Committee of the Committee on Public Policy Studies of the University of Chicago, which produced more than 300 graduates trained in public policy over a 15-year period. In 1988, the Harris Graduate School of Public Policy Studies was established. Course work at the school provides a foundation of statistical and other analytical skills, mentors, internships, leadership training, and informal collegial interactions also prepare students to become able policy analysts and researchers. (see P. Chase-Lansdale, R. Gordon, and K. McLain, 1999 for a discussion of the school from faculty and student perspectives.)

The Harris Professional Development Network

In 1994, Irving Harris determined that the time was right to develop a network of training centers across the country whose primary mission was to expand the numbers of trained professionals in the field of infancy. Over a three-year period, the Harris Professional Development Network of eight training programs in the United States and a consortium of programs in Israel were established. While each program has a unique mission tailored to the needs of its geographic region, its institutional goals, and the expertise of its faculty, all are committed to bringing the frontiers of knowledge and clinical practice to front-line practitioners and leaders.

Collectively, the programs reach over 4,000 persons each year from a range of disciplines involved in infancy, including child development, early childhood education, nursing, occupational therapy, pediatrics, physical therapy, psychiatry, psychology, social work, and special education. Persons participating in the training work in hospitals and in community-based child care, child welfare, early intervention, prevention, and mental health settings. With the facilitation of the Harris Foundation and Zero-to-Three, faculty from the eight centers in the United States and representatives from the Israeli programs meet regularly to provide peer consultation in program development and to discuss training issues of common concern. The following brief descriptions provide an overview of the range of training activities encompassed within the Harris Professional Development Network.

Boston, Massachussetts: Child Development Training and Technical Assistance

Training Institute for Early Child
    Development
Boston Medical Center
Boston University School of Medicine
Boston, Massachusetts

The Boston Institute for Early Child Development at Boston Medical Center has been, in large part, funded through the Harris Foundation. Our mission is to provide training and technical assistance to all who care for young children, with a special focus on the training of health professionals. Child development rotations are now required in accredited pediatric residency training programs in the United States. To meet this new need for training, the Institute (1) develops videotapes, slides, and other curriculum material for directors of developmental and behavioral pediatric training programs and academic pediatric residency programs, (2) trains child development fellows at Boston University School of Medicine to

provide academic leadership in early child development, and (3) trains pediatric practitioners around the country in strategies to promote early literacy through the Reach Out and Read program.

The second focus of the Institute is to provide training to and develop written and videotape materials and training for other frontline providers in the Boston and New England region. Activities include free community evening seminars offered in both English and Spanish, the creation of a University collaborative partnership which sponsors a joint cross-disciplinary graduate course in infant mental health across four of the member institutions, workshops at child care centers and Head Start offices, ongoing mentoring of child care teachers at their site, conferences roundtables facilitated by pediatricians for home and center-based child care providers, and a course for "master clinicians in early intervention" designed to train early intervention specialists to offer consultation and training to their local child care programs. Our goal is to provide all of these groups with a theoretical understanding of early development that informs and enriches their everyday work and inspires them to achieve new levels of expertise.

All professionals must educate parents and caregivers that their relationship with their child, from the moment of birth onward, is the most important contributor to their child's physical, mental and emotional well-being and development. We believe that our work in enhancing the development of the young child promotes resilience by providing a firm foundation upon which all future cognitive and emotional experiences can draw.

Margot Kaplan-Sanoff, Ed.D.
Marilyn Augustyn, MD

Chicago, Illinois: Master's and Certificate Infant Specialist and Early Intervention Training

Irving B. Harris Infant Studies Program
Erikson Institute
Chicago, Illinois

Begun in 1984, the Infant Studies Program has as its primary goal preparation of a cadre of postbaccalaureate and master's prepared infant specialists to work in prevention, early intervention for infants and toddlers with disabilities, family support, infant child care, and child life programs. The core academic specialist program consists of four courses on infant development, family studies, assessment, and early intervention methods and a yearlong supervised internship. Community students take all four courses. Master's students embed the assessment and methods courses within their 38-credit degree program. A Director's Seminar is offered to build the supervisory capacity of internship sites and to nurture the leaders of infant/parent services throughout the city of Chicago. The program was one of the first in Illinois approved by the Illinois Interagency Council on Early Intervention to credential early intervention specialists.

The Harris Grant allowed the program to develop a range of new initiatives: An Advanced Practice Seminar Series for experienced practitioners, specialized course work for infant child care directors and providers and for home visitors, an NICU outreach training program in collaboration with Heidelise Als, Ph.D., Boston Children's Hospital for to up to two Chicago-based Level III units, an Early Childhood Faculty Development Project on the Brain in partnership with the McCormick-Tribune Foundation, and an Infant Mental Health specialization within the Infant Studies Program. The program is moving in the direction of field-based, cohort group education linked to changing training needs in our city.

With Mr. Harris' support the Infant Studies Program has become an ongoing source of professional education for new and experienced practitioners, and program directors as well. Now, over one-third of our Master's students choose the field of infancy—a dramatic increase fueled by the pressing need for infant personnel and the exciting curriculum we can offer.

Linda Gilkerson, Ph.D.
Director, Irving B. Harris Infant Studies
Program

Denver Colorado: Advanced Fellowship Training

University of Colorado Health Sciences
Center
Irving B. Harris Training Program in
Child Development and Infant Mental
Health
Denver, Colorado

The Irving B. Harris Training Program in Child Development and Infant Mental Health is an advanced fellowship program for predoctoral and postdoctoral students in psychology, postdoctoral fellows in child and adolescent psychiatry, and midcareer mental health, social work, and early childhood professionals. It provides didactic and clinical experiences designed to promote expertise in the problems of infancy, toddlerhood, and parenthood. The primary focus of the training is understanding growth from the multiple perspectives of cognitive and developmental theories, attachment theory, psychoanalysis, and family development. The didactic curriculum covers normal infant development, temperament, normal pregnancy and pregnancy loss, high-risk infants and parents, developmental psychopathology (including attachment disorders, failure-to-thrive, and behavioral problems), and the issues of the impact of abuse and neglect. Fellows receive didactic course work in developmentally appropriate assessment, diagnosis and treatment of infants and toddlers, and the treatment of infant-parent psychopathology. Clinical training sites include Early Head Start, Infant Mental Health clinics, partial hospital therapeutic preschools, and programs for addicted mothers and their infants. Other activities include increased involvement in the NICU, consultation to the State Department of Education and Division of Mental Health Birth-to-Three initiatives, community training for mental health and early childhood professionals, and the development of a statewide network of trained infant mental health professionals for whom the Program will provide training and consultation and eventually supervision and consultation by phone, e-mail, and teleconferencing.

There is an important role for advanced professionals with specialized training in child development and infant mental health to serve as consultants, teacher/educators, clinicians and clinical supervisors to help meet the developmental and mental health needs of very young children and their families.

Robert Harmon, MD, Director
Karen Frankel, Ph.D., Associate Director
Irving B. Harris Training Program

Minneapolis/St. Paul, Minnesota: Continuing Education Through University/Community Partnership

University of Minnesota
Irving B. Harris Training Center for
  Infant and Toddler Development
Minneapolis, Minnesota
e-mail: asusman@tc.umn.edu

A native of Minnesota, Irving Harris began to support the Department of Child Psychology at the University of Minnesota in 1990, when he helped to establish two named chairs now held by Byron Egeland, Ph.D. and Alan Sroufe, Ph.D. In the context of the Center for Early Education and Development (CEED), the researchers at the Institute for Child Development have long viewed "giving away" child development as a cornerstone of their community outreach efforts. The Irving B. Harris Training Center for Infant and Toddler Development began in 1996 and is an educational nonprofit center dedicated to the training and continuing education of individuals working in the field of infant and toddler development at all levels. The Harris Center is a University/Community partnership with a twofold mission: (1) to serve as an information resource for the University and the community and (2) to maximize the ability of professionals and organizations to better serve infant and toddler populations. The current mix of projects includes the Harris Visiting Scholar program (David Olds will be the Visiting Scholar in spring 1998), the Harris Forum (a community-wide seminar with the Visiting Scholar), the Harris Seminars (quarterly seminars for supervisors, trainers, and frontline workers), a Training-the-Trainers expansion of Brazelton's Touch-points program, new course development for graduate students and community professionals, and formal curriculum development of Project STEEP, a model for early intervention for families at risk.

> Mr. Harris' leadership and commitment to improving the lives of high-risk children are truly inspirational. He is a pioneer and strong advocate and has helped blaze pathways for progress in understanding and supporting the development of young children. His vision, devotion, and enthusiasm for the field are exceptional.
>
> Byron Egeland, Irving B. Harris Professor Child Psychology and Codirector of the Harris Center
> Richard Weinberg, Director of the Institute of Child Development and Codirector of the Harris Center

New Haven, Connecticut: Service-Based Research and Training

Yale University
Child Study Center
New Haven, Connecticut

The Yale Child Study Center has worked intensively with very young children for more than four decades. A philosophy of service-based research, always carefully studying all

clinical endeavors while actively working in the community, characterizes the Center's work with infants and young children. Exemplified by Dr. Sally Provence's work with infants in institutions and continued in the Center's development of mental health services in preschool and daycare programs, service-based research draws upon the deepest of scholarly and scientific traditions. Research programs for children with autism and related disorders, preschoolers with anxiety and depression, and children with serious medical disorders are among the most active investigative programs in the Center's work with young children. Through the Harris expansion grant, the Center is increasing community consultation to child care and education providers, Head Start, and early intervention programs and is adding a new educational module for early childhood educators, thus creating an "educational/clinical" model of training.

> Irving Harris has been a long-standing friend and supporter of the Center's early childhood programs. His devotion to better care for families and their young children has deeply shaped the Center's enduring efforts on behalf of our youngest patients.
>
> Linda Mayes, M.D.
> Coordinator, Early Childhood Section

New Orleans, Louisiana: Infant Mental Health Training Network

Louisiana State University Medical Center
Harris Center for Infant Mental Health
New Orleans, Louisiana

A major objective of the Harris Center for Infant Mental Health in New Orleans and of infant mental health training, in general, is to raise awareness that even very young infants can have mental health problems and that early identification, intervention, and prevention can have a significant positive impact on their lives and those of their families. The goals of our program are: (1) to develop a critical number of people locally and regionally who are trained to evaluate and treat infants, (2) to develop networks—local, regional, national, and international—to provide support for individuals working with infants, (3) to bring together individuals from different mental health disciplines who will have a set of skills and knowledge to assess and treat infants, and (4) to develop expertise in evaluation and treatment for infants and families at high psychosocial risk. Training activities include didactic seminars, clinical case seminars, and intensive clinical supervision by senior infant mental health professionals. Networking efforts will link the many other systems that come in contact with infants and families who face the complex, interrelated risks of poverty, adolescent parenthood, intergenerational violence, and unsafe neighborhoods. These systems include the judicial system, child welfare, law enforcement, schools, community centers, and day care and early intervention programs.

The growth of the Harris Center for Infant Mental Health in New Orleans has provided the opportunity for us to train mental health professionals from a variety of disciplines in evaluation, assessment, intervention, and treatment with infants and families. Thanks to the vision of Irving Harris, we are particularly excited about being able to expand both infant mental health training and services to high-risk children in underserved areas and to frontline professionals.

Joy D. Osofsky, Ph.D.
Director, Harris Center for Infant Mental Health

New York, New York: Early Childhood Site-Based Psychodynamic Services, Consultation, and Training

Early Childhood Group Therapy Training Program
Child Development Center and Martha K. Selig Educational Institute
Jewish Board of Family and Children's Services

The only one of the Harris Professional Development Network programs geared specifically for preschoolers and their families, the mission of the Early Childhood Group Therapy (ECGT) Training Program is to develop a safety net for troubled young children and their families by teaching an interdisciplinary group of professionals to bring direct and consultative psychodynamic mental health services into preschools and the first years of elementary school. Established in 1966 and enriched by the Harris Foundation beginning in 1994, the individualized, strength-centered, transdisciplinary training and service delivery approach is rooted in birth-to-three principles. The program is a certificate-granting two-year, half-time in-depth training experience consisting of seminars, case conferences, intensive reflective supervision, and a center- or school-based field placement. In it, a variety of mental health and early childhood professionals learn to identify children as young as 2½ as at risk for school failure through classroom observations and then to utilize peer play assessment psychotherapy to assist them. Using resourceful outreach with a wide variety of parents, candidates also provide a range of treatment modalities to families from individual, dyadic, and couples psychotherapy to intermittent and brief therapeutic approaches, home visits, "life space" techniques, and concrete services.

The ECGT Program supports children and families and depathologizes services by embedding direct long- and short-term mental health intervention approaches where the children are every day, at their centers and schools. Simultaneously, candidates offer regularly occurring case and classroom-based consultation to teachers and directors, generating a secure forum in which they reflect upon practice and upon the individual needs of children and families. The continuing, thoughtful focus on developmental/mental health issues child by child and family by family which the candidates learn and pass on promotes more relationally attuned, individualized teaching, not only of children designated for services but of all children in a given classroom.

New York, New York: Infant / Toddler-Parent Psychodynamic Training Network for Midcareer Leaders

Institute for Clinical Studies of Infants, Toddlers and Parents
Child Development Center and Martha K. Selig Educational Institute
Jewish Board of Family and Children's Services

Harris Foundation support made possible the establishment of a certificate-granting, advanced training program for both midcareer mental health professionals and for directors and other senior staff of existing infant-toddler programs in the New York and tristate area. All domains of study at the Institute for Clinical Studies of Infants, Toddlers and Parents (ICS–ITP) are informed by biodevelopmental, psychodynamic-psychoanalytic, and systems perspectives. Established in 1996, ICS–ITP has convened a large multidisciplinary faculty and midcareer candidates from a range of fields and many varied community and private practice settings. Organized into weekly afternoon-through-evening sessions and emphasizing both relational-emotional and physiological-sensory-cognitive developmental lines, the state-of-the-art curriculum includes courses, case conferences, seminars on leadership and program design, and intensive reflective supervision related to both clinical cases and administrative challenges in job assignments or field placements. Clinical treatment, understanding, and process are a central part of the core program. Other concentrations include infant/parent psychotherapy for parents and very young children in a range of diagnostic categories and specialized approaches to children who have regulatory/multisystem delays within the pervasive developmental disorder/autistic spectrum.

One significant mission of the Institute is to inspire a new, broad-based, clinically aware generation of birth-to-three training in existing service and training institutions. In order to accelerate overarching improvements in the state-of-the-field, the Institute has a "Train the Trainers" approach, accepting candidates who are already in or moving toward positions of leadership. The Institute accepts candidates with Ph.D., M.D., M.S.W., or other commensurate degree or experience including nursing, child development, occupational, physical, speech/language and the arts therapies, early childhood, and special education.

> Mr. Harris is helping our nation to inch the state of the field towards the state-of-the-art and, in fact, is moving the state-of-the-art forward at the same time. He, before others, knew that more excellent training is key to this great goal. As he wrote in *Children in Jeopardy* (Yale University Press, 1996), "We must expand the scale of efforts to match the scale of knowledge." Through our own efforts, let us celebrate and honor a man who is no less than a hero for our times.
>
> Rebecca Shahmoon Shanok, M.S.W., Ph.D.
> Director, ECGT and ICS-ITP Training
>   Programs, on the occasion of the First
>   Annual Irving Brooks Harris Lecture on
>   Infancy. New York City, October, 1997

San Francisco, California: Infant-Parent Psychotherapy: Direct Service Training and Consultation

University of California–San Francisco
Infant-Parent Program
San Francisco, CA

Based on a knowledge of infant-toddler development, adult development, and infant-parent interaction, the Infant-Parent Program provides direct service to parents whose relationships with their infants and toddlers are significantly troubled. In addition, the program, through its Day Care Consultants program, provides mental health consultation to child care. The clinical training program accepts 10 to 14 trainees each year from a range of disciplines, including psychiatric residents and child psychiatry fellows, social workers, psychologists, and special educators in early interaction. Those in the first year participate in three weekly seminars: (1) a year long seminar in early development taught by our developmental neuropsychologist and a clinical psychologist, (2) a one-half year seminar on issues surrounding home-visiting, observation, assessment, and infant-parent psychotherapy, and (3) a one-half year seminar on the relevance of psychoanalytic theories to infant-parent work. Each week all staff and trainees participate in a clinical case seminar. All trainees receive extensive supervision. Selected trainees are being prepared to provide mental health consultation to child care, and others are focusing intensively on learning developmental assessment with the developmental psychologist.

All staff at the program train and present locally, regionally, and nationally in the areas of their expertise. All also provide consultation locally to practitioners whose work touches the lives of children, such as pediatricians, child welfare workers, and the courts.

Both the training inside and outside of the program and the consultation illuminate the crucial importance to children's development of their experiences in the matrix of relationships in which they are embedded.

With Irving we firmly believe that both training and consultation regarding the importance of infants' and toddlers' relationships must be provided within relationships that are themselves the embodiments of the principles underlying the work that is to be done.

Jeree Pawl, Ph.D.
Director, Infant-Parent Program

Jerusalem and Tel Aviv, Israel: Collaboration among Departments, Training Institutions, and Government Agencies

The Hebrew University of Jerusalem,
   in partnership with Shaare Zedek
   Medical Center
Early Childhood Training Center
Jerusalem, Israel

The Early Childhood Training Center in Jerusalem provides new forms of interdisciplinary training to developmental psychologists, pediatricians, neonatologists, social workers, public health nurses, occupational, physical, and speech therapists, early childhood caregivers, and other paraprofessionals working with very young children and their families. In addition to the development of a core curriculum, special projects include a two-year, supervision-based program for training caregivers in day care centers, training in early development and the detection of developmental delays and disorders for nurses in public Mother-Child Health Stations, intervention for high-risk infants and their families, in-service education for the legal profession, and a conference workshop on social policy toward children and families.

Charles Greenbaum, Ph.D., Marshall
   Professor of Psychiatry

Arthur Eidelman, M.D., Director,
   Department of Neonatology
Miriam Rosenthal, Paul Baerwald School
   of Social Work and School of
   Education
Marsha Katz, Department of Psychology
Asher Ornoy, Department of Anatomy
   and Cell Biology, School of Medicine

Bar-llan University, Tel Aviv
The Harris Program for Infants, Toddlers
   and Families in Israel (ITF)

This program is a collaboration with the Ministries of Health and Education and the Community Renewal Program. Faculty from the Departments of Education, Psychology, Early Childhood, Physical Education, Educational Technology, and Genetics advise the program, which will provide interdisciplinary training in early childhood at the BA, MA, and Ph.D. levels, as well as professional development and field training and supervision to individuals working in the field. The first annual I. B. Harris symposium in early childhood was held in November 1997. Special projects include training professionals who are working in well-baby clinics and educational specialists for young children with multisystem developmental disorders.

Pnina Klein, Ph.D.
Director, Child Development Programs
Department of Education and
   Psychology

Tel Aviv University
Masters Program in Early Childhood
   Education

Advisors include faculty from the Departments of Psychology and Medicine who specialize in social, cognitive, language, reading, and the emotional development of young children. Masters students receive interdisciplinary training and participate in two field placements.

Sidney Strauss, Ph.D.
Department of Child Development and
Education

The three Israeli interdisciplinary training programs are linked informally and participate in collaborative programs and research projects. In addition, each site works with appropriate government ministries to ensure that training is having an impact on professionals working within state-run health and education systems as well as on policy development.

Conclusion

Adult education involves the transmission of knowledge to all who will try to learn, the integration of knowledge from various sources and disciplines, and the application of knowledge to problems of the day. Irving Harris had the foresight to support the education of those who work with young children and families. He has been an insightful and courageous student of child development who has integrated and applied his own considerable knowledge. The consummate adult learner, Harris makes connections within and between disciplines and seeks to put new findings

about children and families into perspective and ultimately, into policy and practice for professionals and nonspecialists alike.

Irving and Joan Harris are not the only people in their family who are interested in early childhood development. Irving's daughter Roxanne worked in the nursery school while a student at Sarah Lawrence College. His daughter Virginia received a master's degree at Bank Street College of Education and taught preprimary school (her son, Jack Polsky is on the board of trustees of Erikson Institute). His son Bill is the founder of KidsPAC. Daughter-in-law Robie, also a Bank Street alumna, first achieved prominence as an author with *Before You Were Three: How You Began to Walk, Talk, Explore and Have Feelings* (Harris & Levy, 1977). How does a businessman justify long-term funding for higher education? Harris made these observations in 1982:

Having supplied the original capital to start the Erikson Institute in 1966 and having supported Erikson with my own time as well as money these past 16 years I have time and again searched my soul to ask whether it continues to make sense to put money into the training of child development specialists . . . Applying a business approach, (I calculate that if) one child who could have been helped does not get the necessary help and fails, the cost to society will probably run to $300,000 over the lifetime of that child/adult (considering the cost of special education, welfare, crime, disease prison, etc.). . . . I assume that each of our graduates is able to prevent two or three children each year from that sort of future . . . So that is how I analyze the cost and benefits of our subsidies. (Harris, 1987, p. 2)

The kind of professional education that Irving Harris supports is expensive. But it works. As evidence, consider the talented people his innovative outreach programs have drawn into training and the graduates of the schools and educational programs he has founded or helped to support. They are an exceptional group of child development practitioners and leaders, deeply grounded in theory, research, and practice. They are going forth to meet the need that Irving Harris long ago identified—for children to be cared for and educated so that they are whole and capable and have hope for the future.

References

Bloom, B. (1964). *Stability and change in human characteristics.* New York: Wiley.

Burman, E. (1994). *Deconstructing developmental psychology.* New York: Rutledge.

Chase-Lansdale, L., Gordon, R., & McLain, K. (1998). The Irving B. Harris Graduate School of Public Policy Studies: An overview and personal reflections. *Zero to Three:* National Center for Infants, Toddlers, and Families, 18(5), 36–43.

Delpit, L. (1988). The silenced dialogue: Power and pedagogy in educating other people's children. *Harvard Educational Review, 58,* 280–298.

Harris, I. (1982, September 29). Remarks at a luncheon hosted by Continental Illinois National Bank and Trust Company of Chicago, Chicago, IL.

Harris, I. (1987). *Play now or pay later.* Remarks to NCCIP Fifth Biennial National Training Institute, Washington, DC.

Harris, I. B. (1996). *Children in jeopardy.* New Haven: The Yale Child Study Center.

Harris, R. H., & Levy, L. (1977). *Before you were three: How you began to walk, talk, explore and have feelings.* New York: Delacorte Press.

Hunt, J. M. (1961). *Intelligence and experience.* New York: Ronald Press.

Jipson, J. (1991). Extending the discourse on developmental appropriateness: A developmental perspective. *Early Education and Development, 2,* 95–108.

Lubeck, S. (1996). Deconstructing "child development knowledge" and "teacher preparation." *Early Childhood Research Quarterly, 11*(2), 147–168.

Schon, D. A. (1987). *Educating the reflective practitioner.* San Francisco: Jossey-Bass.

Soltis, J. F. (1981). Education and the concept of knowledge. In *Philosophy and education: 80th yearbook of the National Society for the Study of Education* (pp. 161–79). Chicago: The University of Chicago Press.

Stott, F., & Bowman, B. (1996). Child development knowledge: A slippery base for practice. *Early Childhood Research Quarterly, 11*(2), 169–183.

16

Preparing Infant Mental Health Personnel for Twenty-First Century Practice

Susan C. McDonough

16

Introduction

The field of infant mental health has grown markedly in the last decades. Twenty years ago, the majority of infant mental health (IMH) practitioners worked with babies and their caregivers in the family's home, in our professional offices, social service agencies, hospitals, or clinics. While IMH practitioners continue to work in these contexts, many of us increasingly work in such diverse settings as schools, prisons, drug treatment centers, displacement camps, reservations, the bush, or the streets. We find ourselves going to places where the most overburdened world citizens struggle to raise their young children amidst poverty and squalor. The challenge of preparing IMH practitioners to work in the new caregiving contexts is indeed daunting; but I believe success is possible.

Relational Approaches to Personnel Preparation in Infant Mental Health

From the field's earliest beginnings, infant mental health practitioners understood how the infant develops in the context of the caregiving relationship. Specifically, infant behavior cannot be viewed separately from the young child's relationships. During infancy the child's most important relationships are with primary caregivers. More recently, IMH practitioners are recognizing the critical importance of the infant's own caregivers' relationships with the broader social context. These principles provide a nesting of the infant in multiple relational contexts: the baby and his or her primary caregivers, the primary caregivers and extended family members, and the broader social and cultural networks in which these babies, caregivers, and family members live (McDonough, in press).

My goal in this chapter is to illustrate how a relationship-focused orientation can illuminate and guide our training of infant mental health practitioners. To meet this goal I will describe qualities of exemplary training models that incorporate principles of an adult education with relationship-focused training.

Personnel preparation is viewed as an ongoing process of professional development rather than a series of short-term training activities or a program of study that culminates with the award of an academic degree (McDonough, 1981, 1999). This chapter outlines issues relating both to preservice and continuing professional education training initiatives. The chapter primarily addresses the training of infant mental health practitioners. However, much of the information presented also is relevant to administrators, supervisors, resource staff, and support personnel who oversee, mentor, supervise, and aid IMH specialists in their work.

Rather than highlight one particular training model, this chapter delineates aspects of quality education and training experiences found across exemplary programs.

Successful training programs possess both *structural* and *process* elements that contribute to the breadth and depth of the training experience. Structural elements include the specific educational content of the training program. For example, some structural elements include addressing the interface between the developing infant's brain and the influence of the caregiving context, techniques for engaging hard-to-reach families in treatment, and knowledge of developmental psychopathology across the lifespan. The process elements of successful training programs address how the training is delivered. For example, process elements include integrating developmental theory into clinical practice through the use of relationship-focused treatment case illustrations, providing reflective supervision to trainees, and engaging a multidisciplinary faculty in team-teaching course content or in supervising clinical training experiences. Each element will be illuminated further through the chapter's specific training examples.

Infant Mental Health Training Programs

Regardless of our theoretical orientations and our own disciplinary backgrounds, infant mental health training programs strive to prepare practitioners for work with infants, toddlers, and their families in multiple and diverse caregiving contexts. To accomplish this goal, IMH training programs face several challenges. Infant mental health workers need to possess knowledge and demonstrate skills in several disciplinary areas. Ideally, this can occur by providing educational opportunities for trainees to work in interdisciplinary settings and to be mentored by multidisciplinary professionals.

In reality, trainees in these programs often come from various disciplinary backgrounds. This diversity of the knowledge base and practice principles contributes to the ability of many IMH practitioners to work with distinct families in diverse settings. Whether by tradition or professional credential mandate, discipline-specific training programs (i.e., psychology or social work) often require that their trainees are supervised by disciplinary professionals rather than by someone knowledgeable about and skillful in infant mental health training.

The situation is further complicated by the lack of a recognized credential in infant mental health that includes an agreed-upon cluster of training competencies. A finite number of institutions of higher education around the world offer infant mental health training. Consequently, individuals training IMH professionals generally do so with limited knowledge about and exposure to exemplary training models for curricular guidance and direction. As a result, many programs exist solely due to the energy and enthusiasm of seasoned IMH practitioners willing to serve as training instructors, supervisors, and mentors.

Finally, the contexts in which IMH practitioners work are expanding. With those broadening practice contexts come increased demands for more sophisticated knowledge and practice skills in areas ranging from the effects of environmental deprivation on brain growth and development to human rights issues and how to address service inequities for babies and their caregivers with government officials and funding agents. The expanding venues for IMH practitioners to work with vulnerable infants and their overburdened caregivers demand additional skills and specialized training opportunities. Many of our current IMH training programs (including the one I direct) do not place enough emphasis on addressing these critical 21st century social needs. They must do so in the future.

IMH Practitioners Require Transgenerational Relationship Expertise

The field of infant mental health seeks to nurture the development of adult family members in their roles as the child's parents or caregivers. The importance of extended networks of kin, friends, neighbors, service providers, and community has long been recognized as critical to our work. Traditionally, IMH practitioners are well educated in child growth and development and in parent-infant psychotherapy and clinical intervention skills. Some of us, through our disciplinary training, understand development across the lifespan and developmental psychopathology, and feel competent and confident in diagnosing, assessing, and treating adults with developmental problems and mental health concerns. Fewer of us have had opportunities to appreciate how adults learn, adult learning styles, and optimal strategies to enhance adult learning as articulated in adult education texts (Knox, 1999; Bennett, 1998). Much of our relationship-focused IMH work focuses on engaging adults in therapeutic treatments and interventions.

Interestingly, in my 25 years of work in this field, I've never had a baby open the door to let me into his or her family's home, transport him or herself to my office, or call me on the phone to request my help. Yet much of our current IMH practitioner training focuses on the infant and on the primacy of the infant-caregiver relationship. While acknowledging the significance of the early attachment relationship and of the importance of relationship-focused diagnosis, assessment, and treatment, our IMH training programs might be enhanced by what our adult education colleagues can teach us about working more effectively with the adult partners in an infant-caregiver relationship. As the adult relationship partners and other adult family members ultimately decide whether or not to use our services, we need their cooperation and support. Our adult education colleagues also may provide us with useful insights on how to educate fellow disciplinary colleagues, policy makers, funding agencies, and potential donors about the crucial importance of infant mental health.

Structural Elements of IMH Training

Infant mental health trainees can be encouraged to make certain assumptions when working with babies and their families. These beliefs are helpful both in understanding the important roles that family members have in their infant's life and in providing a more generous interpretation of some families' apparently ongoing struggle to nurture and protect their child.

Embrace the position that parents and caregivers are doing the best they know how to do.

Although this sounds quite simple, it can be a challenging concept to put into practice. By emphasizing the phrase "the best they know how to do," one is able to keep open the possibility that the parents can acquire new ways of thinking, coping, behaving, and feeling. It also conveys acceptance and respect of where parents are now without assuming that it is all of which they are capable. Use existing positive parental behavior and attitudes to assist in building feelings of self-confidence in the caregivers.

Address what parents believe to be the problem or issue of concern.

As professionals working with multiproblem families, it is frustrating and often heartbreaking to see parents worry excessively about things they cannot change or fail to take some direct action that could minimize or alleviate difficulty. Sometimes what appears to be a critical family need is not identified as an area of concern by the family. The family may choose to use their resources differently. Acknowledge and accept the family's negative feelings and attributions of child behavior without feeling

541

as if you need to change them immediately or concur in order to maintain your relationship with the family. Often caregivers are seeking to be heard.

Ask the family what you can do to be helpful to them.

At the simplest level, the helping process involves two components: a) a person offers some assistance or aid; and b) another person accepts what is offered. Professionals working with families can increase the likelihood that the offered help will be accepted by encouraging the family to decide what, if any, assistance they desire or need rather than assuming that a clinician-identified problem is the family's source of concern. Promote the role of the parents as decision-makers in the family and protectors of the child by deferring to their expertise as the individuals who know their child "best." Consider the ramifications of "doing for" (including handling the baby) without being asked to do so. Sometimes our "assistance" may be interpreted as the clinician knowing better, taking over, criticizing, or correcting.

Answer questions posed by the family directly; provide information when asked.

Many families come to the helping professional with questions they hope to have answered. Occasionally the information requested by the family may be unknown or unanswerable, or the material requested may be very technical for the family's use. Often families need to have things repeated many times, in many different ways and sometimes by more than one person, be-fore they grasp the meaning of what is being said to them. Even then the family's understanding of the long-term implications of particular circumstances or conditions may change as the family acquires additional information or experiences new insights. Families report that what a professional tells them is not always as important as the manner in which the information is shared.

Discuss with family members under what circumstances they will feel as if they experienced some success in their work with you.

Families who are having difficulties in raising their children or who already have experienced a parenting failure need some reassurance that things are capable of changing. Sometimes articulating a "piece of work" that you and the family hope to accomplish within a relatively short time can empower families to believe that aspects of their life circumstances can change for the better. Involving the family in an ongoing discussion of treatment progress also affords the IMH practitioner with an opportunity to observe how the family attempts to solve problems and prioritize their goals. For example, is the family's notion of "success" dependent upon whether the psychological symptoms of distress go away? Do the families reflect both on internal changes (their feelings, thoughts, beliefs) and behavioral manifestations (child sleeps through the night), or do they reflect only on one kind of changes? Is the family's understanding of successful completion of a piece of work more child-focused, parent-focused, or relational? Responses to questions such as these often provide the IMH practitioner with insight into how to establish the therapeutic alliance with the family. Maintaining and strengthening that alliance often occurs when caregivers feel respected and accepted.

Invite the family to evaluate your work together on a weekly basis.

Involving families in evaluating their own progress assists the IMH practitioner in observing areas of family growth and development and of the family's perceived sense of impasse, resistance, and relapse. If treatment is proceeding positively, the family can share feelings of achievement and accomplishment. If one party is dissatisfied, those feelings can be explored openly and a change or redirection in treatment focus suggested. This weekly monitoring appears to be especially helpful in dealing with the resistant client, whose anger often can be addressed and worked through by providing a regular opportunity for the client to express his or her thoughts and feelings about the treatment process. Because one of the principle partners in the relationship may not be able to speak in his or her own behalf, use your own voice to gain the family's attention and interest by articulating the baby's needs and desires.

Process Elements of IMH Training

Some particular process elements training is included here to illustrate how IMH practitioners can be encouraged to incor-

porate these characteristics into their own work with families.

Work very hard and very quickly to establish a positive working alliance.

When working with families who have a history of unproductive contacts with social service professionals, it is useful to acknowledge where the "system" and those working within it have failed them in the past. Clearly, many overburdened families have spent years struggling mightily to resolve complex life problems. What needs to be conveyed during an initial family meeting is that you, as an IMH practitioner, are asking to join in an alliance with the family rather than assuming that they will join with you. Because disappointment and failure often characterize past dealings with professionals, it seems particularly important to offer concrete assistance that produces some tangible result for the family during your initial family meeting. This may involve arranging a scheduled appointment at the family's convenience rather than during available hours. The message to be conveyed is your intention to work hard toward making this collaborative work experience a productive one for the family.

Convey your professional expertise in an egalitarian and non-judgmental way.

Every family wants to play a meaningful role in their child's life. Often the strategies that overburdened families use are not fulfilling this family desire. Asking the family what they have discovered about what works best and not so well for their own family invites an egalitarian discussion between you and the family. It also offers the possibility for you to share what other families have shared with you about their own successful efforts to adapt and cope. Using other families' life lessons can be a less threatening way for a family to entertain new ideas or to broaden their perspectives about different ways of thinking about issues or trying new ways of behaving.

Use the families' existing nurturing behavior and positive attitudes to help build feelings of self-confidence in the caregivers.

The majority of the families with whom we work are doing the best job they know how to do in caring for their children and themselves. No matter how well intentioned, sometimes a caregiver's "best job" isn't good enough to guarantee the safety and well being of their children. Using existing parental strengths to enhance what capacities the caregivers do possess can foster the family's belief that they can adopt alternative ways of feeling, thinking, and behaving toward their children. It also conveys the IMH practitioner's belief that caregivers can engage in positive parenting behavior while they develop more sensitive nurturing of the children.

Make note of parental attitudes and behavior that you hope to alter or to modify but address only those issues you believe to be of critical importance.

Often overburdened families come with a plethora of problems, issues, and concerns. For these families, everyday life challenges

preoccupy much of their physical and psychic energy. Providing instrumental help, advice, or guidance on how to address a pressing family concern may provide some relief, albeit temporary, for the caregivers. Demonstrating a willingness to work with the family at addressing what they believe to be of critical importance provides concrete evidence of an IMH practitioner's commitment to forming an active working alliance. Many worrisome family issues or inadequate problem-solving strategies are rooted in longstanding family pathology. Once the therapeutic relationship is stronger and the family and IMH practitioner experience some satisfaction and success in working together, additional relationship issues can be tackled.

Use of Videotaping in Training and Ongoing Supervision

Many preservice and continuing professional education training programs use videotaping as a way to enhance trainees' own self-assessment and for use in the ongoing clinical supervision. The use of videotape in training and ongoing supervision allows for salient and objective feedback to the trainees' own behavior and its effect on the family's, infant's, and caregiver's behavior. Through viewing self-selected video samples of their work with the families, the trainees become more aware of what they say and the manner in which they say it, and how what they do can impact, albeit subtly, on the families with whom they are working. This method of self-assessment allows the trainee to focus on the skills that they and their supervisors agree are positive and can be elaborated and extended, and also to pinpoint those practice skills which require redirection and alteration. Archiving videotape segments of the trainee's work throughout the training provides a record of the trainee's emerging practice skills and professional development.

dence for the justification of continuing successful program elements or changing less effective elements.

Summative evaluation techniques serve to assess the impact, efficacy, and adequacy of the overall training program. Information gleaned through this evaluation phase provides useful data for the development of new training initiatives and ideas for how to best deliver this training.

Evaluation of IMH Training

As in many areas of our work, increasingly we are being asked to assess the efficacy and long-term effectiveness of our training initiatives. Well articulated IMH training competencies offer an opportunity for trainees to evaluate their own growing capacities and for their supervisors or mentors to assess the trainee's progress in acquiring the knowledge and practice skills necessary for successful work experience.

The training program's effectiveness can be ascertained through formative and summative evaluations. For example, as individual educational activities occur, data can be collected via trainee self-report questionnaires, observational ratings by the supervisor or mentor, and interviews with the trainees, their supervisors, or the families with whom they work. Information gathered through formative evaluation provides feedback for training program improvement on an ongoing and continuous basis. This evaluative strategy can document areas of program strength and weakness, thereby providing crucial evi-

Recommendations for IMH Personnel Preparation Programs

Based on the information presented in this chapter regarding both preservice and in-service approaches for training IMH practitioners, the following training recommendations are proposed:

- The training of IMH practitioners is best viewed as a continuing educational process from preservice training through ongoing professional development.
- Preservice training competencies are best limited to those that are essential for entry level IMH positions. In-service training and continuing professional educational programs can be used to elaborate and expand existing skills and to develop a more sophisticated and nuanced understanding of theory, practice, self and program evaluation, and social policy implementation.
- The unique combination of conceptual, clinical, and evaluative skills required of an IMH practitioner necessitate a trans-

disciplinary approach to both preservice and continuing professional education.

- Professionals representing the various disciplines involved in work with infants, toddlers, and their caregivers contribute to the richness of IMH training initiatives and should be formally involved in educational programs both at the preservice and continuing professional development levels.
- The acquisition of conceptual knowledge, both at preservice and ongoing professional education levels, is enhanced by supervised practice experiences.
- The efficacy of both preservice and continuing professional development training initiatives can be evaluated by the practitioners' demonstrated performance of IMH training competencies in the natural practice setting—the diverse caregiving contexts in which babies live and practitioners work.
- Cooperative training efforts between personnel preparation institutions (i.e., universities, medical schools, professional organizations) and practice settings (i.e., public and private social service agencies) could mutually benefit from being expanded. In many instances, universities and colleges may need to assume responsibility for initiating and maintaining these partnership opportunities.

References

Benn, R., Elliot, J., & Whaley, P. (1998). *Educating Rita and her sisters: Women and continuing education.* Leicester, England: National Institute of Adult Continuing Education.

Jarvis, P. (1997). *Adult and continuing education: Theory and practice.* London/New York: Routledge.

Knox, A. (1993). *Strengthening adult and continuing education: A global perspective on synergistic leadership.* New York: Jossey-Bass.

McDonough, S. C. (1981). Personnel preparation: Procedures and best practices manual (pp. 27–42). In J. Carter (Ed.), Early Childhood Handicapped: Best practices manual. Springfield, IL: Illinois State Board of Education.

McDonough, S. C. (1996). Post-master certificate program in work with infants, toddlers and their families: Survey of 75 infant mental health certificate graduates. Continuing Professional Education Working Paper #2. Ann Arbor, MI: University of Michigan.

McDonough, S. C. (1999). Engaging difficult to reach families. In C. Zeanah (Ed.), *Handbook of Infant Mental Health: Second edition,* pp. 485–493. New York: Guilford.

Author Index

Abadi, J., 187
Aber, J. L., 339
Abidin, R. R., 427
Achenbach, T., 174
Achenbach, T. M., 88, 90, 92, 427
Adam, E., 21
Adamson, L., 101, 105
Adamson, L. B., 162, 164
Adelson, E., 6, 16, 40, 128, 248, 320
Advisory Committee on Services for Families with Infants and Toddlers, 38
Ahadi, S. A., 409, 415, 500
Aimsworth, M. H., 101
Ainsworth, M. D. S., 40, 247, 281, 287, 326, 344, 409, 412
Akiyama, T., 178, 186
Aksan, N., 8
Alansky, J. A., 494, 502
Alessandri, S. M., 498
Allen, A. B., 355
Allen, B., xii
Allen, J. P., 339
Allen, M. C., 344, 346
Als, H., 39, 69, 101, 105, 166, 181
American Academy of Child and Adolescent Psychiatry, 407, 408, 409, 412, 413, 414, 415, 428
American Psychiatric Association, 24, 264, 424, 430
Amini, F., 410
Anders, F. A., 245, 261
Anders, T., 163, 278
Anders, T. F., 94, 321, 408
Anderson, B. J., 494
Anderson, C. J., 174
Anderson-Goetz, D., 495

Andur, J. R., 351
Angleitner, A., 480
Anisfield, E., 165
Anthony, E. J., 344
Anzalone, M., 416
Anzalone, M. F., 322
Aponte, H. J., 15
Arcus, D., 499
Ards, S., 339
Arnold, R., xii, 355
Ashton, P., 494
Avard, D., 338
Axtmann, A., 38
Ayoub, C. C., 86, 349
Azuma, S. D., 171

Bachelor, A., 290
Bachmann, J. P., 277, 290, 303, 306, 411
Baker, W. L., 408
Baltman, K., 133, 134, 137
Barnard, K., 141
Barnard, K. E., 14, 16, 17, 21, 166, 328
Barnes, H. V., 339, 340
Barnett, W. S., 20
Barocas, R., 347, 409
Baron-Cohen, S., 264
Barr, R., 163, 167, 185
Barrett, D., 174
Barrett, K. C., 410
Barrett, L. C., 497
Basch, M., 446
Bates, J. E., 322, 480, 481, 482, 484, 485, 487, 489, 495, 496, 497, 499, 500, 501, 502, 504
Baumbacher, G., 410
Bayles, K., 496

Bayley, N., 141, 322, 326
Beal, J. A., 165, 174, 180, 185
Beardslee, W. R., 344
Beckwith, L., 171
Beebe, B., 446
Beeghly, M., 161, 171, 174, 175
Behnke, M., 161, 171
Behrman, R. E., 340
Belenkey, M. F., 40
Bell, R. Q., 5, 344
Bell, S., 247
Bell, S. M., 281, 287
Belsky, J., 165, 174, 175, 181, 490, 502
Bemporad, J. V., 344
Benham, A. L., 85, 96, 99
Bennett, L. A., 14
Benoit, D., xiii, 102, 103, 105, 345
Berger, A., 187
Berger, E., 91
Berger, M., 243
Bergman, A., 6, 8, 40, 181
Berney, C., 411
Bernstein, V., 124, 137
Bertacchi, J., 65, 148, 149
Bertenthal, B. I., 86
Bettens, C. G., xii
Beutler, L. E., 21
Bibring, G., 282
Bick, E., 133
Bijleveld, C., 290, 293
Bingham, D., 254
Bingham, R., 407
Bion, W., 446
Birch, H., 103
Birch, H. G., 344, 482, 483
Biringen, Z., 7, 11, 15, 101, 105
Black, M., 446

Author Index

Subject Index

SUBJECT INDEX

alcohol, 171, 173
  abuse, 344, 346, 356, 360
  maternal, 415
alcoholism, 15, 147
alert periods, 163
alert states, 168, 171
alertness, 172, 176, 180
allergy problems, 286
alliance, therapeutic, 183–184
ambivalence, maternal, 261
American Academy of Pediatrics, 87
analyses, sequential, 21
analytic intervention, 17
anesthesia, perinatal, 161
Angel Island, 397
anger, 218, 486, 498
  proneness, 493
Anna Freud Centre, 133
anorexia in infants, 264
ANOVA testing, 290
antisocial behavior, 20, 339
anxiety disorders, 220
  and overprotection, 91–92
anxiety, 220, 280, 282, 344, 353, 418, 425
  of child, 418
  in parents, 89
  of parents with medically ill children, 93–94
  phobic, 353
  resolution, 282
Apgar scores, 167, 415
appearance of child, 419
approach, 484, 489, 498
approach-withdrawal systems, 482, 483, 491
arousal level regulation, 86
Asperger's syndrome, 226, 227
assertiveness, 217, 218
  family, 411
assessment
  approaches, 130
  basic principles, 131–132
  child, 46
  children with medical conditions, 81–117
  clinical, 211–217
    of the child, 98–99
  community-based programs, 335–368
  developmental, 46
    components of, 99
  dimensions for parenting competence, 111
  disorders, 251–253
  family-centered, 411–412
  father, 450
  frequency and time, 132
  historical significance, 133–134
  infant and caregiver, 131–132
  infant disorders, 203–238

infant psychopathology, challenges and methods,
    239–265
  instruments, 100, 140–142, 286–288
    parental perceptions of medically ill children,
      90–93
  integrated formal and informal approaches, 128
  intervention-centered, 403–436
    clinical observation, 417–426
  interviewing, 142–145
  methods, 255–265
  mother, 450
  motor skills, 425–426
  object, 243–251
  observation and listening, 119–155
  parent involvement, 98
  parenting skills, 110–112
  partnership of parents and practitioner, 132 (see
    trust)
  process, 359–366
  process for medically ill children, 93
  psychometric properties, 100
  risk factors, 251
  setting, 132
  socioemotional competence, 100–107
  standardized measures, 99–107
  as successful intervention, 433–434
  supervision, 148–149
  temperament, 477–504
    laboratory approaches, 497–450
    multidimensional approaches, 497–498
    naturalistic approaches, 494–497
    psychobiological approaches, 499–500
    questionnaire approaches, 486–494
    scripted observations, 496–497
  training in infant mental health, 325–326
assimilation, cognitive, 8
asthma, 86
attachment, 107, 166, 246, 247, 252, 322, 410, 416, 427
  children with medical conditions, 88
  differentiation, 101
  disorders, 320
  figures, special, 416
  insecure, 344
  paradigm, xii, 281
  pattern, 253
    of children with medical conditions, 89
  relationships, 244, 451
  security, 345–346
  system, 410
  theory, xii, 6, 446
    and family systems, xii
attachment-exploration phenomena, xi
attention span, 484, 485, 491
attention, 415, 416, 427, 485, 499
  autonomic cost, 175